T0328307

ROUTLEDGE HANDBOOK OF SPORT AND EXERCISE SYSTEMS GENETICS

Technological advances over the last two decades have placed genetic research at the forefront of sport and exercise science. It provides potential answers to some of contemporary sport and exercise's defining issues and throws up some of the area's most challenging ethical questions, but to date, it has rested on a fragmented and disparate literature base. The *Routledge Handbook of Sport and Exercise Systems Genetics* constitutes the most authoritative and comprehensive reference in this critical area of study, consolidating knowledge and providing a framework for interpreting future research findings.

Taking an approach which covers single gene variations, through genomics, epigenetics, and proteomics, to environmental and dietary influences on genetic mechanisms, the book is divided into seven sections. It examines state-of-the-art genetic methods, applies its approach to physical activity, exercise endurance, muscle strength, and sports performance, and discusses the ethical considerations associated with genetic research in sport and exercise.

Made up of contributions from some of the world's leading sport and exercise scientists and including chapters on important topical issues such as gene doping, gender testing, predicting sport performance and injury risk, and using genetic information to inform physical activity and health debates, the handbook is a vital addition to the sport and exercise literature. It is an important reference for any upper-level student, researcher, or practitioner working in the genetics of sport and exercise or exercise physiology, and crucial reading for any social scientist interested in the ethics of sport.

J. Timothy Lightfoot is the Omar Smith Endowed Chair in Kinesiology and the Director of the Sydney and JL Huffines Institute for Sports Medicine and Human Performance at Texas A&M University in College Station, Texas (USA) and holds the rank of Professor of joint appointments on the Texas A&M Genetics Faculty and the Texas A&M Institute for Genome Sciences and Society. His research focus has been the genetic factors that regulate daily physical activity. He is an Associate Editor of *Medicine and Science in Sports and Exercise*. He was a founding member of the National Exercise Clinical Trials Network and is a Fellow of the American College of Sports Medicine.

Monica J. Hubal is an Associate Professor of Kinesiology at Indiana University–Purdue University Indianapolis, USA. She is also an Adjunct Associate Professor of Cellular and

Integrative Physiology, a research scientist in the Diabetes Translational Research Center and is affiliated with the Indiana Center for Musculoskeletal Health at the Indiana University School of Medicine. Her research focuses on understanding the systems biology of emergent cardiometabolic disease and the mechanisms driving response to various interventions. She was a principal investigator in the Research Center for Genetic Medicine at the Children's National Medical Center. She is an Associate Editor for *Medicine and Science in Sports and Exercise* and *Exercise and Sport Sciences Reviews* and is a Fellow of the American College of Sports Medicine.

Stephen M. Roth is a Professor of Kinesiology and Associate Dean at the University of Maryland in College Park, USA. He has researched the genetic aspects of exercise and sport for over 15 years. He is an author or co-author of over 90 peer-reviewed articles, book chapters, and books. He served as an Associate Editor for *Medicine and Science in Sports and Exercise* and *Exercise and Sport Sciences Reviews*. He is a Fellow of the National Academy of Kinesiology and the American College of Sports Medicine.

ROUTLEDGE HANDBOOK OF SPORT AND EXERCISE SYSTEMS GENETICS

Edited by J. Timothy Lightfoot, Monica J. Hubal,
and Stephen M. Roth

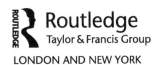

Routledge
Taylor & Francis Group

LONDON AND NEW YORK

First published 2019 by Routledge

2 Park Square, Milton Park, Abingdon, Oxon, OX14 4RN

605 Third Avenue, New York, NY 10017

Routledge is an imprint of the Taylor & Francis Group, an informa business

First issued in paperback 2020

British Library Cataloguing-in-Publication Data
A catalogue record for this book is available from the British Library

Library of Congress Cataloging-in-Publication Data
Names: Lightfoot, J. Timothy, editor. | Hubal, Monica J., editor. |
Roth, Stephen M., 1973– editor.
Title: Routledge handbook of sport and exercise systems genetics /
Edited by J. Timothy Lightfoot, Monica J. Hubal, and Stephen M. Roth.
Other titles: Handbook of sport and exercise systems genetics
Description: Abingdon, Oxon ; New York, NY : Routledge, 2019. |
Includes bibliographical references and index.
Identifiers: LCCN 2018051636 | ISBN 9781138504851 (hardback) |
ISBN 9781315146287 (ebook)
Subjects: LCSH: Sports–Physiological aspects–Research. |
Exercise–Physiological aspects–Research. | Human genetics–Research. |
Athletic performance–Physiological aspects–Research.
Classification: LCC RC1235 .R683 2019 | DDC 612/.044–dc23
LC record available at https://lccn.loc.gov/2018051636

ISBN: 978- 1-138-50485-1 (hbk)
ISBN: 978-0-367-73131-1 (pbk)

Typeset in Bembo
by Newgen Publishing UK

CONTENTS

Contents

LIST OF FIGURES

LIST OF TABLES

LIST OF CONTRIBUTORS

Philip J. Atherton, PhD
MRC-ARUK Centre for Musculoskeletal
Ageing Research & NIHR Nottingham
BRC University of Nottingham, School of
Medicine
Royal Derby Hospital
Derby, UK

Joshua J. Avila, PhD
Department of Health and Kinesiology
Texas A&M University
College Station, TX, USA

Jacob L. Barber, MS
Department of Exercise Science
Arnold School of Public Health
University of South Carolina
Columbia, SC, USA

Matthew D. Barberio, PhD
Center for Genetic Medicine Research
Children's National Medical Center
Washington, DC, USA

Frank W. Booth, PhD
Department of Biomedical Sciences
College of Veterinary Medicine
University of Missouri
Columbia, MO, USA

Claude Bouchard, PhD
Boyd Professor, John W. Barton Sr. Chair in
Genetics and Nutrition
Human Genomics Laboratory
Pennington Biomedical Research Center,
Baton Rouge, LA, USA

Molly Bray, PhD
Professor and Susan T. Jastrow Chair for
Excellence in Nutritional Sciences
Chair, Department of Nutritional Sciences
College of Natural Sciences
The University of Texas at Austin
Austin, TX, USA

Jessica Cegielski, MSc
MRC-ARUK Centre for Musculoskeletal
Ageing Research & NIHR Nottingham
BRC University of Nottingham, School of
Medicine
Royal Derby Hospital
Derby, UK

Malcolm Collins, PhD
Division of Exercise Science and Sports
Medicine
Department of Human Biology
Faculty of Health Sciences
University of Cape Town
Cape Town, South Africa

Lauren M.L. Corso, MS
Department of Kinesiology
College of Agriculture, Health and Natural
Resources
University of Connecticut
Storrs, CT, USA

Sean M. Courtney, PhD
Department of Health and Kinesiology
Texas A&M University
College Station, TX, USA

Eco de Geus, PhD
Head of the Department of Biological
Psychology
Human Behavioral and Movement Sciences
Vrije Universiteit Amsterdam
Amsterdam, Netherlands

David Epstein
Former reporter for ProPublica and Sports
Illustrated,
author of *The Sports Gene* and *Range*

Nir Eynon
Institute for Health and Sport
Victoria University, and
Murdoch Children's Research Institute
The Royal Children Hospital
Melbourne, Australia

David P. Ferguson, PhD, RCEP
Assistant Professor
Director of the Neonatal Nutrition and
Exercise Research Lab
Department of Kinesiology
College of Education
Michigan State University
East Lansing, MI, USA

Ebony C. Gaillard, BS
Laboratory of Systems Physiology
Department of Kinesiology
UNC Charlotte
Charlotte, NC, USA

Fleur C. Garton, PhD
Murdoch Children's Research Institute
Royal Children's Hospital
Victoria, Australia

Benjamin D.H. Gordon, PhD, CEP
Department of Exercise & Rehabilitative
Sciences
Slippery Rock University
Slippery Rock, PA, USA

Jorge Z. Granados, MS
Department of Health and Kinesiology
College of Education and Human
Development
Texas A&M University
College Station, TX, USA

Kolter B. Grigsby, PhD
Department of Biomedical Sciences
College of Veterinary Medicine
University of Missouri
Columbia, MO, USA

Dustin S. Hittel, PhD
Cumming School of Medicine
University of Calgary
Calgary, Alberta, Canada

Reuben Howden, PhD
Laboratory of Systems Physiology
Department of Kinesiology
UNC Charlotte
Charlotte, NC, USA

Peter J. Houweling, PhD
Murdoch Children's Research Institute
Royal Children's Hospital
Victoria, Australia

Monica J. Hubal, PhD, FACSM
Department of Kinesiology
School of Health and Health Sciences
Affiliate – Indiana Center for
Musculoskeletal Health
Affiliate – Diabetes Translational
Research Center
Indiana University – Purdue University at
Indianapolis
Indianapolis, IN, USA

Macsue Jacques, BSc
Institute for Health and Sport
Victoria University
Melbourne, Australia

Jaakko Kaprio, MD, PhD
Professor of Genetic Epidemiology
Department of Public Health, Faculty of
Medicine
& Institute for Molecular Medicine FIMM
University of Helsinki
Helsinki, Finland

Peter T. Katzmarzyk, PhD
Pennington Biomedical Research Center
Louisiana State University
Baton Rouge, LA, USA

Scott A. Kelly, PhD
Associate Professor
Department of Zoology
Ohio Wesleyan University
Delaware, OH, USA

Taylor J. Kelty, PhD
Department of Biomedical Sciences
College of Veterinary Medicine
University of Missouri
Columbia, MO, USA

William J. Kraemer, PhD
Department of Human Sciences
The Ohio State University
Columbus, OH, USA

Shanie Landen, BSc
Institute for Health and Sport
Victoria University
Melbourne, Australia

Ayland C. Letsinger, BS
Department of Health and Kinesiology
College of Education and Human
Development
Texas A&M University
College Station, TX, USA

J. Timothy Lightfoot, PhD, FACSM, RCEP, CES
Omar Smith Endowed Chair in Kinesiology
Director, Sydney and JL Huffines Institute for
Sports Medicine and Human Performance
Department of Health and Kinesiology
College of Education and Human
Development
Texas A&M University
College Station, TX, USA

Jill Livingston, MLS
Homer Babbidge Library
Health Sciences
University of Connecticut
Storrs, CT, USA

José Maia, PhD
Faculty of Sport
University of Porto
Porto, Portugal

Michael P. Massett, PhD
Department of Health and Kinesiology
Texas A&M University
College Station, TX, USA

Kathryn N. North
Murdoch Children's Research Institute
The Royal Children's Hospital
Melbourne, Australia

Jane K. McDevitt, PhD
Temple University
Department of Kinesiology
Philadelphia, PA, USA

Andy Miah, PhD
University of Salford
Salford, UK

Mindy Millard-Stafford, PhD
Exercise Physiology Laboratory
School of Biological Sciences
Georgia Institute of Technology
Atlanta, GA, USA

Verner Møller, PhD
Department of Public Health
Aarhus University
Aarhus, Denmark

Rasmus Bysted Møller, PhD
Department of Public Health
Aarhus University
Aarhus, Denmark

Colin N. Moran, PhD
Physiology, Exercise and Nutrition
Research Group
University of Stirling
Stirling, UK

John Nauright, PhD
University of North Texas
Denton, TX, USA

Linda S. Pescatello, PhD, FACSM, FAHA
Board of Trustees Distinguished Professor of
Kinesiology
Department of Kinesiology
College of Agriculture, Health and Natural
Resources
The Institute for Systems Genomics
University of Connecticut
Storrs, CT, USA

Emidio E. Pistilli, PhD
Department of Human Performance –
Exercise Physiology
West Virginia University
Morgantown, WV, USA

Herman Pontzer, PhD
Department of Evolutionary Anthropology
Duke University
Durham, NC, USA

John C. Quindry, PhD, FACSM
Department Chair, Associate Professor, IHI
Cardiovascular Research Fellow
Department of Health and Human
Performance
University of Montana
Missoula, MT, USA

Masouda Rahim, PhD
Division of Exercise Science and Sports
Medicine
Department of Human Biology
Faculty of Health Sciences
University of Cape Town
Cape Town, South Africa

David A. Raichlen, PhD
School of Anthropology
University of Arizona
Tucson, AZ, USA

Nicholas A. Ratamess, PhD
Department of Health and Exercise Science
The College of New Jersey
Ewing, NJ, USA

Justin S. Rhodes, PhD
Associate Professor
Department of Psychology
Beckman Institute for Advanced Science and
Technology
University of Illinois
Urbana-Champaign, IL, USA

Penny K. Riggs, PhD
Associate Professor of Functional Genomics
Department of Animal Science
College of Agriculture and Life Sciences
Texas A&M University
College Station, TX, USA

Michael D. Roberts, PhD
School of Kinesiology
Auburn University
Auburn, AL, USA

Stephen M. Roth, PhD
Department of Kinesiology
School of Public Health
University of Maryland
College Park, MD, USA

Gregory N. Ruegsegger, PhD
Division of Endocrinology, Diabetes, and
Nutrition
Department of Medicine
Mayo Clinic
Rochester, MN, USA

Lucas P. Santos, MSc
Cardiology and Cardiovascular Sciences
Faculty of Medical Sciences
Federal University of Rio Grande do Sul
Porto Alegre, Brazil

Mark A. Sarzynski, PhD
Department of Exercise Science
Arnold School of Public Health
University of South Carolina
Columbia, SC, USA

Emily E. Schmitt, PhD
Assistant Professor
Division of Kinesiology and Health
College of Health Sciences
University of Wyoming
Laramie, WY, USA

Jaime Schultz, PhD
Department of Kinesiology
Pennsylvania State University
State College, PA, USA

Alison V. September, PhD
Division of Exercise Science and Sports
Medicine
Department of Human Biology
Faculty of Health Sciences
University of Cape Town
Cape Town, South Africa

Jane T. Seto, PhD
Murdoch Children's Research Institute, and
Department of Paediatrics
University of Melbourne
The Royal Children's Hospital
Melbourne, Australia

Mark Tarnopolsky, MD, PhD
Department of Pediatrics and Medicine
McMaster University
Hamilton, Ontario, Canada

Beth A. Taylor, PhD
Department of Kinesiology
College of Agriculture, Health and Natural
Resources
University of Connecticut
Storrs, CT, and
Department of Preventive Cardiology
Hartford Hospital
Hartford, CT, USA

Martine Thomis, PhD
KU Leuven
Faculty of Movement and Rehabilitation
Sciences
Department of Movement Sciences Physical
Activity
Sports & Health Research Group
Tervuursevest Leuven, Belgium

Ryan T. Tierney, PhD
Temple University
Department of Kinesiology
Philadelphia, PA, USA

Matthijs D. van der Zee, MSc
PhD candidate, Department of Biological
Psychology
Human Behavioral and Movement Sciences
Vrije Universiteit Amsterdam
Amsterdam, Netherlands

Heather L. Vellers, PhD, RCEP
Assistant Professor of Exercise Physiology
Department of Kinesiology and Sport
Management
Texas Tech University
Lubbock, TX, USA

Andrew C. Venezia, PhD
Department of Exercise Science and Sport
The University of Scranton
Scranton, PA, USA

Jakob L. Vingren, PhD
Department of Kinesiology
Health Promotion and Recreation
University of North Texas
Denton, TX, USA

Sarah Voisin, PhD
Institute for Health and Sport
Victoria University
Melbourne, Australia

Guan Wang, PhD
Collaborating Centre of Sports Medicine
University of Brighton
Eastbourne, UK

James T. Webber, AS, BS, MA
School of Anthropology
University of Arizona
Tucson, AZ, USA

David K. Wiggins, PhD
George Mason University
Fairfax, VA, USA

Daniel J. Wilkinson, PhD
MRC-ARUK Centre for Musculoskeletal
Ageing Research & NIHR Nottingham
BRC University of Nottingham, School of
Medicine
Royal Derby Hospital
Derby, UK

Alun G. Williams, PhD
Sports Genomics Laboratory
Manchester Metropolitan University
Manchester, UK

Matthew T. Wittbrodt, PhD
Exercise Physiology Laboratory
School of Biological Sciences
Georgia Institute of Technology
Atlanta, GA, USA

FOREWORD

David Epstein

Since writing *The Sports Gene*, a book about genetics and athleticism for a lay audience, I've had the pleasure of discussing genes and exercise with a broader swath of humanity than I ever expected. A theme emerged in those conversations: every important aspect of an individual's personality and all of their proud accomplishments, they are certain, are purely functions of their unalloyed free will and expert decision-making; whenever they get really sick, that is purely genetic.

Interestingly, human intuition might more closely approximate the opposite of the truth. Evidence for important genetic contributions to personality is so voluminous that it is encoded in the so-called *first law* of behavioral genetics: "All human behavioral traits are heritable." That is not strictly true – if a Japanese couple moves to England and raises a daughter there, she will speak English but may inherit no Japanese – but it isn't far off. Meanwhile, we are facing an epidemic of common diseases – metabolic syndrome, obesity, diabetes – that were hardly even on the radar a few generations ago.

Sixty years ago, the number of Americans with diabetes was about equal to the population of Detroit. Today, that number is equal to the population of the 15 largest cities in the country combined. Throw in the number of Americans with prediabetes, and you'd have the 14th largest country in the world. To belabor the point, 1.3% of the global population is made up of Americans who are diabetic or likely to be diabetic within 5 years. And the US is merely leading the charge. A peloton of other countries is giving game chase. Needless to say, nothing changed in humanity's gene pool overnight to make so many people sick. Rather, our environment changed. Evolution did not prepare us for such rapid social change. The combination of supermarket culture and the knowledge economy have made for the perfect maladaptive storm: a practically limitless supply of food for a population of desk jockeys.

I was mulling over exactly this issue in my Brooklyn apartment in 2012 when Hurricane Sandy swept through. I decided to pass the time (until the electricity went out) watching the Disney film *WALL-E*, which one of the editors of this book (JTL) had recommended to me. (All in the name of science, of course.) It's a feel-good movie, to be sure, but I found part of it more harrowing than the hurricane. Smuggled inside a lovable Disney cartoon is a Philip K. Dick-esque sci-fi premonition. In the film, humans live aboard a spaceship, which they move through in what look like hovering La-Z-Boys. They need not even unglue their faces from hovering screens to summon robots with jumbo beverages. The bulbous space citizens have let their lower limbs atrophy, so when one falls out of his chair, an emergency message alerts him that he should not attempt to move. The message of modern society hasn't been quite so frank, but the results are trending in the same direction.

WALL-E crystallized an important question for me: Does the fact that the most pressing health concerns facing society are due to environmental change mean that there is no sense in bringing our ingenuity to bear to investigate the genetics of physical activity, and inactivity? In my opinion, absolutely not. The public is inundated with "nature versus nurture" headlines, but scientists know that without both genes and environments, there are no outcomes. Neither one can be understood in isolation.

Consider height, as easily measurable and intuitively heritable a trait as exists. In developed-world populations, variance in height between adults is typically 80–90% heritable. Nobody would argue that height does not have an important genetic component. And yet, visit a developing nation and you can see that height need not run in families. Ultimately, the work of scientists studying exercise genetics will hopefully help society learn how to ensure that physical inactivity need not run in families. Perhaps that will occur through a deeper understanding of the genetic mechanisms that regulate physical activity and how that knowledge can be used to create the most effective environmental interventions. That is, after all, the primary reason for studying genetics related to health and performance: to figure out how best to change the environment. Writing about genetics, I have frequently been asked (usually by fellow journalists and social scientists) why anyone should bother studying genetics since an individual cannot change their genes. I think the answer is simple: we need to understand what differences between people are real – and not intuition or folklore; which of those are important for outcomes we care about; and, finally, how to use that knowledge to get optimal outcomes for every individual.

Someday, perhaps, we can even go beyond tailoring environmental interventions. With developments such as the gene-editing technology CRISPR, there is, at least theoretically, the possibility of tailoring the genome. Alas, as anyone who has been paying attention to the last 15 years of research has noticed, the field might as well adopt a motto that Laura Hercher, director of research in human genetics at Sarah Lawrence College, NY, uses as her Twitter bio: *Genetics. It turned out to be more complicated than we thought.* In 2015, a team of psychologists and economists proposed a fourth law of behavioral genetics. (There were three already.) Their proposed law stated: "A typical human behavioral trait is associated with very many genetic variants, each of which accounts for a very small percentage of the behavioral variability." A corollary, it would seem, is that it will be extremely hard *ever* to use gene editing technology to shape a complex trait, because there are so many genetic variants contributing (not to mention nongene components of DNA, and other factors).

Except, several case studies in sports genetics have demonstrated how a single, powerful mutation can completely alter a phenotype. While reporting *The Sports Gene*, I tracked down Eero Mäntyranta, then an elderly but vigorous reindeer farmer in the Arctic region of Finland. In the 1960s, he was one of the best endurance athletes in the world – a seven-time Olympic medalist in cross-country skiing who won the 15 km in 1964 by a margin unequaled before or since. Twenty years after he retired, Finnish geneticists identified a mutation in his erythropoietin receptor gene (*EPOR*) that caused a massive overproduction of red blood cells. Another member of the family with the mutation was also an Olympic gold medalist, and a third was a world junior champion. Nobody in the family without the mutation was an accomplished ski racer. More recently, I was contacted by a self-taught amateur geneticist with two rare genetic diseases who thought she spotted one in an Olympic medalist sprinter. Together, we convinced the sprinter, Priscilla Lopes-Schliep, to take a genetic test, and it turned out she had an *LMNA* gene mutation that caused her to have lipodystrophy coupled with extreme muscle growth.

Finally, there is the so-called German Superbaby, with two mutated myostatin genes. Myostatin is a topic covered later in this book. As a teaser, Superbaby's mother is the only adult I'm aware of in the scientific literature with a single myostatin mutation, and she was a professional sprinter.

Any time a single mutation can have such a large effect, it is a potential gene-editing target. That also means that it is a potential gene-doping target. It might seem silly to contemplate gene doping when traditional methods of doping are so effective, but if sports history has proven anything, it is that whatever it is and whether it works or not, someone is going to try it. (And that someone is going to make big news and influence public perception if they get caught.) I'm glad to see that gene doping is one of the topics in this book, because it is one segment of an important discussion about gene editing and gene therapy in general. One of my favorite things about sports is that they provide a unique entry point into thorny ethical discussions that extend well beyond the field, to all of society. And this is an ethical discussion we need to have, sooner rather than later. For the most part, though, hopefully society-wide genetic alteration is something to be concerned about only in the longer term.

Right now, I hope, we can focus on accruing knowledge that will help make for impactful environmental interventions. If the health benefits of physical activity came in pill form, I think it's safe to say there is not a single healthcare provider who would not prescribe it. It is hard to imagine a body of evidence for anything that is more compelling than the evidence for the virtues of exercise. And yet, that evidence isn't having the widespread impact that, say, information about the harms of smoking has had. One need only look at cancer statistics to see that in the latter half of the 20th century, deaths related to smoking swamped all other forms of cancer. There is a 20-year lag between smoking rates and cancer deaths, and the current decline in deaths is not due to a med-tech victory in the "War on Cancer," but rather it is in large part the result of successful public health messaging about tobacco. Today, we are reaping the rewards of a decline in smoking rates that began decades ago. Unfortunately, messaging about the benefits of exercise appears to be less effective than warnings about the dangers of smoking. It suggests to me that addiction to inactivity in our society is more complex and stubborn than cigarette addiction.

That is an important reason for a systems approach to this research, and to a volume like this one. As scientists are increasingly forced to hyperspecialize, they necessarily tend to look at smaller pieces of a large puzzle. A cardiologist used to be the height of medical specialization, and now there are cardiologists who study only cardiac valves, with the muscle and electricity of the heart outside their purview. That is necessary for advancing the frontier of knowledge, but entails the risk of seeing the entire world through cardiac valve-colored glasses. Scientists run the risk of ending up like the ancient people Tolstoy wrote of who see only the figurehead on the prow of an approaching vessel and assume that it must be the motive force behind the ship. A reference book like this, which puts an incredible diversity of background information (and the associated citations) in one place, is a gift to the field. (Not to mention to curious layfolk, like the author of this foreword.)

It also ensures that we won't mistake the figurehead on the front of the ship, or any other single component, for the only important piece driving a complex phenomenon. That is important, because the work discussed in this book is ultimately about the most difficult and, I think, most important public health challenge in the developed world. Let this book be a call to interdisciplinary-research arms for an absolutely critical area of science.

PREFACE

As Monica, Steve, and I worked on this volume over the past 2 years, we all feel privileged to be a part of the growing foundation of sport and exercise systems genetics. All three of us, through luck, good timing, and/or inspiration, were fortunate to get into this field during its early days, when we were all primarily doing applied exercise physiology. The optimism that surrounded the general field of genetics at that time, as well as the belief that genetics would help us solve intractable health problems, led all of us to paddle hard enough to catch the front of the exercise genetics wave. Since that time, we have been fortunate to have many publications regarding the role of genetics and genomics in exercise as well as fortunate to have held funding from national granting agencies to investigate the role of genetics and genomics in determining exercise or activity responses. All three of us have also been called upon many times to be both scientific reviewers as well as associate editors dealing specifically with genetics articles submitted to national scientific journals. Through these experiences, we have had the opportunity to witness and be a part of the explosion over the past 25 years in knowledge regarding the genetics and genomics of sport and exercise.

While one of us (SR) had previously published books in this area, all three of us had separately realized that the amount of people wanting to work in the field was outstripping the available reference material. There are fine volumes available, but these are all several years old and, in this field, knowledge is moving quickly which outdates books rapidly. Additionally, all three of us have given numerous talks about specific areas within the field and during these talks we have found much curiosity, interest, and desire from colleagues to bring their efforts and expertise to the communal collaborative space that we are calling sport and exercise systems genetics. As such, there has always been a question about what to read to acquire a good background in the field and other than the few dated volumes available, there has been little to suggest. Thus, when we were approached by Routledge about developing this book, we jumped at the chance to help establish a reference manual in this fast-moving field; one that we acknowledge will at best serve as a marker of the available knowledge at this time and one that will require updates and revisions in the future to stay current.

Certainly, another aspect of this project which attracted us was the opportunity to bring together the thoughts of the finest minds in the world in these areas – scientists and writers who have contributed significantly to scientific thought in these areas, as well as new and upcoming scientists who are already making an impact. A perusal of the author list will show you that we are welcoming some bright newcomers to the field – e.g., Dr. David Ferguson at Michigan State University who has provided the only global proteomic scans available of the genetic mechanisms associated with physical activity as well as a novel method of transiently silencing genes in healthy animals – as well as hearing from established authors in the field, such as Dr. Claude Bouchard from Pennington Biomedical Center, who with over 1100 peer-reviewed articles to his name, really blazed the path for this field. These two examples are just representatives of the bright and curious minds that agreed to populate this volume with their knowledge and we profusely thank them and all of those that have helped write the individual chapters.

As editors, we want to thank our original Routledge development editor William Bailey who initiated and believed in this project, as well as Rebecca Connor who got us through the contract stages and all the Routledge internal processes. On our side, we want to thank Katie Feltman from the American College of Sports Medicine who gave us invaluable advice in the early stages of the proposal and contract development. As we drew closer to the end, as happens at times, both William Bailey and Rebecca Connor moved on to other projects and the book was ably picked up and carried over the goal line by David Varley and Megan Smith whom we thank both for their guidance, patience, and multiple conversations regarding "discoverability" of book chapters in this age of online digital literature discovery.

Lastly, as an editorial group, we want to thank you the reader for taking the time to read this book. We hope that you'll share it with your colleagues and make suggestions to us on how to improve future editions. What topics to include in this type of volume is a question that only those in the field – or those coming into the field – can help us with. In the end, this volume and future editions will only be stronger if the community helps us develop it.

As individuals, we each have many people to thank for their support as we developed this volume and it is only correct that we recognize those folks at the beginning of this volume:

- From Tim: I must thank my two co-editors Steve and Monica for keeping us on track with this book as well as all my genetics colleagues over the years who have patiently "tutored" me in the fine and sometimes not-so-fine points of genetics. Those colleagues include people like Drs. Steve Kleeberger, Larry Leamey, Daniel Pomp, and Ted Garland, Jr. Further, a huge thanks goes out to all my colleagues and students that have journeyed with me on all our "genetics adventures" including Drs. Mike Turner, Reuben Howden, Robin Fuchs-Young, Weston Porter, and Mike Massett. Lastly, the most thanks go to my wonderful and brilliant wife Faith who has had to put up with me babbling about SNPs and proteins at the dinner table for years; her support and encouragement is one of the pillars of my life (and my writing!).

- From Monica: It seems like just yesterday that my PhD mentor, Dr. Priscilla Clarkson, wandered into my tiny graduate student office and asked me if I wanted to play with some new research "toys" called muscle GeneChips that were being used in Dr. Eric Hoffman's laboratory. Never one to resist new toys, that day led me down a path (including a postdoctoral stint in the Hoffman laboratory and time as a junior faculty in his department) that balanced my background in applied muscle physiology with systems biology and genetics. As Tim mentioned earlier, the timing of getting to work within this emerging field of molecular exercise physiology brought me so many exciting opportunities, for which I am eternally thankful. For those, I have to thank Drs. Clarkson and Hoffman, along with other colleagues and collaborators, including Drs. Bill Kraus, Paul Thompson, and Joe Houmard, among many others, along with my fellow trainees and, later, my mentees. Finally, it has been a great pleasure working with Tim and Steve on this project and I appreciate being a part of such a great collaborative project.

- From Steve: I am indebted to the many colleagues I've had over the years, including several in this volume, who have helped push my work to be better. A few names in particular stand out, including Drs. Jim Hagberg, Robert Ferrell, and Ben Hurley, without whom I doubt very much genetics would have been a landing place for me. And years before that, Drs. Brian Sharkey and Brent Ruby sparked my interest in the field of exercise physiology as an undergraduate at the University of Montana. My students and technicians were the folks who pushed the science day-to-day and I'm grateful to be able to watch their successes and hope I played a part in the good work they are now doing. I've enjoyed my time working on this volume with Tim and Monica and thank them very much for their efforts.

INTRODUCTION

J. Timothy Lightfoot, Monica J. Hubal, and Stephen M. Roth

There is little doubt that humans have entered the "genetic" age, where the effort to understand and alter humanity's basic underlying code has become foremost in the minds of many scientists while many media outlets have declared the "21st century will be the age of genetics" (e.g., 2). The advances made in sequencing the human genome in the early 2000s – as well as other species' genomes – promised "to help convert this growing knowledge into treatments that can lengthen and enrich lives" (1). Since the early 2000s, information regarding pieces of the "genetic story" have continued to be revealed with continued hope that precision medicine – or treatments tailored to each of us based on our underlying genetic code – will become commonplace.

The idea that our underlying genetic code plays a role in sport and exercise performance is not a new one but, with access to a growing number of molecular tools associated with genetics, has become of greater interest and the topic of a burgeoning new discipline within exercise science. This text is meant to serve as a handbook – a reference marker if you like – for where this burgeoning discipline is today. As such, this reference marker is a foundation that includes most of what is known about the genetics of exercise and sports, written by the scientists who have discovered and developed much of that foundation over the past 40 years.

It may be logically asked, why use the term "systems genetics" to describe the various genetically related mechanisms involved in exercise characteristics? Our use of the term "systems genetics" is one indication of the tremendous changes that have occurred over the past 20 years in the field traditionally called "genetics." Formerly, "genetics" was used to refer to any factor/mechanism that was related to the heritability and function/structure of inheritance mechanisms. With the tremendous expansion of knowledge in this area, the term "genetics" is now more often used to refer to the action and mechanisms of single genes, while a newer term – "genomics" – is used in relation to the action and mechanisms of several genes in combination (3). In discussing whether to use "genetics" or "genomics" to describe the general content of this book, we believed that we needed to use a broader term that encompassed all mechanisms that arose from genetic and genomic pathways, as well as those mechanisms that were influenced by potential interactions between genetic, biological, and environmental factors. When we consulted with three geneticists (yes, they still call themselves that), each with extensive publication records regarding this issue, all three basically advised that we could use whatever term we thought was most appropriate. Thus, to encompass the diversity that is present in the field today, we choose to use the term "systems genetics" to indicate all mechanisms, processes, and interactions that influence the heritable characteristics of an organism. Applying this description to exercise and sport resulted in "sport and exercise systems genetics" which we define as "all heritable mechanisms, processes, and interactions that impact the capability and performance of sport and exercise." We believe that after reading this book, you will understand why it is well accepted that most exercise and sport characteristics (i.e., phenotypes) are influenced by not only classical genetic mechanisms, but also interactions among these mechanisms, other bio-logical systems, and what we know today as epigenetic influences.

As science in systems genetics has advanced, the media has warmed to the topic, resulting in more awareness by the public of news with genetic findings. Most of us are familiar with the increasing number of "Scientists Find Gene that Causes [*Insert Disease/Characteristics Here*]" types of articles that have been written since 2000, many of which may not be valid. Indeed, most scientists who work in the genetics world would immediately spot at least two problems with the hypothetical headline just mentioned. However, mistaken concepts aside, the public awareness of advances in genetics has caused an increase in awareness of the *possibility* of gen-etic involvement in sport and exercise performance among many exercise professionals. Indeed, there is a whole sub-field concerned with using genetic results to predict sport capability in athletes, especially child athletes (Drs. Venezia and Roth review this issue in Chapter 31). Thus, as research in genetics has grown, so has the interest in applying research findings to exercise and sports, as well as the interest from commercial companies in profiting from this knowledge.

The growing research interest in sport and exercise systems genetics, from our observa-tion, has led two types of science professionals to come into the field. One is the classically trained geneticist who views sport and exercise as interesting physiological and psychological perturbations to which s/he can apply their systems genetics knowledge. The other type of science professional, of which the three editors are all examples of, are traditionally trained exercise physiologists who see systems genetics as a way to understand the variation in response observed in humans engaged in acute or chronic exercise. This book targets both populations of science professionals to provide a review of the current knowledge on what is known about systems genetics across various areas of exercise and sport. Due to the dynamic nature of both systems genetics and exercise science, we anticipate that this volume, rather than being a static foundational reference manual, will also grow and change through future editions.

The structure of the book revolves around separate topical sections, each of which comprises multiple chapters. Four of these topical sections form the core of the book by focusing on gen-etic findings in the common forms of sport and exercise. These four core sections are prefaced by a section on general systems genetics concepts and capped off by a section on the ethics of employing systems genetics in exercise and sport settings. The four core sport and exer-cise sections address physical activity, exercise endurance and trainability, muscle strength and trainability, and sport performance. Within these sections, the reader will find a diversity of approaches and methodologies that have been used to explore not only whether there are gen-etic influences on these core areas, but also what genetic mechanisms regulate these core areas. While these four core sections comprise the crux of the sport- and exercise-related findings, the beginning and ending sections are no less important, especially in the context of today's systems genetics climate. The opening section deals with general systems genetics concepts and serves as a conceptual foundation for the rest of the book, as well as providing a succinct overview of the tremendous strides in systems genetics since 2000. Further, the concluding section deals with the ethics of applying these genetic findings to sport and performance. These types of ethical considerations are critical as we face – as practitioners – questions regarding talent selection, gene doping, and even gene editing.

To begin the book, we are honored to have a Foreword which sets the stage for why systems genetics in sports and exercise is important, written by Mr. David Epstein who – to our knowledge – is the only author to have written a sports genetics book that appeared on the *New York Times* best-seller list. After the six primary sections of the book, we have a closing section that includes a "last words chapter" as well as a conclusion chapter. With this last section, we have attempted to set the stage for future research in the field. The "last words chapter" was graciously written by Dr. Claude Bouchard, who is easily the most published and cited scientist in our field and whom many of us consider the "godfather" of exercise genetics. All in all, we believe that the structure of the book provides the most comprehensive coverage of this field to date and we are so thankful for all the authors who agreed to participate.

One of the challenges in writing about a relatively new area of scientific investigation – and especially a field that is at the intersection of two dynamic and rapidly changing disciplines – is that there are many more questions than there are good data and studies available to answer those questions. As such, one of the limitations of this book is that there are several areas where some existing science is available, but by no means a substantial enough base to provide solid conclusions at this time. We believe the general topics falling into this category currently are:

- the role of epigenetics in determining exercise responses;
- the role of miRNA – both circulating and tissue based – in regulating exercise responses;
- the role of genetics in determining the limits of performance; and
- the role of genetics in modulating performance psychology.

This list is by no means all inclusive, but represents a sampling of the topics about which we kept saying, "Wow, it'd be great if there was enough information on this topic for a chapter!" We do believe that there will be enough information in these areas in the future to address them in revised editions and would welcome scholars willing to join the author team and accept the challenge of describing those topics!

One area that we wanted to approach in this volume, but could not find any authors willing to tackle the topic (even after almost 9 months of the three of us searching), regarded the technical aspects of gene therapy in relation to the potential for gene doping. Given the tremendous interest and research with CRISPR-Cas9 systems, as well as existing work with *in vivo* gene silencing techniques, there have been suggestions that the use of these technologies in an exercise/sports environment may be imminent and even appropriate (see Chapters 32 and 33 in this volume). Some of these techniques are applied in Chapter 9 in this volume, but the uses described are purely from an animal hypothesis-testing approach. We hope that future volumes of this handbook will address this topic more fully because shining light on the topic is one of the few ways to prevent use and abuse of these technologies in the exercise and sports arena.

As we have worked on this volume, the new knowledge that is becoming apparent through the genetic approaches to exercise is quite exciting. Sport and exercise systems genetics encompass two disciplines that are individually rapidly growing and adding new theories and perspectives to their canon, while at the same time, intersecting to add substantially to each other. As such, we are proud to present this volume that summarizes where the field is at this moment. Perhaps more importantly, we are most excited to have the following chapters give us a benchmark so we can look forward to the discoveries that lie ahead.

References

1. **Collins FS**. Remarks at the Press Conference Announcing Sequencing and Analysis of the Human Genome. February 12, 2001. www.genome.gov/10001379/february-2001-working-draft-of-human-genome-director-collins/ [Accessed December 18, 2018.]
2. **Editorial Board**. March of science: the 21st century will be the age of genetics. *Independent* November 6, 2013.
3. **World Health Organization**. WHO definitions of genetics and genomics. www.who.int/genomics/geneticsVSgenomics/en/. [Accessed January 1, 2018.]

SECTION 1

General systems genetics

Introduction

With the completion of the first human genome sequence in 2000, scientific and public interest increased in regard to the impact of genetics on a wide variety of physiological traits. Sport and exercise traits were no exception, with many in the public and in science questioning the role that "genetics" played in both sport and exercise performance. However, because most sport and exercise scientists had/have little in the way of genetics background and training, catching up and keeping up with the rapid changes occurring in genetics continues to be a major challenge for the application of genetics to sport and exercise questions. Thus, the following four chapters aim to provide a foundation for the systems genetics concepts and techniques that are described and discussed in the remainder of the book.

As it should be with a general foundational section, the set of chapters that make up this section is wide ranging with each written by an acknowledged international leader in the field. The first chapter, written by Dr. Frank Booth and co-workers, encompasses a broad overview of why considering systems genetics is important, with the consistent context of the chapter focused on the personal and health cost of physical inactivity.

Maybe more than any other scientific discipline, the conceptual and theoretical framework of genetics has undergone massive changes in the past 20 years. Much of the genetics many of us learned before 2000 is obsolete and so the second chapter, by Dr. Penny Riggs, is a review of the major changes in genetics since the sequencing of the human genome, with an emphasis on the new concepts such as miRNA and epigenetics that can and should be applied to exercise and sport.

Physiologists do not often consider how the individual's genetic makeup could alter the responses that are observed during experiments, when in fact the genetic framework of an individual (or animal) can lead to marked differences during an experiment. Therefore, appropriate modeling systems are critical in genetic studies, so Chapter 3 provides an overview of the common human modeling systems used in genetic studies by Dr. Jaakko Kaprio.

Lastly, understanding the mechanisms and modeling are important, but most scientists agree that if we cannot apply the results to a population in general, then our science has difficulty making a difference. That is why the section finishes with a critical chapter by Dr. Molly Bray dedicated to how we can apply systems genetics to translational models and everyday life, with Dr. Bray using physical activity as the exercise phenotype described.

We believe that these four chapters will provide a great foundation for the rest of the book. You will find that the basic concepts covered in these chapters will be returned to repeatedly throughout the rest of the book as specific exercise and sport situations are dealt with. Due to the foundational nature of these chapters, we are grateful that these scientific thought leaders all agreed to participate. Enjoy!

1

WHY STUDY THE SYSTEMS GENETICS OF SPORT AND EXERCISE?

Frank W. Booth, Taylor J. Kelty, Kolter B. Grigsby,
and Gregory N. Ruegsegger

Introduction

This chapter is tilted toward the authors' perspective of the future of exercise science in contrast to our recent reviews (8, 9, 44) which were more focused on the retrospective side of exercise mechanisms. Both types of reviews can be controversial. However, perspective reviews distinguish themselves in that they are based more upon an opinion of the future, and less on data from the literature. As such, the future being unpredictable, the authors' comments could be considered to provide backgrounds for future research considerations as well as the rest of the chapters of this volume.

Exercise systems genomics

This section bookends the final contributed chapter of the book, which is written by the founder of the field of exercise genomics, Claude Bouchard. Bouchard's tremendous foresights allowed him to establish exercise systems genetics in humans three decades before systems genetics was recognized as a field. Bouchard began phenotyping exercise as early as 1976 (14), when he correlated variables with skeletal maturity and chronological age in 8–18-year-old boys. A 1980 paper (12) was about estimates of sibling correlations and genetic/heritability estimates in a number of French-Canadian families which was extended in 1983 by an overall review of the genetics of physiological fitness (13). Furthermore, Bouchard pioneered the integration of exercise training and genetics in his classical Heritage family study (10, 11). In 2007, the term "systems genomics" began being popularized (35) to include Bouchard's older science of "exercise genomics." In 1999, he already had performed sufficient studies to conclude that trainability of VO_2max had a significant genetic component based upon considerable heterogeneity in degree of increase in VO_2max following the same endurance-training program in 481 sedentary, adult Caucasians from 98 two-generation families. With the establishment of exercise genomics and exercise systems genomics, a wide variety of exercise characteristics can be viewed through the lens of exercise systems genetics.

One example of exercise systems genetics is that contracting skeletal muscle releases peptides (termed myokines (22, 39)) into capillaries. The myokines then circulate to a distant site (i.e., cells, tissues, or organs) where they initiate a cascade to have a subsequent biochemical effect at that site (25, 37). The first investigator to identify a molecule that fitted the criteria to have an endocrine-like function from skeletal muscle was Pedersen, whose lab reported in 1994 that blood interleukin (IL)-6 increased during exercise (52). Then, in 2003, Pedersen proposed, "IL-6 and other cytokines, which are produced and released by skeletal muscles, exerting their effects in other organs of the body, should be named 'myokines'" (38). IL-6 is now the prototype myokine emulating skeletal muscle-to-organ crosstalk, or systems genetics. Recently, Whitham et al. (54) reported that many circulating proteins are packaged within extracellular vesicles that also perform tissue crosstalk during exercise to produce systemic biological effects. Our notion is that components in the extracellular vesicles could form another candidate for the therapeutic manipulation of some of the thousands of positive molecular benefits of exercise.

The challenge of understanding the above example was reflected in a 2017 opinion piece where 16 invited experts presented their viewpoints on the status and future of systems genetics (5). The experts' consensus opinion was: "deciphering genotype to phenotype relationships is a central challenge of systems genetics and will require understanding how networks and higher-order properties of biological systems underlie complex traits" (5). The authors' interpretation of systems genetics in relationship to physical activity and physical inactivity will be considered in the next section.

Exercise presents a high stress; however, the body is able to survive by maintaining its homeostasis during performance

Exercise is stress. Stress has numerous definitions. The operational definition for stress used herein is an increased blood cortisol concentration. As such, maximal exercise effort is one of the greatest stressors to the body. An underlying reason for intense exercise, and thus intense stress, was postulated by Charles Darwin. On a statistical basis, those who are physically unfit are more likely to be eliminated prior to their being able to reach reproductive age. Herbert Spencer coined the phrase "survival of the fittest." It is unlikely that the pre-adolescent individual of 5000 years ago, who never had the capability to perform physical activity, could have survived to puberty to perpetuate their genes to the next generation. Thus, their gene pool would be extinguished and not passed on to the next generation (21). Today, the elimination of infectious diseases allows most individuals in developed communities to live to puberty and have the ability to pass their genes to the next generation, while having less than the maximal fitness of their distinct ancestors. Thus, the notion can be raised whether "survival of the fitness" by natural selection to infectious organisms has been bypassed, allowing individual survival to pass a "less fit" gene pool to stress on to the next generation. Simultaneously, during the same era, we have the notion that children and adolescents who are physically playing less will have a lower development of lifetime physical fitness, which could mean that they are passing epigenetic changes for weaker maximal aerobic and strength fitness to their offspring. The lifetime consequence of such changes in physical fitness would become apparent when your friends must enter assisted care living while you do not. Along this line, we previously reviewed in greater detail our interpretation of exercise and Darwin's writings (7).

Exercise systems genetics versus inactivity systems genetics

Exercise systems genetics identifies the genes that: 1) prevent chronic disease, 2) treat for loss of function due to lack of sufficient exercise, and 3) increase sports performance. For definition purposes related to the previous sentence, a National Institutes of Health (NIH) website (2) defines the Common Fund $170-million research program:

> The Molecular Transducers of Physical Activity in Humans' effort to uncover the molecular changes that occur in response to movement is expected to transform clinical medicine's use of physical activity as a *treatment* and *preventive* strategy. Although researchers have demonstrated that physical activity is good for us in many ways, they know little about the molecules that *cause* these improvements.

We interpret the mission of this NIH Common Fund Program to be to look for molecules that cause the "treatment and preventive strategies" of physical activity. In this sense, the NIH Program has made an important distinction. Stein and Bollister (47) in 2006 made the statement, "Anabolic and catabolic pathways are usually separate." They compared two lists of mRNAs in papers by Lecker et al. (31) and by Fluck (23) that showed "virtually no overlap" in skeletal muscle mRNAs for atrophy and for recovery from atrophy, respectively. Taken together, future research will need to recognize that gene changes during exercise training may not be identical to gene changes when athletes and those who are physically active "take time off" to recover from "the season," recover from injury, or switch sports where some genes may play a role in detraining while others play a role in training. An example of detraining while continuing to train is that VO_2max fell for 22 years between the mid 20s and later 40s in men whose training volume declined over 22 years (50). However, the two men in the same study who were able to maintain their exercise volume unchanged over the 22 years had no decline in their VO_2max (50). In an animal model, the Booth lab showed that lifetime VO_2peak occurred at 19 weeks of age in female rats (45, 49), which in the same rats was independent from their lifetime peak in voluntary running distance that happened at their younger age of 8–9 weeks, implying the mechanisms for these two lifetime events could be different. In humans, a study of 23 females and males who trained one leg for 3 months, detrained for 9 months, and then retrained both legs for 3 months (33) found 3404 gene isoforms in the vastus lateralis muscle, mainly associated with oxidative function, after the first training. All training changes in these mRNAs were absent after 9 months of detraining. The experiment's investigators concluded, "No coherent evidence of a skeletal muscle transcriptome memory was observed, even though there were some data indicating a training–induced memory mechanism … These findings show the great need for highly controlled studies of repeated exercise training."

Physical inactivity is a necessary reference group to show healthy exercise effects – and turns out to be a very unhealthy comparison!

The effect of exercise can be better elucidated by exercise in the absence of gravity. Weight–bearing exercise is necessary to prevent bone loss. Nongravity ("lack of pounding of bones upon impact") exercise such as cycling is associated with a seven times increased likelihood to have spine osteopenia than running (41). Weightlessness of spaceflight causes 10 years of bone atrophy to occur in 1 year (53). The cardiovascular system experiences a tenfold faster loss of functional capacity in space (53). In comparison with ground-based models of weightlessness, the decline of 27% in VO_2max when aging from 20 to 60 years old was comparable with the 26% loss that the same men experienced after 20 days of continuous (24 hours/day) bed rest at the age of 20 (34). The above examples of short-term (days to 1 year) drastic reductions in physical activity leading to dramatic losses of physiological function provide insight into subtle reductions in physical activity over decades. Failure to have more than 150 minutes of weekly exercise over periods of decades leads to the increased risk of 40 chronic diseases and a premature end to life (44).

A biased positive look to the future

One of the charges to the authors of this review that came from an editor of this book was to give a 30,000-foot view.

A projection into where technology seems to be taking physical inactivity

Until now, most genetic studies have focused on a single gene or gene clusters that dictate a single trait in a phenotype. However, with technological advances, it is now possible to look at a phenotype as a dynamic system utilizing the entire genome. Systems genetics integrates transcriptomics, proteomics, and metabolomics for the different physiological systems to gain a more complete understanding of a phenotype.

First, let us examine how systems genetics has developed until now. Human skeletal muscle has over 6000 expressed genes leading to more than 600 secreted proteins (37). Training is able to alter over 3000 of these gene isoforms (33), producing hundreds of different proteins in skeletal muscle (36), leading to over 200 metabolites secreted into the bloodstream (15), all of which contribute to the rise of a specific phenotype. Therefore, identification of a single athlete-model phenotype with traditional single gene methods will prove very difficult, if not impossible. Conversely, an approach using systems genetics could reproduce the phenomics of the athlete, leading to the potential of improved exercise performance through gene manipulation.

The benefits of systems genetics do not just benefit champion athletes, but are useful for the entire population. Studies associate physical inactivity with multiple negative health consequences (8, 32). Two key approaches can be used to fight physical inactivity: 1) to identify the underlying genetics that produce a physically inactive phenotype, and 2) to look at the underlying mechanisms of physical inactivity that contribute to the negative health effects. Importantly, mechanisms of physical inactivity and physical activity are sometimes different (9). Applying the holistic approach of systems genetics to physical inactivity could generate novel gene therapies that either could prevent a physically inactive phenotype from beginning in the first place, or could prevent the negative health consequences birthed by physical inactivity (27, 44).

Multiple, biased, concerned looks to the future

New technology is often based upon reducing physical activity

New technologies will continue to remove physical activity from daily living. To counter loss of physical activity because of new technology, a molecular understanding of both the motivation to keep active and to counter motivation to be inactive will be needed. One example of a new technology that will reduce physical activity is artificial intelligence. At one end of the spectrum, artificial intelligence can scan massive amounts of data and not only give the specific output, but also store that data to be called on in future problems, giving it a vast potential to revolutionize public health (29). Ironically, however, these advancements in technology could also render much of the physical work done by the public unnecessary. Studies around the world have shown that the public and even children are becoming more physically inactive (9, 20, 43), while technology is advancing and becoming more accessible to the public (26, 40). This leads to a question to be answered: Will advancing technology (e.g., artificial intelligence) worsen the pandemic of physical inactivity worldwide, and thus worsen chronic diseases? In summary, advancements in technology are unlikely to stop so we must find another approach to survive by maintaining appropriate physical activity levels for a healthy lifestyle. Stated alternatively, a need exists to stay healthy through physical activity while our lives are getting easier.

Inheritance of low voluntary running behavior

One concern for the future to be expressed is whether physical inactivity will produce adverse transgenerational epigenetic changes. Stated alternatively, do the offspring of physically inactive parents inherit some of their parents' consequential epigenetic changes due to physical inactivity and therefore remain predisposed to physical inactivity behavior themselves? One example of precedence to support the viability of such a hypothesis now exists. Rapid, human-wide, epigenetic changes in the last 30 years of the 20th century exist in the form of an increased type 2 diabetes prevalence in Arizonian Pima Indians. In the 10–14-year-old age group of Arizonian Pima Indians, type 2 diabetes increased in boys in the 1967–1976 time period from 0% to 1.4% in the 1987–1996 time period. In girls, the increase was from 0.72% in 1967–1976 to 2.88% in 1987–1996. Dabelea et al. (17), in reference to the above-mentioned increase in Arizonian Pima Indians concluded that "a vicious cycle related to an increase in the frequency of exposure to diabetes *in utero* appears to be an important feature of this epidemic."

Arizonian Pima Indians separated geographically from Mexican Pima Indians approximately 300 BC by moving to what is now Arizona (17). Schulz and Chaudhari (46) have reviewed the lifestyle changes that began in about 1900 in the Arizonian Pima Indians after they were forced to switch from their Mexican agricultural lifestyle to a Western diet and a sedentary lifestyle. The change occurred because white settlers diverted water that supported the Pimas' agriculture, forcing them to eventually move to a US government-run reservation where they no longer worked for their food. Schulz and Chaudhari (46) commented on the event, stating "The timing of this significant change in lifestyle and livelihood coincides with the development of diabetes among the Arizona Pimas." In contrast, the Mexican Pima Indian cohort remained farming in Mexico, where they did not experience an increase in prevalence in type 2 diabetes during the same time period. Importantly, the increased type 2 diabetes prevalence occurred within Arizonian Pima Indians during a few generations of experiencing the new Western lifestyle. Pima Indians have now been shown to be one of the world's populations most susceptible to environmentally induced type 2 diabetes (50% in adults).

Does epigenetics play a role in type 2 diabetes and in physical inactivity?

Epigenetics could play a role in the growing incidence of type 2 diabetes, as described in a recent review paper (18). The above-mentioned points lead us to the research question of whether physical inactivity, which was associated with the Arizionian Pima's development of type 2 diabetes, also caused transgenerational epigenetic changes that accentuates greater behavior of motivation to be physically inactive, which is unknown.

Low voluntary running animal model to mimic increased human inactivity

To begin to tie the above-discussed human studies into future generations, animal studies have the potential to model the state of human inactivity, which arguably occurred when machines began replacing human physical labor over a century ago. In 2009, we began the selective breeding of rats for the phenotype of low voluntary running to mimic the loss of human physical labor/work. Our experimental design was modeled after the selective breeding models of Garland (48) and of Britton and Koch (30). The female and the male with the lowest voluntary running distance from each litter of 13 families were selected to be the breeding pair for the next generation of breeding using a scheduled order of breeding. Our initial findings in 2012 were that the newly bred rats voluntarily ran the same distances in each of the first five generations of selective breeding compared to their wild-type ancestors. However, litters in the sixth generation voluntarily ran significantly lower distances than their wild-type founders (42). In 2018, we rescued about one-third of the voluntary running distance lost by selective breeding by a transient overexpression of the protein kinase inhibitor alpha (*PKIA*) gene, which was delivered within an adeno-associated virus by a localized injection into the nucleus accumbens (24). The observation supported the existence of genes with low voluntary physical activity functions. In 2013, den Hoed et al. (19) reported that genes with sedentary functions were present in the more sedentary pair of 772 pairs of monozygotic and dizygotic twins. The recognition that genes exist for physical inactivity changes physical inactivity from being classified by the US government as a "risk factor" for chronic diseases to an "actual cause" of chronic diseases. Eventually, because genes cause physical inactivity, physical inactivity will need to be considered as a disease that causes chronic diseases and aging.

The high economic costs of physical inactivity are contributing in their small way to the bankruptcy of our children's future cost of living

Why must economics be a vital part of an exercise systems genetics review? To provide some potential answers to the question, this paragraph provides six sets of facts. First, with accelerometers as the measurement vehicle, only 1 out of 20 US adults meet the US guidelines (51). Alternatively stated, 19 out of 20 US adults do not meet the US physical activity guidelines. Thus, in our opinion, 19 out of 20 US adults are not likely obtaining the health benefits from exercise. Second, US healthcare costs of 17.9% of gross domestic product are the highest in the world, compared to a range of 9.6–12.4% in a select group of the ten highest-income countries (6). The US Congressional Budget Office (CBO) data shows that spending on major healthcare programs which accounts for 28% of federal noninterest spending as of 2017 would increase to 40% in 2047 (1). The CBO states: "The aging of the population and excess cost growth are reasons for the sharp rise projected for spending on Social Security and the major federal healthcare programs over the next 30 years" (1). Third, the US ranks 43rd (4) and 45th (3) in life expectancy. Fourth, the average US life expectancy decreased for the past 2 years (55) – is the lack of exercise a contributor to loss of life expectancy? Fifth, Carlson et al. (16) of the CDC reported, "Overall, 11.1% (95% CI: 7.3, 14.9) of aggregate, annual, healthcare expenditures were associated with inadequate physical activity (i.e., inactive and insufficiently active designations)." Sixth, we used the 11.1% annual cost in the previous sentence from Carlson et al. (16) to estimate the accumulated annual costs of physical inactivity. In 2016, $3.3 trillion was the total US health costs, or $10,348/person. Thus taking 11.1% as the fraction of total healthcare cost, physical inactivity in the US cost $366 billion in 2016. To obtain a better appreciation of the magnitude of $366 billion, the next comparisons are made: 1) US healthcare costs for physical inactivity was $1132/individual; 2) 8 years' worth of healthcare costs for physical inactivity would pay for 1 year of total healthcare; and 3) 1 year's cost of physical inactivity in 2016 would pay for 9.8 annual NIH budgets at $37.3 billion each.

As we noted in 2012, there is one potential solution to the problem (8). Kersh and Morone (28) wrote, "Public health crusades are typically built on a scientific base … In any event, medical knowledge in itself is rarely enough to stimulate a political response. Rather, the key to its impact lies in the policy entrepreneurs who spread the medical findings" (28). Thus, we suggest that a more impactful method to appeal to the policy entrepreneurs is to explain the impact of exercise, sport, and physical inactivity on the economy, as we did earlier.

What systems genetics could do for humans

Systems genetics can be appreciated for its potential future molecular explanations regarding the basis for the biological beauty that underwrites the living machinery in animals and humans to provide them with a continuous sub-conscious, homeostatic maintenance of their existence. Furthermore, regulatory systems invoke physiological reinforcements to allow molecular adaptations to new environments by lowering homeostatic disruptions. Alternatively phrased as a question: "What is the ensemble within the orchestra of genes in organs throughout the organism that permit survival to restrict the stress of exercise within homeostatic limits?" Upon answering this question, the next challenge will be to determine how to slow the unrelenting reduction in maximal capacities of physiological systems whose demise is not compatible with continued life because one or more of the dwindling capacities of organ and system capacities to maintain homeostasis is exceeded. When we gain a firm grasp on the systems genetics that regulate both exercise and sport responses, we will be one step closer to answering the aforementioned question.

Acknowledgements: Supported by the University of Missouri (FWB, TJK, KBG, and GNR).

References

1. **Congressional Budget Office**. *The 2017 Long-Term Budget Outlook.* Washington, DC: Congressional Budget Office, 2017.
2. **National Institute of Health**. Frequently asked questions. In: Molecular Transducers of Physical Activity in Humans. Bethesda, MD: National Institute of Health, 2016.
3. **World Population Review**. Life expectancy by country 2017. www.worldpopulationreview.com/countries/life-expectancy-by-country/, 2017.
4. **Central Intelligence Agency**. *The World Factbook.* Washington, DC: Central Intelligence Agency, 2018.
5. **Baliga NS, Bjorkegren JL, Boeke JD, Boutros M, Crawford NP, Dudley AM, Farber CR, Jones A, Levey AI, Lusis AJ, Mak HC, Nadeau JH, Noyes MB, Petretto E, Seyfried NT, Steinmetz LM, and Vonesch SC.** The state of systems genetics in 2017. *Cell Systems* 4: 7–15, 2017.
6. **Bauchner H and Fontanarosa PB.** Health care spending in the United States compared with 10 other high-income countries: What Uwe Reinhardt might have said. *JAMA* 319: 990–992, 2018.
7. **Booth FW, Chakravarthy MV, and Spangenburg EE.** Exercise and gene expression: physiological regulation of the human genome through physical activity. *The Journal of Physiology* 543: 399–411, 2002.
8. **Booth FW, Roberts CK, and Laye MJ.** Lack of exercise is a major cause of chronic diseases. *Comprehensive Physiology* 2: 1143–1211, 2012.
9. **Booth FW, Roberts CK, Thyfault JP, Ruegsegger GN, and Toedebusch RG.** Role of inactivity in chronic diseases: evolutionary insight and pathophysiological mechanisms. *Physiological Reviews* 97: 1351–1402, 2017.
10. **Bouchard C.** Genomic predictors of trainability. *Experimental Physiology* 97: 347–352, 2012.
11. **Bouchard C, An P, Rice T, Skinner JS, Wilmore JH, Gagnon J, Pérusse L, Leon AS, and Rao DC.** Familial aggregation of VO(2max) response to exercise training: results from the HERITAGE Family Study. *Journal of Applied Physiology (Bethesda, MD: 1985)* 87: 1003–1008, 1999.

12. **Bouchard C, Demirjian A**, and **Mongeau E.** Sibling correlations and genetic estimates for selected blood variables in French Canadian children. *Human Genetics* 54: 259–263, 1980.

13. **Bouchard C** and **Malina RM.** Genetics of physiological fitness and motor performance. *Exercise and Sport Sciences Reviews* 11: 306–339, 1983.

14. **Bouchard C, Malina RM, Hollmann W**, and **Leblanc C.** Relationships between skeletal maturity and submaximal working capacity in boys 8 to 18 years. *Medicine and Science in Sports* 8: 186–190, 1976.

15. **Burke MF, Dunbar RL**, and **Rader DJ.** Could exercise metabolomics pave the way for gymnomimetics? *Science Translational Medicine* 2: 41–35, 2010.

16. **Carlson SA, Fulton JE, Pratt M, Yang Z**, and **Adams EK.** Inadequate physical activity and health care expenditures in the United States. *Progress in Cardiovascular Diseases* 57: 315–323, 2015.

17. **Dabelea D, Hanson RL, Bennett PH, Roumain J, Knowler WC**, and **Pettitt DJ.** Increasing prevalence of type II diabetes in American Indian children. *Diabetologia* 41: 904–910, 1998.

18. **Davegardh C, Garcia-Calzon S, Bacos K**, and **Ling C.** DNA methylation in the pathogenesis of type 2 diabetes in humans. *Molecular Metabolism*, 14: 12–25, 2018.

19. **den Hoed M, Brage S, Zhao JH, Westgate K, Nessa A, Ekelund U, Spector TD, Wareham NJ**, and **Loos RJ.** Heritability of objectively assessed daily physical activity and sedentary behavior. *The American Journal of Clinical Nutrition* 98: 1317–1325, 2013.

20. **Duan J, Hu H, Wang G**, and **Arao T.** Study on current levels of physical activity and sedentary behavior among middle school students in Beijing, China. *PloS One* 10: e0133544, 2015.

21. **Eaton SB** and **Eaton SB.** An evolutionary perspective on human physical activity: Implications for health. *Comparative Biochemistry and Physiology Part A, Molecular & Integrative Physiology* 136: 153–159, 2003.

22. **Febbraio MA** and **Pedersen BK.** Contraction-induced myokine production and release: is skeletal muscle an endocrine organ? *Exercise and Sport Sciences Reviews* 33: 114–119, 2005.

23. **Fluck M, Schmutz S, Wittwer M, Hoppeler H**, and **Desplanches D.** Transcriptional reprogramming during reloading of atrophied rat soleus muscle. *American Journal of Physiology – Regulatory, Integrative and Comparative Physiology* 289: R4–R14, 2005.

24. **Grigsby KB, Ruegsegger GN, Childs TE**, and **Booth FW.** Overexpression of protein kinase inhibitor alpha reverses rat low voluntary running behavior. *Molecular Neurobiology*, 2018. doi: 10.1007/s12035-018-1171-0.

25. **Hojman P, Gehl J, Christensen JF**, and **Pedersen BK.** Molecular mechanisms linking exercise to cancer prevention and treatment. *Cell Metabolism* 27: 10–21, 2018.

26. **Johnson GM.** Internet use and child development: The techno-microsystem. *Australian Journal of Educational and Developmental Psychology* 10: 32–43, 2010.

27. **Kelly SA, Villena FP**, and **Pomp D.** The "Omics" of voluntary exercise: Systems approaches to a complex phenotype. *Trends in Endocrinology and Metabolism* 26: 673–675, 2015.

28. **Kersh R** and **Morone J.** The politics of obesity: Seven steps to government action. *Health Affairs (Project Hope)* 21: 142–153, 2002.

29. **Kiefer AW, Pincus D, Richardson MJ**, and **Myer GD.** Virtual reality as a training tool to treat physical inactivity in children. *Frontiers in Public Health* 5: 349, 2017.

30. **Koch LG** and **Britton SL.** Artificial selection for intrinsic aerobic endurance running capacity in rats. *Physiological Genomics* 5: 45–52, 2001.

31. **Lecker SH, Jagoe RT, Gilbert A, Gomes M, Baracos V, Bailey J, Price SR, Mitch WE**, and **Goldberg AL.** Multiple types of skeletal muscle atrophy involve a common program of changes in gene expression. *FASEB Journal* 18: 39–51, 2004.

32. **Lee IM, Shiroma EJ, Lobelo F, Puska P, Blair SN**, and **Katzmarzyk PT.** Effect of physical inactivity on major non-communicable diseases worldwide: an analysis of burden of disease and life expectancy. *The Lancet* 380: 219–229, 2012.

33. **Lindholm ME, Giacomello S, Werne Solnestam B, Fischer H, Huss M, Kjellqvist S**, and **Sundberg CJ.** The impact of endurance training on human skeletal muscle memory, global isoform expression and novel transcripts. *PLoS Genetics* 12: e1006294, 2016.

34. **McGavock JM, Hastings JL, Snell PG, McGuire DK, Pacini EL, Levine BD**, and **Mitchell JH.** A forty-year follow-up of the Dallas Bed Rest and Training study: The effect of age on the cardiovascular response to exercise in men. *The Journals of Gerontology Series A, Biological Sciences and Medical Sciences* 64: 293–299, 2009.

35. **Morahan G** and **Williams RW.** Systems genetics: The next generation in genetics research? *Novartis Foundation Symposium* 281: 181–188; discussion 188–191, 208–189, 2007.

36. **Padrao AI**, **Ferreira R**, **Amado F**, **Vitorino R**, and **Duarte JA.** Uncovering the exercise-related proteome signature in skeletal muscle. *Proteomics* 16: 816–830, 2016.

37. **Pedersen BK** and **Febbraio MA.** Muscles, exercise and obesity: Skeletal muscle as a secretory organ. *Nature Reviews Endocrinology* 8: 457–465, 2012.

38. **Pedersen BK**, **Steensberg A**, **Fischer C**, **Keller C**, **Keller P**, **Plomgaard P**, **Febbraio M**, and **Saltin B.** Searching for the exercise factor: Is IL-6 a candidate? *Journal of Muscle Research and Cell Motility* 24: 113–119, 2003.

39. **Petersen AM** and **Pedersen BK.** The anti-inflammatory effect of exercise. *Journal of Applied Physiology* (Bethesda, MD: 1985) 98: 1154–1162, 2005.

40. **Prensky M.** Digital natives, digital immigrants part 1. *On the Horizon* 9: 1–6, 2001.

41. **Rector RS**, **Rogers R**, **Ruebel M**, and **Hinton PS.** Participation in road cycling vs running is associated with lower bone mineral density in men. *Metabolism: Clinical and Experimental* 57: 226–232, 2008.

42. **Roberts MD**, **Gilpin L**, **Parker KE**, **Childs TE**, **Will MJ**, and **Booth FW.** Dopamine D1 receptor modulation in nucleus accumbens lowers voluntary wheel running in rats bred to run high distances. *Physiology & Behavior* 105: 661–668, 2012.

43. **Roman B**, **Serra-Majem L**, **Ribas-Barba L**, **Perez-Rodrigo C**, and **Aranceta J.** How many children and adolescents in Spain comply with the recommendations on physical activity? *The Journal of Sports Medicine and Physical Fitness* 48: 380–387, 2008.

44. **Ruegsegger GN** and **Booth FW.** Health benefits of exercise. *Cold Spring Harbor Perspectives in Medicine* 8: a029694, 2018.

45. **Ruegsegger GN**, **Toedebusch RG**, **Braselton JF**, **Childs TE**, and **Booth FW.** Left ventricle transcriptomic analysis reveals connective tissue accumulation associates with initial age-dependent decline in Vo2peak from its lifetime apex. *Physiological Genomics* 49: 53–66, 2017.

46. **Schulz LO** and **Chaudhari LS.** High-risk populations: The Pimas of Arizona and Mexico. *Current Obesity Reports* 4: 92–98, 2015.

47. **Stein TP** and **Bolster DR.** Insights into muscle atrophy and recovery pathway based on genetic models. *Current Opinion in Clinical Nutrition and Metabolic Care* 9: 395–402, 2006.

48. **Swallow JG**, **Carter PA**, and **Garland T**, Jr. Artificial selection for increased wheel-running behavior in house mice. *Behavior Genetics* 28: 227–237, 1998.

49. **Toedebusch RG**, **Ruegsegger GN**, **Braselton JF**, **Heese AJ**, **Hofheins JC**, **Childs TE**, **Thyfault JP**, and **Booth FW.** AMPK agonist AICAR delays the initial decline in lifetime-apex Vo2 peak, while voluntary wheel running fails to delay its initial decline in female rats. *Physiological Genomics* 48: 101–115, 2016.

50. **Trappe SW**, **Costill DL**, **Vukovich MD**, **Jones J**, and **Melham T.** Aging among elite distance runners: a 22-yr longitudinal study. *Journal of Applied Physiology* (Bethesda, MD: 1985) 80: 285–290, 1996.

51. **Troiano RP**, **Berrigan D**, **Dodd KW**, **Masse LC**, **Tilert T**, and **McDowell M.** Physical activity in the United States measured by accelerometer. *Medicine and Science in Sports and Exercise* 40: 181–188, 2008.

52. **Ullum H**, **Haahr PM**, **Diamant M**, **Palmo J**, **Halkjaer-Kristensen J**, and **Pedersen BK.** Bicycle exercise enhances plasma IL-6 but does not change IL-1 alpha, IL-1 beta, IL-6, or TNF-alpha pre-mRNA in BMNC. *Journal of Applied Physiology* (Bethesda, MD: 1985) 77: 93–97, 1994.

53. **Vernikos J** and **Schneider VS.** Space, gravity and the physiology of aging: parallel or convergent disciplines? A mini-review. *Gerontology* 56: 157–166, 2010.

54. **Whitham M**, **Parker BL**, **Friedrichsen M**, **Hingst JR**, **Hjorth M**, **Hughes WE**, **Egan CL**, **Cron L**, **Watt KI**, **Kuchel RP**, **Jayasooriah N**, **Estevez E**, **Petzold T**, **Suter CM**, **Gregorevic P**, **Kiens B**, **Richter EA**, **James DE**, **Wojtaszewski JFP**, and **Febbraio MA.** Extracellular vesicles provide a means for tissue crosstalk during exercise. *Cell Metabolism* 27: 237–251.e234, 2018.

55. **Woolf SH** and **Aron L.** Failing health of the United States. *BMJ* 360: k496, 2018.

2

EXPANSION OF KNOWLEDGE AND ADVANCES IN GENETICS FOR QUANTITATIVE ANALYSES

Penny K. Riggs

Introduction

During the nearly two decades since completion of the Human Genome Project, breakthroughs in technologies and analytical approaches, along with deeper understanding of the genome, have resulted in advanced research tools. Because of this progress, research efforts can be directed toward clarifying the genetic mechanisms that affect physiological responses to exercise activity and performance. This chapter broadly introduces genetic concepts that have emerged since the beginning of the millennium. In addition to exploring new-found aspects of genome function and regulation, the role of multigenic traits and the challenges in determining causality following identification of genetic associations are also addressed.

The Human Genome Project

Following debates and discussion among scientists, policymakers, and other interested parties during the early 1980s, a strategy developed for conducting the Human Genome Project, which was anticipated to be a 15-year endeavor. With US congressionally authorized funding, the Department of Energy (DOE) and the National Institutes of Health (NIH) agreed to participate in making the project a reality (15). A final component of funding was appropriated in 1989 to establish the National Center for Human Genome Research (PLN 101–166 (55)). The Center, now known as the National Human Genome Research Institute (NHGRI), along with the DOE Joint Genome Institute, provided "headquarters" for the daunting project that officially began in October 1990. Lively accounts of events leading up to the project give detailed looks into the personalities, policies, and substantial discussion that preceded the project's implementation (13, 66).

Over the next decade, the Human Genome Project was *on* in the US, and in conjunction with international partners. Technological advances in methodology and computing, and corporate competition spurred on the process. With the turn of the century, the first draft of the genome sequence was declared complete, and in February 2001, the International Human Genome Project team (29) and the Celera Genomics team (74) independently published the first sequence assembly drafts of the human genome. Completion of the draft brought some surprise and generated discussion. That the structure of the genome contained far fewer genes than anticipated was unexpected (12). Political and ethical concerns for the use of genomic information (32), and controversy over competing approaches to the project (9) brought much attention and new legislation such as The Genetic Information Nondiscrimination Act (50). However, enthusiasm for using this "great gift to humanity" (31) ensued, and the rapid pace of advancements in knowledge and tools since 2000 is nothing short of amazing.

Advances in sequencing

In 2004, the euchromatic portion of the human genome sequence was finished and the "near-complete" human genome sequence was ready to use (28). Genomes of other species, beginning with the mouse (48), became available as well. Since then, rapid progress in technology has greatly altered the landscape. As Shendure and colleagues (67) note, automation and continual improvements in fluorescence-based methods led to near-maximum efficiency and cost reduction for Sanger sequencing strategies. However, the completion of the human genome sequence was only the beginning for the genome sequencing era. Next-generation sequencing (NGS) technologies appeared on the market during the 2000s as several companies developed different approaches for "massively parallel sequencing" methods. During this time, sequencing throughput accelerated exponentially. Strengths and limitations of various methods (8) and thorough reviews of the historical timeline are published elsewhere (46, 57, 67). By 2015, the cost of genome sequencing approached the once far-fetched cost of $1000 USD per genome (49), and much anticipated third-generation sequencing (5, 64) technologies that enable single molecule sequencing also became available. One of these methods, nanopore sequencing, identifies nucleotides based on the electrical disturbance created as an enzyme ratchets movement of a nucleic acid molecule through a nanopore (37, 42). This process, commercialized by Oxford Nanopore Technologies Limited (Oxford, UK), has resulted in small, portable sequencing devices that produce long sequence reads, such as the minION device shown in Figure 2.1 that has now been utilized to successfully generate an entire human genome sequence (17, 30). A smaller device designed for use with a smart phone is reportedly in development as of August

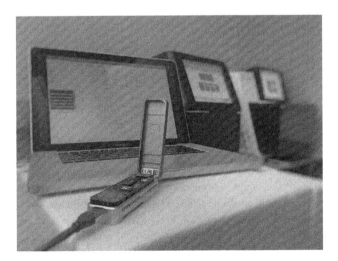

Figure 2.1 An example of a hand-held minION sequencer in use in a laboratory setting.
Source: Photo provided by Andrew E. Hillhouse, Texas A&M University Institute of Genome Sciences and Society.

2018. The availability of such a device means the ability to generate sequence data anytime, anywhere, and at an affordable cost, has been realized. However, challenges still remain in storing, analyzing, and comprehending these data.

Association studies

For many decades, researchers made maps of gene locations to use as tools for finding the genes that were responsible for diseases, defects, or phenotypic traits of interest (58). As genomic sequence data from more individuals became available, variations between individuals were identified. The database of sequence variants – single nucleotide polymorphisms (SNPs) – could be used for identifying genomic regions associated with measurable phenotypic traits affected by multiple genes. The regions, known as quantitative trait loci (QTL), could be detected in populations when the genes or sequences responsible for phenotype variation segregated within the population studied, and SNP markers were distributed across the map at sufficient density. With knowledge of family structure, each SNP could be tested statistically for association with the trait of interest (10, 38).

As genome sequencing became more accessible, SNP markers reflecting common genetic variation accumulated more rapidly. With a goal to find genes related to health and disease, the International HapMap Consortium was formed to collect and characterize human variation on a large scale. In phase II of the project, more than 3 million SNPs from 270 people from four geographic regions were characterized (71). This HapMap resource was soon replaced after the 1000 Genomes Project was completed and produced a map of variation from 2504 people from 26 populations (68, 70). Similarly, genome resources were accumulated for mice and numerous other species (34). With abundant characterized SNPs, and improvements in microarray platforms for conducting hundreds of thousands of assays simultaneously, the traditional genetic linkage studies gave way to genome-wide association studies (GWAS) as a popular approach for associating genomic regions with quantitative, physical traits of interest (16, 35, 52, 56, 60). Publication of GWAS rose rapidly and has held at a fairly steady state in recent years (Figure 2.2), although individual studies continue to increase in size. Connecting genetic variation with complex, quantitative traits remains challenging because many genetic variations, each with small effects, influence overall phenotype.

A GWAS approach takes advantage of knowledge of common genetic variation across the genome and requires only that the SNP be in linkage disequilibrium with the causal variant. No prior knowledge of the genome map location is required for identification of a variant responsible for a trait of interest (27). However, meaningful GWAS results require careful study design, sufficient SNP density and population frequency, and sample numbers of a size to achieve suitable statistical power for analysis (27, 54). Although powerful, this approach has not been without controversy and debate has occurred about whether GWAS experiments could return value worth the cost (76). The probability of success for GWAS is affected by several factors including the number of loci that influence a trait, allele frequency within the population, the effect on phenotype, the size of the sample population, the SNP panel composition, and how well the phenotype can be accurately measured (77). Depending on effect size and minor allele frequency, minimum sample sizes for detecting SNP–trait associations could range from a few hundred to more than 100 million (77). Thus, an investigator's choice of analytical tools and models, as well as treatment of rare variants, pleiotropic effects, and means for validation must also be carefully considered (19, 25, 53). For complex physiological phenotypes, GWAS might be expected to result in variable rates of success. In 2007, one of the earliest large GWAS investigated seven diseases, with 2000 individuals for each case, along with a set of 3000

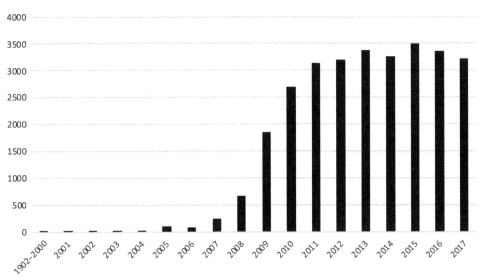

Figure 2.2 The Medline database was queried with the keyword search terms "genome wide association" or "genome-wide association studies" and publication numbers per year are plotted in this graph.

control individuals (72). Several significant associations at new regions of the genome offered insight into mechanisms underlying disease. These early studies and subsequent data have also supported the idea that complex traits are highly polygenic, and the path from association to causation is often slow and complex (2). Despite drawbacks, Bouchard described the usefulness of GWAS in exercise studies (4) and Meyre (47) argued for continued investment in appropriately designed studies, complemented by whole-genome sequencing and sequence imputation, citing the impact of a large meta-analysis of diabetes-related GWAS publications (65).

Exercise, physical activity, and sport-related GWAS studies are, to some extent, only beginning. For example, Sarzynski and colleagues (62) identified four SNP loci associated with triglyceride response to exercise training, as well as gene expression (transcriptomic) variants that may contribute to variability in lipid response. In another study, Verweij et al. examined heart rate response during and after exercise (75). The GWAS analyses returned 23 loci associated with heart rate response resulting in 36 candidate causal genes for further investigation. Many of the identified candidates play a role in neuron biology, and led the authors to new hypotheses regarding the role of the autonomic nervous system in heart rate recovery, as well as new directions for investigating sudden cardiac death. Several investigators are also beginning to consider the entire body of association results for specific applications (41, 63, 78). Frau and colleagues (22) undertook a systems genetics analysis to identify genetic variation from multiple GWAS for type 2 diabetes as well as 12 additional traits that are associated comorbidities. To do so, they combined GWAS results, an examination of cross-trait effects, and gene network analyses to identify a set of 38 genetic variants associated with type 2 diabetes as well as its comorbidities. These types of studies lay a strong foundation for investigating the genetic mechanisms by which exercise and sport can play a role in overall health and disease prevention. In addition, mouse model systems have also proven useful for identifying genetic loci associated with voluntary physical activity (36, 40), as well as responses to exercise training (44).

Noncoding sequences

Noncoding RNA and antisense sequences

One outcome of various genome projects, and ensuing genetic analyses, is the discovery that the genome is far more complex than may have been anticipated. At one time, descriptions of "junk DNA" (51) and the discovery of far fewer than expected genes within the human genome caused surprise. As interrogation of the genome has progressed, a variety of genomic regulatory elements and transcribed RNAs that do not encode gene products have revealed that genome function is much more complicated than the "Central Dogma" of DNA to messenger RNA to protein. This truth is observed in the outcome of GWAS. For example, the landmark Wellcome Trust study in 2007 revealed a previously unidentified, strong association between coronary artery disease (CAD) and a region of chromosome 9p21 (72). The associated SNPs were located in a noncoding region of the DNA, and have strong associations with CAD in multiple populations. Yet, in 2018, the causal mechanism of this sequence with CAD remains unknown despite progress that has led to subsequent identification of more than 150 loci associated with CAD risk (11). A noncoding RNA transcript, *XIST*, was identified as key to inactivation of the X-chromosome in female mammals (6, 7). In the case of callipyge sheep, affected animals exhibit muscular hypertrophy of the loin and hindquarters, but not all muscles, due to a single SNP in an intergenic region of the sheep genome (21, 69). This SNP results in altered expression of both sense and antisense transcripts, with additional parent-of-origin effects. Although the mutation is well known, the mechanisms by which postnatal muscle growth is altered are not completely understood. Even with knowledge of the genome sequence, understanding how that sequence is converted to phenotype remains a complex problem.

MicroRNAs

Small (~17–27 nucleotides) RNA molecules known as microRNAs, or miRNAs, can function as a type of molecular rheostat to modulate gene expression during various physiological processes. MicroRNAs can act on entire networks of genes, vastly increasing the complexity of genetic mechanisms (33). Skeletal muscle phenotypes can be regulated by miRNAs, whose differential expression within muscle may reflect response to exercise or even variation in activity (14, 43). In human and mouse experiments, Gastebois et al. (23) demonstrated that expression of a miRNA, miR-148b, played a role in decreased insulin sensitivity following a transition from physical activity to inactivity. This miRNA was previously shown to be associated with muscle catabolism (79), and the investigators found that inactivity resulted in increased miR-148b and downregulation of its target genes, resulting in reduced insulin responsiveness. In another study, Lew and colleagues conducted an extensive review of how exercise can modulate miRNA activity in molecular networks to protect cardiac function in diabetic patients. They proposed that miRNAs, shown to be induced by exercise and to have cardioprotective effects, could serve as biomarkers for determining optimal exercise strategies for diabetic patients (39).

Exosomes

Functional miRNAs are cleaved from longer precursor molecules, and the remaining "passenger strand" molecule was thought to be degraded. However, in an investigation into mechanisms of cardiac fibrosis in response to stress, and subsequent heart failure, Bang and colleagues discovered that cardiac fibroblasts excreted microvesicles known as exosomes (3). They found that under stress conditions, fibroblast exosomes containing the miR-21 passenger strand miRNA (miR-21★) acted on cardiac myocytes, and miR-21★ altered gene expression that ultimately led to hypertrophic growth. This study is just one example of how miRNA regulatory function can contribute orders of complexity to genetic studies of exercise-related physiological functions. Additional studies have found that physical exercise can cause skeletal muscle to release exosomes containing miRNAs into the bloodstream (24), potentially functioning as trans-acting regulators on other tissues. As noted in a discussion of exercise-induced circulating miRNAs, a current challenge is to move toward understanding the functional role of these regulatory molecules in skeletal muscle adaptation, and other physiological effects that occur in response to physical activity (61).

Epigenetics

In addition to variation in the sequence of the genetic code contained in the genome, epigenetic modifications that enable heritable alterations in phenotype without changes in DNA sequence must also be considered (1). Modification of the histone proteins by methylation, acetylation, and other processes, as well as methylation of stretches of guanines and cytosines in the genome (CpG islands) can alter gene activity (often in a repressive fashion in the case of methylation). Following the pattern of other genome mapping projects, the Epigenomics Roadmap Project established complete epigenomes for 111 reference human genomes (59). Epigenetic modifications occur in early development during the differentiation of specific cell types. Epigenetics is also a component of fetal programming, in which the fetal environment can have long-term effects on a developing fetus, as well as its offspring. This phenomenon gained much attention in studies of the Dutch famine birth cohort, whose mothers had experienced starvation (18, 26). In this study, those who were subjected to prenatal famine had altered methylation of the *IGF2* gene in comparison with their siblings who were born later during less severe conditions.

Exercise has been shown to affect epigenetic processes. An early study of histone modification following bouts of cycling exercise demonstrated a global increase in acetylation of H3K36 (45). An increase in transcriptional elongation is a typical response to this histone modification. In one extensive review that documents exercise-induced epigenetic effects, induced DNA methylation and histone acetylation or methylation was shown to result in modifications important for learning, memory, and cognition (20). Another meta-analysis of literature to examine the direct and indirect impact of exercise on cancer-related biochemical pathways was conducted by Thomas et al. (73). In this study, the authors categorized the published direct effects on the activity of several biological pathways that likely have a positive impact on health. They also examined current literature that has demonstrated postexercise epigenetic alterations including histone modifications, DNA methylation, and telomere length. While these studies provide valuable information, the review highlights specific areas where clear understanding of the biological consequences of exercise biochemistry falls short.

Summary

The completion of the Human Genome Project represented the opening of a door into a whole new realm of genetic technologies and advances that have continued to expand during the past two decades. Along with the advances have come many more questions and enormous quantities of data. What remains is how to best conduct sound experiments to interrogate and analyze these data, and to move from genetic variation to causal mechanisms that shape phenotypes of interest. With careful study designs and tools at hand, the interaction of genetics with exercise and sport activity can be better understood and utilized for improving overall health and well-being.

References

1. **Allis CD** and **Jenuwein T.** The molecular hallmarks of epigenetic control. *Nat Rev Genet* 17: 487, 2016.
2. **Angel JM, Abel EL, Riggs PK, McClellan SA,** and **DiGiovanni J.** Fine mapping reveals that promotion susceptibility locus 1 (*Psl1*) is a compound locus with multiple genes that modify susceptibility to skin tumor development. *G3 (Bethesda)*, 4: 1071–1079, 2014.
3. **Bang C, Batkai S, Dangwal S, Gupta SK, Foinquinos A, Holzmann A, Just A, Remke J, Zimmer K, Zeug A, Ponimaskin E, Schmiedl A, Yin X, Mayr M, Halder R, Fischer A, Engelhardt S, Wei Y, Schober A, Fiedler J,** and **Thum T.** Cardiac fibroblast-derived microRNA passenger strand-enriched exosomes mediate cardiomyocyte hypertrophy. *J Clin Invest* 124: 2136–2146, 2014.
4. **Bouchard C.** Overcoming barriers to progress in exercise genomics. *Exerc Sport Sci Rev* 39: 212–217, 2011.
5. **Branton D, Deamer DW, Marziali A, Bayley H, Benner SA, Butler T, Di Ventra M, Garaj S, Hibbs A, Huang X, Jovanovich SB, Krstic PS, Lindsay S, Ling XS, Mastrangelo CH, Meller A, Oliver JS, Pershin YV, Ramsey JM, Riehn R, Soni GV, Tabard-Cossa V, Wanunu M, Wiggin M,** and **Schloss JA.** The potential and challenges of nanopore sequencing. *Nat Biotechnol* 26: 1146–1153, 2008.
6. **Brockdorff N, Ashworth A, Kay GF, McCabe VM, Norris DP, Cooper PJ, Swift S,** and **Rastan S.** The product of the mouse Xist gene is a 15 kb inactive X-specific transcript containing no conserved ORF and located in the nucleus. *Cell* 71: 515–526, 1992.
7. **Brown CJ, Hendrich BD, Rupert JL, Lafrenière RG, Xing Y, Lawrence J,** and **Willard HF.** The human XIST gene: Analysis of a 17 kb inactive X-specific RNA that contains conserved repeats and is highly localized within the nucleus. *Cell* 71: 527–542, 1992.
8. **Buermans HPJ** and **den Dunnen JT.** Next generation sequencing technology: Advances and applications. *Biochim Biophys Acta* 1842: 1932–1941, 2014.
9. **Butler D.** Publication of human genomes sparks fresh sequence debate. *Nature* 409: 747, 2001.
10. **Churchill GA** and **Doerge RW.** Empirical threshold values for quantitative trait mapping. *Genetics* 138: 963–971, 1994.
11. **Clarke SL** and **Assimes TL.** Genome-wide association studies of coronary artery disease: Recent progress and challenges ahead. *Curr Atheroscler Rep* 20: 47, 2018.
12. **Claverie J-M.** What if there are only 30,000 human genes? *Science* 291: 1255–1257, 2001.
13. **Cook-Deegan RM.** The Human Genome Project: The formation of federal policies in the United States, 1986–1990. In: *Biomedical Politics*, edited by Hanna KE and Institute of Medicine (US) Committee to Study Biomedical Decision Making. Washington, DC: National Academy Press, 1991, p. 99–168.
14. **Dawes M, Kochan KJ, Riggs PK,** and **Lightfoot JT.** Differential miRNA expression in inherently high- and low-active inbred mice. *Physiol Rep* 3: e12469, 2015.
15. **DeLisi C.** Santa Fe 1986: Human genome baby-steps. *Nature* 455: 876, 2008.
16. **Dewan A, Liu M, Hartman S, Zhang SS, Liu DT, Zhao C, Tam PO, Chan WM, Lam DS, Snyder M, Barnstable C, Pang CP,** and **Hoh J.** HTRA1 promoter polymorphism in wet age-related macular degeneration. *Science* 314: 989–992, 2006.
17. **Eisenstein M.** An ace in the hole for DNA sequencing. *Nature* 550: 285, 2017.
18. **El Hajj N, Schneider E, Lehnen H,** and **Haaf T.** Epigenetics and life-long consequences of an adverse nutritional and diabetic intrauterine environment. *Reproduction* 148: R111–R120, 2014.
19. **Evangelou E** and **Ioannidis JPA.** Meta-analysis methods for genome-wide association studies and beyond. *Nat Rev Genet* 14: 379, 2013.
20. **Fernandes J, Arida RM,** and **Gomez-Pinilla F.** Physical exercise as an epigenetic modulator of brain plasticity and cognition. *Neurosci Biobehav Rev* 80: 443–456, 2017.

21. **Fleming-Waddell JN, Olbricht GR, Taxis TM, White JD, Vuocolo T, Craig BA, Tellam RL, Neary MK, Cockett NE,** and **Bidwell CA.** Effect of DLK1 and RTL1 but not MEG3 or MEG8 on muscle gene expression in callipyge lambs. *PLoS One* 4: e7399, 2009.

22. **Frau F, Crowther D, Ruetten H,** and **Allebrandt KV.** Type-2 diabetes-associated variants with cross-trait relevance: Post-GWAs strategies for biological function interpretation. *Mol Genet Metab* 121: 43–50, 2017.

23. **Gastebois C, Chanon S, Rome S, Durand C, Pelascini E, Jalabert A, Euthine V, Pialoux V, Blanc S, Simon C,** and **Lefai E.** Transition from physical activity to inactivity increases skeletal muscle miR-148b content and triggers insulin resistance. *Physiol Rep* 4: e12902, 2016.

24. **Guescini M, Canonico B, Lucertini F, Maggio S, Annibalini G, Barbieri E, Luchetti F, Papa S,** and **Stocchi V.** Muscle releases alpha-sarcoglycan positive extracellular vesicles carrying miRNAs in the bloodstream. *PLoS One* 10: e0125094, 2015.

25. **Hackinger S** and **Zeggini E.** Statistical methods to detect pleiotropy in human complex traits. *Open Biol* 7: 170125, 2017.

26. **Heijmans BT, Tobi EW, Stein AD, Putter H, Blauw GJ, Susser ES, Slagboom PE,** and **Lumey LH.** Persistent epigenetic differences associated with prenatal exposure to famine in humans. *Proc Natl Acad Sci U S A* 105: 17046–17049, 2008.

27. **Hirschhorn JN** and **Daly MJ.** Genome-wide association studies for common diseases and complex traits. *Nat Rev Genet* 6: 95, 2005.

28. **International Human Genome Sequencing Consortium.** Finishing the euchromatic sequence of the human genome. *Nature* 431: 931–945, 2004.

29. **International Human Genome Sequencing Consortium, Lander ES, Linton LM, Birren B, Nusbaum C, Zody MC, Baldwin J, Devon K, Dewar K, Doyle M, FitzHugh W, Funke R, Gage D, Harris K, Heaford A, Howland J, Kann L, Lehoczky J, LeVine R, McEwan P, McKernan K, Meldrim J, Mesirov JP, Miranda C, Morris W, Naylor J, Raymond C, Rosetti M, Santos R, Sheridan A, Sougnez C, Stange-Thomann Y, Stojanovic N, Subramanian A, Wyman D, Rogers J, Sulston J, Ainscough R, Beck S, Bentley D, Burton J, Clee C, Carter N, Coulson A, Deadman R, Deloukas P, Dunham A, Dunham I, Durbin R, French L, Grafham D, Gregory S, Hubbard T, Humphray S, Hunt A, Jones M, Lloyd C, McMurray A, Matthews L, Mercer S, Milne S, Mullikin JC, Mungall A, Plumb R, Ross M, Shownkeen R, Sims S, Waterston RH, Wilson RK, Hillier LW, McPherson JD, Marra MA, Mardis ER, Fulton LA, Chinwalla AT, Pepin KH, Gish WR, Chissoe SL, Wendl MC, Delehaunty KD, Miner TL, Delehaunty A, Kramer JB, Cook LL, Fulton RS, Johnson DL, Minx PJ, Clifton SW, Hawkins T, Branscomb E, Predki P, Richardson P, Wenning S, Slezak T, Doggett N, Cheng JF, Olsen A, Lucas S, Elkin C, Uberbacher E,** et al. Initial sequencing and analysis of the human genome. *Nature* 409: 860–921, 2001.

30. **Jain M, Koren S, Miga KH, Quick J, Rand AC, Sasani TA, Tyson JR, Beggs AD, Dilthey AT, Fiddes IT, Malla S, Marriott H, Nieto T, O'Grady J, Olsen HE, Pedersen BS, Rhie A, Richardson H, Quinlan AR, Snutch TP, Tee L, Paten B, Phillippy AM, Simpson JT, Loman NJ,** and **Loose M.** Nanopore sequencing and assembly of a human genome with ultra-long reads. *Nat Biotechnol* 36: 338, 2018.

31. **Jasny BR** and **Kennedy D.** The human genome. *Science* 291: 1153–1153, 2001.

32. **Jeffords JM** and **Daschle T.** Political issues in the genome era. *Science* 291: 1249–1251, 2001.

33. **Jeffries CD, Fried HM,** and **Perkins DO.** Additional layers of gene regulatory complexity from recently discovered microRNA mechanisms. *Int J Biochem Cell Biol* 42: 1236–1242, 2010.

34. **Kirby A, Kang HM, Wade CM, Cotsapas C, Kostem E, Han B, Furlotte N, Kang EY, Rivas M, Bogue MA, Frazer KA, Johnson FM, Beilharz EJ, Cox DR, Eskin E,** and **Daly MJ.** Fine mapping in 94 inbred mouse strains using a high-density haplotype resource. *Genetics* 185: 1081–1095, 2010.

35. **Klein RJ, Zeiss C, Chew EY, Tsai JY, Sackler RS, Haynes C, Henning AK, SanGiovanni JP, Mane SM, Mayne ST, Bracken MB, Ferris FL, Ott J, Barnstable C,** and **Hoh J.** Complement factor H polymorphism in age-related macular degeneration. *Science* 308: 385–389, 2005.

36. **Kostrzewa E, Brandys MK, van Lith HA,** and **Kas MJH.** A candidate syntenic genetic locus is associated with voluntary exercise levels in mice and humans. *Behav Brain Res* 276: 8–16, 2015.

37. **Laszlo AH, Derrington IM, Ross BC, Brinkerhoff H, Adey A, Nova IC, Craig JM, Langford KW, Samson JM, Daza R, Doering K, Shendure J,** and **Gundlach JH.** Decoding long nanopore sequencing reads of natural DNA. *Nat Biotechnol* 32: 829, 2014.

38. **Lebreton CM** and **Visscher PM.** Empirical nonparametric bootstrap strategies in quantitative trait loci mapping: conditioning on the genetic model. *Genetics* 148: 525–535, 1998.

39. **Lew JKS, Pearson JT, Schwenke DO,** and **Katare R.** Exercise mediated protection of diabetic heart through modulation of microRNA mediated molecular pathways. *Cardiovasc Diabetol* 16: 10, 2017.

40. **Lightfoot JT, Turner MJ, Pomp D, Kleeberger SR,** and **Leamy LJ.** Quantitative trait loci for physical activity traits in mice. *Physiol Genomics* 32: 401–408, 2008.

41. **Lin X, Eaton CB, Manson JE,** and **Liu S.** The genetics of physical activity. *Curr Cardiol Rep* 19: 119, 2017.

42. **Madoui MA, Engelen S, Cruaud C, Belser C, Bertrand L, Alberti A, Lemainque A, Wincker P,** and **Aury JM.** Genome assembly using nanopore-guided long and error-free DNA reads. *BMC Genomics* 16: 327, 2015.

43. **Margolis LM, Lessard SJ, Ezzyat Y, Fielding RA,** and **Rivas DA.** Circulating MicroRNA are predictive of aging and acute adaptive response to resistance exercise in men. *J Gerontol A Biol Sci Med Sci* 72: 1319–1326, 2017.

44. **Massett MP, Avila JJ,** and **Kim SK.** Exercise capacity and response to training quantitative trait loci in a NZW X 129S1 intercross and combined cross analysis of inbred mouse strains. *PLoS One* 10: e0145741, 2016.

45. **McGee SL, Fairlie E, Garnham AP,** and **Hargreaves M.** Exercise-induced histone modifications in human skeletal muscle. *J Physiol* 587: 5951–5958, 2009.

46. **McGinn S** and **Gut IG.** DNA sequencing – spanning the generations. *N Biotechnol* 30: 366–372, 2013.

47. **Meyre D.** Give GWAS a chance. *Diabetes* 66: 2741–2742, 2017.

48. **Mouse Genome Sequencing Consortium, Chinwalla AT, Cook LL, Delehaunty KD, Fewell GA, Fulton LA, Fulton RS, Graves TA, Hillier LW, Mardis ER, McPherson JD, Miner TL, Nash WE, Nelson JO, Nhan MN, Pepin KH, Pohl CS, Ponce TC, Schultz B, Thompson J, Trevaskis E, Waterston RH, Wendl MC, Wilson RK, Yang S-P, An P, Berry E, Birren B, Bloom T, Brown DG, Butler J, Daly M, David R, Deri J, Dodge S, Foley K, Gage D, Gnerre S, Holzer T, Jaffe DB, Kamal M, Karlsson EK, Kells C, Kirby A, Kulbokas Iii EJ, Lander ES, Landers T, Leger JP, Levine R, Lindblad-Toh K, Mauceli E, Mayer JH, McCarthy M, Meldrim J, Meldrim J, Mesirov JP, Nicol R, Nusbaum C, Seaman S, Sharpe T, Sheridan A, Singer JB, Santos R, Spencer B, Stange-Thomann N, Vinson JP, Wade CM, Wierzbowski J, Wyman D, Zody MC, Birney E, Goldman N, Kasprzyk A, Mongin E, Rust AG, Slater G, Stabenau A, Ureta-Vidal A, Whelan S, Ainscough R, Attwood J, Bailey J, Barlow K, Beck S, Burton J, Clamp M, Clee C, Coulson A, Cuff J, Curwen V, Cutts T, Davies J, Eyras E, Grafham D, Gregory S, Hubbard T, Hunt A, Jones M, Joy A, Leonard S,** et al. Initial sequencing and comparative analysis of the mouse genome. *Nature* 420: 520–562, 2002.

49. **National Human Genome Research Institute.** The cost of sequencing a human genome. www.genome.gov/27565109/the-cost-of-sequencing-a-human-genome/ 2016. Accessed July 19, 2018.

50. **National Human Genome Research Institute.** Legislative history of GINA. www.genome.gov/27568535/legislative-history-of-gina/ 2017. Accessed August 19, 2018.

51. **Ohno S** and **Yomo T.** The grammatical rule for all DNA: Junk and coding sequences. *Electrophoresis* 12: 103–108, 1991.

52. **Ozaki K, Ohnishi Y, Iida A, Sekine A, Yamada R, Tsunoda T, Sato H, Sato H, Hori M, Nakamura Y,** and **Tanaka T.** Functional SNPs in the lymphotoxin-α gene that are associated with susceptibility to myocardial infarction. *Nat Genet* 32: 650, 2002.

53. **Palmer C** and **Pe'er I.** Statistical correction of the Winner's Curse explains replication variability in quantitative trait genome-wide association studies. *PLoS Genet* 13: e1006916, 2017.

54. **Pearson TA** and **Manolio TA.** How to interpret a genome-wide association study. *JAMA* 299: 1335–1344, 2008.

55. **Public Law Number 101–156.** H.R. 3566. Departments of Labor, Health and Human Services, and Education, and related agencies appropriations. 101st Congress of the United States, 1989.

56. **Rankinen T, An P, Pérusse L, Rice T, Chagnon YC, Gagnon J, Leon AS, Skinner JS, Wilmore JH, Rao DC,** and **Bouchard C.** Genome-wide linkage scan for exercise stroke volume and cardiac output in the HERITAGE Family Study. *Physiol Genomics* 10: 57–62, 2002.

57. **Reuter Jason A, Spacek DV,** and **Snyder Michael P.** High-throughput sequencing technologies. *Molecular Cell* 58: 586–597, 2015.

58. **Riggs PK** and **Gill CA.** Molecular mapping and marker-assisted breeding for muscle growth and meat quality. In: *Applied Muscle Biology and Meat Science*, edited by Du M and McCormick RJ. Boca Raton: CRC Press, 2009, p. 287–310.

59. **Roadmap Epigenomics Consortium, Kundaje A, Meuleman W, Ernst J, Bilenky M, Yen A, Heravi-Moussavi A, Kheradpour P, Zhang Z, Wang J, Ziller MJ, Amin V, Whitaker JW, Schultz MD, Ward LD, Sarkar A, Quon G, Sandstrom RS, Eaton ML, Wu Y-C, Pfenning A, Wang X, ClaussnitzerYaping Liu M, Coarfa C, Alan Harris R, Shoresh N, Epstein CB, Gjoneska E, Leung D, Xie W, David Hawkins R, Lister R, Hong C, Gascard P, Mungall AJ, Moore R, Chuah E, Tam A, Canfield TK, Scott Hansen R, Kaul R, Sabo PJ, Bansal MS, Carles A, Dixon JR, Farh K-H, Feizi S, Karlic R, Kim A-R, Kulkarni A, Li D, Lowdon R, Elliott G, Mercer TR, Neph SJ, Onuchic V, Polak P, Rajagopal N, Ray P, Sallari RC, Siebenthall KT, Sinnott-Armstrong NA, Stevens M, Thurman RE, Wu J, Zhang B, Zhou X, Abdennur N, Adli M, Akerman M, Barrera L, Antosiewicz-Bourget J, Ballinger T, Barnes MJ, Bates D, Bell RJA, Bennett DA, Bianco K, Bock C, Boyle P, Brinchmann J, Caballero-Campo P, Camahort R, Carrasco-Alfonso MJ, Charnecki T, Chen H, Chen Z, Cheng JB, Cho S, Chu A, Chung W-Y, Cowan C, Athena Deng Q, Deshpande V, Diegel M, Ding B, Durham T, Echipare L, Edsall L, Flowers D**, et al. Integrative analysis of 111 reference human epigenomes. *Nature* 518: 317–330, 2015.

60. **Rosenthal A.** Editorial overview. Genomics and proteomics. *Curr Opin Mol Ther* 1: 669–670, 1999.

61. **Russell AP** and **Lamon S.** Exercise, skeletal muscle and circulating microRNAs. *Prog Mol Biol Transl Sci* 135: 471–495, 2015.

62. **Sarzynski MA, Davidsen PK, Sung YJ, Hesselink MK, Schrauwen P, Rice TK, Rao DC, Falciani F,** and **Bouchard C.** Genomic and transcriptomic predictors of triglyceride response to regular exercise. *Br J Sports Med* 49: 1524–1531, 2015.

63. **Sarzynski MA, Ghosh S,** and **Bouchard C.** Genomic and transcriptomic predictors of response levels to endurance exercise training. *J Physiol* 595: 2931–2939, 2017.

64. **Schadt EE, Turner S,** and **Kasarskis A.** A window into third-generation sequencing. *Hum Mol Genet* 19: R227–R240, 2010.

65. **Scott RA, Scott LJ, Mägi R, Marullo L, Gaulton KJ, Kaakinen M, Pervjakova N, Pers TH, Johnson AD, Eicher JD, Jackson AU, Ferreira T, Lee Y, Ma C, Steinthorsdottir V, Thorleifsson G, Qi L, Van Zuydam NR, Mahajan A, Chen H, Almgren P, Voight BF, Grallert H, Müller-Nurasyid M, Ried JS, Rayner NW, Robertson N, Karssen LC, van Leeuwen EM, Willems SM, Fuchsberger C, Kwan P, Teslovich TM, Chanda P, Li M, Lu Y, Dina C, Thuillier D, Yengo L, Jiang L, Sparso T, Kestler HA, Chheda H, Eisele L, Gustafsson S, Frånberg M, Strawbridge RJ, Benediktsson R, Hreidarsson AB, Kong A, Sigurðsson G, Kerrison ND, Luan Ja, Liang L, Meitinger T, Roden M, Thorand B, Esko T, Mihailov E, Fox C, Liu C-T, Rybin D, Isomaa B, Lyssenko V, Tuomi T, Couper DJ, Pankow JS, Grarup N, Have CT, Jørgensen ME, Jørgensen T, Linneberg A, Cornelis MC, van Dam RM, Hunter DJ, Kraft P, Sun Q, Edkins S, Owen KR, Perry JRB, Wood AR, Zeggini E, Tajes-Fernandes J, Abecasis GR, Bonnycastle LL, Chines PS, Stringham HM, Koistinen HA, Kinnunen L, Sennblad B, Mühleisen TW, Nöthen MM, Pechlivanis S, Baldassarre D, Gertow K, Humphries SE, Tremoli E, Klopp N, Meyer J, Steinbach G,** et al. An expanded genome-wide association study of type 2 diabetes in Europeans. *Diabetes* 66: 2888–2902, 2017.

66. **Shapiro R.** *The Human Blueprint: The Race to Unlock the Secrets of our Genetic Script.* New York: St. Martin's Press, 1991.

67. **Shendure J, Balasubramanian S, Church GM, Gilbert W, Rogers J, Schloss JA,** and **Waterston RH.** DNA sequencing at 40: past, present and future. *Nature* 550: 345–353, 2017.

68. **Sudmant PH, Rausch T, Gardner EJ, Handsaker RE, Abyzov A, Huddleston J, Zhang Y, Ye K, Jun G, Hsi-Yang Fritz M, Konkel MK, Malhotra A, Stütz AM, Shi X, Paolo Casale F, Chen J, Hormozdiari F, Dayama G, Chen K, Malig M, Chaisson MJP, Walter K, Meiers S, Kashin S, Garrison E, Auton A, Lam HYK, Jasmine Mu X, Alkan C, Antaki D, Bae T, Cerveira E, Chines P, Chong Z, Clarke L, Dal E, Ding L, Emery S, Fan X, Gujral M, Kahveci F, Kidd JM, Kong Y, Lameijer E-W, McCarthy S, Flicek P, Gibbs RA, Marth G, Mason CE, Menelaou A, Muzny DM, Nelson BJ, Noor A, Parrish NF, Pendleton M, Quitadamo A, Raeder B, Schadt EE, Romanovitch M, Schlattl A, Sebra R, Shabalin AA, Untergasser A, Walker JA, Wang M, Yu F, Zhang C, Zhang J, Zheng-Bradley X, Zhou W, Zichner T, Sebat J, Batzer MA, McCarroll SA, The Genomes Project C, Mills RE, Gerstein MB, Bashir A, Stegle O, Devine SE, Lee C, Eichler EE,** and **Korbel JO.** An integrated map of structural variation in 2,504 human genomes. *Nature* 526: 75–81, 2015.

69. **Takeda H, Caiment F, Smit M, Hiard S, Tordoir X, Cockett N, Georges M,** and **Charlier C.** The callipyge mutation enhances bidirectional long range DLK1-GTL2 intergenic transcription in cis. *Proc Natl Acad Sci U S A* 103: 8119–8124, 2006.

70. **The Genomes Project Consortium, Auton A, Abecasis GR, Altshuler DM, Durbin RM, Abecasis GR, Bentley DR, Chakravarti A, Clark AG, Donnelly P, Eichler EE, Flicek P, Gabriel SB, Gibbs RA, Green ED, Hurles ME, Knoppers BM, Korbel JO, Lander ES, Lee C, Lehrach H, Mardis ER, Marth GT, McVean GA, Nickerson DA, Schmidt JP, Sherry ST, Wang J, Wilson RK, Gibbs RA, Boerwinkle E, Doddapaneni H, Han Y, Korchina V, Kovar C, Lee S, Muzny D, Reid JG, Zhu Y, Wang J, Chang Y, Feng Q, Fang X, Guo X, Jian M, Jiang H, Jin X, Lan T, Li G, Li J, Li Y, Liu S, Liu X, Lu Y, Ma X, Tang M, Wang B, Wang G, Wu H, Wu R, Xu X, Yin Y, Zhang D, Zhang W, Zhao J, Zhao M, Zheng X, Lander ES, Altshuler DM, Gabriel SB, Gupta N, Gharani N, Toji LH, Gerry NP, Resch AM, Flicek P, Barker J, Clarke L, Gil L, Hunt SE, Kelman G, Kulesha E, Leinonen R, McLaren WM, Radhakrishnan R, Roa A, Smirnov D, Smith RE, Streeter I, Thormann A, Toneva I, Vaughan B, Zheng-Bradley X, Bentley DR, Grocock R, Humphray S, James T, Kingsbury Z, Lehrach H, Sudbrak R,** et al. A global reference for human genetic variation. *Nature* 526: 68–74, 2015.

71. **The International HapMap Consortium, Frazer KA, Ballinger DG, Cox DR, Hinds DA, Stuve LL, Gibbs RA, Belmont JW, Boudreau A, Hardenbol P, Leal SM, Pasternak S, Wheeler DA, Willis TD, Yu F, Yang H, Zeng C, Gao Y, Hu H, Hu W, Li C, Lin W, Liu S, Pan H, Tang X, Wang J, Wang W, Yu J, Zhang B, Zhang Q, Zhao H, Zhao H, Zhou J, Gabriel SB, Barry R, Blumenstiel B, Camargo A, Defelice M, Faggart M, Goyette M, Gupta S, Moore J, Nguyen H, Onofrio RC, Parkin M, Roy J, Stahl E, Winchester E, Ziaugra L, Altshuler D, Shen Y, Yao Z, Huang W, Chu X, He Y, Jin L, Liu Y, Shen Y, Sun W, Wang H, Wang Y, Wang Y, Xiong X, Xu L, Waye MMY, Tsui SKW, Xue H, Wong JT-F, Galver LM, Fan J-B, Gunderson K, Murray SS, Oliphant AR, Chee MS, Montpetit A, Chagnon F, Ferretti V, Leboeuf M, Olivier J-F, Phillips MS, Roumy S, Sallée C, Verner A, Hudson TJ, Kwok P-Y, Cai D, Koboldt DC, Miller RD, Pawlikowska L, Taillon-Miller P, Xiao M, Tsui L-C, Mak W, Qiang Song Y, Tam PKH, Nakamura Y, Kawaguchi T, Kitamoto T, Morizono T, Nagashima A,** et al. A second generation human haplotype map of over 3.1 million SNPs. *Nature* 449: 851–861, 2007.

72. **The Wellcome Trust Case Control Consortium, Burton PR, Clayton DG, Cardon LR, Craddock N, Deloukas P, Duncanson A, Kwiatkowski DP, McCarthy MI, Ouwehand WH, Samani NJ, Todd JA, Donnelly P, Barrett JC, Burton PR, Davison D, Donnelly P, Easton D, Evans D, Leung H-T, Marchini JL, Morris AP, Spencer CCA, Tobin MD, Cardon LR, Clayton DG, Attwood AP, Boorman JP, Cant B, Everson U, Hussey JM, Jolley JD, Knight AS, Koch K, Meech E, Nutland S, Prowse CV, Stevens HE, Taylor NC, Walters GR, Walker NM, Watkins NA, Winzer T, Todd JA, Ouwehand WH, Jones RW, McArdle WL, Ring SM, Strachan DP, Pembrey M, Breen G, St Clair D, Caesar S, Gordon-Smith K, Jones L, Fraser C, Green EK, Grozeva D, Hamshere ML, Holmans PA, Jones IR, Kirov G, Moskvina V, Nikolov I, O'Donovan MC, Owen MJ, Craddock N, Collier DA, Elkin A, Farmer A, Williamson R, McGuffin P, Young AH, Ferrier IN, Ball SG, Balmforth AJ, Barrett JH, Bishop DT, Iles MM, Maqbool A, Yuldasheva N, Hall AS, Braund PS, Burton PR, Dixon RJ, Mangino M, Stevens S, Tobin MD, Thompson JR, Samani NJ, Bredin F, Tremelling M, Parkes M, Drummond H, Lees CW, Nimmo ER, Satsangi J, Fisher SA, Forbes A, Lewis CM,** et al. Genome-wide association study of 14,000 cases of seven common diseases and 3,000 shared controls. *Nature* 447: 661–678, 2007.

73. **Thomas RJ, Kenfield SA,** and **Jimenez A.** Exercise-induced biochemical changes and their potential influence on cancer: A scientific review. *Br J Sports Med* 51: 640–644, 2017.

74. **Venter JC, Adams MD, Myers EW, Li PW, Mural RJ, Sutton GG, Smith HO, Yandell M, Evans CA, Holt RA, Gocayne JD, Amanatides P, Ballew RM, Huson DH, Wortman JR, Zhang Q, Kodira CD, Zheng XH, Chen L, Skupski M, Subramanian G, Thomas PD, Zhang J, Gabor Miklos GL, Nelson C, Broder S, Clark AG, Nadeau J, McKusick VA, Zinder N, Levine AJ, Roberts RJ, Simon M, Slayman C, Hunkapiller M, Bolanos R, Delcher A, Dew I, Fasulo D, Flanigan M, Florea L, Halpern A, Hannenhalli S, Kravitz S, Levy S, Mobarry C, Reinert K, Remington K, Abu-Threideh J, Beasley E, Biddick K, Bonazzi V, Brandon R, Cargill M, Chandramouliswaran I, Charlab R, Chaturvedi K, Deng Z, Francesco VD, Dunn P, Eilbeck K, Evangelista C, Gabrielian AE, Gan W, Ge W, Gong F, Gu Z, Guan P, Heiman TJ, Higgins ME, Ji R-R, Ke Z, Ketchum KA, Lai Z, Lei Y, Li Z, Li J, Liang Y, Lin X, Lu F, Merkulov GV,**

Milshina N, Moore HM, Naik AK, Narayan VA, Neelam B, Nusskern D, Rusch DB, Salzberg S, Shao W, Shue B, Sun J, Wang ZY, Wang A, Wang X, Wang J, Wei M-H, Wides R, Xiao C, Yan C, et al. The sequence of the human genome. *Science* 291: 1304–1351, 2001.

75. **Verweij N, van de Vegte YJ**, and **van der Harst P.** Genetic study links components of the autonomous nervous system to heart-rate profile during exercise. *Nat Communications* 9: 898, 2018.

76. **Visscher Peter M, Brown Matthew A, McCarthy Mark I**, and **Yang J.** Five years of GWAS discovery. *Am J Hum Genet* 90: 7–24, 2012.

77. **Visscher PM, Wray NR, Zhang Q, Sklar P, McCarthy MI, Brown MA**, and **Yang J.** 10 years of GWAS discovery: Biology, function, and translation. *Am J Hum Genet* 101: 5–22, 2017.

78. **Williams CJ, Williams MG, Eynon N, Ashton KJ, Little JP, Wisloff U**, and **Coombes JS.** Genes to predict VO(2max) trainability: a systematic review. *BMC Genomics* 18: 831, 2017.

79. **Zhang J, Fu SL, Liu Y, Liu YL**, and **Wang WJ.** Analysis of microRNA expression profiles in weaned pig skeletal muscle after lipopolysaccharide challenge. *Int J Mol Sci* 16: 22438–22455, 2015.

3

HUMAN SYSTEMS GENETIC MODELING USED IN EXERCISE

Jaakko Kaprio

Introduction

Nearly all human characteristics and behaviors run in families, that is to say, relatives and people living together tend to resemble each other more than two individuals chosen at random from the same population. Such characteristics can be structural (height, bone structure, obesity) or physiological (muscle strength), behavioral (physical activity), or life-course related (such as number of children or lifespan). Correspondingly, abnormal conditions and disease often also run in families. Familial aggregation is thus a well-established observation, but the nature and causes of it depends on the trait in question. Familial aggregation is also well known for physical activity and exercise characteristics (2, 5, 21; see also Chapter 6). Given that there are multiple modes of physical activity and exercise, this chapter uses physical activity traits as the primary phenotypes in the examples described below.

Genetic modeling is a method to test hypotheses about the causes of familial aggregation and to seek understanding of its mechanisms. Until recently, the role of genetic factors was inferred on the basis of indirect evidence from family relationships – greater resemblance between genetically close persons was taken as evidence for genetic evidence but was not proof of it. Indeed, among humans, almost all the literature on the role of genetic factors in physical activity comes from modeling of family data, including special family designs such as twins. Modern molecular genetic methods are only now, in the past few years, providing robust, direct evidence for genetic factors to account for interindividual differences in human exercise and physical activity in the population at large.

This chapter will not go deeply into the theoretical framework or detailed modeling of quantitative genetics or molecular genetics. For this the reader is referred to textbooks and review articles that cover these aspects more thoroughly and some suggested further reading is provided at the end of the chapter. Further, Table 3.1 provides commonly accepted definitions of the most frequently used terms in this area. The chapter will cover family and twin designs, as they have been integral in providing evidence for genetic factors, while the chapter will conclude by summarizing molecular genetic designs, particularly the genome-wide association study (GWAS) and its recent developments. A couple of very new studies are reviewed to show how GWAS is being applied to exercise and physical activity.

Table 3.1 Definitions of selected terms

Additive genetic variance: The component of variance of a phenotype that is attributable to the additive effect of both alleles at all relevant loci

Allele: One of two or more states in which either copy of a gene can exist. This can be a single base-pair difference or a more extensive change in the genomic sequence

Assortative mating: A tendency for individuals with similar genotypes to mate

Genetic variance due to dominance: The component of variance of a phenotype that is attributable to the interactions between alternative alleles at a locus over all relevant loci

Epistatic genetic variance: The component of variance of a phenotype that is attributable to the interactive effect of two or more genes

Shared environmental variance: The component of variance of a phenotype that is attributable to the experiences and exposures shared by family members making them more similar over the expected similarity based on their degree of gene relatedness

Unshared environmental exposure: The component of variance of a phenotype that is attributable to all environmental factors specific to the individual considered, and includes also measurement error

---

Source: Based partly on the "Glossary" of Thomas DC. *Statistical methods in genetic epidemiology.* Oxford University Press, New York 2004, see "Further reading."

Study of families

What are families?

The core biological and social unit for studies of families consists of two parents, who have one or more offspring. They are thus biologically related due to transmission of shared chromosomes and genes from parents to their children. Parents and their children are defined as first-degree relatives, and through other biological relatives, more extensive biological relationships can be identified. These include grandparents, aunts and uncles, and cousins as second-degree relatives. By sharing genes in common, family members can be assumed to resemble each other due to genes affecting the structures and functions that underlie physical activity.

We may further characterize the nuclear family as consisting of parents and children who share the same environment for varying amounts of time. In an idealized situation, both parents raise their children together, creating a family environment with common material conditions (such as a shared home and finances), time spent together, and common rearing and family values. This family environment then acts throughout the development of the child into adolescence and at least until the child moves out of the parental home. One can then assume that the children would adopt behaviors, such as sports, that their parents engage in. The children would also adopt common parental values (e.g., the value of exercise). Thus, the parents and children resemble each other due to the nature of the time they spend together. Together with the effect of shared genes, shared social influences within families can result in familial aggregation. Overall, nongenetic environmental influences are more important during the time family members share a common household, i.e., during childhood and adolescence, but these influences can be maintained in later life either socially or even through epigenetic mechanisms. If we study nuclear families (parents and children), we can observe familial aggregation, but cannot be confident in ascribing where it arises from – is it common genes, shared exposures and experiences, or both?

In human society, there is a lot of variation in the structure and function of family units. This variation has also provided opportunities for research designs that help to distinguish the effects of genes from the rearing environment. The most used of these has been the twin study and its extensions. However, there are increasing numbers of diverse family relationships, such as single-parent families in which the other parent has been present for only a short period of the child's life, if at all. On the other hand, blended families consist of a couple, the children they have had together, and their children from previous relationships. Such families offer opportunities but also considerable challenges for study of the behavioral determinants of physical activity and engagement in sports.

Family studies focused on first-degree relatives assess only overall "familiality," i.e., the proportion of variance attributable to both genetic and nongenetic familial influences as well as their interactions (8). Family studies can include nuclear families (parents and their offspring) or more-extended pedigrees (grandparents, parents, offspring, aunts, uncles, cousins, etc.). Exceptionally large multigenerational pedigrees can be studied with very distantly related persons descendant from early ancestors even some centuries back (6) – such as studies conducted among the Amish, Mormons, Icelanders, and other geographically defined isolates with very little immigration until recent times. In larger pedigrees, there is more scope for distinguishing genetic and nongenetic factors, but most have focused on diseases and other conditions and there appears to be a dearth of studies of exercise characteristics in these large pedigrees.

Quantifying family data

For quantitative, continuous traits, familial correlations can be estimated for pairs of relatives. The intraclass correlation coefficient estimates the degree of resemblance between two family members of the same generation (such siblings or cousins), while interclass correlation estimates the degree of resemblance between two family members from different generations (such as parents and children, and grandparents and children). Higher values of these correlations are evidence of more familial resemblance; first-degree relatives are expected to show larger correlations than second-degree relatives.

Categorical traits such as the presence or absence of participation in a selected sport, or ordered categories such as the level of activity (e.g., asked as inactive, moderately active, or very active) can be analyzed using a threshold model of liability (1). In the model, the liability to the behavior is assumed to be normally distributed, and there are certain latent cut points that distinguish one category from the next. The latent liability is assumed to arise from multiple causative factors, each with a small effect, either genetic or environmental, which then give rise to the variation in liability in the population. The model precludes major genes with large effects, but these have not been found for physical activity or other exercise characteristics. The assumption of bivariate normality (for a relative pair) can be tested when there are three or more categories of the study variable, and the familial resemblance is then computed using a polychoric correlation. For a binary trait, the assumption cannot be tested.

In order to understand the roots of family aggregation, it is necessary to distinguish between effects arising from the rearing environment, and those arising from shared genes. By studying nuclear families alone, this is very difficult. For example, a recent major meta-analysis (26) of 112 studies of parent–child physical activity derived estimates ranging from 0.19 for mother–son pairs to 0.29 for father–son pairs, with parent–daughter correlations taking intermediate values. As parents and children share 50% of their segregating genes, the parent–offspring correlation can be doubled to yield an upper-bound estimate of the proportion of variance ascribed to genetic factors (i.e., 38–58% of the population variance ascribed to genetic factors) under the assumption that nongenetic factors play no role. However, the actual role of genetic factors may be much smaller, and social modeling, as proposed by the authors, might be more meaningful.

Without further information from other relative types, we cannot estimate the true proportion of variance accounted for by genetic effects in nuclear families. One option is to extend family studies to second-degree relatives. However, biologically less-related family members (such as aunts and nephews or cousins) are also less likely to have spent time in a common rearing environment, not permitting incisive study of relative contribution of genes and rearing environment. Until the advent of modern molecular genetics and the ability to genotype millions of genetic variants in large samples, adoption, twin, and twin-family designs were almost the only way to provide more insight about the relative contribution of genetic and nongenetic contributions to familiality. Therefore, in order to disentangle genes and experience, we have studied special family groups: twins who share experiences but differ in shared genes, or adoptees and their biological and foster parents who differ in their shared experience.

Twin studies

There is a massive twin literature on human behaviors and traits of all kinds as summarized in a recent comprehensive review article (17) indicating that nearly all studied traits have some degree of genetic influence, but environmental influences are also ubiquitous. Thus, twin studies have been the workhorse of behavioral genetic studies of exercise and physical activity.

Biology of twins and twinning

The biology of twinning and twins is complex. Genetically, two types of twins exist in humans. First, monozygotic (MZ) twins, as the result of an early division of the zygote into two individuals share the same genomic sequence and hence are genetically identical, thus often called identical twins. Whole-genome sequencing indicates that at most only a handful of base-pair differences are seen between twins in young MZ pairs, but with age and in certain conditions they do accumulate somatic mutations and other changes that may account for discordance between twins (12, 27). Other external influences can act on them *in utero* to create phenotypic differences. A notable potential source is the variation in pregnancy experiences. MZ twins, depending on the timing of the division of the zygote, may develop with their own chorion and placenta, or share the same placenta and chorion either with or without a common amnion. There is little available evidence that these placentation differences affect the results of twin studies of exercise behaviors, but few studies have rigorously assessed this due to a lack of reliable placentation information. After birth, multiple factors can generate both similarities and differences between the MZ twins.

Dizygotic (DZ) twinning is more heritable than MZ twinning and arises from the simultaneous release and fertilization of two eggs. Thus, DZ twins are genetically full siblings and each twin has their own placenta during pregnancy. Twin pregnancies result in the birth of the two individuals, generally with lower birth weight and shorter gestation than singletons. Despite the lower birth weight, twins catch up with singletons in development quickly, and as adults are very similar to singletons in mortality and virtually all behavior measures that have been examined. This supports the generalizability of twin study results to the general population.

The classical twin model

The realization of the existence of two types of twins more than a century ago has led to comparison of the similarity of MZ versus DZ twins for estimates on the role and relative contribution of genetic factors to interindividual differences in behavior. If both types of pairs are overall more similar than two individuals chosen at random, this is evidence for familial aggregation. The absence of differences in mean similarity of MZ versus DZ co-twins suggests the absence of genetic influences. As MZ twins share the same genomic sequence and DZ twins share only 50% of their segregating genes on average, then in the presence of genetic factors, MZ twins would be expected to resemble each other for the trait in question more than DZ twins.

This inference about the role of genetic factors from the twin model holds under certain basic assumptions. The first is that the environmental variances in MZ and DZ pairs are equal, i.e., that MZ and DZ twins are equally correlated in the exposure to environmental experiences and factors that are relevant for the behavior being studied. This assumption has been found to hold generally (9). Differences could arise from placentation and *in utero* effects, or from differential parental treatment of MZ versus DZ twins. Assessment of relevant exposures and their similarity in MZ and DZ pairs is needed to test the assumption, and violation of the assumption may give rise to spuriously high estimates of genetic effects. The analysis is particularly challenging as it has been shown that measures of what are often considered environmental exposures may also have a genetic component to them. For example, smoking is considered to be an environmental exposure, and actual cigarette smoke is a true environmental toxicant exposure. However, there are interindividual differences in the amount smoked by smokers that relate to genetic differences (3).

The other key assumption of the twin model is the random mating of the parents with respect to the behavior being studied. It is assumed that the DZ pairs, like full siblings, share 50% of their segregating genes. However, if the parents resemble each other more than expected in a particular characteristic and the characteristic has a genetic basis, then this would make the siblings more similar than expected under random mating. For example, if both parents are elite athletes, the biological characteristics underlying that elite ability may be expected to be enriched in their children. This assortative mating then biases the family and twin models.

Basic concepts of the twin model

The twin model assumes that we are dealing with behaviors in which the genetic component is due to multiple genes, each of quite small effect. For example, new studies with molecular genetic approaches indicate that this is indeed the case for physical activity behaviors and major genes with large effects are rare or nonexistent (25). Twin study designs, basic analyses, and modeling approaches are reviewed elsewhere (4, 18, 23).

As indicated above, the genetic similarity of MZ twins is expected to be twice that of DZ twins, and so the expected genetic correlation for additive effects of MZ pairs is unity (1.0) and that of DZ twins is 0.5; for a derivation of the expectation and the underlying genetics, please see, for example, Neale and Cardon (1992) or Thomas (2003) (see "Further reading"). This source of variation in the phenotype is known as additive genetic variance (A) and it is that part of genetic effects that is transmitted from parents to offspring. Genetic effects may also be due to dominance (D), i.e., the sum of all nonlinear effects of alleles at a locus. The expected genetic correlation reflecting dominance effects is unity in MZ but only 0.25 in DZ and sibling-pairs, and this is known as genetic variance due to dominance; *dominance effects do not contribute to parent–offspring similarity*. Finally, there may be gene–gene interactions (i.e., epistasis) affecting phenotypes, but the classical twin model assumes that these are not present.

Nongenetic variance in a trait is divided into that shared by the twin siblings, i.e., those experiences and exposures that make them similar – termed environmental effects in common (C), and those that are not shared, i.e., unique to each twin (E). These are distinguished by whether the effects of the experiences and exposures are shared and have equal effects on both twins, not by the actual environmental factor. Also, measurement error and random effects are part of E (i.e., unique environment exposure), so E is included in all models.

The univariate twin model

Figure 3.1 provides a path diagram of a twin model for estimation of A, C, and E effects, commonly known as the ACE model. Based on the expectations listed above, it is possible to model data from MZ and DZ twin pairs to derive estimates of the relative contribution of genetics. This model also yields an estimate of the heritability of a trait, defined as the proportion of total variance for a trait accounted for by genetic factors. This heritability estimate may be A/A+C+E but sometimes also A+D/A+D+E. Heritability is a relative measure, so changes in the environmental variance can change it even when no genetic changes occur. Also, heritability is not a fixed characteristic of the behavior, but rather a population-level estimate taken at a given time in a given population. For an extensive discussion of the concept of heritability, there are two excellent reviews (14, 24).

Modeling permits evaluation of which models best account for the observed variance in a trait, providing the best statistical fit. Thus, we can evaluate which of several models fits the data when a single behavior is looked at. The simplest model is unique environment (E), thus rejecting all evidence for familial effects; this model rarely happens. An AE model would specify that the pattern of twin similarity in MZ and DZ models fits a purely polygenic additive model with environmental effects unique to each twin. It would have no shared environmental effects (C) and no genetic effects due to dominance (D). The alternative models (CE, ACE, and ADE) can also be specified and tested. By comparing the fit of two models, such as ACE and AE, one

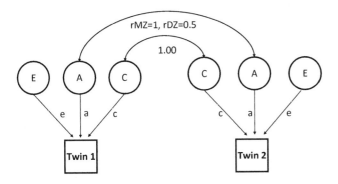

Figure 3.1 Univariate twin model path diagram for decomposition of variance into additive genetic factors (A), environmental factors shared by the twins (i.e., are in common C), and environmental factors unique (E) to each twin. The three latent variables A, C, and E affect the measured phenotypes (as shown by single-headed arrows) of twin 1 and twin 2 (the rectangles). The C effects are by definition fully correlated in both monozygotic (MZ) and dizygotic (DZ) twin pairs, while the expectation of the degree of additive genetic relatedness is unity (1.00) in MZ pairs and 0.5 in DZ pairs under the assumptions of random mating of the parents for the trait in question and satisfaction of the equal environments assumption. In a model accounting for nonadditive effects, C is replaced by D (effects due to dominance), and the expected correlation for D is 1.00 in MZ pairs and 0.25 in DZ pairs. The regression coefficients (a, c, e) provide information on the degree of relationship between the latent and observed. In the ACE model, the observed correlation for MZ pairs has an expected value (based on the paths through A and C of both twins) of $a^2 + c^2$, and for DZ pairs $1/2a^2 + c^2$. Solving these two equations provides a crude estimate of the additive genetic variance (a^2).

can decide whether shared environment (C) effects are statistically needed to account for the data. Very often the pattern of MZ and DZ correlations is used as a starting point to guide the modeling – in a univariate case the choice is often straightforward, but not for multivariate models. Customized software for conducting twin modeling is available, but it is recommended to seek the advice and guidance of an experienced statistical geneticist knowledgeable about the model, particularly if one aims to conduct multivariate models. A number of postgraduate courses in statistical genetics, behavioral genetics, or genetic epidemiology are regularly offered that include twin modeling.

Multivariate twin models

At present, many types of multivariate and longitudinal quantitative genetic models are possible. The simplest form is to run the univariate model in strata of the data, say, separately among young and old participants or among women and men, to see if the variance components A, C, and E differ between strata. Twin models can address sources of sex differences in more detail if data on opposite-sex twins have been collected. The so-called sex-limitation models ask whether different sets of genes influence the behavior in men and women. If the observed correlation for the behavior is much lower in opposite-sex (male–female) DZ pairs than in same-sex DZ pairs of either sex, this result can indicate that there are sex-specific effects. For example, such effects were observed in the very large twin analysis of physical activity in the GenomEUtwin study by Stubbe et al. (21).

Multivariate models permit answering questions about the degree of shared genetic or environmental effects across related traits or over time. For example, do the same genetic and environmental effects affect physical activity in adolescence and adulthood, providing more detail on the contributors to stability and change of the behavior than can be obtained from standard longitudinal surveys and follow-up studies of unrelated individuals? While genes do not change in structure over time, their expression and activity do. These alterations in expression and activity permit novel genetic effects to arise as people age and develop. Another multivariate question may address whether two or more facets of exercise behavior are correlated due to shared genes or due to shared nongenetic influences. Such genetic correlations have been estimated until recently solely by family and twin data (15), but now molecular genetic data can provide more information on the genetic structure of related phenotypes through GWAS studies (see later section). This information can then guide phenotype development, in terms of combining or otherwise constructing variables with the most genetic information.

A basic starting point for multivariate modeling is the Cholesky decomposition or lower-triangle model. Figure 3.2 provides a schematic of the model, and the legend to the figure provides more details. An advantage of the model is that it is solvable and provides a saturated model against which models with fewer parameters and/or paths can be tested. Also, it is easy to apply to data sets if variables or measurement points of the same variable are relatively few. The model produces genetic and environmental correlation matrices of the study variables, which can then be compared to the genetic correlations derived from GWAS analyses. Because the model decomposes variances in each component from left to right into more restricted factors, the ordering of variables is important to consider.

This schematic illustrates a full model and can be used to derive matrices of the genetic and environmental correlations between variables. These may represent different variables, such as levels of physical activity during work, leisure, and sports (9) or the same variable at different points in time; for an illustrative full model of four measures of physical activity from adolescence to young adulthood see Figure 1 in Aaltonen et al. (1)

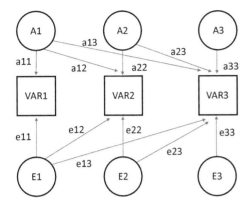

Figure 3.2 Schematic diagram of the essential feature of the Cholesky decomposition multivariate model. The figure shows an AE model applied to three variables (VAR1, VAR2, VAR3) for which twin data are available. The univariate twin model in Figure 3.1 is extended so that paths from the latent genetic (A) and environmental (E) variation also cover relationships between variables. Paths a11, a22, and a33 represent variable-specific effect of genes on the trait (variable), and correspondingly a12 denotes the degree to which genetic effects affecting VAR1 also affect VAR2, and so on. The corresponding relationships hold for the environmental effects.

In addition, the full model can be tested against models that specify selected values for the paths. For example, setting path a12 to zero would test whether there a significant genetic correlation between VAR1 and VAR2.

For longitudinal models using the Cholesky approach, time/age is the natural ordering given that all factors impact only on current and later time points. Given its nature, the Cholesky decomposition can accommodate different patterns of change but is not directly falsifiable. In longitudinal contexts, the Cholesky model provides information about the relative contribution of genetic and environmental factors to the tracking of trait. Thus, it is a useful starting point for analyses when little is known about the longitudinal process and contributing variables. From this exploratory tool one can expand to other longitudinal models such as the simplex model or the longitudinal growth model (7). The longitudinal growth model allows us to ask whether genetic factors contribute to variation in both initial level as well as rate of change of the study variable and are those correlated. In other words, do the same genes influence both initial level (say, initial fitness) and rate of change (improvement in fitness over a training period)? In contrast to the Cholesky decomposition, the longitudinal growth model enables predictions on future time points.

Multivariate models may also be much more specific in their construct. Among the best known are the common pathways model and the independent pathways model. The common pathways model specifies that there is one common latent trait through which the genetic and environment variances act. For example, there may be four or more correlated physical activity measures. In the common pathway model, the latent variable has regression paths to all measured variables, and this common latent variable is then decomposed into genetic and environmental factors. Thus, unlike the Cholesky, the genetic and environmental components do not act directly on the variables but run through the common latent variable. In addition, each variable has residual genetic and environmental components to them. The common pathway model is a useful tool for measurement construction and theory development (for more details, see Neale and Cardon (1992) in "Further reading"). The independent pathway model can be considered a special case of the common pathway model. It posits three latent variables for A, C, and E effects, such that they all correlate with the measured variables. Other models that have been developed for use with twin data include the direction of causation model, a sibling inter-action model, and models to assess rater bias (for more details, see Neale and Cardon (1992) in "Further reading"). The latter can be used to assess the effect of having two more raters provide information on several family members, typically parents reporting on both twins.

Finally, these models permit assessment of gene–environment interactions, asking whether a known exposure modifies the impact of genetic variation. An example is the well-replicated finding that physical activity buffers the impact of genes on obesity; among sedentary persons, genes account for a much larger fraction of variance in body mass index (BMI) than among physically active persons. This observation from twin studies (16) has now been extensively corroborated using measured genotypes associated with BMI (11, 20).

MZ discordant pairs to study causal associations

When studying the association of a putative risk factor or exposure on an outcome, the asso-ciation may be causal, i.e., implying that reducing the exposure would lead to a reduction in the outcome. Alternatively, it can be due to confounding. Measurement of known confounders and adjustment for them in statistical models has been the standard approach in observational epidemiology, be they cohort or case–control studies. However, not all confounders are known or can be measured. Genetic factors underlying athletic ability may be shared with genetic effects on obesity. Thus, the association of exercise with weight gain may be causal or it may be accounted for by known and unknown confounders. As exercise itself is, in part, heritable and now that genes for various aspects of exercise behavior are beginning to be identified, there is potentially confounding due to shared genes, as illustrated by the very latest molecular genetic studies.

A study design to examine nongenetic (possibly causal) associations that control for genetic variation uses exposure-discordant twin pairs. As MZ twins share the same genomic sequence, all difference between the twins arise from nongenetic causes, taken very broadly to include all small random events. If we can identify twin pairs in which one exercises and the other does not, then a test of the causal hypothesis of the association between exercise and weight gain would be to study weight development in a large number of such pairs discordant for exercise. If the MZ co-twins who are physically inactive have significantly more weight gain than their co-twins who are active, strong evidence would be provided to support a causal hypothesis. The design controls for genetic background, but also for sex and age effects as well as the exposures that both twins have shared, such as numerous childhood and adolescent exposures from their common childhood home. The challenge in such studies is often finding sufficient numbers of pairs who are truly discordant. Exposing one twin to an experimental intervention while keeping the other twin as a control is a strong design that combines twins with an intervention. Another design is to examine the children of discordant pairs, to see if the discordance is trans-mitted in equal measures to the children of DZ pairs (biologically cousins) and of MZ pairs (biologically half-siblings but socially cousins).

Adoption studies

Theoretically, adoption studies are a very powerful design for disentangling genetic and nongenetic influences. A biological parent–adoptee correlation, when the adopted child has been raised since birth by unrelated adoptive parents, is strong evidence for genetic effects.

However, in practice the adoption may not have occurred immediately after birth, and exposures during pregnancy may be transmitted epigenetically later into life. Adoptive parent–adoptee correlations are indicators of the effects of the rearing environment. Adoption studies of physical activity and related traits are rare.

Twin family designs

A central limitation of the twin design is that it does not directly tell about the transmission of effects from one generation to the next. Therefore, there are a number of designs combining family and twins, where the twins can be either in the offspring generation or as parents. Including two generations permits one to not only model the transmission of the study trait from parents to offspring, but also to include the relationship of the parents. As discussed above, the twin model assumes that there is random mating with respect to the trait being studied. When this is not the case, the twin model results may be biased. Parents may resemble each other more than expected if they come from a microenvironment that is more homogeneous than in the general population. This could, for example, be a religious affiliation, social strata (of deprivation, for example), or geographical locality. This results in what is known as social homogamy, whereby the parents are more alike for social reasons rather than genetic. If spouses have chosen their mates on the basis of their actual personal characteristics, this phenotypic assortment means that there is also some degree of genetic relatedness. For example, spouses have more similar heights than expected, i.e., height shows phenotypic assortment and this would increase the expected genetic relatedness with respect to height in their offspring. One concern in two-generational studies results from the fact that the parents and offspring are often studied at different ages, and the actual behavior may have different genetic and environmental determinants at different ages; simple adjustment for age may not suffice. Ideally, the study behavior should be assessed at the same age in that case, but that may mean waiting for several decades in a longitudinal study of such families. Three-generation studies are even rarer (2).

Genome-wide association studies

In contrast to family studies, molecular genetic studies permit the study of the role of genetic factors in unrelated persons. Until the sequencing of the human genome, the available tools were limited and findings regarding the genetic basis of physical activity sparse and inconsistent. Some candidate genes have been put forward and studied, but on their basis, it has not been possible to assess how much human genetic variation actually contributes to interindividual differences in exercise ability, physical activity, and related phenotypes (19). In the past decade, the experimental design of GWAS has led to increasing findings on the role of specific genes and genetic variation overall in many diseases as well as normal physiological and behavioral traits. Peter Visscher and his colleagues reviewed recently the first 10 years of GWAS discoveries (25).

The design of GWAS is fairly straightforward as current genotyping technologies permit the efficient and cheap genotyping of hundreds of thousands of genetic variants, mostly SNPs, across the human genome. These serve as markers for blocks of DNA that are mostly inherited together and therefore there is no need to fully sequence all the genomes under study. GWAS is informative of a large fraction of human genetic variation and permits identification of small regions of association. Advances in technology, statistical genetics, and genomic biology have permitted researchers to make strong advances in the use of GWAS for understanding population and complex-traits genetics and the biology of the conditions. Two central advances have been the availability of ever larger sample sizes on the one hand, and better characterized phenotypes on the other. Unlike studies done on obesity, diabetes, height, and education which have yielded hundreds of genetic loci linked to these traits, the study of physical activity has been challenging, and until recently very little progress in GWAS of physical activity was achieved (19).

Using data on nearly half a million persons from the UK Biobank (22), Tikkanen et al. identified 64 loci associated with handgrip strength that replicated using 223,315 individuals for discovery and 116,610 for replication. The strongest association was with *FTO*, a locus first associated with obesity. The handgrip loci findings extended those reported earlier in the CHARGE consortium (13) and will help to understand the reasons for variation in handgrip strength in the population. We can expect that as other objectively measured indices of exercise characteristics such as time spent on various physical activities become available for genomic studies, more loci will be found due to more accuracy in the studied phenotype. The genome-wide significant loci for handgrip strength accounted for only 1.7% of variance in measured physical activity, but overall common variants accounted for some 13% of variance. This is substantial but considerably less than implied by twin and family studies.

The UK Biobank data was also at the core of another large GWAS study (10) that extended the analyses with data from the ARIC study, with robust findings for eight loci for moderate to vigorous physical activity. The strongest associations were seen with *APOE*, a lipid and dementia-associated gene, and with *CADM2*, previously associated with risk-taking behaviors. The authors also found that the physical activity measures show genetic correlations with educational attainment and various obesity-related traits. In summary, large-scale GWAS of self-reported and objectively measured physical activity traits are now producing the first consistent and replicated associations with a handful of genes. They also show that the common genetic variants overall account for as little as 10% of the variance in these traits, a share that may rise somewhat as more variants are genotyped and imputed more accurately and phenotyping improves. Finally, the examined physical activity GWAS analyses reveal expected genetic correlations with other traits such as education, obesity, and risk-taking behaviors.

The future in the era of molecular genetics

When considering overall genetic influences, it should be kept in mind that heritability of a trait in a population is not necessarily static. For example, if important, influential environmental and behavioral exposures change over time and explain more or less of the population variance in a trait. As such, with all else being equal, there will be inverse variations in the heritability of the trait. In addition, heritability of a trait may vary by sex and age and other covariates. While heritability is an important concept related to the overall magnitude of genetic versus environmental influences on a trait at the population level, it must be recognized that there is a highly complex interplay between genetic and environmental factors, as is seen in epigenetics and gene expression, for example.

Beyond heritability estimates, classic twin studies with multivariate analyses have allowed the examination of shared genetic influences between phenotypes to test hypotheses regarding shared etiologies or possible pathways of genetic influences on clinical phenotypes. Finally, molecular genetics are now bringing a host of new approaches and tools to better understand the genetic architecture of exercise characteristics and gain insights to relevant biological processes.

Further reading

Knopik VS, Neiderhiser JM, DeFries JC, Plomin R. *Behavioral Genetics* (7th ed.). New York: Worth, 2017.

Lynch M, Walsh B. *Genetics and Analysis of Quantitative Traits*. Sunderland, MA: Sinauer, 1998.

Neale BM, Ferreira M. AR, Medland SE and Posthuma D. *Statistical Genetics: Gene Mapping Through Linkage and Association*. New York: Taylor & Francis, 2008.

Neale MC, Cardon LR. *Methodology for Genetic Studies of Twins and Families*. NATO ASI series D: Behavioural and Social Sciences, Vol. 67. Dordecht: Kluwer, 1992.

Thomas DC. *Statistical Methods in Genetic Epidemiology*. New York: Oxford University Press, 2004.

References

1. **Aaltonen S, Ortega-Alonso A, Kujala UM**, and **Kaprio J.** Genetic and environmental influences on longitudinal changes in leisure-time physical activity from adolescence to young adulthood. *Twin Research and Human Genetics* 16: 535–43, 2013.

2. **Aarnio M, Winter T, Kujala UM**, and **Kaprio J.** Familial aggregation of leisure-time physical activity – a three generation study. *International Journal of Sports Medicine* 18: 549–56, 1997.

3. **Benowitz NL.** Nicotine addiction. *New England Journal of Medicine* 362: 2295–2303, 2010.

4. **Boomsma D, Busjahn A**, and **Peltonen L.** Classical twin studies and beyond. *Nature Reviews Genetics* 3: 872–82, 2002.

5. **de Geus EJ, Bartels M, Kaprio J, Lightfoot JT**, and **Thomis M.** Genetics of regular exercise and sedentary behaviors. *Twin Research and Human Genetics* 17: 262–71, 2014.

6. **Kaplanis J, Gordon A, Shor T, Weissbrod O, Geiger D, Wahl M, Gershovits M, Markus B, Sheikh M, Gymrek M, Bhatia G, MacArthur DG, Price AL**, and **Erlich Y.** Quantitative analysis of population-scale family trees with millions of relatives. *Science* 360: 171–175, 2018.

7. **Kaprio J** and **Silventoinen K.** Advanced methods in twin studies. *Methods in Molecular Biology* 713: 143–52, 2011.

8. **Kendler KS** and **Neale MC.** "Familiality" or heritability. *Archives of General Psychiatry* 66: 452–3, 2009.

9. **Kendler KS, Neale MC, Kessler RC, Heath AC**, and **Eaves LJ.** A test of the equal-environment assumption in twin studies of psychiatric illness. *Behavior Genetics* 23: 21–7, 1993.

10. **Klimentidis YC, Raichlen DA, Bea J, Garcia DO, Wineinger NE, Mandarino LJ, Alexander GE, Chen Z**, and **Going SB**. Genome-wide association study of habitual physical activity in over 377,000 UK Biobank participants identifies multiple variants including CADM2 and APOE. *International Journal of Obesity* 42: 1161–1176, 2018.

11. **Kilpeläinen TO, Qi L, Brage S, Sharp SJ, Sonestedt E, Demerath E, Ahmad T, Mora S, Kaakinen M, Sandholt CH, Holzapfel C, Autenrieth CS, Hyppönen E, Cauchi S, He M, Kutalik Z, Kumari M, Stančáková A, Meidtner K, Balkau B, Tan JT, Mangino M**, et al. Physical activity attenuates the influence of FTO variants on obesity risk: a meta-analysis of 218,166 adults and 19,268 children. *PLoS Medicine* 8: e1001116, 2011.

12. **Martin N, Boomsma D**, and **Machin G.** A twin-pronged attack on complex traits. *Nature Genetics* 17: 387–92, 1997.

13. **Matteini AM, Tanaka T, Karasik D, Atzmon G, Chou WC, Eicher JD, Johnson AD, Arnold AM, Callisaya ML, Davies G, Evans DS, Holtfreter B, Lohman K, Lunetta KL, Mangino M, Smith AV, Smith JA, Teumer A, Yu L, Arking DE, Buchman AS, Chibinik LB**, et al. GWAS analysis of handgrip and lower body strength in older adults in the CHARGE consortium. *Aging Cell* 15: 792–800, 2016.

14. **Mayhew AJ** and **Meyre D.** Assessing the heritability of complex traits in humans: methodological challenges and opportunities. *Current Genomics* 18: 332–340, 2017.

15. **Mustelin L, Joutsi J, Latvala A, Pietiläinen KH, Rissanen A**, and **Kaprio J.** Genetic influences on physical activity in young adults: a twin study. *Medicine and Science in Sports and Exercise* 44: 1293–301, 2012.

16. **Mustelin L, Silventoinen K, Pietiläinen K, Rissanen A**, and **Kaprio J.** Physical activity reduces the influence of genetic effects on BMI and waist circumference: a study in young adult twins. *International Journal of Obesity* 33: 29–36, 2009.

17. **Polderman TJ, Benyamin B, de Leeuw CA, Sullivan PF, van Bochoven A, Visscher PM**, and **Posthuma D.** Meta-analysis of the heritability of human traits based on fifty years of twin studies. *Nature Genetics* 47: 702–9, 2015.

18. **Posthuma D, Beem AL, de Geus EJ, van Baal GC, von Hjelmborg JB, Iachine I**, and **Boomsma DI.** Theory and practice in quantitative genetics. *Twin Research* 6: 361–76, 2003.

19. **Sarzynski MA, Loos RJ, Lucia A, Pérusse L, Roth SM, Wolfarth B, Rankinen T**, and **Bouchard C.** Advances in exercise, fitness, and performance genomics in 2015. *Medicine and Science in Sports and Exercise* 48: 1906–16, 2016.

20. **Shungin D, Deng WQ, Varga TV, Luan J, Mihailov E, Metspalu A; GIANT Consortium, Morris AP, Forouhi NG, Lindgren C, Magnusson PKE, Pedersen NL, Hallmans G, Chu AY, Justice AE, Graff M, Winkler TW, Rose LM, Langenberg C, Cupples LA, Ridker PM, Wareham NJ**, et al. Ranking and characterization of established BMI and lipid associated loci as candidates for gene-environment interactions. *PLoS Genetics* 13: e1006812, 2017.

21. **Stubbe JH, Boomsma DI, Vink JM, Cornes BK, Martin NG, Skytthe A, Kyvik KO, Rose RJ, Kujala UM, Kaprio J, Harris JR, Pedersen NL, Hunkin J, Spector TD**, and **de Geus EJ.** Genetic influences on exercise participation in 37,051 twin pairs from seven countries. *PLoS One* 1: e22, 2006.

22. **Tikkanen E, Gustafsson S, Amar D, Shcherbina A, Waggott D, Ashley EA**, and **Ingelsson E.** Biological insights into muscular strength: Genetic findings in the UK Biobank. *Scientific Reports* 8: 6451, 2018.

23. **van Dongen J, Slagboom PE, Draisma HH, Martin NG**, and **Boomsma DI.** The continuing value of twin studies in the omics era. *Nature Reviews Genetics* 13: 640–53, 2012.

24. **Visscher PM, Hill WG**, and **Wray NR.** Heritability in the genomics era – concepts and misconceptions. *Nature Reviews Genetics* 9: 255–66, 2008

25. **Visscher PM, Wray NR, Zhang Q, Sklar P, McCarthy MI, Brown MA**, and **Yang J.** 10 Years of GWAS discovery: Biology, function, and translation. *American Journal of Human Genetics* 101: 5–22, 2017.

26. **Yao CA** and **Rhodes RE.** Parental correlates in child and adolescent physical activity: A meta-analysis. *International Journal of Behavioral Nutrition and Physical Activity* 12: 10, 2015.

27. **Ye K, Beekman M, Lameijer EW, Zhang Y, Moed MH, van den Akker EB, Deelen J, Houwing-Duistermaat JJ, Kremer D, Anvar SY, Laros JF, Jones D, Raine K, Blackburne B, Potluri S, Long Q, Guryev V, van der Breggen R, Westendorp RG, 't Hoen PA, den Dunnen J, van Ommen GJ**, et al. Aging as accelerated accumulation of somatic variants: whole-genome sequencing of centenarian and middle-aged monozygotic twin pairs. *Twin Research and Human Genetics* 16: 1026–32, 2013.

4

THE TRANSLATION OF SYSTEMS GENETICS OF EXERCISE TO EVERYDAY LIFE

Molly Bray

Introduction

Whether in the context of cardiovascular fitness, weight loss/maintenance, metabolic disease risk, or mental health, the benefits of physical activity and exercise for most individuals are undeniable. Conversely, physical inactivity is among the leading causes of death in the US, second only to tobacco use (5). Sedentary behavior has been shown to have a significant dose–response effect in increasing risk for cardiovascular disease, type 2 diabetes, obesity, and all-cause mortality (47, 71). In adults aged 40–69 years, almost 10% of deaths have been attributed directly to insufficient levels of physical activity (14). Despite the health benefits associated with physical activity, many individuals find it difficult to maintain participation in regular physical activity, regardless of their interest or intent. Approximately 25% of adults do not engage in any leisure-time physical activity (45), and only 21% of adults meet the 2008 physical activity guidelines of 2.5 or more hours per week, with the lowest prevalence of physical activity participation among Hispanics and non-Hispanic black individuals (16). How might an understanding of the genetic underpinnings of physical activity and exercise response be used to improve intervention efficacy and turn the rising tide of sedentarism in the world? A primary goal of exercise genomics is to determine what makes a person "naturally" physically active and to use this knowledge to help others to achieve this natural state through enhanced interventions and more efficacious and personalized exercise prescription.

Theoretical foundations of exercise interventions

Physical activity and exercise are complex behaviors driven by both extrinsic and intrinsic factors. Attitudes, perceived barriers, enjoyment, self-efficacy, and self-motivation have all been associated with exercise adherence (9, 18, 46, 63). Various theoretical frameworks explain the association between these concepts and exercise adherence or dropout in different ways. According to social-cognitive theory, those who have high self-efficacy about physical activity would perceive fewer barriers to their physical activity or be less influenced by them, be more likely to act on their expectations of desirable outcomes of being physically active (i.e., extrinsic motives), and be more likely to enjoy physical activity (intrinsic motives; 3, 4). Self-determination theory and schema theory are complementary to social-cognitive theory and suggest that intrinsic motives for physical activity and a physically active self-identity, which develop during late adolescence and young adulthood, interact with physical and social environments to influence physical activity (54). The transtheoretical model proposes that when people try to increase their physical activity, they use neurocognitive processes to move through stages of change (48). The theory of reasoned action states that behaviors are initially determined by intentions, which are in turn driven by both extrinsic motives for physical activity, such as social affiliation and appearance, and intrinsic motives, such as physical competence and enjoyment (15). Most interventions targeted at improving health through changes in diet and/or physical activity are grounded in behavior theory, which can be useful for formulating strategies for changing behavior but generally lack a biological component. Exercise genomics can inform intervention studies by identifying the genes and pathways that underlie and drive the theoretical behavior.

A common observation among exercise and physical activity intervention studies is a high level of initial compliance and concomitant positive responses to exercise, followed by poor long-term adherence and eventual dropout. Many exercise programs have reported a 50–60% dropout rate within the first 3–6 months (19, 20, 67). Variables reported to be associated with exercise dropout include age, education, sex, ethnicity, previous activity, dietary habits, smoking, occupation, and social support, but no single variable explains all the variance in subject attrition (9, 12, 52, 63, 66). Additional research has shown that exercise dropouts are more likely to have higher body fat and body weight than those who continue with an exercise program (28); conversely, participants who are physically active and have a moderate level of aerobic fitness are the most likely to continue to exercise (66). Rothman (53) notes that behavior change differs from behavior maintenance or adherence. Factors driving the initiation of a behavior are strongly linked to anticipated positive effects, while the factors contributing to behavior maintenance are strongly dependent upon perceived satisfaction with the outcome of the behavioral change (53). Though multiple psychological and physical traits have been identified that may be predictive of exercise and physical activity behavior, what is lacking in these investigations is the incorporation of putative biological drivers of behavior, such as neural signaling and metabolism that may be revealed through genetic studies.

Translating exercise genomics into practice

As described above, behavioral theories can provide a strong foundation for the development of physical activity-based interventions. As shown in Figure 4.1, understanding the biological processes that underlie observed behavior gleaned from genetic studies has the potential to greatly enhance intervention efficacy through: 1) improvement of exercise adherence; 2) optimization of exercise prescriptions; and 3) early identification of individuals at risk for dropout. In terms of exercise adherence, genetic studies can be used to identify the neural pathways that influence motivation, persistence, and attitudes toward exercise. To optimize exercise prescription, genes identified for physical activity may reveal new information about biological processes that enhance or inhibit positive physiological responses to exercise, which in turn influence exercise adherence. Genetic variation may also explain the variability in response to environmental changes. For example, while strategies such as modifying the built environment to encourage physical activity are important at a community level, genetic information may reveal how and why some individuals are drawn to use environmental resources such as parks, cycle lanes, and trails and some are not. Importantly, genetic information may be extremely useful in identifying those individuals who may be at risk for dropout or nonresponse and, thus, may need more encouragement or instruction to successfully incorporate physical activity as a lifestyle.

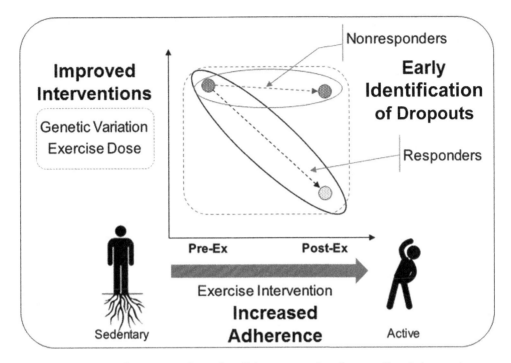

Figure 4.1 Genetic information can be used to: 1) improve exercise adherence; 2) optimize exercise prescriptions; and 3) identify individuals at risk for dropout.

Using genetic information to enhance exercise adherence

Like most dietary interventions, exercise programs are generally effective when people stick to them, and the best way to increase intervention efficacy is through improved adherence. Adherence can be defined as completion of or compliance with a prescribed protocol or course of action. As described above, attitudes and beliefs play a substantial role in physical activity behavior and exercise dropout, and at least some of the heritability of physical activity may represent genetic variation associated with the neural processing underlying exercise attitudes and adherence. Huppertz and colleagues examined the heritability of attitudes toward exercise in adult twin pairs, with a focus on six domains: perceived benefits; lack of skills, support, and/or resources; time constraints; lack of energy; lack of enjoyment; and embarrassment (34). All attitude domains were significantly correlated with exercise behavior and exhibited significant heritability. Interestingly, the highest heritabilities observed were for intrinsic factors such as lack of enjoyment (males: 0.47; females: 0.44), embarrassment (males: 0.42; females: 0.49), and lack of skills (males: 0.45; females: 0.48), while external factors such as time constraints and perceived benefits were more strongly explained by environmental factors in both men and women (0.70–0.79). Together, these attitudes explained 28% of variance in exercise behavior (34). Heritability studies provide support for a genetic basis for the psychological constructs associated with physical activity, and ultimately, it is important to identify the genes and pathways underlying the genetic basis of physical activity behavior in order to make more informed decisions about how to intervene.

Altering physical and behavioral traits through selective animal breeding is one of the most powerful experimental approaches for demonstrating that a trait is genetic. Genes that underlie voluntary physical activity in animals or humans likely influence both physical (e.g., exercise performance and ability) and psychological (e.g., motivation, adherence) components of exercise behavior, which reinforce each other in a feed-forward manner (35). As described in Chapter 5, a number of animal models have been created with extremely high levels of physical activity, with rodents running both further and faster than their wildtype counterparts (17, 21). Interestingly, animals bred to be physically active demonstrate increased signs of stress when the running wheel is removed, enhanced preference for running in lieu of other activities, and increased neuronal activity associated with physical activity, supporting the hypothesis that neurocognitive traits can be selected for in the breeding process (51). Though a limited number of syntenic quantitative trait loci regions between mouse and human have been identified through gene mapping studies in selectively bred animals, it is surprising how little overlap has been reported, although critical differences in study design may have contributed to this lack of replication (38). The lack of replication for genes identified in animal studies points to the tremendous importance of considering genetic background, environmental cues and conditions, stress, and other mental states when assessing physical activity behavior.

Many genes have been identified that appear to regulate both spontaneous and planned physical activity, as well as exercise response. As outlined in Chapter 8, genes identified to date provide compelling evidence that physical activity behavior is under substantial neural control. Variation within the dopaminergic, serotonergic, and endocannabinoid systems may alter satisfaction, pleasure, and reward derived from exercise and physical activity, and in turn, influence persistence in physical activity behavior. In support of this hypothesis, Bryan et al. demonstrated that affective state, perceived exertion, mood, and heart rate were a function of whether and how long a person had been performing an acute bout of exercise and that changes in these attitudes were mediated by a variant (Val66Met, rs6265) in the brain-derived neurotropic factor (*BDNF*) gene (11). Positive affect increased with greater duration of acute exercise, and carriers of the *BDNF* Met66 allele showed a more pronounced increase in positive affect compared to Val/Val homozygotes. Increases in heart rate during exercise were also associated with both alterations in mood and variation in *BDNF*, suggesting that affective mood may be influenced by the interaction between physiologic changes and genetic variation (11). In a follow-up study, the *BDNF* Met66 allele was also associated with intrinsic motivation for exercise, with carriers being more likely to remain on the treadmill, even when given the option to discontinue the exercise session (13).

Although many studies have examined the interaction between genes and physical activity/exercise on disease risk, energy balance, and exercise response, few studies have been specifically designed to examine how genetic variation influences exercise adherence. Thompson et al. examined an insertion/deletion (I/D) polymorphism in the angiotensin-converting enzyme (*ACE*) gene for an association with exercise response and adherence, which was defined by session attendance in a progressive aerobic exercise-training program. While the *ACE* I/D polymorphism was not associated with exercise response (in terms of aerobic fitness, anthropometrics, or blood pressure), adherence to the exercise training protocol was significantly higher in I carriers than in D homozygotes (61). No differences were observed in average exercise intensity between the I/D genotypes, however, suggesting that simply accounting for attendance without considering other parameters of the workout sessions does not sufficiently define adherence (61). The Training Interventions and Genetics of Exercise Response (TIGER) study was developed to investigate the genetic underpinnings of exercise adherence and response in young adults (55). A total of 3665 subjects in the study underwent 15 weeks of aerobic exercise training, for three days per week for at least 30 minutes at an intensity between 65%

and 85% of maximum heart rate reserve. Every exercise session was documented and tracked using computerized heart rate monitors. Compliance with the study protocol was quantified by adjusting the duration of each exercise session by the average intensity of the session and summing over all sessions to create a total score of exercise intensity-minutes, called the heart rate physical activity score (HRPAS) (44). Exercise adherence was defined as meeting the minimum prescribed HRPAS. HRPAS is also considered a measure of exercise tolerance, since it is a function of how hard and how long the participants exercised within the range of the exercise prescription. Whole-genome association analysis using HRPAS as a primary outcome identified SNPs in ten genes that exceeded a genome-wide significance of $P < 10^{-4.5}$, including the fructosamine 3 kinase related protein (*FN3KRP*), brain-derived neurotropic factor (*BDNF*), fat mass and obesity related transcript (*FTO*), receptor interacting serine/threonine kinase 2 (*RIPK2*), ATP binding cassette subfamily B member 11 (*ABCB11*), brain and reproductive organ-expressed (*BRE*), zinc fingers and homeoboxes 3 (*ZHX3*), insulin degrading enzyme (*IDE*), tubulin folding cofactor D (*TBCD*), and centrosomal protein 112 (*CEP112*) genes (30). Pathways contributing to lipid metabolism, neural signaling, muscle contraction, and adiposity were significantly represented by SNPs with a nominal $P < 0.0001$. The strongest single gene association with exercise adherence/tolerance was for *FN3KRP* ($P < 10^{-11}$), which functions in gene regulation through deglycation of target proteins (60). Though no other studies to date have reported associations between *FN3KRP* and physical activity or exercise, it has been identified in gene mapping studies for multiple cardiometabolic risk traits (body mass index, waist, hip, systolic blood pressure) (7, 56), and allele-specific expression of *FN3KRP* driven by miR-34a is associated with variation in hemoglobin A1c levels (29), supporting its role in glycation-based regulation. The functional role of the *FN3KRP* gene in exercise adherence is not yet known, and it is possible that it is in disequilibrium with other functional genes or regulatory sequence.

At the far end of the exercise adherence spectrum is exercise addiction. Similar to other types of addiction, exercise addiction is associated with increasing tolerance, withdrawal anxiety, lack of control, and reduction of other activities (27). As described in earlier chapters, exercise is known to excite areas of the brain and systems associated with pleasure and reward, such as dopamine, endorphins, and cannabinoids, in a manner similar to that of addictive substances. Genes that have been associated with physical activity, including serotonin receptor 2A (*HTR2A*), serotonin receptor 1B (*HTR1B*), dopamine receptor D2 (*DRD2*), and dopamine receptor D4 (*DRD4*), have also been associated with alcohol, cocaine, and opioid dependence (31). Strategies to reduce addictive behavior in other areas may inform the conversion of exercise addicts to a normal level of adherence. In addition, such studies also have the potential to reveal important mechanisms that motivate behavior.

What is currently lacking in terms of genetic studies of exercise adherence are prospective studies of individuals selected on genotype and powered to detect a difference between genotype groups to validate association studies. One difficulty in identifying genes for exercise adherence retrospectively in existing cohorts is that subjects are often urged to remain in the intervention by extrinsic rewards or motivation such as monetary compensation and/or prompting and encouragement from study investigators, which may influence the natural process of attrition. To identify and replicate genes for exercise adherence, studies should be performed in which optimal exercise interventions are provided and subjects are allowed to drop from the study without external interference. In addition, future genetic studies should examine the interaction between genes and other factors, such as those listed above, that have been associated with exercise dropout to simultaneously characterize the multivariate predictors of exercise adherence.

Using genetic information to enhance exercise prescription and intervention

Currently, exercise prescription is a largely a one-size-fits-all undertaking, with the argument being that "exercise is good for everyone." Nevertheless, significant variability has been observed in response to exercise training, with some individuals experiencing negative, rather than positive effects of exercise, depending on the outcome being studied (10). As identified in other chapters, numerous genes have been associated with physical activity and exercise behavior, providing potential targets for developing gene-based exercise prescriptions. In addition, the interaction between genes and exercise has been robustly demonstrated to influence response to exercise training for multiple traits (muscular strength and power, cardiorespiratory fitness and endurance performance, body weight and adiposity, insulin and glucose metabolism, lipid and lipoprotein metabolism, and hemodynamic traits) (57). As with many other complex traits, the genes identified to date explain only a small proportion of the total variability in the exercise-related outcomes studied, and many have suggested that much larger cohorts than those currently being examined are needed to robustly develop a set of genetic variants that can predict exercise adherence and response (24).

In developing interventions targeted at improving health behaviors, the systems genetics of exercise points to the fact that genes play a plausible role in influencing many components of health behaviors. Reiss and colleagues note that genes can modify how individuals respond to the social and physical environments by influencing response to environmental stress, sensitivity to changes in the environment, compatibility with the environment, and environment-specific responses (50). Thus, changing the built environment to promote physical activity may cause stress in some individuals and excitement or challenge in others. For example, the serotonin system, which has been shown to be involved in physical activity behavior, has also been implicated in differential cardiovascular reactivity in response to social stress (65), providing a potential link between physical activity behavior and environmentally induced stress. Making assumptions that individuals who do not take advantage of such environmental alterations are simply lazy or unmotivated ignores a potential key biological underpinning of inactivity.

While animal studies provide evidence that disrupting candidate genes may influence physical activity and other metabolic traits, few human studies have been designed to directly test the effects of exercise training by selecting subjects based on genotype. In a study by Thompson and colleagues, balanced groups of subjects were selected based on their apolipoprotein E (*APOE*) genotype to have sufficient power to detect differences in lipid response to exercise training (62). The investigators were able to demonstrate significant differences between genotype groups in exercise response, not only in lipid traits (total cholesterol/high-density lipoprotein ratio, low-density lipoprotein/high-density lipoprotein ratio) but also in aerobic capacity, with significantly lower VO_2max in subjects with the 3/3 genotype compared to the other genotype groups (62).

Similar to other studies, the BDNF signaling pathway emerged as a central factor linking multiple other pathways, and highlighting neural signaling as a target for exercise adherence in the TIGER study (30). BDNF provides an example of the potential use of genetic information to guide the development of behavioral exercise interventions as well as to direct the use of exercise and physical activity for therapy for other types of conditions. BDNF is a neurotrophin that has been shown to play a central role in neuronal plasticity and long-term potentiation associated with learning and memory (40). The Val66Met variant in the *BDNF* gene has been associated with depression and multiple neurodegenerative disorders (e.g., Parkinson's disease, multiple sclerosis, Alzheimer's disease; 37, 59), in addition to physical activity. Importantly, both acute and chronic aerobic exercise have been shown to increase peripheral *BDNF* expression (33), and exercise has been shown to attenuate the negative effects of BDNF sequence variation on memory loss, depression, and hippocampal atrophy (23). Increases in BDNF expression associated with exercise training have been proposed as one potential mechanism for the action of exercise in reducing depressive symptoms, enhancing self-esteem, improving mood and sleep, and increasing resilience to stress (25, 33), making *BDNF* not only a plausible candidate gene but also a likely target for intervention. One way to apply this knowledge would be to use BDNF as a marker to identify individuals who are sensitive to the effects of exercise versus those who are not. This could involve measuring plasma levels of BDNF or measuring gene variants in *BDNF*; given new technologies for characterizing genetic variation, the latter might be the easier of the two. As in the Thompson study (62), subjects could be selected based on BDNF protein levels or genotype, and then examined for exercise response and adherence *a priori*. Such a strategy would represent a translational approach to a critical issue in exercise research.

Using genetic information to identify individuals at risk for exercise dropout

Of all the ways in which genetic information may be utilized to improve health, genetic risk prediction is among the most straightforward. Genetic risk alleles/scores have been shown to inform risk prediction for cardiovascular disease (e.g., markers at 9p21 for incident coronary artery disease), cancer (e.g., *BRCA1* and *BRCA2* for breast cancer), venous thromboembolism (e.g., factor V Leiden), drug response (e.g., multilocus risk score at *NAT2*, *CYP2D6*, *CYP2C19*, *CYP2C9*, and *CYP4F2* for coumarin response), Alzheimer's disease (e.g., *APOE*), and others (32, 39, 68, 70), with large-effect alleles providing the most reproducible and stable predictions of disease risk. Nevertheless, for complex diseases and traits, such as exercise adherence or dropout, in which multiple small-effect variants likely explain most of the variance, genetic prediction has been less robust. Despite the fact that many genome-wide association study (GWAS) findings have been convincingly replicated, Marigorta and colleagues caution that even when combining all functional SNPs for a complex trait into a genetic risk score, the ability to predict risk is limited by the heritability of the trait (43). Nevertheless, GWAS data could be combined with other types of "omics" data (e.g., transcriptome, methylome, metabolome, and phenome) to better understand biological interactions and more robustly predict behavioral outcomes like exercise adherence and dropout.

In the TIGER study (described previously), the *FTO* gene was associated with exercise adherence, with combinations of any three risk-raising alleles in the *FTO* locus more than doubling exercise dropout risk (odds ratio=2.22; 95% confidence interval: 1.45–3.40) (30). In a follow-up study, subjects were selected based on genetic risk score for *FTO* (less than three risk-raising alleles or more than six risk-raising alleles), and differences in gene expression from leukocytes before and after exercise and between groups were examined. After controlling for multiple testing, the diacylglycerol kinase zeta (*DGKZ*) gene was found to be significantly differentially expressed between pre- and postexercise time points in the high-risk group ($P < 0.04$) (22). Interestingly, *DGKZ* has been implicated in muscle hypertrophy, insulin sensitivity, energy metabolism, and addictive behavior (8, 42, 69), providing a plausible biological mechanism for its potential action in exercise adherence. How the effect of DGKZ is modified by variation in *FTO* is not yet known.

To date, exercise and physical activity have been primarily assessed as behavioral/lifestyle means of reducing genetic risk for metabolic diseases, rather than in the context of genetic risk for the behaviors themselves. For example, the *FTO* gene is one of the most highly replicated findings in obesity genetics (26, 58), and it has also repeatedly been reported that physical activity attenuates the increased risk associated with deleterious *FTO* variation (1, 49, 64). Physical activity has been shown to substantially reduce multigenic disease risk for obesity and coronary heart disease (36, 41) and to be more important in determining risk than genetic factors for type 2 diabetes (2, 6). These examples demonstrate that health behaviors are important in the context of genetic risk and that people are not "doomed" by their DNA sequence. Because healthy behaviors such as diet and exercise can offset the risk-raising effect of gene variation, it is more important than ever to develop a better understanding of the factors that influence exercise adherence.

Conclusion

The systems genomics approach has been extremely effective in identifying genes associated with physical activity behavior and exercise response, many of which have been robustly replicated. The list of potential candidate genes associated with physical activity behavior and exercise response is extensive and growing with each new study. Genes identified to date point to a strong neural basis for exercise behavior that is supported by studies of the genetics of exercise adherence. To translate the findings from exercise and physical activity studies to intervention and practice, statistical replication should be followed by functional analysis in the laboratory along with well-powered studies in humans to test the effects and interactions of genotype *a priori*. The message that "exercise and physical activity are good for everyone" has clearly not been effective in promoting physical activity, and a stronger basis in biology is needed to devise more efficacious and personalized exercise interventions and prescriptions. Given the success of genetic risk prediction in many areas and the increasing ease with which genetic data can be collected, it is reasonable to envision a straightforward genetic testing protocol that can be used to identify individuals at risk for dropout or nonresponse.

Acknowledgement: Thanks to Matthew Lehrer, MS, for his tremendous help with summarizing the references for this chapter.

References

1. **Andreasen CH, Mogensen MS, Borch-Johnsen K, Sandbaek A, Lauritzen T, Sorensen TI, Hansen L, Almind K, Jorgensen T, Pedersen O**, and **Hansen T.** Non-replication of genome-wide based associations between common variants in INSIG2 and PFKP and obesity in studies of 18,014 Danes. *PLoS One* 3: e2872, 2008.
2. **Ardisson Korat AV, Willett WC**, and **Hu FB.** Diet, lifestyle, and genetic risk factors for type 2 diabetes: A review from the Nurses' Health Study, Nurses' Health Study 2, and Health Professionals' Follow-up Study. *Curr Nutr Rep* 3: 345–354, 2014.
3. **Bandura A.** Health promotion by social cognitive means. *Health Educ Behav* 31: 143–164, 2004.
4. **Bandura A.** *Social Foundations of Thought and Action: A Social Cognitive Theory.* Englewood Cliffs, NJ: Prentice Hall, 1986.
5. **Bauer UE, Briss PA, Goodman RA**, and **Bowman BA.** Prevention of chronic disease in the 21st century: elimination of the leading preventable causes of premature death and disability in the USA. *Lancet* 384: 45–52, 2014.
6. **Bellou V, Belbasis L, Tzoulaki I**, and **Evangelou E.** Risk factors for type 2 diabetes mellitus: An exposure-wide umbrella review of meta-analyses. *PLoS One* 13: e0194127, 2018.
7. **Benton MC, Lea RA, Macartney-Coxson D, Carless MA, Goring HH, Bellis C, Hanna M, Eccles D, Chambers GK, Curran JE, Harper JL, Blangero J**, and **Griffiths LR.** Mapping eQTLs in the Norfolk Island genetic isolate identifies candidate genes for CVD risk traits. *Am J Hum Genet* 93: 1087–1099, 2013.
8. **Benziane B, Borg ML, Tom RZ, Riedl I, Massart J, Bjornholm M, Gilbert M, Chibalin AV**, and **Zierath JR.** DGKzeta deficiency protects against peripheral insulin resistance and improves energy metabolism. *J Lipid Res* 58: 2324–2333, 2017.

9. **Booth ML, Owen N, Bauman A, Clavisi O,** and **Leslie E.** Social-cognitive and perceived environment influences associated with physical activity in older Australians. *Prev Med* 31: 15–22, 2000.

10. **Bouchard C** and **Rankinen T.** Individual differences in response to regular physical activity. *Med Sci Sports Exerc* 33: S446–S451; discussion S452–S443, 2001.

11. **Bryan A, Hutchison KE, Seals DR,** and **Allen DL.** A transdisciplinary model integrating genetic, physiological, and psychological correlates of voluntary exercise. *Health Psychol* 26: 30–39, 2007.

12. **Buckworth J** and **Wallace LS.** Application of the transtheoretical model to physically active adults. *J Sports Med Phys Fitness* 42: 360–367, 2002.

13. **Caldwell Hooper AE, Bryan AD,** and **Hagger MS.** What keeps a body moving? The brain-derived neurotrophic factor val66met polymorphism and intrinsic motivation to exercise in humans. *J Behav Med* 37: 1180–1192, 2014.

14. **Carlson SA, Adams EK, Yang Z,** and **Fulton JE.** Percentage of deaths associated with inadequate physical activity in the United States. *Prev Chronic Dis* 15: E38, 2018.

15. **Chatzisarantis N** and **Brickell T.** Functional significance of psychological variables that are included in the theory of planned behaviour: A self-determination theory approach to the study of attitudes, subjective norms, perceptions of control and intentions. *Eur J Soc Psychol* 28: 303–322, 1998.

16. **Centers for Disease Control.** Facts about physical activity. www.cdc.gov/physicalactivity/data/facts.htm, 2014.

17. **Copes LE, Schutz H, Dlugosz EM, Acosta W, Chappell MA,** and **Garland T,** Jr. Effects of voluntary exercise on spontaneous physical activity and food consumption in mice: Results from an artificial selection experiment. *Physiol Behav* 149: 86–94, 2015.

18. **Dishman RK.** Biologic influences on exercise adherence. *Res Q Exerc Sport* 52: 143–159, 1981.

19. **Dishman RK.** Exercise compliance: A new view for public health. *Phys Sportsmed* 14: 127–145, 1986.

20. **Dishman RK** and **Ickes W.** Self-motivation and adherence to therapeutic exercise. *J Behav Med* 4: 421–438, 1981.

21. **Dlugosz EM, Chappell MA, McGillivray DG, Syme DA,** and **Garland T,** Jr. Locomotor trade-offs in mice selectively bred for high voluntary wheel running. *J Exp Biol* 212: 2612–2618, 2009.

22. **Dong F, Vazquez A, Dishman R, O'Connor P, Jackson A, Fernandez J,** and **Bray M.** The interaction between FTO variation and exercise in influencing gene expression and DNA methylation. In preparation.

23. **Erickson KI, Miller DL,** and **Roecklein KA.** The aging hippocampus: interactions between exercise, depression, and BDNF. *Neuroscientist* 18: 82–97, 2012.

24. **Eynon N, Voisin S, Lucia A, Wang G,** and **Pitsiladis Y.** Preface: Genomics and biology of exercise is undergoing a paradigm shift. *BMC Genomics* 18: 825, 2017.

25. **Fox KR.** The influence of physical activity on mental well-being. *Public Health Nutr* 2: 411–418, 1999.

26. **Frayling TM.** Genome-wide association studies provide new insights into type 2 diabetes aetiology. *Nat Rev Genet* 8: 657–662, 2007.

27. **Freimuth M, Moniz S,** and **Kim SR.** Clarifying exercise addiction: Differential diagnosis, co-occurring disorders, and phases of addiction. *Int J Environ Res Public Health* 8: 4069–4081, 2011.

28. **Gale JB, Eckhoff WT, Mogel SF,** and **Rodnick JE.** Factors related to adherence to an exercise program for healthy adults. *Med Sci Sports Exerc* 16: 544–549, 1984.

29. **Ghanbari M, Franco OH, de Looper HW, Hofman A, Erkeland SJ,** and **Dehghan A.** Genetic variations in microRNA-binding sites affect microRNA-mediated regulation of several genes associated with cardio-metabolic phenotypes. *Circ Cardiovasc Genet* 8: 473–486, 2015.

30. **Herring M, Vazquez A, Dong F, Dishman R, O'Connor P, Jackson A,** and **Bray M.** Genome-wide association for exercise adherence and tolerance in the TIGER study. In preparation.

31. **Herring MP, Sailors MH,** and **Bray MS.** Genetic factors in exercise adoption, adherence and obesity. *Obes Rev* 15: 29–39, 2014.

32. **Huang SS, Liu Y, Jing ZC, Wang XJ,** and **Mao YM.** Common genetic risk factors of venous thromboembolism in Western and Asian populations. *Genet Mol Res* 15: 15017644, 2016.

33. **Huang T, Larsen KT, Ried-Larsen M, Moller NC,** and **Andersen LB.** The effects of physical activity and exercise on brain-derived neurotrophic factor in healthy humans: A review. *Scand J Med Sci Sports* 24: 1–10, 2014.

34. **Huppertz C, Bartels M, Jansen IE, Boomsma DI, Willemsen G, de Moor MH,** and **de Geus EJ.** A twin-sibling study on the relationship between exercise attitudes and exercise behavior. *Behav Genet* 44: 45–55, 2014.

35. **Kelly SA** and **Pomp D.** Genetic determinants of voluntary exercise. *Trends Genet* 29: 348–357, 2013.

36. **Khera AV, Emdin CA, Drake I, Natarajan P, Bick AG, Cook NR, Chasman DI, Baber U, Mehran R, Rader DJ, Fuster V, Boerwinkle E, Melander O, Orho-Melander M, Ridker PM,** and **Kathiresan S.** Genetic risk, adherence to a healthy lifestyle, and coronary disease. *N Engl J Med* 375: 2349–2358, 2016.

37. **Kishi T, Yoshimura R, Ikuta T,** and **Iwata N.** Brain-derived neurotrophic factor and major depressive disorder: Evidence from meta-analyses. *Front Psychiatry* 8: 308, 2017.

38. **Kostrzewa E** and **Kas MJ.** The use of mouse models to unravel genetic architecture of physical activity: A review. *Genes Brain Behav* 13: 87–103, 2014.

39. **Labos C** and **Thanassoulis G.** Genetic risk prediction for primary and secondary prevention of atherosclerotic cardiovascular disease: An update. *Curr Cardiol Rep* 20: 36, 2018.

40. **Leal G, Comprido D,** and **Duarte CB.** BDNF-induced local protein synthesis and synaptic plasticity. *Neuropharmacology* 76: 639–656, 2014.

41. **Li S, Zhao JH, Luan J, Ekelund U, Luben RN, Khaw KT, Wareham NJ,** and **Loos RJ.** Physical activity attenuates the genetic predisposition to obesity in 20,000 men and women from EPIC-Norfolk prospective population study. *PLoS Med* 7: e1000332, 2010.

42. **Mancino S, Burokas A, Gutierrez-Cuesta J, Gutierrez-Martos M, Martin-Garcia E, Pucci M, Falconi A, D'Addario C, Maccarrone M,** and **Maldonado R.** Epigenetic and proteomic expression changes promoted by eating addictive-like behavior. *Neuropsychopharmacology* 40: 2788–2800, 2015.

43. **Marigorta UM, Rodriguez JA, Gibson G,** and **Navarro A.** Replicability and prediction: Lessons and challenges from GWAS. *Trends Genet* 34: 504–517, 2018.

44. **Miller FL OCD, Herring MP, Sailors MH, Jackson AS, Dishman RK, Bray MS.** Exercise dose, exercise adherence, and associated health outcomes in the TIGER study. *Med Sci Sports Exerc*, 46: 69–75, 2013.

45. **Moore LV, Harris CD, Carlson SA, Kruger J,** and **Fulton JE.** Trends in no leisure-time physical activity – United States, 1988–2010. *Res Q Exerc Sport* 83: 587–591, 2012.

46. **Oman RF** and **King AC.** Predicting the adoption and maintenance of exercise participation using self-efficacy and previous exercise participation rates. *Am J Health Promot* 12: 154–161, 1998.

47. **Patterson R, McNamara E, Tainio M, de Sa TH, Smith AD, Sharp SJ, Edwards P, Woodcock J, Brage S,** and **Wijndaele K.** Sedentary behaviour and risk of all-cause, cardiovascular and cancer mortality, and incident type 2 diabetes: A systematic review and dose response meta-analysis. *Eur J Epidemiol*, 33: 811–829, 2018.

48. **Prochaska JO, Velicer WF, Rossi JS, Goldstein MG, Marcus BH, Rakowski W, Fiore C, Harlow LL, Redding CA, Rosenbloom D,** and et al. Stages of change and decisional balance for 12 problem behaviors. *Health Psychol* 13: 39–46, 1994.

49. **Rampersaud E, Mitchell BD, Pollin TI, Fu M, Shen H, O'Connell JR, Ducharme JL, Hines S, Sack P, Naglieri R, Shuldiner AR,** and **Snitker S.** Physical activity and the association of common FTO gene variants with body mass index and obesity. *Arch Intern Med* 168: 1791–1797, 2008.

50. **Reiss D, Leve LD,** and **Neiderhiser JM.** How genes and the social environment moderate each other. *Am J Public Health* 103 Suppl 1: S111–S121, 2013.

51. **Rhodes JS, Garland T, Jr,** and **Gammie SC.** Patterns of brain activity associated with variation in voluntary wheel-running behavior. *Behav Neurosci* 117: 1243–1256, 2003.

52. **Ross CE.** Walking, exercising, and smoking: Does neighborhood matter? *Soc Sci Med* 51: 265–274, 2000.

53. **Rothman AJ.** Toward a theory-based analysis of behavioral maintenance. *Health Psychol* 19: 64–69, 2000.

54. **Ryan R** and **Deci E.** Self-determination theory and the facilitation of intrinsic motivation, social development, and well-being. *Am Psychologist* 55: 68–78, 2000.

55. **Sailors MH, Jackson AS, McFarlin BK, Turpin I, Ellis KJ, Foreyt JP, Hoelscher DM,** and **Bray MS.** Exposing college students to exercise: the Training Interventions and Genetics of Exercise Response (TIGER) study. *J Am Coll Health* 59: 13–20, 2011.

56. **Sajuthi SP, Sharma NK, Chou JW, Palmer ND, McWilliams DR, Beal J, Comeau ME, Ma L, Calles-Escandon J, Demons J, Rogers S, Cherry K, Menon L, Kouba E, Davis D, Burris M, Byerly SJ, Ng MC, Maruthur NM, Patel SR, Bielak LF, Lange LA, Guo X, Sale MM, Chan KH, Monda KL, Chen GK, Taylor K, Palmer C, Edwards TL, North KE, Haiman CA, Bowden DW, Freedman BI, Langefeld CD,** and **Das SK.** Mapping adipose and muscle

tissue expression quantitative trait loci in African Americans to identify genes for type 2 diabetes and obesity. *Hum Genet* 135: 869–880, 2016.

57. **Sarzynski MA, Loos RJ, Lucia A, Perusse L, Roth SM, Wolfarth B, Rankinen T,** and **Bouchard C.** Advances in exercise, fitness, and performance genomics in 2015. *Med Sci Sports Exerc* 48: 1906–1916, 2016.

58. **Scuteri A, Sanna S, Chen WM, Uda M, Albai G, Strait J, Najjar S, Nagaraja R, Orru M, Usala G, Dei M, Lai S, Maschio A, Busonero F, Mulas A, Ehret GB, Fink AA, Weder AB, Cooper RS, Galan P, Chakravarti A, Schlessinger D, Cao A, Lakatta E,** and **Abecasis GR.** Genome-wide association scan shows genetic variants in the FTO gene are associated with obesity-related traits. *PLoS Genet* 3: e115, 2007.

59. **Shen T, You Y, Joseph C, Mirzaei M, Klistorner A, Graham SL,** and **Gupta V.** BDNF polymorphism: A review of its diagnostic and clinical relevance in neurodegenerative disorders. *Aging Dis* 9: 523–536, 2018.

60. **Szwergold BS.** Fructosamine-6-phosphates are deglycated by phosphorylation to fructosamine-3,6-bisphosphates catalyzed by fructosamine-3-kinase (FN3K) and/or fructosamine-3-kinase-related-protein (FN3KRP). *Med Hypotheses* 68: 37–45, 2007.

61. **Thompson PD, Tsongalis GJ, Ordovas JM, Seip RL, Bilbie C, Miles M, Zoeller R, Visich P, Gordon P, Angelopoulos TJ, Pescatello L,** and **Moyna N.** Angiotensin-converting enzyme genotype and adherence to aerobic exercise training. *Prev Cardiol* 9: 21–24, 2006.

62. **Thompson PD, Tsongalis GJ, Seip RL, Bilbie C, Miles M, Zoeller R, Visich P, Gordon P, Angelopoulos TJ, Pescatello L, Bausserman L,** and **Moyna N.** Apolipoprotein E genotype and changes in serum lipids and maximal oxygen uptake with exercise training. *Metabolism* 53: 193–202, 2004.

63. **Trost SG, Owen N, Bauman AE, Sallis JF,** and **Brown W.** Correlates of adults' participation in physical activity: Review and update. *Med Sci Sports Exerc* 34: 1996–2001, 2002.

64. **Vimaleswaran KS, Li S, Zhao JH, Luan J, Bingham SA, Khaw KT, Ekelund U, Wareham NJ,** and **Loos RJ.** Physical activity attenuates the body mass index-increasing influence of genetic variation in the FTO gene. *Am J Clin Nutr* 90: 425–428, 2009.

65. **Way BM** and **Taylor SE.** A polymorphism in the serotonin transporter gene moderates cardiovascular reactivity to psychosocial stress. *Psychosom Med* 73: 310–317, 2011.

66. **Wier LT** and **Jackson AS.** Factors affecting compliance in the NASA/Johnson Space Center fitness programme. *Sports Med* 8: 9–14, 1989.

67. **Wilson K** and **Brookfield D.** Effect of goal setting on motivation and adherence in a six-week exercise program. *Int J Sport Exercise Physiol* 7: 89–100, 2009.

68. **Wunderle M, Olmes G, Nabieva N, Haberle L, Jud SM, Hein A, Rauh C, Hack CC, Erber R, Ekici AB, Hoyer J, Vasileiou G, Kraus C, Reis A, Hartmann A, Schulz-Wendtland R, Lux MP, Beckmann MW,** and **Fasching PA.** Risk, prediction and prevention of hereditary breast cancer – large-scale genomic studies in times of big and smart data. *Geburtshilfe Frauenheilkd* 78: 481–492, 2018.

69. **You JS, Dooley MS, Kim CR, Kim EJ, Xu W, Goodman CA,** and **Hornberger TA.** A DGKzeta-FoxO-ubiquitin proteolytic axis controls fiber size during skeletal muscle remodeling. *Sci Signal* 11: eaao6847, 2018.

70. **Zhang G** and **Nebert DW.** Personalized medicine: Genetic risk prediction of drug response. *Pharmacol Ther* 175: 75–90, 2017.

71. **Zhang Y, Liu J, Yao J, Ji G, Qian L, Wang J, Zhang G, Tian J, Nie Y, Zhang YE, Gold MS,** and **Liu Y.** Obesity: Pathophysiology and intervention. *Nutrients* 6: 5153–5183, 2014.

SECTION 2

Systems genetics of physical activity

Introduction

Over the last 25 years, it has been accepted that physical activity is a public health issue. In literally hundreds of thousands of well-conducted studies, physical activity or physical inactivity has been linked with positive or negative health outcomes, respectively. However, as noted several times in the coming chapters, global physical activity levels measured in almost every population are much less than is appropriate for positive health benefits despite the tremendous educational efforts that have been made worldwide to encourage physical activity. This disconnect – between knowing that we must be active and not being active – is at the root of the six chapters in this section. Specifically, these chapters comprehensively consider what is known about the systems genetics of physical activity, ranging from the basic question of whether genetic systems regulate physical activity to how the environment may affect the genetic systems regulating physical activity.

The section starts with a consideration of the basic question "Do genetics regulate physical activity level?" This critical question must be answered before further mechanistic studies and application can be considered. Perhaps surprisingly, this question has probably generated more studies than any other systems genetics question in the exercise and sport science disciplines. Chapter 5, written by Dr. Scott Kelly, tackles the question of whether genetics regulate physical activity in animal models and provides an initial hypothesis that both central and peripheral mechanisms are involved. This chapter is followed by one written by Matthijs van der Zee and Dr. Eco De Geus, that carries the question into human models and results in some elegant theoretical models showing that there are enough data to support a systems genetics regulation of physical activity levels. With the foundation from Chapters 5 and 6, we are then open to consider other important aspects of genetic regulation of physical activity. Chapter 7, written by Dr. J. Timothy Lightfoot, Ayland Letsinger, and Jorge Granados, consider what factors might have resulted in the evolution of genetic control of physical activity – in other words, why should genetics regulate physical activity? In Chapter 8, Dr. Justin Rhodes begins the discussion of where the genetic mechanisms that control physical activity are located, with an examination of the data that point to potential genetic mechanisms in the brain that regulate physical activity. Another approach to the "Where are the mechanisms located?" question is presented in Chapter 9 by Dr. David Ferguson that focuses on potential peripheral genetic regulating mechanisms of activity. While this book is focused on systems genetics, most scientists understand that the environment can interact with and play a role in regulating genetic mechanisms. Thus, Drs. Heather Vellers and Emily Schmitt in Chapter 10 address the possibility that if physical activity is regulated by genetic mechanisms, perhaps these genetic mechanisms can be altered by unique environmental exposures which lead to alterations in physical activity.

In total, these chapters provide a comprehensive review of the literature and thinking on the systems genetics regulation of physical activity. We are pleased that these chapters have been written by those investigators most involved and published in the topic, and as such, the chapters provide the most current ideas and theories on the topic. As a result, we hope that these chapters provide a foundation and starting point for increased investigation and identification of the critical controlling genetic factors of physical activity.

5

IS PHYSICAL ACTIVITY REGULATED BY GENETICS? EVIDENCE FROM ANIMAL MODELS

Scott A. Kelly

What is physical activity in an animal model?

As in human populations, physical activity can represent a range of behaviors in animal models. Consequently, context matters when discussing the genetic regulation of physical activity. For example, assessing exercise endurance in rodents typically utilizes forced running on a motorized treadmill equipped with a shock grid for a negative stimulus (48). Alternatively, assessing daily movement distance may involve measuring the number of revolutions an animal voluntarily turns a running wheel in a given amount of time (16). These two types (forced vs. voluntary) of physical activity are a result of, and result in, at least some variation in physiological and molecular responses. And, most relevant to this chapter, these exercise types may be regulated by different genetic architectures or genomic mechanisms. I emphasize this early in the text because results (e.g., genetic mapping, transcriptomic, and proteomic) across animal models and between studies may appear inconsistent, and, in part, this lack of replication may simply be a reflection of measuring different phenotypes, however subtle. This is especially pronounced within the broad category of voluntary physical activity, where subtypes are numerous (e.g., wheel running, home-cage activity, open-field activity, spontaneous physical activity, and nonexercise activity thermogenesis). So, context certainly matters when comparing results obtained from a variety of measures, but may not be as important if we are broadly looking for genetic regulation of physical activity that transcends specific activity types (i.e., a set of master activity regulators). Thus, in this chapter, I will attempt to provide examples in the context of specific measurements.

I will not attempt to describe each of the voluntary activity types listed above given that operational definitions and methodology of the measurements have been previously reviewed (12, table 1 in 19). Given that this chapter will not attempt to be exhaustive, I will primarily discuss the evidence for the genetic regulation of physical activity in the context of studies utilizing voluntary wheel running. For more exhaustive reviews covering a range of activity types in both rodents and humans, there are numerous studies available (12, 19, 22, 30, 31). This chapter will focus on voluntary wheel running as an activity measure because of the importance it has played in the early understanding of the genetic regulation of physical activity, and its hypothesized parallels to human exercise behavior.

Running wheels have long been used to measure voluntary activity in rodents (44), although precisely why rodents engage in wheel-running behavior and how applicable it is to human voluntary exercise has been rightly debated. In an exhaustive review of wheel-running behavior, Sherwin (42) concluded that "wheel running has no directly analogous naturally occurring behavior, it is (sometimes) performed for its own sake per se rather than as a redirected or substitute activity, and studies on motivation show that wheel running is self-reinforcing and perceived by animals as 'important'." Sherwin (42) further argued that wheel-running behavior is most likely an "artefact of captive environments," but regardless is "one of great interest to behavioural science." Counter to Sherwin's contention that wheel-running behavior is an artifact of captive environments, Meijer and Robbers (34) demonstrated that when running wheels are placed in nature, mice not only utilize them but also do so in bout lengths that match captive mice. Eikelboom (7), in a response to Sherwin (42), argued: "Many similarities exist between this intrinsically motivated human exercise and the wheel running seen in animals, so analyzing them together may lead to theories explaining both." Regardless, it can probably be agreed upon that voluntary wheel-running behavior requires ability and motivation, can be self-reinforcing, and as described by Novak et al. (37), "is not solely reflective of the tendency to be physically active, but is a complex and dynamic behavior that interacts with genetics and the environment." For these reasons, I, and others have argued that voluntary wheel-running behavior in rodents adequately models human voluntary exercise behavior. However, a notable discrepancy between human and rodent voluntary physical activity occurs between the sexes. In human populations, males tend to engage in more physical activity, while among rodents, females tend to be more active. The cause of this discrepancy has been discussed elsewhere (2; and see Chapter 10). It is also important to note that when discussing the genetic architecture of voluntary wheel-running behavior I am referencing the predisposition to initiate physical activity and not the response to exercise or trainability (e.g., 41), although it is certainly possible the architectures may overlap and/or interact.

Heritability

"Are the individual differences in spontaneous activity inherent?" (40). Although others had suggested that behaviors might be regulated by "internal drives" (e.g., 39), Rundquist (40) appears to be the first to have expressly designed an experiment to answer the question pertaining to voluntary wheel-running activity. Rundquist (40) used the qualifier "spontaneous" to distinguish between an internal drive as opposed to external motivators (presumably environmental factors) of activity. In an attempt to answer the question, Rundquist (40) selectively bred rats for 12 generations utilizing rotating drums, a design previously utilized by Stewart (44). The rotating drums were solid surface running wheels with the home cage suspended inside the drum (see Figure 1 in 44). Rundquist (40) commented on the "unbelievable" interindividual variation observed through the course of selective breeding and noted that he handled "a male rat which travelled approximately *sixty feet* in fifteen days, and at the other extreme, a female which travelled over *two hundred miles* during the same period." After 12 generations of selective breeding, Rundquist (40) concluded that: "It is, then, quite safe to ascribe the major role in the production of the individual differences in this activity to inheritance." A logical follow-up to Rundquist (40), and at least partially the focus of the following studies, was to ask how much of the total variance observed in voluntary physical activity is attributable to the genetic variance – or, what is the exact "heritability" of voluntary wheel running?

Festing (10) quantified voluntary activity in 26 mouse strains, exposing them to wheels (85 mm in diameter) over a 48-hour (5 mice from each of 23 strains) and 7-day (6 mice from each of 27 strains) period. In each experiment, mean daily activity was calculated (revolutions per 24 hours in thousands). Despite high individual variation, Festing (10) observed statistically significant interstrain differences in wheel activity in both experiments, with closely related strains having similar activity levels. Lerman et al. (26) examined the genetic variability in voluntary exercise in seven inbred mouse strains. Running duration and distance was examined over a 2-week period using running wheels (11.5 cm diameter) placed inside individual cages. Lerman et al. (26) observed statistically significant interstrain differences in wheel running duration, distance, and speed. Lerman et al. (26), using the coefficient of genetic determination (g^2), estimated broad-sense heritability to be 0.42, 0.39, and 0.24 for running duration, distance, and average speed, respectively. Lightfoot et al. (27), using 13 strains of mice, also estimated broad-sense heritability of wheel-running activity. Lightfoot et al. (27) monitored wheel (127 mm) running for 21 consecutive days. Heritability estimates, using the coefficient of genetic determination (g^2), were 0.18 for average daily distance (km), 0.25 for average daily exercise time or duration (minutes), and 0.14 for average daily exercise velocity (m/minute). When examining heritability among female mice only, estimates were 0.12 (distance), 0.12 (duration), and 0.44 (velocity). For males estimates were 0.31 (distance), 0.44 (duration), and 0.49 (velocity).

Coming full circle, back to the approach used by Rundquist (40), the most convincing case that physical activity is a heritable trait in rodents (i.e., exhibits significant narrow-sense heritability or, significant additive variance) resulted from an artificial selection experiment for high levels of voluntary wheel running in mice (45). The work was initiated by Theodore Garland Jr. and colleagues, is currently ongoing, and has resulted in over 150 publications to date characterizing the morphological, physiological, and behavioral traits that have evolved in concert with high levels of voluntary activity. The replicated selection experiment began from a base population of outbred Hsd:ICR mice (*Mus domesticus*). Utilizing 224 mice (112 male, 112 female) eight closed lines (i.e., once established, individuals were only bred within a line) were generated. Four replicate lines were selectively bred for high voluntary wheel running (high running lines, HR) and four lines were maintained as controls (C lines). The C lines were exposed to the same experimental protocol as the HR lines but were bred without regard to the amount of wheel running. Individual mice, at 6–8 weeks of age, were given access to running wheels (1.12 m circumference, 35.7 cm diameter) for 6 days and the mean number of total revolutions on days 5 and 6 was the criterion for which the HR lines were selectively bred. After ten generations, realized heritability estimates, adjusted for within-family selection, ranged from 0.18–0.32 across the four HR lines, with an average of 0.28. By generation 16, selection had resulted in an approximate 2.5- to 3.0-fold increase in total revolutions per day in HR lines (four replicates) as compared to the control lines (C lines, four replicates). At generation 16, the difference in number of revolutions was primarily caused by HR mice running faster rather than for more minutes each day, but the relative importance of the two components differed between the sexes with males showing a significant increase in amount of time spent running (45). Recent work by Garland and colleagues has demonstrated variable selection signatures ("genomic regions showing excessive differentiation between treatments") in each of the four HR replicate lines (49). These findings support the hypothesis that physical activity is a phenotype that may be amenable to multiple independent evolutionary solutions (discussed further in Chapter 7).

Although estimates vary (Table 5.1), the studies just described have conclusively shown that voluntary wheel running (and its components) in rodents is a heritable behavior. Additionally, the heritability estimates in these studies match those of human populations (see Chapter 6 and references therein). The remainder of this chapter, while reinforcing the heritability of voluntary wheel-running behavior, will focus on identifying specific chromosomal regions and potential candidate genes responsible for physical activity.

Table 5.1 Heritability estimates of voluntary wheel-running traits in three different mouse models

Trait[*]	Heritability estimate	Reference
Running distance	0.39	Lerman et al. (27)
	0.18	Lightfoot et al. (28)
	0.28[**]	Swallow et al. (46)
Running duration	0.42	Lerman et al. (27)
	0.25	Lightfoot et al. (28)
	0.14[**]	Swallow et al. (46)
Running speed	0.24	Lerman et al. (27)
	0.14	Lightfoot et al. (28)
	0.28[**]	Swallow et al. (46)

[*] Generalized categories. See text for additional methodological details (e.g., wheel size, number of measurement days, etc.)

[**] Represent narrow-sense heritability estimates. Running duration and average running speed are estimated using a midparent offspring regression and are not adjusted for within-family artificial selection.

Genetic architecture

Genetic mapping

To date, numerous, quantitative trait loci (QTL) which are chromosomal regions correlating with variation in a phenotype, have been mapped for a variety of physical activity traits utilizing several different mouse models. Regardless of the exact physical activity trait or mouse model, the ultimate goal of these studies is to identify specific genes and mutations within these regions controlling the behavior of interest. These approaches have relied on second-generation intercrosses between inbred populations (F_2), backcrosses (BC), advanced intercross lines (AIL), and large panels of recombinant inbred lines (e.g., the Collaborative Cross (CC)). Below, I will discuss studies that have successfully utilized each of these approaches to identify QTL underlying voluntary wheel running behavior in mice. As stated at the beginning of this chapter, physical activity can be very broadly defined and the following examples are not meant to be representative of the entirety of the behavior. And, indeed, there have been QTL identified for other physical activity traits such as home-cage activity (14), open-field behavior (6), and treadmill running (4, 48). By focusing on a few representative studies, all targeting the same behavior, direct comparisons, although difficult in isolated mapping populations, are made somewhat easier when the phenotype is narrowly defined to voluntary wheel running.

Lightfoot et al. (28) documented the first QTL controlling voluntary wheel running in a F_2 population. The F_2 population ($n=310$) was generated from previously characterized high-active (C57L/J) and low-active (C3H/HeJ) inbred strains (27). F_2 mice were given access to a running wheel (solid-surface, 145 mm diameter) for 21 consecutive days and average running distance (km), duration (minutes), and speed (m/minute) were calculated. As is frequently observed in rodent models of exercise (2), F_2 female mice ran greater distances, for a longer period of time, and at greater speeds than males. Using 129 single nucleotide polymorphisms (SNPs) evenly spaced across the genome, four statistically significant (5% experiment-wise threshold) QTL were identified underlying the variation in running distance (*DIST13.1*), duration (*DUR13.1*), and speed (*SPD9.1, SPD13.1*). Three of the QTL colocalized to the same region of chromosome 13 and each of these three accounted for approximately 6% of the total phenotypic variation in a given trait with an additional running speed QTL (*SPD9.1*), located on chromosome 9, accounting for 11.3% of the total phenotyple. All four of these QTL were replicated with additional haplotype mapping. In addition to the four statistically significant QTL, Lightfoot and colleagues identified 14 suggestive (5% chromosome-wise threshold) QTL underlying the voluntary exercise traits. None of the QTL identified significantly interacted with sex. Despite a relatively small population size and low marker density, this original mapping study was highly impactful. Lightfoot et al. (28) reinforced that voluntary locomotion was a heritable trait and the additive genetic components matched narrow-sense heritability estimates from prior studies (for comparison see 45). Additionally, for the first time, specific chromosomal regions underlying the variation in voluntary exercise traits were identified. Although the chromosomal regions identified were large, the results facilitated functional hypotheses (by Lightfoot and others) about the role of specific genes underlying these QTL in the biological regulation of activity.

Following on the work of Lightfoot and colleagues, Nehrenberg et al. (36) utilized a BC population (n=384) initiated between mice selectively bred for high voluntary wheel running (HR) and the inbred strain C57BL/6J, an average runner among inbred strains (27). The HR mice utilized to create the F_1 population originated from one of the four replicated selection lines and were fixed for a recessive mutation causing an approximately 50% reduction in hindlimb muscle mass (the "mini-muscle" phenotype (MM)) (20). F_1 male mice were backcrossed to HR female parents producing a population of 384 mice with a 50:50 ratio of normal to MM phenotypes. BC mice were given access to a running wheel (nonsolid surface, circumference=1.1 m) for 6 consecutive days. Mean values of distance (m), time (minutes), average speed (m/minute), and maximum speed in any one-minute running interval (m/minute), were calculated for days 5 and 6 of the 6-day test. These values were calculated and chosen for mapping, as the mean number of total revolutions on days 5 and 6 was the criterion for which the HR line was selectively bred (45). In the BC population, female mice ran more than males and mice with the MM allele ran faster and further than mice without the mutation (13). In the BC population, using 154 evenly spaced genome-wide SNPs, statistically significant QTL were detected for average running speed (chromosome 7) and maximum running speed (chromosomes 6 and 7), while none were detected for running distance or duration. Additionally, a sex-specific QTL, for the male subpopulation, was detected for running time on chromosome 2. Nehrenberg et al. (37) reinforced that QTL for voluntary wheel could be detected and that, in at least one case, the QTL can be sex specific. The absence of replication of the findings of the Lightfoot study (28) was also a major contribution. As pointed out by Nehrenberg et al. (36), the lack of replication reinforced the importance of differences in measurement methods (e.g., different running wheels, different days of wheel access), general laboratory-to-laboratory variation, age differences at the time of measurement, differences in genetic background of mice utilized, and differences in the genetic cross design (F_2 vs. BC).

Continuing to build on the work of the previous two studies, Kelly et al. (16) generated an AIL between one HR line and the inbred strain C57BL/6J (B6). Although Kelly et al. (16) utilized a different replicate HR line, the AIL was an opportunity to attempt to replicate the findings of previously identified QTL in a nearly similar genetic background used by Nehrenberg et al. (36). The AIL also allowed for the theoretical reduction in confidence intervals surrounding any mapped QTL, thus allowing greater inference of potential candidate genes underlying loci. AILs are generated through random intercrossing over multiple generations to accumulate recombination events and provide increased mapping resolution compared with F_2 and BC populations (5). The progenitor lines utilized by Kelly and colleagues underwent a reciprocal breeding protocol to produce a F_1 generation and the subpopulations (HR♀ × B6♂ and B6♀ × HR♂) were subsequently kept separate (15). Following the F_3 generation, a large G_4 population (N=815) was utilized to measure a variety of phenotypes related to voluntary exercise behavior (16) and body composition prior to and following exercise (17). G_4 individuals were given access to running wheels for 6 consecutive days and revolutions were recorded in 1-minute intervals for 23–24 hours of each day. Mice were genotyped using 764 fully informative SNPs evenly spaced across the genome. As expected, the additional mating through generations three and four resulted in an approximate threefold genetic map expansion (averaged across all chromosomes) and increased mapping resolution. One of the two reciprocal crosses (B6♀ × HR♂) was maintained through a G_{10} and subsequent phenotyping and mapping (with 2058 fully informative SNPs) was performed in an attempt to replicate QTL identified in the G_4.

In the G_4 population, 32 significant and 13 suggestive QTL were identified underlying voluntary wheel-running behavior. These QTL collectively represented running distance (total daily revolutions), time spent running (i.e., cumulative 1-minute intervals in which at least one revolution was recorded), average speed (total revolutions/time spent running), and maximum speed (highest number of revolutions in any 1-minute interval within a 24-hour period). Additionally, the QTL were representative of the slope (i.e., trajectory of running on a temporal scale) and intercept (i.e., starting point of temporal trajectory) of a linear regression across all 6 days of running. The primary conclusions of Kelly and colleagues (16) were threefold. First, reinforcing the findings of Lightfoot et al. (28) and Nehrenberg et al. (36), the genetic architecture underlying voluntary wheel-running behavior is complex and most likely governed by many genes, each having a relatively small effect. The largest QTL effect discovered in the AIL accounted for only 6.6% of the total phenotypic variation. Second, QTL were often unique to single days of running, a phenomena not examined by the Lightfoot (28) or Nehrenberg (36) studies, but later replicated by Leamy and colleagues (24). This was especially pronounced when comparing the initial days (1 and 2) of wheel exposure with the remaining days (3–6). Third, QTL associated with the trajectory of running across all 6 days (quantified by the slope of a linear regression) largely did not colocalize with chromosomal regions identified on individual days. Kelly and colleagues concluded that their results "reinforce a genetic basis for the predisposition to engage in voluntary exercise," but unique regions may govern "initiation, continuation, and temporal pattern of voluntary activity in mammals" (16).

As a follow-up to the G_4 study, a similar study was repeated on one (B6♀ × HR♂) of the two reciprocal crosses in the G_{10} population (25). In theory, replication of the G_4 QTL would be high and confidence intervals would be reduced even further, increasing the likelihood of identifying a narrowed set of candidate genes. Leamy et al. (25) discovered that, on average, QTL confidence intervals were reduced from 23 Mb in the G_4 to 11.3 Mb in the G_{10} population. However, there was only a 40% replicate rate of QTL in the G_{10} compared to the G_4. Several potential explanations for the lack of replication are discussed by Leamy et al. (25), the most likely being that one-half of the G_{10} mice were fed a high-fat diet, whereas all G_4 mice were fed a standard diet. A small sample size and lack of statistical power prevented mapping with G_{10} individuals only fed a standard diet.

Despite the contribution of novel QTL discoveries in the studies presented above, limitations persist. First, the above studies (and others not identified here) have failed to consistently replicate individual loci. Perhaps this is not surprising given the subtle, but important interstudy differences, and the infinitesimal regulation of complex traits such as physical activity (11). But, it does make it difficult for future studies to target prioritized regions. Second, the studies typically identify QTL with large confidence intervals (e.g., 11 Mb or larger) containing potentially hundreds of candidates, again, making it difficult to prioritize functional genes and their physiological effects. Third, given the relatively limited genetic background of the strains utilized, the broad applicability of the findings may be limited. The final two QTL studies discussed below have specifically attempted to minimize the size of the confidence intervals using large populations and high marker densities. They also attempt to address the lack of genetic diversity in the previous studies by utilizing populations representative of multiple inbred and recently wild derived strains.

Mathes et al. (33) utilized CC mice to identify QTL for wheel-running distance on days 5 and 6 and days 11 and 12 of a 12-day exposure to voluntary running wheels (the same wheel model utilized by Kelly et al. (16)). The CC are a large panel of recombinant inbred mouse lines derived from a genetically diverse set of eight founder strains, thus providing high levels of broadly representative phenotypic and genetic diversity (1). Within the CC mapping population, wheel-running variation exceeded that observed in the eight founder strains and ranged from about 1 km per night up to about 16 km per night on days 5 and 6 of a 12-day test. The maximum values for the CC mice were comparable to those observed in mice selectively bred for high voluntary wheel running (HR mice discussed above). Mathes et al. (33) identified only one statistically significant QTL for mean running distance on days 11 and 12, but this QTL accounted for 17% of the phenotypic variation. In a separate population, haplotype association mapping across 38 inbred strains failed to replicate the findings of the CC (29), but did identify three significant QTL for running distance among the entire population on chromosomes 12, 18, and 19. Additionally, five sex-specific QTL were identified among males (chromosomes 5, 6, 8 (distance), and 6 (speed)), and four among females (chromosomes 8 and 11 (running distance), 11 (running speed), and X (running duration)). Given the genetic diversity present in the two studies previously described (30, 33), there is undoubtedly a greater ability to generalize the results to additional mouse models and translate the findings to human populations. Indeed, Lightfoot et al. (30) discuss the encouraging overlap between their findings, other mouse studies discussed above (16, 36), and the findings of human studies (e.g., 3, 43). Additionally, some QTL identified by Lightfoot et al. (29) had narrow confidence intervals containing as few as eight predicted genes, facilitating the identification of potential candidates regulating physical activity behavior. Mathes et al. (33) were also able to identify candidate genes within QTL, but by using a complementary expression (eQTL) approach.

Fine-mapping approaches

As discussed above, the identification of chromosomal regions containing QTL has been successful, but the identification of genes underlying these regions that regulate voluntary exercise behavior has been more difficult. One approach to identify potential candidate genes has been to combine QTL mapping with gene expression analysis, or the mapping of eQTL. Limitations to this approach are discussed elsewhere (47), but are primarily associated with the tendency to favor *cis* eQTL over *trans* eQTL and low microarray probe density. In short, expression level of individual transcripts is treated as the phenotype, and variation in expression levels is correlated with chromosomal regions (as in QTL mapping). Genes that are mapped under loci for previously identified QTL and are locally controlled (*cis*-acting eQTL) are prioritized.

Using a G_4 AIL population (discussed earlier), Kelly et al. (18, 21) examined the transcriptome in both brain and muscle tissue. These two tissues were chosen as voluntary physical activity has been shown to be composed of both motivation (neurobiological) and ability (muscular). Both of these studies (18, 21) identified eQTL colocalizing with previously identified wheel-running QTL. In brain tissue, Kelly et al. (18) discussed six plausible candidate genes

(*Insig2, Socs2, DBY, Arrdc4, Prcp, IL15*) and in muscle (21) three (*Insig2, Prcp, Sparc*) that potentially may play a role in regulating voluntary activity. These candidates were chosen based on the strength of the effect observed, their known biological functions, and their correlation with distance run, time spent running, or speed of running. However, in each of these studies there were many additional eQTL mapped under wheel-running QTL that were not discussed. For example, in brain tissue, on average, 30 eQTL were mapped under each of 43 previously identified wheel-running QTL. Although this approach does narrow the list of candidate genes it still leaves many more to sift through than is desired.

More commonplace than eQTL approaches is the examination of the global transcriptome using mouse models exhibiting discordant phenotypes. Significant differential gene expression (typically in physiologically relevant tissues) between groups with different phenotypes is then used to prioritize potential candidate genes underlying the phenotype. If genes that are significantly differentially expressed happen to fall under previously identified QTL then even higher priority is given. For example, Mathes et al. (32) examined gene expression in the dorsal striatum and nucleus accumbens in mice selectively bred for high voluntary wheel running or for obesity. Mathes et al. (32) chose these target tissues and these strains of mice to determine how dopamine may potentially contribute to opposing phenotypes. Mathes et al. (32) found significant differences in gene expression between the strains in both brain areas within the dopamine pathway, concluding that central reward pathways are important in both obesity and excessive exercise.

Although both of the above approaches have been successful, neither predicts the protein products that result from the identified genes. Proteomic approaches, however, do identify proteins associated with a particular phenotype. Proteomic approaches have been utilized to identify end-protein expression, in both brain and muscle tissue, in high- and low-active inbred strains of mice (8, 9). Ferguson et al. (8) examined protein expression in the soleus and extensor digitorum longus muscles and found higher expression of proteins relating to calcium regulation and the Krebs cycle pathways in high-active mice. Low-active mice overexpressed proteins associated with cytoskeletal structure and electron transport pathways. Furthermore, transient knockdown of proteins annexin A6 and calsequestrin 1 protein of high-active mice significantly reduced physical activity levels. Taken together Ferguson et al. (8) conclude, "each pattern contributes to the peripheral capability to be either high- or low-active ..." and "specific mechanisms regulate activity leading to the high- or low activity status of the animal." In a follow-up study on the nucleus accumbens, Ferguson et al. (9) identified seven differentially expressed proteins associated with neural stress (stress 70 protein and V type proton ATPase catalytic subunit A) and metabolism (creatine kinase B, succinyl-CoA ligase), overexpressed in the low- and high-active strains respectively. Ferguson et al. (9) also reinforce the systems approach outlined in Figure 4 of Pomp et al. (38), suggesting that protein signatures should be a part of efforts to identify mechanisms regulating physical activity.

Future directions

The studies described here and elsewhere have clearly demonstrated that voluntary physical activity (wheel running) in rodent models is a heritable behavior. These studies have also identified chromosomal regions underlying the behavior. However, overall, there has been very little progress identifying the specific genes and variants underlying identified QTL. The identification of these genes and understanding how they function physiologically to regulate activity levels must be a priority of future investigations. Once specific genes are identified, studies can begin to examine whether or not these genes also directly impact disease states through pleiotropy. Exacerbating this challenge is that studies thus far have demonstrated that the genetic architecture regulating physical activity is exceedingly complex (e.g., 23). The genetic architecture of exercise behavior has been shown to be population specific (or mouse model-dependent) with very low replication of QTL across populations and even within populations. The "next-generation" mouse models (e.g., Collaborative Cross and Diversity Outbred populations) will hopefully alleviate the need to create isolated mapping populations and be used universally in studies attempting to uncover the genetic architecture of exercise behavior. Whether or not interstudy replication of QTL increases and translation to human populations becomes easier with these new mouse models remains unanswered.

Not only does the genetic architecture of physical activity vary by population, but it also interacts with environmental factors such as sex, age, and diet, each of which may also directly influence the predisposition to engage in voluntary activity. The overall complexity of the genetic, environmental, and interactive effects on the predisposition to voluntarily exercise is depicted in Figure 5.1 and elsewhere with accompanying references (19). As was stated at the beginning of the chapter, physical activity is not a single trait, and the context in which we discuss the genetic architecture matters. Highlighting this fact is that at least two studies (16, 24) have demonstrated that the genetic architecture underlying a specific type of activity (voluntary wheel running) shifts over the course of an exercise regimen (or wheel exposure period). These findings may inform clinicians as to why individuals vary in their willingness to initiate and adhere to prescribed exercise programs. These findings also reinforce the point that the genetic regulation of activity depends not just on the type of activity, but when the activity occurs relative to the rest of the activity. Further research is needed to establish the genetic factors contributing to the temporal stability of voluntary exercise levels.

In this chapter, I focused on the genetic architecture of voluntary wheel running. There are many studies that have examined the genetic architecture of other physical activity types. Although I have stressed narrowly defining the type of physical activity when comparing studies, I also want to emphasize the importance of trying to discover a common genetic architecture across all physical activity types. To my knowledge, there is little overlap in the genetic regions

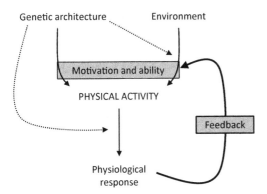

Figure 5.1 Voluntary physical activity is simultaneously influenced by genetic architecture, the environment, and gene-by-environment interactions. As a result of physical activity there is typically a physiological response, the magnitude of which may itself be influenced by the genome. And, this physiological response may "feedback" to increase or decrease subsequent physical activity. This feedback (negative or positive) may act through the two components that comprise voluntary physical activity behavior, motivation, and ability.

identified across activity types (e.g., home-cage activity, open-field activity, wheel running, and treadmill running), but I am also unaware of a study that has intentionally sought to map loci across a broad range of behaviors in a single population. A related outstanding question is whether the same genes are responsible for both elevated activity and inactivity and, if different, if is there an imbalance in the number of genes that regulate each. The importance of pursuing these unanswered questions cannot be overstated given the relative decline in human activity (e.g., 46) and the potential human-health impact of this decline (e.g., 35).

References

1. **Aylor DL, Valdar W, Foulds-Mathes W, Buus RJ, Verdugo RA, Baric RS, Ferris MT, Frelinger JA, Heise M, Frieman MB, Gralinski LE, Bell TA, Didion JD, Hua K, Nehrenberg DL, Powell CL, Steigerwalt J, Xie Y, Kelada SN, Collins FS, Yang IV, Schwartz DA, Branstetter LA, Chesler EJ, Miller DR, Spence J, Liu EY, McMillan L, Sarkar A, Wang J, Wang W, Zhang Q, Broman KW, Korstanje R, Durrant C, Mott R, Iraqi FA, Pomp D, Threadgill D, de Villena FP, Churchill GA.** Genetic analysis of complex traits in the emerging Collaborative Cross. *Genome Res* 21: 1213–1222, 2011.
2. **Bowen RS, Turner MJ, Lightfoot JT.** Sex hormone effects on physical activity levels: why doesn't Jane run as much as Dick? *Sports Med* 41: 73–86, 2011.
3. **Cai G, Cole SA, Butte N, Bacino C, Diego V, Tan K, Goring HH, O'Rahilly S, Farooqi IS, Comuzzie AG.** A quantitative trait locus on chromosome 18q for physical activity and dietary intake in Hispanic children. *Obesity* 14: 1596–1604, 2006.
4. **Courtney SM, Massett MP.** Identification of exercise QTL using association mapping in inbred mice. *Physiol Genomics* 44: 948–955, 2012.
5. **Darvasi A, Soller M.** Advanced intercross lines, an experimental population for fine genetic mapping. *Genetics* 141: 1199–1207, 1995.
6. **Delprato A, Algeo MP, Bonheur B, Bubier JA, Lu L, Williams RW, Chesler EJ, Crusio WE.** QTL and systems genetics analysis of mouse grooming and behavioral responses to novelty in an open field. *Genes Brain Behav* 16: 790–799, 2017.
7. **Eikelboom R.** Human parallel to voluntary wheel running: exercise. *Anim Behav* 57: F11–F12, 1999.
8. **Ferguson DP, Dangott LJ, Schmitt EE, Vellers HL, Lightfoot JT.** Differential skeletal muscle proteome of high- and low-active mice. *J Appl Physiol* 116: 1057–1067, 2014.
9. **Ferguson DP, Dangott LJ, Vellers HL, Schmitt EE, Lightfoot JT.** Differential protein expression in the nucleus accumbens of high- and low-active mice. *Behav Brain Res* 291: 283–288, 2015.
10. **Festing MFW.** Wheel activity in 26 strains of mouse. *Lab Anim* 11: 257–258, 1977.
11. **Fisher RA.** *The Genetical Theory of Natural Selection.* Oxford: Oxford University Press, 1930.
12. **Garland T Jr, Schutz H, Chappell MA, Keeney BK, Meek TH, Copes LE, Acosta W, Drenowatz C, Maciel RC, van Dijk G, Kotz CM, Eisenmann JC.** The biological control of voluntary exercise, spontaneous physical activity, and daily energy expenditure in relation to obesity: human and rodent perspectives. *J Exp Biol* 214: 206–229, 2011.
13. **Hannon RM, Kelly SA, Middleton KM, Kolb EM, Pomp D, Garland T Jr.** Phenotypic effects of the mini-muscle allele in a large HR × C57BL/6J mouse backcross. *J Hered* 99: 349–354, 2008.
14. **Kas MJH, de Mooij-van Malsen JG, de Krom M, van Gassen KLI, van Lith HA, Olivier B, Oppelaar H, Hendriks J, de Wit M, Groot Koerkamp MJA, Holstege FCP, van Oost BA, de Graan PNE.** High-resolution mapping of a novel genetic locus regulating voluntary physical activity in mice. *Genes Brain Behav* 11: 113–24, 2012.
15. **Kelly SA, Nehrenberg DL, Hua K, Gordon RR, Garland T Jr, Pomp D.** Parent-of-origin effects on voluntary exercise levels and body composition in mice. *Physiol Genomics* 40: 111–120, 2010.
16. **Kelly SA, Nehrenberg DL, Peirce JL, Hua K, Steffy BM, Wiltshire T, Pardo-Manuel de Villena F, Garland T Jr, Pomp D.** Genetic architecture of voluntary exercise in an advanced intercross line of mice. *Physiol Genomics* 42: 190–200, 2010.
17. **Kelly SA, Nehrenberg DL, Hua K, Garland T Jr, Pomp D.** Exercise, weight loss, and changes in body composition in mice: phenotypic relationships and genetic architecture *Physiol Genomics* 43: 199–212, 2011.

18. **Kelly SA, Nehrenberg DL, Hua K, Garland T** Jr, **Pomp D.** Functional genomic architecture of predisposition to voluntary exercise in mice: Expression QTL in the brain. *Genetics* 191: 643–654, 2012.

19. **Kelly SA, Pomp D.** Genetic determinants of voluntary exercise. *Trends Genet* 29: 348–357, 2013.

20. **Kelly SA, Bell TA, Selitsky SR, Buus RJ, Hua K, Weinstock GM, Garland T** Jr, **de Villena FPM, Pomp D.** A novel intronic single nucleotide polymorphism in the myosin heavy polypeptide 4 gene is responsible for the mini-muscle phenotype characterized by major reduction in hind-limb muscle mass in mice. *Genetics* 195: 1385–1395, 2013.

21. **Kelly SA, Nehrenberg DL, Hua K, Garland T** Jr, **Pomp D.** Quantitative genomics of voluntary exercise in mice: Transcriptional analysis and mapping of expression QTL in muscle. *Physiol Genomics* 46: 593–601, 2014.

22. **Kostrzewa E, Kas MJ.** The use of mouse models to unravel genetic architecture of physical activity. *Genes Brain Behav* 13: 87–103, 2014.

23. **Leamy LJ, Pomp D, Lightfoot JT.** An epistatic genetic basis for physical activity traits in mice. *J Hered* 99: 639–646, 2008.

24. **Leamy LJ, Pomp D, Lightfoot JT.** A search for quantitative trait loci controlling within-individual variation of physical activity traits in mice. *BMC Genet* 11: 83, 2010.

25. **Leamy LJ, Kelly SA, Hua K, Pomp D.** Exercise and diet affect quantitative trait loci for body weight and composition traits in an advanced intercross population of mice. *Physiol Genomics* 44: 1141–1153, 2012.

26. **Lerman I, Harrison BC, Freeman K, Hewett TE, Allen DL, Robbins J, Leinwand LA.** Genetic variability in forced and voluntary endurance exercise performance in seven inbred mouse strains. *J Appl Physiol* 92: 2245–2255, 2002.

27. **Lightfoot JT, Turner MJ, Daves M, Vordermark A, Kleeberger SR.** Genetic influence on daily wheel running activity level. *Physiol Genomics* 19: 270–276, 2004.

28. **Lightfoot JT, Turner MJ, Pomp D, Kleeberger SR, Leamy LJ.** Quantitative trait loci (QTL) for physical activity traits in mice. *Physiol Genomics* 32: 401–408, 2008.

29. **Lightfoot JT, Leamy L, Pomp D, Turner MJ, Fodor AA, Knab A, Bowen RS, Ferguson D, Moore-Harrison T, Hamilton A.** Strain screen and haplotype association mapping of wheel running in inbred mouse strains. *J Appl Physiol* 109: 623–634, 2010.

30. **Lightfoot JT.** Current understanding of the genetic basis for physical activity. *J Nutr* 141: 526–530, 2011.

31. **Lightfoot JT, De Geus EJC, Booth FW, Bray MS, den Hoed M, Kaprio J, Kelly SA, Pomp D, Saul MC, Thomis MA, Garland T** Jr, **Bouchard C.** Biological/genetic regulation of physical activity level: consensus from GenBioPAC. *Med Sci Sports Exerc* 50: 863–873, 2018.

32. **Mathes WF, Nehrenberg DL, Gordon R, Hua K, Garland T** Jr, **Pomp D.** Dopaminergic dysregulation in mice selectively bred for excessive exercise or obesity. *Behav Brain Res* 210: 155–163, 2010.

33. **Mathes WF, Aylor DL, Miller DR, Churchill GA, Chesler EJ, de Villena FP, THreadgill DW, Pomp D.** Architecture of energy balance traits in emerging lines of the Collaborative Cross. *Am J Physiol Endocrinol Metab* 6: E1124–1134, 2011.

34. **Meijer JH, Robbers Y.** Wheel running in the wild. *Proc Biol Sci* 281: 20140210, 2014.

35. **Mokdad AH, Marks JS, Stroup DF, Gerberding JL.** Actual causes of death in the United States, 2000. *JAMA* 291: 1238–1245, 2004.

36. **Nehrenberg DL, Wang S, Hannon RM, Garland T** Jr, **Pomp D.** QTL underlying voluntary exercise in mice: interactions with the "mini-muscle" locus and sex. *J Hered* 101: 42–53, 2010.

37. **Novak CM, Burghardt PR, Levine JA.** The use of a running wheel to measure activity in rodents: Relationship to energy balance, general activity, and reward. *Neurosci Biobehav Rev* 36: 1001–1014, 2012.

38. **Pomp D, Nehrenberg D, Estrada-Smith D.** Complex genetics of obesity in mouse models. *Annu Rev Nutr* 28: 331–345, 2008.

39. **Richter CP.** Animal behavior and internal drives. *Q Rev Biol* 2: 307–343, 1927.

40. **Rundquist EA.** Inheritance of spontaneous activity in rats. *J Comp Psych* 16: 415–438, 1933.

41. **Sarzynski MA, Ghosh S, Bouchard C.** Genomic and transcriptomic predictors of response levels to endurance exercise training. *J Physiol* 595: 2931–2939, 2017.

42. **Sherwin CM.** Voluntary wheel running: a review and novel interpretation. *Anim Behav* 56: 11–27, 1998.

43. **Simonen R, Rankinen T, Perusse L, Rice T, Rao DC, Chagnon Y, Bouchard C.** Genome-wide linkage scan for physical activity levels in the Quebec Family study. *Med Sci Sports Exerc* 35: 1355–1359, 2003.

44. **Stewart CC.** Variations in daily activity produced by alcohol and by changes in barometric pressure and diet, with a description of recording methods. *Am J Physiol* 1: 40–56, 1898.

45. **Swallow JG, Carter PA, Garland T** Jr. Artificial selection for increased wheel-running behavior in house mice. *Behav Genet* 28: 227–237, 1998.

46. **Troiano RP, Berrigan D, Dodd KW, Masse LC, Tilert T, Mcdowell M.** Physical activity in the United States measured by accelerometer. *Med Sci Sports Exerc* 40: 181–188, 2008.

47. **Verdugo RA, Farber CR, Warden CH, Medrano JF.** Serious limitations of the QTL microarray approach for QTL gene discovery. *BMC Biol* 8: 96, 2010.

48. **Ways JA, Smith BM, Barbato JC, Ramdath RS, Pettee KM, DeRaedt SJ, Allison DC, Koch LG, Lee SJ, Cicila GT.** Congenic strains confirm aerobic running capacity quantitative trait loci on rat chromosome 16 and identify possible intermediate phenotypes. *Physiol Genomics* 29: 91–97, 2007.

49. **Xu S, Garland T** Jr. A mixed model approach to genome-wide association studies for selection signatures, with application to mice bred for voluntary exercise behavior. *Genetics* 207: 785–799, 2017.

6

IS PHYSICAL ACTIVITY REGULATED BY GENETICS? EVIDENCE FROM STUDIES IN HUMANS

Matthijs D. van der Zee and Eco de Geus

Introduction

Physical activity (PA) is a broad concept containing a variety of different human behaviors that share the common denominator of expected beneficial effects on mental and somatic health (1). Typically, daily PAs take up about 30% of total energy expenditure and reflect a mixture of obligatory activities related to transportation, work, or household chores and self-chosen PA behaviors including sports and exercise activities in leisure time. Objective measurements of daily PA in studies conducted in Europe and the US have confirmed the existence of large individual differences in activity levels (26, 27). These differences are observed in men and women alike, and persist after stratifying for age which is known to have a strong effect on average PA level (49).

To increase the success of intervention on this important health behavior, much research has been devoted to the causes of the individual differences seen in PA in the general population. In this chapter, we focus on the role played by genetic factors. Broadly, the genetic research on PA phenotypes can be classified into a) twin studies that partition the observed variance in PA phenotypes into environmental and genetic components based on well-established biometric models of human inheritance (48), and b) gene-finding studies that use either candidate gene-based approaches based on the known biological role of proteins (e.g., in neurotransmission) or agnostic whole-genome searches using genome-wide microsatellite (linkage) or single nucleotide polymorphism (SNP) markers to detect genomic loci harboring variants associated with PA. We will summarize the current evidence from each of these types of studies to address the question of whether PA is regulated by genetics.

Twin studies

PA behaviors appear to "run in the family," for example, the chance of one family member being a regular exerciser increases the chance of all other family members to be, or to become, an exerciser. Familial aggregation of PA can be investigated by computing correlations among relatives such as siblings, and parents and their offspring. However, siblings among each other, and parents and their offspring, share not just half of their genes, they also share a household, socioeconomic status, the neighborhood, and various other aspects of belonging to the same family or living in the same neighborhood (the so-called shared environment), including parenting behaviors, family functioning, shared peers, etc.

Twin studies can separate the two mechanisms of familial aggregation by comparing the resemblance in monozygotic (MZ) or identical twins to the resemblance in dizygotic (DZ) or fraternal twins (48). When twins are reared together, the amount of this sharing of the family environment is the same for MZ and DZ twins. The important difference between MZ and DZ twins is that the former share most, if not all, of their genotypes, whereas the latter share on average only half of the genotypes segregating in that family. If the resemblance in PA within MZ pairs is larger than that in DZ pairs, this suggests that additive genetic factors (A) influence PA. If MZ resemblance is more than double as large, it suggests the influence of nonadditive (D) genetic factors. Additive genetic factors represent the sum of all linear effects of the genetic loci that influence the trait of interest. Nonadditive factors include dominance and epistatic interaction effects. If, however, the resemblance in PA in DZ twins is as large as it is in MZ twins, this points to shared environmental factors (C) as the cause of twin resemblance. Furthermore, the extent to which MZ twins do not resemble each other is ascribed to the unique environmental factors (E). These include all person-specific experiences such as differential jobs or lifestyles, accidents or other life events, and in childhood, differential treatment by the parents, going to different schools, and having nonshared friends and peers. Measurement error will also be subsumed by the unique environmental factor. For more details on the modeling of twin and family resemblance, see Chapter 3.

We have previously reviewed all twin and family studies on the heritability of total PA and regular sports and exercise behaviors in childhood or adolescent samples (50). In younger children, the shared environmental factors (C) explain the largest part of the variation in PA. However, the importance of these shared environmental factors decreases in adolescence and young adulthood, where genetic effects become the dominant factor explaining individual differences in both total PA and regular sports and exercise behaviors. A sample size–weighted meta-analysis showed PA heritability estimates of 20% (95% confidence interval (CI) 13–27%) in children, 35% (95% CI 17–52%) in early adolescents, and 53% (95% CI 47–59%) in late adolescents. This increase in heritability ran in parallel to a gradual decrease in the importance of shared environmental factors, which are the main cause of individual differences in PA and exercise behavior in young childhood, but then gradually become overwhelmed by the importance of genetic factors during adolescence. Using longitudinal follow-up of twins from childhood to adolescence, we showed that the increase in heritability, at least for voluntary exercise behaviors, was due to a strong increase in the genetic variance in the course of adolescence that was not paired to a similar increase in environmental variance (31). Whether the trend of increasing heritability is continued or curbed in young, middle, or late adulthood remains to be established.

Sufficient studies in adult twins (>18 years of age) have now accrued to allow a similar meta-analytic approach and to arrive at solid estimates of additive genetic and shared environmental variance for PA phenotypes in adulthood. We searched publications in the English language on human subjects in PubMed and Web-of-Science from January 1980 to December 2017 using the keywords ("Physical Activity" OR Exercise OR Sports OR Lifestyle) AND (Genetic OR Genes OR Linkage OR QTL OR Twin OR Family OR Familial OR Heritability) AND "Humans" [MeSH terms]. From the 850 putative papers, title and abstract analysis was used to select only those publications reporting MZ and DZ/sib correlations (in at least 30 complete pairs) and/or estimates of (non-)additive genetic, shared, and/or unique environmental variance components. Reference sections of selected papers were used to identify additional papers missed by these search terms. We then removed samples reporting on twins with a mean age less than 18. Next we removed partly overlapping datasets from the same twin cohorts. When the same phenotype was used in largely the same age group, we only used the study reporting the largest dataset, which typically would be the most recent study. A final set of 27 adult twin studies (2, 3, 8, 11, 14–16, 20–24, 29–32, 34, 35, 40, 44, 45, 46, 47, 51, 53, 54, 58) were selected by the above search criteria.

Physical activity phenotypes

In the final set of 27 adult twin studies, we encountered a large variation in measurement instruments and PA measures used. By far the largest common denominator was the use of survey-based methods using subjective PA reporting on self or family members. In large population-based twin registries, surveys are often considered the only feasible strategy. However, subjective reporting of PA is vulnerable to distortion due to recall error and reporting biases (25). It is particularly difficult to estimate both the duration and frequency of PAs that are light to moderate in intensity, including common activities such as walking and standing, or household activities (5). For total PA and light to moderate PA, objective measurement strategies using indirect calorimetry, the doubly labeled water method, or movement sensors (60) are therefore superior.

When the focus is not on the detection of total PA, but when people are asked to report moderate to vigorous PA, specifically when confined to structured activities in leisure time, self-reporting seems to fare much better (10). The cognitive salience of such intensive PAs is higher than light to moderate intense activities occurring as part of daily routine. Reliability of self-reporting further increases when a restriction is made to the reporting of regular exercise and sports behaviors in leisure time. In our own research, for instance, we have shown a high short-term test–retest reliability (17, 55) as well as substantial tracking over longer periods of time for the weekly volume of voluntary exercise behavior (31).

Our meta-analysis was organized into the main domains of PA that we encountered in the literature: total physical activity (TPA), moderate to vigorous physical activity (MVPA, including separate measures for moderate or vigorous PA where applicable), leisure-time physical activity (LTPA), and voluntary exercise behavior (VEB). The first two categories (TPA and MVPA) cover activities that are only partly under the individual's control, whereas the latter two (LTPA and VEB) cover PA that is largely voluntary in nature. We excluded PA measures that deliberately excluded sports and exercise activities (e.g., Baecke's nonexercise-related PA index), measures exclusively reporting on PA in the occupational setting (e.g., Baecke's Work/ School index), and measures of daily activities of low intensity (e.g., accelerometer derived time spent in low LPA).

To convert the measured PA behaviors into an actual summary metric for use in the genetic analyses, again a breadth of different strategies has been used. Most studies adopt an estimation of the total energy expenditure by PA as their focus. Estimation of energy expenditure is usually based on published compendia (4) that convert each activity into equivalents of the resting energy expenditure (1 MET, approximately 1 kcal/kg/hour). For VEB, most studies use a strategy akin to what we do in the Netherlands Twin Register, where we use an open format that allows reporting all sports and exercise activities that are performed for at least 3 months a year and then record duration, frequency, and intensity of each reported activity. Typically, activities are censored that do not reach a minimal threshold of intensity such as fishing or chess. Exercise related to swimming, sailing, or skiing that are restricted to the annual holidays is discarded. Physical education classes are also discarded as they are poorly standardized and the activities are not voluntary. Energy expenditure in all leisure-time VEB is then summed across all valid exercise activities in a weekly MET-hour score by taking the sum of the products of their weekly frequency, average duration, and MET score.

Another major difference across studies is the type of scale used to quantify PA. Continuous interval scales seem most optimal in terms of statistical power but quite often either ordinal categories (e.g., tertiles of MET-hours weekly; frequency of LTPA as once per month, once per week, every day) or even nominal dichotomies (YES/NO regular exerciser; YES/NO adheres to PA guidelines) were used. This use of dichotomies and categories is mostly inspired by the frequency distribution of some of the LTPA and VEB phenotypes. For instance, moderate to vigorous PA in leisure time is very skewed. Likewise, many individuals do not engage in voluntary exercise behavior (zero score) and even in those who do the amount of exercise can still show a skewed distribution. Often no transformation is available that converts such mixed distributions to a normal distribution. For these phenotypes, therefore, the use of ordinal categories or a dichotomy can be meaningful. A liability threshold model can then be used in the genetic analysis to recapture the normal distribution of the latent "liability to be a (vigorous) exerciser."

Meta-analyses

To assess heritability and influence of common environmental factors in the four PA categories mentioned previously, meta-analysis on A and C estimates was conducted across twin studies. Within the 27-study database, the A and C estimates and their standard errors were often reported separately for males and females. However, if the A and C estimates were reported only for males and females combined, we assigned the same estimates to the male and female part of the sample, adjusting the N to reflect the number of male or female twins. Most studies used age and sex as covariates, but additional covariates were sometimes used too, including socioeconomic status, body mass index, or fitness. When multiple estimates were generated for different covariate compositions, we opted to use the estimates only correcting for age and sex effects on mean PA level. In these studies, structural equation-based variance decomposition modeling was by far the most used analytic strategy. Unless stated otherwise, the results from the most parsimonious structural equation model were used in the meta-analysis. This model was most often an AE or ACE model. If the AE model was used, C was set to zero. No studies reported a model with nonadditivity (D).

For each of the four PA phenotypes, the estimates for A and C were computed in a sample-size weighted meta-analysis across all available studies for males and females separately. Inverse variance weighting was not possible because not all studies provided either standard errors of the estimates or 95% CIs from which the standard errors could be approximated. Forest plots in Figures 6.1 and 6.2 present the characteristics and the A and C estimates per study, and the meta-analytic results per PA phenotype. Study characteristics are as follows: country, whether males and females were combined in A and C estimation, whether PA measurement was through surveys (SUBJ) or experimental (OBJ), type of scale used (DIchotomy, CATegorical, or CONtinuous), mean age, and sex-specific sample size. The estimates for A and C are listed in the forest plots as a function of mean sample age.

Results for total physical activity

For the meta-analysis of TPA (see Figures 6.1 and 6.2) a total of six studies using eight phenotypes was available, most using an objective measure to quantify PA, and all combining males and females. The meta-analytic heritability estimate was 48% for females and 51% for

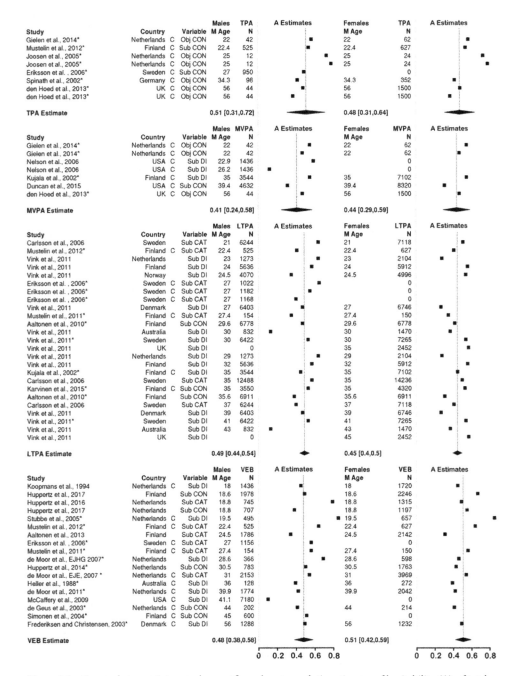

Figure 6.1 Forest plot containing study-specific and meta-analytic estimates of heritability (A) of total physical activity (TPA), moderate to vigorous activity (MVPA), leisure-time physical activity (LTPA), and voluntary exercise behavior (VEB), for males and females. Estimates include results from subjective (Sub), and objective (Obj), continuous (CON), categorical (CAT), and dichotomous (DI) variables. ★=studies where an AE model was fitted. C=estimates from a combined male and female sample.

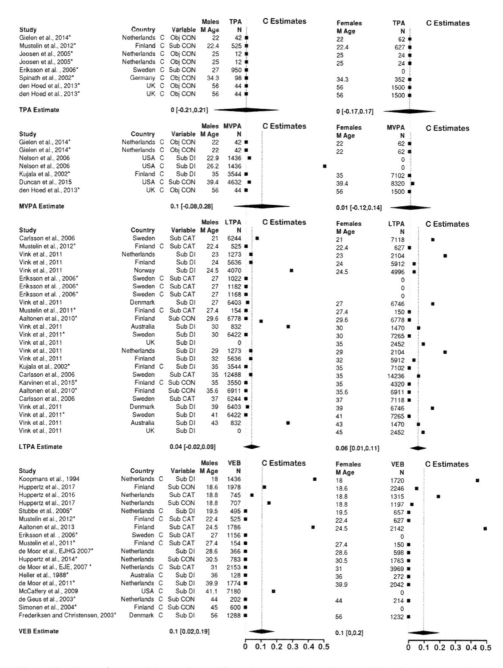

Figure 6.2 Forest plot containing study-specific and meta-analytic estimates of shared environmental contribution (C) to the variance in total physical activity (TPA), moderate to vigorous activity (MVPA), leisure-time physical activity (LTPA), and voluntary exercise behaviour (VEB), for males and females. Estimates include results from subjective (Sub), and objective (Obj), continuous (CON), categorical (CAT), and dichotomous (DI) variables. ★=studies where an AE model was fitted. C=estimates from a combined male and female sample.

males. Largest heritability estimates were found by Joosen et al. (34) who used the most reliable methods, namely the doubly labeled water method and more than 14 days of accelerometer recording, albeit in the smallest sample. The two survey methods using the Baecke questionnaire yielded results comparable to the objective methods. No evidence for common environmental effects was found.

Results for moderate to vigorous physical activity

For the meta-analysis of MVPA (see Figures 6.1 and 6.2) a total of five studies using seven phenotypes was available, all combining males and females. The meta-analytic heritability estimate was 44% for females and 41% for males. Comparable heritability was found for objective and subjective measures. Somewhat deviant results were found in the 26-year-old Add Health study participants (47). Using a 7-day recall questionnaire to obtain a dichotomy of MVPA frequency that indicated whether participants met national PA recommendations (>5 bouts/week), lower heritability was paired to the only evidence for a shared household effect on MVPA (50%).

Results for leisure-time physical activity

We used eight twin studies for the meta-analysis of LTPA (see Figures 6.1 and 6.2) reporting on more than 200,000 twins from seven countries. The meta-analytic heritability estimate was 49% for males and 45% for females with narrow confidence intervals (95% CI upper − lower=~10%) reflecting little heterogeneity. LTPA was only available from self-report measures in these very large epidemiological samples. In two countries, Norway and Australia, evidence for common environmental impact on LTPA was found (~28%). Comparing sample sizes, the absence of a large C in other twin studies cannot be attributed to low power.

Results for voluntary exercise behavior

VEB was also measured exclusively by survey or interview measures. A total of 15 different studies using 14 unique samples/measures yielded a meta-analytic heritability estimate of 48% for males and 51% for females (see Figure 6.1) with mild heterogeneity (95% CI upper − lower=~20%). Some evidence for common environmental effects were found, mostly driven by the younger samples (~10%, see Figure 6.2) with a particularly strong C effect in the young adult Finnish twins (43% males, 49% females).

Gene-finding studies

The above meta-analyses show that genetic variants play a key role in adult PA, whether it is total daily PA as measured with objective means (e.g., accelerometers), or self-reported voluntary sports and exercise activities in leisure time. We now turn to the gene-finding studies aiming to detect the actual "PA genes". For this, we have to use a narrative approach because not enough replication is currently available for any single locus to consider meta-analysis. The majority of gene-finding studies on TPA, MVPA, LTPA, and VEB have used a candidate gene approach. The use of this approach was predicated on the expectation that individual genetic variants would be associated with complex behavioral traits at a magnitude that would be small but detectable with hundreds, or a few thousand individuals. The advent of large international consortia performing meta-analyses on genome-wide association results for many complex behavioral traits in samples as large as hundreds of thousands of participants has found this expectation to be untenable. The risk contributed by any single variant is tiny rather than just small, with only an increase of ~0.05 standard deviation per risk allele at best, necessitating much larger sample sizes to be able to detect them (59). Based on these types of concerns regarding candidate gene studies using small samples, we focus here mainly on the data-driven genome-wide approach in linkage and genome-wide association studies (GWAS).

Linkage

The three genome-wide linkage studies (7, 19, 52) performed to date have only produced suggestive hits, in keeping with their modest sample sizes (767 <N <1120). In the Quebec family study, Simonen et al. (52) reported linkage for TPA (13q22–q31), MVPA (4q28.2, 7p11.2, 9q31.1, 13q22–q31), and VEB (11p15 and 15q13.3). Interestingly, the latter 15q linkage region contains the *GABRG3* gene in which a SNP (rs8036270) was found to be significantly associated with VEB in GWAS on a combined sample of 2622 Dutch and European American middle-aged adults (18). Significant association with *GABRG3* was replicated for LTPA in older adults in a GWAS in 10,684 European and 11,093 African Americans (42) although with different SNPs (rs72707657, rs12438610, rs12902711, rs12595253). The *GABRG3* gene may be involved in the aversive effects of exercise-induced fatigue because high expression levels of the *GABRG3* gene was found after a bout of exhaustive exercise (36). However, a GWAS in 13,980 Japanese older adults did not find significant association with any SNPs in the *GABGR3* gene region and the gene also did not surface in the other two GWAS.

In the Viva La Familia study (7), physical inactivity, recorded as the percentage time in sedentary activity, significantly mapped to markers D18S1102–D18S64 in the chromosome 18q21 region where the *MC4R* gene resides. An additional suggestive linkage signal for TPA was detected in the same region. *MCR4* had been implicated in smaller-scaled candidate gene studies (9, 43) but it failed to replicate in any of the five GWAS, two of which explicitly tested it as a candidate gene (i.e., at lower P-value). In the Viva La Familia study, a further linkage signal was found for MVPA in the region at 9q31.1, which harbors the *RN7SK* gene. A SNP (rs7023003) near this gene produced a suggestive (P <10^{-5}) association with TPA in 8454 Korean participants (38). However, the same *RN7SK* SNP was explicitly but unsuccessfully tested for replication in Japanese participants (28) and the gene also did not surface in the other two GWAS.

Finally, in a sample from the Netherlands Twin Register (19), a suggestive linkage with exercise participation was found in all subjects on chromosome 19p13.3 (LOD 2.18). A SNP (rs12462609) in this region, located in the *CACNA1A* gene, was associated with vigorous PA in 261,055 older adult participants in the UK Biobank (39), and with TPA in 8454 older adult Koreans (38) whereas another SNP (rs111901094) in *GATAD2A* in the 19p13 linkage region was associated with VEB in the UK Biobank participants (39). The 19p13 region did not generate a significant or suggestive signal in the other two GWAS (28, 42). In summary, genes suggested from linkage regions (*GABRG3, MCR4, RN7SK, CACNA1A*) have not held up systematically when tested as candidate genes in GWAS.

Genome-wide association

Five GWAS (18, 28, 38, 39, 42) conducted for exercise behavior or related PA phenotypes were available at the time of writing. The three smallest GWAS (2632 <N <11,093) did not detect significant associations after the required stringent correction for the multiple testing burden that is inherent in the agnostic genome-wide approach (18, 38, 42). However, some genes listed as receiving suggestive evidence based on more lenient thresholds ($P < 10^{-5}$) showed interest-generating patterns of replication across multiple studies. For example, a suggestive association of VEB was found in Dutch and American participants of European descent (18) for an eQTL (rs12612420) that influences the expression of the *DNAPTP6* gene. This association was replicated *(P=0.0092)* in 16,026 Japanese participants (28).

Suggestive evidence for an association between VEB and the *PAPSS2* gene in Dutch and American participants (18) was replicated in 11,903 African American participants (42) for LTPA, although for different SNPs (rs10887741 vs. rs1819162). The *PAPSS2* gene has been linked to maximal exercise capacity (49) which may be a factor influencing the motivation to engage in voluntary exercise (12). Explicit testing of an association between VEB and *PAPSS2* in 13,980 Japanese participants, however, did not produce a significant replication (28). Suggestive evidence for an association with LTPA was found for rs116550874 at 1p36.23, and rs3792874, rs3792877, rs3792878, rs79173796 at 5q31.1 ($P < 8.61 \times 10^{-7}$) in 11093 African Americans and for rs28524846 at 14q23.3 ($P < 1.30 \times 10^{-6}$) in 10,684 European Americans (42). The authors point to the *ENO1*, *SLC22A5*, and *PDLIM4* genes as potential sources of the association signal at 1p36. *ENO1* encodes a glycolytic enzyme and the integral membrane protein SLC22A5 is associated with skeletal myopathy, whereas the PDLIM4 protein is involved in the pathway of actin cytoskeleton remodeling, and bone and skeletal muscle development. The rs28524846 SNP at 14q23 is an eQTL for *MPP5* and *APT6V1D* in nerve tissue, with the MPP5 protein known to regulate myelinating Schwann cells and *ATP6V1D* related to synaptic vesicle cycle and ATPase activity.

Encouragingly, the two largest GWAS to date did successfully detect genome-wide significant associations with PA. In a Japanese sample ($N=16,016$), Hara et al. (28) identified an association *(Pmeta=2.2×10^{-9})* between LTPA and rs10252228, a SNP located in the intergenic region between the *NPSR1* and *DPY19L1* genes. Although functional links of intergenic SNPs to nearby genes should be interpreted with caution, Hara et al. (28) point out that the product of the *NPSR1* and that of the *DNAPTP6* genes previously found by the GWAS of de Moor et al. (18) are both involved in pulmonary function. Variants in *NPSR1* have been shown to be associated with asthma-related phenotypes, and *DNAPTP6* could be involved in bronchodilator response via the downregulation of ß2-adrenergic receptors. Impairments of pulmonary function could be a barrier to the adoption of (vigorous) PA.

In the UK Biobank ($N=380,492$), Klimentidis et al. (39) detected genome-wide significant genetic associations with touchscreen-survey based measures of MVPA. After applying corrections for work-related PA and an indicator of socioeconomic status, associations with MVPA were found at rs429358 (*APOE*), rs169504 (*PBX2*), rs4129572 (*EXOC4*), rs3094622 (*RPP21*), rs181220614 (*ARHGEF26-AS1*), rs149943 (*ZNF165*), and rs2988004 (*PAX5*). Intriguingly, the Alzheimer disease risk allele (E4) of the *APOE* gene was associated with higher levels of MVPA. As noted by Klimentidis et al. (39), *APOE* e4 carriers had a more favorable response to exercise, for instance, as suggested by a study showing larger aerobic fitness in response to training (56). This is in keeping with the theoretical notion that individuals who have higher exercise ability and/or trainability will find it easier to adopt regular exercise as a lifestyle (12, 13, 41).

From the UK Biobank self-reports (39), two dichotomous measures of more vigorous PA were defined: VPA by classifying participants as engaged in vigorous PA if they spend more than 25 minutes on activities "that make you sweat or breathe hard" for 3 or more days a week and VEB by classifying participants as regular vigorous exercisers if they spend more than 15 minutes on 2 or more days a week doing strenuous sports or other exercises. Significant genetic association for VPA was found at rs1248860 (*CADM2*), rs2764261 (*FOXO3*), rs3781411 (*CTBP2*), rs12707131 (*EXOC4*), and rs328919 (*DPY19L1*) and for VEB at rs62253088 (*CADM2*), rs166840 (*AKAP10*), rs10946808 (*HIST1H1D*), rs75930676 (*SIPA1L1*), and rs4865656 (*LOC642366*). In addition, accelerometer data were available in just over 91,000 participants. From up to 7 days of accelerometer wear, overall acceleration was obtained as a measure of TPA and the fraction of accelerations >425 *mg* as a measure of VPA, yielding significant associations at rs55657917 (*CRHR1*) and rs185829646 (*ANKRD22*) for TPA and rs743580 (*PML*) and rs6433478 (*CIR1*) for VPA.

The *CADM2* gene, primarily expressed in the brain, surfaced in the UK Biobank study as a gene influencing vigorous sports and exercise-related PA. Previously this gene had been linked to risk-taking behavior and extraversion (6) as well as executive function (33). This shows a remarkable parallel to results reported in the largest candidate study to date by van der Mee et al. (57) where a polygenic dopaminergic risk score that summed the increaser alleles in *COMT* and *DAT1* for *both* executive function and reward sensitivity was associated with the volume of externally paced sports and exercise activities. Possibly, *CADM2*, like these dopaminergic genes operates through a "double whammy" of increased reward value of exercise and increased sports skills.

Conclusion

Although the gradual rise in heritability of PA seen in adolescence is not continued in adulthood, it is clear that genetic factors remain a major contributor to individual differences in adult PA behaviors. In the reports on over 283,904 adult twins, we find that about half of the variance in the four PA phenotypes can be explained by genetic factors (males 48%; 95% CI 44–52%; females 47%; 95% CI 44–50%). The substantial contribution of the shared environment (C) to childhood PA seems to have largely dissipated in adulthood (males and females 6%; 95% CI 3–10%). There is generally a good correspondence in estimates across individual studies even when they use samples from different countries or measures. For TPA and MVPA, objective measurement showed slightly higher genetic estimates than subjective measurement, but the differences are not striking. Major sex differences in genetic architecture of LTPA and VEB seemed to be absent; for TPA and MVPA estimates, the verdict is still out as analyses were mostly based on combined male/female samples.

The extant studies using a candidate gene, linkage, or whole-genome association approach have yielded a number of genes and variants worth careful monitoring in future gene-finding efforts. Previously, three biological themes have emerged as a potential source for "physical activity genes" from theory: (1) the brain circuitry related to motivational and affective aspects of PA; (2) the brain circuitry involved in the maintenance of energy intake/expenditure balance; and (3) the physiological determinants of the ability to perform (intense and/or prolonged) PA, ideally at an above average level (12, 13, 41). Many of the variants reviewed above do seem to fit these theoretical notions, but we issue a note of caution that this may partly reflect our deep desire (and uncanny ability) to make sense of data by "reasoning towards" our theoretical models. Rigorous replication followed by experimental validation (in animal models) is direly needed. However, the experience from many other complex behavioral traits allows us to end upbeat: once very large samples are amassed in international meta-analytic consortia, we can confidently expect large progress in our understanding of how PA is regulated by genetics.

References

1. **World Health Organization**. *Global Recommendations on Physical Activity for Health*, Switzerland: World Health Organization, 2010.

2. **Aaltonen S, Ortega-Alonso A, Kujala UM**, and **Kaprio J.** Genetic and environmental influences on longitudinal changes in leisure-time physical activity from adolescence to young adulthood. *Twin Res Hum Genet* 16: 535–543, 2013.

3. **Aaltonen S, Ortega-Alonso A, Kujala UM**, and **Kaprio J.** A longitudinal study on genetic and environmental influences on leisure time physical activity in the Finnish Twin Cohort. *Twin Res Hum Genet* 13: 475–481, 2010.

4. **Ainsworth BE, Haskell WL, Herrmann SD, Meckes N, Bassett DR**, Jr., **Tudor-Locke C, Greer JL, Vezina J, Whitt-Glover MC**, and **Leon AS.** 2011 Compendium of Physical Activities: a second update of codes and MET values. *Med Sci Sports Exerc* 43: 1575–1581, 2011.

5. **Bassett DR**, Jr, **Cureton AL**, and **Ainsworth BE.** Measurement of daily walking distance-questionnaire versus pedometer. *Med Sci Sports Exerc* 32: 1018–1023, 2000.

6. **Boutwell B, Hinds D, 23andMe Research Team, Tielbeek J, Ong KK, Day FR**, and **Perry JRB.** Replication and characterization of CADM2 and MSRA genes on human behavior. *Heliyon* 3: e00349, 2017.

7. **Cai GW, Cole SA, Butte N, Bacino C, Diego V, Tan K, Goring HH, O'Rahilly S, Farooqi IS**, and **Comuzzie AG.** A quantitative trait locus on chromosome 18q for physical activity and dietary intake in Hispanic children. *Obesity (Silver Spring)* 14: 1596–1604, 2006.

8. **Carlsson S, Andersson T, Lichtenstein P, Michaelsson K**, and **Ahlbom A.** Genetic effects on physical activity: Results from the Swedish twin registry. *Med Sci Sports Exerc* 38: 1396–1401, 2006.

9. **Cole SA, Butte NF, Voruganti VS, Cai G, Haack K, Kent JW** Jr, **Blangero J, Comuzzie AG, McPherson JD**, and **Gibbs RA.** Evidence that multiple genetic variants of MC4R play a functional role in the regulation of energy expenditure and appetite in Hispanic children. *Am J Clin Nutr* 91: 191–199, 2010.

10. **Craig CL, Marshall AL, Sjostrom M, Bauman AE, Booth ML, Ainsworth BE, Pratt M, Ekelund U, Yngve A, Sallis JF**, and **Oja P.** International physical activity questionnaire: 12-country reliability and validity. *Med Sci Sports Exerc* 35: 1381–1395, 2003.

11. **de Geus EJ, Boomsma DI**, and **Snieder H.** Genetic correlation of exercise with heart rate and respiratory sinus arrhythmia. *Med Sci Sports Exerc* 35: 1287–1295, 2003.

12. **de Geus EJ** and **de Moor MHM.** Genes, exercise, and psychological factors. In: *Genetic and Molecular Aspects of Sport Performance*, edited by Bouchard C and Hoffman EP. Chichester: Wiley, 2011, p. 294–305.

13. **de Geus EJ** and **de Moor MHM.** A genetic perspective on the association between exercise and mental health. *Ment Health Phys Act* 1: 53–61, 2008.

14. **de Moor MH, Posthuma D, Hottenga JJ, Willemsen G, Boomsma DI**, and **de Geus EJ.** Genome-wide linkage scan for exercise participation in Dutch sibling pairs. *Eur J Hum Genet* 15: 1252–1259, 2007.

15. **de Moor MH, Stubbe JH, Boomsma DI**, and **de Geus EJ.** Exercise participation and self-rated health: do common genes explain the association? *Eur J Epidemiol* 22: 27–32, 2007.

16. **de Moor MH, Willemsen G, Rebollo-Mesa I, Stubbe JH, de Geus EJ**, and **Boomsma DI.** Exercise participation in adolescents and their parents: Evidence for genetic and generation specific environmental effects. *Behav Genet* 41: 211–222, 2011.

17. **de Moor MH** and **de Geus, EJ**. Genetic influences on exercise behavior. In: *Lifestyle Medicine*, edited by Rippe JM. Boca Raton, FL: Taylor & Francis Group, 2012, p. 1367–1378.

18. **de Moor MH, Liu YJ, Boomsma DI, Li J, Hamilton JJ, Hottenga JJ, Levy S, Liu XG, Pei YF, Posthuma D, Recker RR, Sullivan PF, Wang L, Willemsen G, Yan H, de Geus EJ**, and **Deng HW.** Genome-wide association study of exercise behavior in Dutch and American adults. *Med Sci Sports Exerc* 41: 1887–1895, 2009.

19. **de Moor MH, Posthuma D, Hottenga JJ, Willemsen AHM, Boomsma DI**, and **de Geus EJC.** Genome-wide linkage scan for exercise participation in Dutch sibling pairs. *Eur J Hum Genet* 15: 1252–1259, 2007.

20. **den Hoed M, Brage S, Zhao JH, Westgate K, Nessa A, Ekelund U, Spector TD, Wareham NJ**, and **Loos RJ.** Heritability of objectively assessed daily physical activity and sedentary behavior. *Am J Clin Nutr* 98: 1317–1325, 2013.

21. **Duncan GE, Cash SW, Horn EE,** and **Turkheimer E.** Quasi-causal associations of physical activity and neighborhood walkability with body mass index: a twin study. *Prev Med* 70: 90–95, 2015.

22. **Eriksson M, Rasmussen F,** and **Tynelius P.** Genetic factors in physical activity and the equal environment assumption – the Swedish young male twins study. *Behav Genet* 36: 238–247, 2006.

23. **Frederiksen H** and **Christensen K.** The influence of genetic factors on physical functioning and exercise in second half of life. *Scand J Med Sci Sports* 13: 9–18, 2003.

24. **Gielen M, Westerterp-Plantenga MS, Bouwman FG, Joosen AM, Vlietinck R, Derom C, Zeegers MP, Mariman EC,** and **Westerterp KR.** Heritability and genetic etiology of habitual physical activity: A twin study with objective measures. *Genes Nutr* 9: 415, 2014.

25. **Hagstromer M, Ainsworth BE, Oja P,** and **Sjostrom M.** Comparison of a subjective and an objective measure of physical activity in a population sample. *J Phys Act Health* 7: 541–550, 2010.

26. **Hagstromer M, Troiano RP, Sjostrom M,** and **Berrigan D.** Levels and patterns of objectively assessed physical activity – a comparison between Sweden and the United States. *Am J Epidemiol* 171: 1055–1064, 2010.

27. **Hansen BH, Kolle E, Dyrstad SM, Holme I,** and **Anderssen SA.** Accelerometer-determined physical activity in adults and older people. *Med Sci Sports Exerc* 44: 266–272, 2012.

28. **Hara M, Hachiya T, Nishida Y, Shimanoe C, Tanaka K, Sutoh Y,** and **Shimizu A.** Genome-wide association study of leisure-1 time exercise behavior in Japanese adults. *Med Sci Sports Exerc*, 2018.

29. **Heller RF, O'Connell DL, Roberts DC, Allen JR, Knapp JC, Steele PL,** and **Silove D.** Lifestyle factors in monozygotic and dizygotic twins. *Genet Epidemiol* 5: 311–321, 1988.

30. **Huppertz C, Bartels M, de Geus EJ, van Beijsterveldt CEM, Rose RJ, Kaprio J,** and **Silventoinen K.** The effects of parental education on exercise behavior in childhood and youth: A study in Dutch and Finnish twins. *Scand J Med Sci Sports* 27: 1143–1156, 2017.

31. **Huppertz C, Bartels M, de Zeeuw EL, van Beijsterveldt CEM, Hudziak JJ, Willemsen G, Boomsma DI,** and **de Geus EJ.** Individual differences in exercise behavior: Stability and change in genetic and environmental determinants from age 7 to 18. *Behav Genet* 46: 665–679, 2016.

32. **Huppertz C, Bartels M, Jansen IE, Boomsma DI, Willemsen G, de Moor MH,** and **de Geus EJ.** A twin-sibling study on the relationship between exercise attitudes and exercise behavior. *Behav Genet* 44: 45–55, 2014.

33. **Ibrahim-Verbaas CA, Bressler J, Debette S, Schuur M, Smith AV, Bis JC, Davies G, Trompet S, Smith JA, Wolf C,** et al. GWAS for executive function and processing speed suggests involvement of the CADM2 gene. *Mol Psychiatry* 21: 189–197, 2016.

34. **Joosen AM, Gielen M, Vlietinck R,** and **Westerterp KR.** Genetic analysis of physical activity in twins. *Am J Clin Nutr* 82: 1253–1259, 2005.

35. **Karvinen S, Waller K, Silvennoinen M, Koch LG, Britton SL, Kaprio J, Kainulainen H,** and **Kujala UM.** Physical activity in adulthood: Genes and mortality. *Sci Rep* 5: 18259, 2015.

36. **Kawai T, Morita K, Masuda K, Nishida K, Sekiyama A, Teshima-Kondo S, Nakaya Y, Ohta M, Saito T,** and **Rokutan K.** Physical exercise-associated gene expression signatures in peripheral blood. *Clin J Sport Med* 17: 375–383, 2007.

37. **Kemper HC, Twisk JW,** and **van Mechelen W.** Changes in aerobic fitness in boys and girls over a period of 25 years: Data from the Amsterdam Growth And Health Longitudinal Study revisited and extended. *Pediatr Exerc Sci.* 25: 524–35, 2013.

38. **Kim J, Kim J, Min H, Oh S, Kim Y, Lee AH,** and **Park T.** Joint identification of genetic variants for physical activity in Korean population. *Int J Mol Sci* 15: 12407–12421, 2014.

39. **Klimentidis YC, Raichlen DA, Bea J, Garcia DO, Mandarino LJ, Alexander GE, Chen Z,** and **Going SB.** Genome-wide association study of habitual physical activity in over 377,000 UK Biobank participants identifies multiple variants including CADM2 and APOE. *Int J Epidemiol*, 42: 1161–1176, 2018.

40. **Kujala UM, Kaprio J,** and **Koskenvuo M.** Modifiable risk factors as predictors of all-cause mortality: The roles of genetics and childhood environment. *Am J Epidemiol* 156: 985–993, 2002.

41. **Lightfoot JT, de Geus EJ, Booth FW, Bray MS, den Hoed M, Kaprio J, Kelly SA, Pomp D, Saul MC, Thomis MA, Garland T,** Jr, and **Bouchard C.** Biological/genetic regulation of physical activity level: Consensus from GenBioPAC. *Med Sci Sports Exerc* 50: 863–873, 2017.

42. **Lin X, Chan KK, Huang Y-T, Luo X, Liang L, Wilson J, Correa A, Levy D,** and **Liu S.** Genetic determinants for leisure-time physical activity. *Med Sci Sports Exerc* 50: 1620–1628, 2018.

43. **Loos RJF, Rankinen T, Tremblay A, Pérusse L, Chagnon Y,** and **Bouchard C.** Melanocortin-4 receptor gene and physical activity in the Québec Family Study. *Int J Obes* 29: 420–428, 2004.

44. **McCaffery JM, Papandonatos GD, Bond DS, Lyons MJ,** and **Wing RR.** Gene X environment interaction of vigorous exercise and body mass index among male Vietnam-era twins. *Am J Clin Nutr* 89: 1011–1018, 2009.

45. **Mustelin L, Joutsi J, Latvala A, Pietilainen KH, Rissanen A,** and **Kaprio J.** Genetic influences on physical activity in young adults: A twin study. *Med Sci Sports Exerc* 44: 1293–1301, 2012.

46. **Mustelin L, Latvala A, Pietilainen KH, Piirila P, Sovijarvi AR, Kujala UM, Rissanen A,** and **Kaprio J.** Associations between sports participation, cardiorespiratory fitness, and adiposity in young adult twins. *J Appl Physiol* 110: 681–686, 2011.

47. **Nelson MC, Gordon-Larsen P, North KE,** and **Adair LS.** Body mass index gain, fast food, and physical activity: effects of shared environments over time. *Obesity (Silver Spring)* 14: 701–709, 2006.

48. **Plomin R, DeFries JC, Knopik V,** and **Niederheiser J.** *Behavioral Genetics.* New York: Worth, 2013.

49. **Rico-Sanz J, Rankinen T, Rice T, Leon AS, Skinner JS, Wilmore JH, Rao DC,** and **Bouchard C.** Quantitative trait loci for maximal exercise capacity phenotypes and their responses to training in the HERITAGE Family Study. *Physiol Genomics* 16: 256–260, 2004.

50. **Schutte NM, Bartels M,** and **de Geus EJ.** Genetics of physical activity and physical fitness. In: *Oxford Textbook of Children's Sport and Exercise Medicine* (3rd ed.), edited by Armstrong N and van Mechelen W. New York: Oxford University Press, 2017, p. 293–302.

51. **Simonen R, Levalahti E, Kaprio J, Videman T,** and **Battie MC.** Multivariate genetic analysis of lifetime exercise and environmental factors. *Med Sci Sports Exerc* 36: 1559–1566, 2004.

52. **Simonen RL, Rankinen T, Perusse L, Rice T, Rao DC, Chagnon Y,** and **Bouchard C.** Genome-wide linkage scan for physical activity levels in the Quebec family study. *Med Sci Sports Exerc* 35: 1355–1359, 2003.

53. **Spinath FM, Wolf H, Angleitner A, Borkenau P,** and **Riemann R.** Genetic and environmental influences on objectively assessed activity in adults. *Pers Individ Dif* 33: 633–645, 2002.

54. **Stubbe JH, Boomsma DI,** and **De Geus EJ.** Sports participation during adolescence: A shift from environmental to genetic factors. *Med Sci Sports Exerc* 37: 563–570, 2005.

55. **Stubbe JH, de Moor MH, Boomsma D,** and **de Geus EJ.** The association between exercise participation and well-being: A co-twin study. *Prev Med* 44: 148–152, 2006.

56. **Thompson PD, Tsongalis GJ, Seip RL, Bilbie C, Miles M, Zoeller R, Visich P, Gordon P, Angelopoulos TJ, Pescatello L, Bausserman L,** and **Moyna N.** Apolipoprotein E genotype and changes in serum lipids and maximal oxygen uptake with exercise training. *Metabolism* 53: 193–202, 2004.

57. **van der Mee DJ, Fedko IO, Hottenga JJ, Ehli EA, van der Zee MD, Ligthart L, van Beijsterveldt TCEM, Davies GE, Bartels M, Landers JG,** and **de Geus, EJC.** Dopaminergic genetic variants and voluntary externally paced exercise behavior. *Med Sci Sports Exerc* 50: 700–708, 2017.

58. **Vink JM, Boomsma DI, Medland SE, de Moor MH, Stubbe JH, Cornes BK, Martin NG, Skytthea A, Kyvik KO, Rose RJ, Kujala UM, Kaprio J, Harris JR, Pedersen NL, Cherkas L, Spector TD,** and **de Geus EJ.** Variance components models for physical activity with age as modifier: A comparative twin study in seven countries. *Twin Res Hum Genet* 14: 25–34, 2011.

59. **Visscher PM, Wray NR, Zhang Q, Sklar P, McCarthy MI, Brown MA,** and **Yang J.** 10 Years of GWAS discovery: Biology, function, and translation. *Am J Hum Genet* 101: 5–22, 2017.

60. **Westerterp KR.** Physical activity and physical activity induced energy expenditure in humans: Measurement, determinants, and effects. *Fron Psychol* 4: 90, 2013.

7

THE EVOLUTION OF GENETIC MECHANISMS CONTROLLING PHYSICAL ACTIVITY

J. Timothy Lightfoot, Ayland C. Letsinger, and Jorge Z. Granados

Introduction

As reviewed in earlier chapters, there is an extensive literature that suggests that physical activity is genetically regulated, even though the mechanisms controlling this genetic influence have not been definitively identified. While there are multiple groups working to understand how genetically linked mechanisms may regulate physical activity, there have been few efforts devoted to understanding how these mechanisms originally developed in humans. Two alternative explanations can be proposed toward this end: 1) the genetic mechanisms that control physical activity were just "built-in" to all mammals as part of the basic set of physiological controllers; or 2) the genetic mechanisms that control physical activity evolved over time due to drift, selection, or mutation (54). The former explanation does not hold if it is assumed that humans evolved from single-celled organisms originally, which is the so-called universal common ancestry (UCA) theory. The UCA theory was initially proposed by Darwin (18) and is currently accepted by most evolutionary biologists with recent quantitative results supporting UCA over a variety of competing, alternative hypotheses (60). If then the genetic mechanisms regulating physical activity evolved over time in mammals, what combination of drift, selection, and mutation resulted in genetic control of activity? Further, if the physical activity regulating genetic mechanisms evolved, which – if any – potential external factors may have contributed to this evolution?

To a large extent, these questions devolve to the following: Why would animals – including humans – have moved? Why were they active? And why would humans have evolved mechanisms that regulated how much movement was performed? There is no doubt that the physiologies of all mammals are made for locomotion of some kind, whether it be walking, running, galloping, trotting, and/or swimming, but why move? There is a long history of psychological research into the reason for human motivation, with some of the best-known work by Maslow (46) suggesting that at the root of motivation is the need to fulfill basic needs such as hunger, safety, waste removal, and sex among others. Indeed, as related to physical activity, early anthropological observations in hunter/gatherer tribes suggested that with fulfillment of nutrient demands, individuals in these tribes were not necessarily physically active (35). Further, an argument can be made that physical activity-induced caloric expenditure above the minimum necessary for collecting nutrition in an environment of limited dietary resources would be adverse to the survival of the individual and communal unit. However, if the genetic regulation of physical activity developed in an inverse relationship to food availability as we have postulated elsewhere (i.e., less food, more activity to find food; or more food, less need for activity) (41), it is uncertain why humans still have the drive to be active given the current food abundance (in general). While Maslow (46) specifically cautioned against applying his theory to animals, why are some animal species (e.g., rodents) still active when they are safe and have an *ad libitum* diet available? For example, we have previously highlighted several different strains of inbred mice that run long distances on a daily basis (~7–12 km/day) in just such conditions (38) with mice in the wild also choosing to run voluntarily on a running wheel (47). These types of observations have led us to further consider why humans (and animals) would have evolved mechanisms to control daily physical activity or if this type of activity control is just a byproduct of the pursuit of basic needs.

The reader may wonder what use this type of inquiry would have. After all, it is extremely difficult to experimentally test any potential selection pressure or mutation that may have caused these activity-regulating mechanisms to evolve (however, it should be noted that Garland and Kelly have published methods to invoke experimental evolution in rodents that could be used in some experimental conditions) (25). As such, at best, any answers derived from considering how physical activity genetic regulating mechanisms evolved may be considered "educated speculation." To this point, Washburn and Lancaster (62) noted:

> In speculations of this kind, it is well to keep the purpose of the speculation and the limitation of the evidence in mind. Our aim is to understand human evolution. What shaped the course of human evolution was a succession of successful adaptations, both biological and cultural. These may be inferred in part from the direct evidence of the archeological record. But the record is very incomplete … As we go farther back in time, there is less evidence and the biological and cultural difference becomes progressively greater. Yet it was in those remote times that the human way took shape, and it is only through speculation that we may gain some insights into what the life of our ancestors may have been.

In this case, insights into how genetic mechanisms controlling activity evolved may be useful in two ways: 1) these insights may prove informative in describing and understanding the actual genetic mechanisms that regulate activity, which at this point are fairly ambiguous; and 2) these insights may either support or undermine the use of animal models in working to understand human genetic regulation of activity. In regard to the former, given the lack of definitive identified genetic mechanisms that control physical activity (42), any information regarding potential mutations or selection pressures that led to the development of activity-regulating mechanisms could help better direct research trying to identify these mechanisms. For example, we had previously suggested that food availability could have been a potential selection pressure for the development of the genetic regulation of physical activity (41). This suggestion has led us to investigate whether food availability controls physical activity, with a multitude of studies showing that moderate caloric restriction increases activity in a wide variety of mammals (e.g., 27, 66) and recent studies showing that caloric overfeeding decreases physical activity significantly (average decrease ~62%) (61).

Perhaps a more critical reason to consider the evolutionary factors for the development of physical activity genetic regulators is to determine whether the animal models that have been extensively used in this field of investigation are actually valid models of the genetic control of human activity. For example, we have written extensively in other papers (38) as to why we believe that a mouse wheel-running model is a valid model of human physical activity. Briefly, mouse wheel-running mimics the physiological conditions that occur in humans during voluntary exercise, wheel-running activates the same neural transmitters (unlike forced treadmill activity in rodents), and most importantly, humans and mice self-select similar exercise intensities when voluntarily running. If the genetic mechanisms controlling physical activity in humans evolved before the basic mammalian species split – for example, it is estimated that mice and humans split on the evolutionary tree approximately 62–100 million years ago (8, 30) – then any insights gleaned from mice as to the genetic mechanisms responsible for physical activity regulation would be potentially translatable to humans (and the converse would be true as well) (39). Therefore, while perhaps not as empirically testable as other hypotheses in the field of genetic regulation of physical activity, the exploration of potential factors that led to the evolution of genetic controllers of physical activity could be used to direct research investigations.

A common question that arises is whether the evolutionary factors that drove the development of the genetic mechanisms controlling physical activity are similar to those that drove the development of genetic mechanisms that may control exercise endurance. While we have directly addressed that question in other papers (e.g., 41), others have written extensively regarding potential evolutionary selection pressures that arose approximately 50,000 years ago to drive the development of exercise endurance (11). As such, the current literature suggests the genetic mechanisms that control physical activity and those that control exercise endurance, while perhaps related, are distinct mechanisms that probably arose at different times. For example, it has been shown that the genomic quantitative trait loci (QTL) associated with exercise endurance (e.g., 10, 17, 43, 56) and physical activity (e.g., 19, 38, 40) do not overlap or colocalize in either human or animal models. Additionally, it has been shown repeatedly that exercise endurance and activity levels are weakly correlated in humans (both adults and children) and animal models (34, 36). Lastly, genetic regulation of physical activity appears to include an additional central drive-controlling element (42) that has not been included in discussions of genetic regulation of exercise endurance. Thus, while there may be some phenotypic overlap, given the differing QTL sets, the lack of a strong correlation between physical activity level and exercise endurance, as well as the probably different regulating mechanisms, the consideration of the development of genetic mechanisms regulating physical activity level should be treated separately from those genetic mechanisms controlling exercise endurance (for a discussion of the evolution of exercise endurance, see Chapter 11).

In the majority of cases, selection pressures are often erroneously considered the only factors involved in evolution. However, it is well established that evolution occurs as a result of some combination of selection pressures, random genetic drift, and/or mutation events that are dependent upon a variety of factors including population size (54). However, our previous writings on the evolution of physical activity genetic regulation – and those in the exercise endurance areas – have primarily been focused on potential selection pressures. Thus, the first section below will consider potential selection pressures acting on physical activity requirements, while the concepts of potential random drift and/or mutation will be returned to in the latter section of the chapter as we take up the consideration of when these mechanisms evolved.

Potential selection pressures driving the development of genetic regulation of physical activity

In many cases, potential selection pressures are the first factors that are considered when investigating the reasons for evolution of a trait. While selection pressures may not be the reason for the evolution of a trait (as discussed above), there are several potential pressures that have been previously discussed as relating directly to physical activity. Here we provide a brief overview of these potential selection pressures and current data arguing for or against their inclusion in future discussions,

Daily energy expenditure as a selection pressure

We had previously observed that energy expenditure (EE) may have been a potential selection pressure in the evolution of physical activity (41). In our earlier data, there were no significant differences in daily EEs (corrected by weight) between pre-technology farmers and hunter-gatherer populations, with both populations having higher daily EE than Western populations. This analysis was flawed, having not accounted for Kleiber's law (31), whereas metabolic rates are scaled to mass by a reciprocal of ¾. The application of Kleiber's law has been illustrated recently by Pontzer and colleagues in several articles (e.g., 50, 52) where they have shown that regardless of population – pre-technology farmer, hunter-gatherer, or Western population – total daily energy expenditures (TEEs) are largely similar even though daily physical activity levels are significantly different. Similar observations had been made earlier by Westerterp and Speakman (63), but these observations were fully empirically validated by Pontzer and colleagues (53) and later extended to several different mammalian species (50). Therefore, given that daily EEs were probably not different between various populations of early humans, it is likely that daily EE was not a selection pressure for the evolution of physical activity control mechanisms.

Food accessibility as a selection pressure

Interestingly, Pontzer has suggested that daily EE, rather than being dependent on daily activity, is homeostatically controlled (50). Pontzer and colleagues suggest that homeostatic control of daily EE in each mammalian species is largely set by both evolutionary and ontogenetic responses to specific influences (50, 52). One specific influence in setting EE suggested by Pontzer and colleagues is chronic food availability (49). The hypothesis that food availability played a role in the evolution of EE homeostasis, is congruent with our own suggestions of food availability playing a role in the development of the genetic mechanisms that control daily physical activity (41).

Our earlier hypothesis that food availability would have been a selection pressure contributing to the evolution of the genetic regulation of physical activity was based on the copious literature showing an inverse relationship between physical activity and food availability. It is well established that moderate reductions in caloric intake significantly increase physical activity in several animal species (e.g., 27, 66), with suggestions that the same responses occur in humans (14). Conversely, two human studies have indirectly suggested that overfeeding significantly decreased physical activity in specific situations (37, 57). Supporting these studies, are recent direct observations that have shown that inbred mice placed on a chronic (9–11-week) high-fat, high-sugar diet decreased daily voluntary wheel-running distance by 70% in males and by 57% in female mice (61). This decreased physical activity remained as long as the mice were exposed to the altered diet; chronic exposure to a running wheel after the chronic dietary exposure did not correct the activity inhibition. Further, the overfeeding-induced activity reduction remained even with exogenous sex hormone supplementation, eliminating overfeeding-induced changes in sex hormones as a potential mechanism for this physical activity reduction (61). These conclusions are supported by earlier, more limited studies that also showed that overfeeding reduced physical activity in rodents (9, 23, 55). Thus, while the mechanisms linking caloric intake with physical activity regulation are unclear, it is clear that food availability is linked to the control of physical activity. Given that food availability has been linked with the evolution of the homeostatic control of daily EE (49), it is also possible that food availability was a selection pressure involved with the evolution of physical activity genetic control mechanisms.

Logic difficulties exist with the argument that food availability is inversely related to physical activity (i.e., decreased food availability=increased activity and vice versa). The logical inconsistencies would occur if food supply were extremely limited and activity was high; from an individual standpoint, activity would be an energy wasteful mechanism which could not be corrected given local food availability. From a community standpoint, increased physical activity would strain the energy resources available to sustain the larger populations. When faced with a decrease in energy resources, the individual/community necessarily has to increase its foraging areas in the hope of finding new energy resources. The necessity to increase the foraging range – the so-called patch-leaving problem (59) – would require a higher physical activity drive. A naturally occurring example of decreased food availability/altered physical activity in nature is seen within ungulates (such as deer) and members of Carnivora (such as wolves) populations with larger animals having larger home ranges (24). In a study conducted on 49 different large mammals, Garland reported that members of carnivora also tended to have larger home ranges when compared to ungulate/herbivore mammals, suggesting that the diversity in home range may be due to food availability (24). This suggestion supports observations from hunter/gatherer populations that foraging ranges increased as local food supplies dwindled until it was more efficient to move the community center to a location with greater food supplies (35). Thus, availability of food may have necessarily impacted physical activity, especially early in the evolution of *Homo sapiens*, so that individuals with greater daily activity were more successful at obtaining food and as a result were at an advantage for reproductive success. There are several studies in other mammalian species suggesting that food availability can be a selection pressure for physiological adaptations. For example, Ariettaz and colleagues (3) showed that within two sibling species of mouse-ear bats, food availability over 13 years of observations within each species niche drove alterations in life-history strategies. Thus, given the linkage between food availability and the regulation of physical activity, as well as existing literature demonstrating that food availability can drive adaptation, it is possible that food availability was a selection pressure that influenced the activity patterns of early mammals.

Mechanisms by which food availability could have been a selection pressure for physical activity control mechanisms are unclear and require further investigation. The adaptations could have been as simple as those animals that were active during times of decreased food availability found more food and thus, were more likely to reproduce, a situation similar to what has been observed in cliff swallows (12). Another hypothesized mechanism that could be applied to understanding how food availability was selective for physical activity control is based on neuroeconomics and the dopamine thrift theory first proposed by Beeler and colleagues (5, 6). The dopamine thrift theory (4) and the later application of neuroeconomics suggest that availability of resources (in this case food) modifies the dopamine response to help the animal determine whether to be active or not to find food (7). As noted, further investigation is needed to determine potential mechanisms through which food availability drove the regulation of physical activity.

Duration of exercise as a potential selection pressure

Recently, it has been suggested that humans evolved faster metabolisms to feed our larger brains in conjunction with an enhanced energy-storing capability through higher levels of adipose tissue and more efficient means of utilizing fat as a fuel source (51). However, this evolutionary trait came with the risk of starvation if the food was not plentiful, especially when humans began to use agriculture to supply food versus hunting and foraging. While many factors played a role in whether a pre-technology farmer would be able to raise adequate foodstuffs, certainly one of the more critical success factors was the willingness of the farmer to be active for the large amounts of time pre-technology agriculture required.

We have previously shown (41) that on a daily basis, males and females across several pre-technology agricultural societies were at least three to five times more active than hunter-gatherers and modern western societies (Figure 7.1) even if their total daily EE (53) were the same. Given these parameters, the farmers' physical activity intensity would have had to be lower to allow for the lengthy duration of physical activity. The lower intensity and longer duration of physical activity would have required the pre-technology farmers to favor fat rather than carbohydrates as a fuel source to fulfill the physical activity energy requirements of agriculture. Thus, we hypothesize that there was a selective advantage in being able to use fat to provide energy for long periods of physical activity at relatively low intensities in successful farmers. Therefore, with the advent of agriculture approximately 11,000 years ago (1), this long duration/low-intensity physical activity requirement, coupled with the more efficient storage of fat in humans (53), may have been a significant selection pressure on physical activity regulating mechanisms. It is unclear how the requirement for longer duration/lower intensity physical activity would have driven the selection of mechanisms regulating physical activity. However, applying the work of Beeler and colleagues regarding dopamine drift (7), the longer duration/lower intensity selection pressure could have exerted a neuroeconomic stimulus such that the dopaminergic mechanisms provided a decreased cost sensitivity resulting in a stimulus for extended activity. Those farmers who had dopamine systems that provided the appropriate cost/benefit ratio in dopamine signaling would have been more likely to be successful and thus, reproduce. However, regardless of how longer duration/lower activity intensities may have driven selection of physical activity regulation, given the relatively recent widespread adoption of agriculture (~11,000 years ago), variants in the genome to regulate physical activity should have developed at approximately the same time as the advent of agriculture.

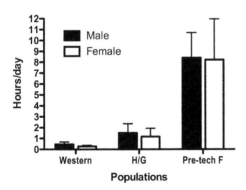

Figure 7.1 Hours per day spent in moderate or vigorous activity per day. Pre-technology farmers were three to five times more active than Western and hunter-gatherer populations. H/G=hunter-gatherer populations; Pre-tech F=pre-technology farmers.
Source: Adapted from data in 41.

Age of associated alleles

Determining the mutation age of alleles associated with physical activity regulation would provide information allowing further consideration of which, if any, processes were involved in the evolution of genetic control of physical activity. For example, if the onset of farming/agriculture was a selection pressure in the development of physical activity regulation, then it would be expected that the genomic alleles associated with activity would be approximately 11,000 years old (1). With the use of physical activity-associated single nucleotide polymorphisms (SNPs) as well as techniques to estimate when alleles mutated (22, 29), it is possible to approximate when physical activity-related SNPs became prominent.

To date, there are four known human-based genome-wide association studies (GWAS) and seven candidate gene studies that have identified physical activity-associated SNPs (13, 16, 19, 26, 32, 44, 45, 64). Within these human-based studies, there are 104 significant SNPs identified as being associated with physical activity. When genomically mapped, these 104 SNPs are in a variety of genomic locations with differing coding outcomes: six are located in exons, 49 are located in introns, one is in a three-prime untranslated region (3′ UTR, potential RNA stabilization), two are considered upstream of a gene (potential promoter/enhancer), three are considered downstream of a gene (potential transcription unit/terminator), and 43 are intergenic. Thus, of the 104 unique physical activity-related SNPs, only the six exon-located SNPs may lead to direct alterations of proteins from that gene. Using an age estimation technique (22) for the average mutation age of the exon-located SNPs, they appeared approximately 478.4 ± 327.5 thousand years ago (kya) in African Americans and 542.1 ± 369.4 kya in European Americans (Figure 7.2). With a total range of 200–1000 kya, these origins are at least as old as the commonly accepted time of emergence of anatomically modern humans (15, 48, 58) and predate the speculated time-frame of when exercise endurance evolved (11) by 4- to 20-fold, suggesting that the activity-associated protein-coding SNPs have been conserved throughout modern human evolution. In fact, the age of the physical activity-related protein-coding SNPs (ranging from 210.5 to 785.2 kya) is considerably older than the average estimated age of all 6515 exon-located human SNPs determined thus far (47.6 ± 1.5 kya African Americans; 34.2 ± 0.9 kya European Americans) (22). Further, the estimated ages of the physical activity-related SNPs would suggest that genetic control of physical activity evolved before the onset of agriculture (~11 kya) (1). However, considering just the age of the physical activity-associated exon-located SNPs, it is unclear whether these SNPs and their relationship to physical activity occurred as the result of one evolutionary event or as an accumulation of many different evolutionary events.

While we have only been able to date the physical activity-associated protein-coding SNPs, when ages can be estimated for the nonprotein-coding activity-related SNPs, a more refined age estimation of the evolution of physical activity regulation will be possible. Additionally, age-dating the nonprotein-coding activity-related SNPs may provide additional information as to whether the evolution of physical activity occurred as one or multiple events. As a very limited illustration of how this nonprotein-coding information may alter our concept of when genomic control of physical activity evolved, consider the estimated mutation age of the only nonprotein-coding physical activity-associated SNP available. Using linkage disequilibrium decay (29), the intron variant rs7910002 of the *DNAJC1* gene was predicted to have developed 7.8 kya, similar in time to the advent of agriculture (1). Thus, including the estimated age of this nonprotein-coding variant suggests that the evolution of the genetic regulation of physical activity may have occurred in multiple eras, with the basic protein-coding genomic variants arising early in the development of modern humans, and further genomic alterations occurring later, possibly in response to various environmental pressures. Further refinement

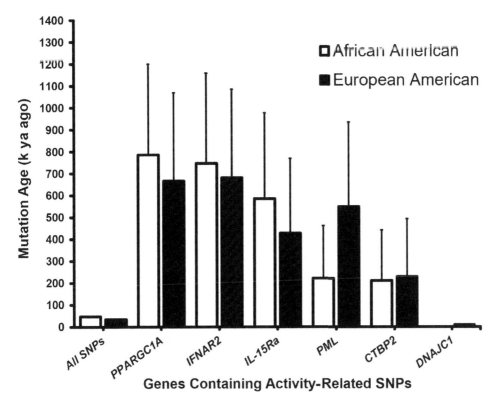

Figure 7.2 Estimated mutation age of SNPs correlated to physical activity. Genes listed on the x-axis contain SNPs related to physical activity. "All SNPs" refers to the 6517 exon-located SNPs in the study by Fu et al. (22).

of the estimates of when genetic control of physical activity arose will be supported by future determination of any additional physical activity-associated SNPs as well as the identification of the actual mechanisms involved.

A secondary purpose of estimating the age of physical activity-associated SNPs is to determine whether animal models are likely to have similar genetic mechanisms underlying the regulation of physical activity. For example, given that the evolutionary divergence of humans and chimpanzees has been estimated to have occurred between 6.23–7.07 million years ago (mya; 8, 30), our estimates of when human activity-related SNPs evolved (average of ~478–542 kya) suggest humans may not share the same genetic regulators of activity as do primates. Using a similar approach, given that the evolutionary split between humans and mice has been estimated to have occurred approximately 62–100 mya (8, 30), suggests there may be different genetic mechanisms controlling activity in humans and mice. However, we urge extreme caution in interpreting these limited data to indicate the absence of similarities between genetic regulation of activity in humans and other species. In particular, the extremely small set of associated genomic SNPs, the lack of understanding regarding all the genetic factors regulating physical activity (e.g., miRNA, epigenetics), the uncertainty of whether physical activity genetic regulation arose with one event or multiple events, and whether genomic SNPs actually indicate all genetic mechanisms involved in physical activity regulation (20, 21), significantly weaken any cross-species application of our SNP-age data.

Table 7.1 Human, Neanderthal, and chimpanzee allele comparisons of physical activity phenotypes

rs ID	Gene	Effect allele[a]	Neanderthal[b]	Ancestral allele[c]	Allele frequency[d]
rs1051393	**IFNAR2**	**Not given**	**DDDDAD:0D1A**	**G>A/G/T**	**0.003/38/62**
rs16933006	Closest *RPL7P3*	C	AAADAA:0D2A	A>A/C	82/17
rs6025590	CTCFL	G	DAAAA_:0D1A	G>A/G	27/73
rs6454672	CNR1	C	AADAAA:1D0A	T>C/T	15/85
rs8066276	ACE	T	DAD_DA:0D1A	C>C/T	38/62
rs2267668	**PPARD**	**A**	**DDDDAA:0D1A**	**A>A/G**	**85/15**
rs1638525	**AKAP10**	**G**	**DADDAD:0D1A**	**G>C/G**	**61/39**
rs35622985	MMS22L	G	AAAADA:0D1A	G>A/G	27/73
rs1959759	DCAF5	A	ADDDAA:0D2A	A>A/G	18/82
rs10851869	PML	T	D_A_AA:0D1A	C>C/T	43/56
rs10145335	**Closest C14ord177**	**G**	**DDDDAD:0D1A**	**A>A/G**	**20/80**
rs113351744	Closest *LINC01029*	G	AADAAA:0D1A	G>A/G	2/98
rs12460611	Closest *CCNE1*	A	AA_DAA:0D3A	A>A/G	83/17

a Allele associated with higher amount of physical activity.

b First six characters represent the allele present in Human Reference San, Yoruba, Han, Papuan, and French populations, A=ancestral, D=derived, or _ if not known. Following the colon is the amount of derived or ancestral alleles in Neanderthal genomes. Bold suggests a selective sweep may have occurred in the *Homo sapiens* lineage.

c The first character represents the chimpanzee reference allele followed by human alleles.

d Allele frequency=UCSC allele frequencies of human genome found in Ancestral Allelew column.

Due to the overlap of the historical timelines of *Homo sapiens* and *Homo neanderthalensis* and the suggested gene flow (i.e., interbreeding) between the two species (33), it is possible to compare allele frequencies to determine if any physical activity-associated SNPs underwent positive selection (i.e., selective sweeps) between the two species (28). Presence of a selective sweep would suggest that a particular SNP provided increased survivability or reproductive fitness for *Homo sapiens*. Thus, we compared modern-day human SNPs related to physical activity to Neanderthal genotypes analyzed by Green et al. (28) using the chimpanzee reference genome to characterize ancestral genes. Due to incomplete genetic reading and high mutation rates at CpG sites in the Neanderthal DNA, we can only determine signs of selective sweeps for 29 of the 104 physical activity-related SNPs. Of these 29 SNPs, four (rs1051393 exon in *IFNAR2*, rs2267668 intron in *PPARD*, rs1638525 intron of *AKAP10*, and rs10145335 intergenic region near *C14ord177*) were among the top 5% strongest signals of selective sweeps among a total of 3,202,190 substitutions and 69,029 indels sequenced (Table 7.1). The strength of these selective sweeps suggest strong positive selection pressures in *Homo sapiens'* history compared to Neanderthals for these particular mutations, i.e., *Homo sapiens* were more likely to inherit these physical activity-related SNPs. Thus, selective sweeps that have occurred since the divergence of *Homo sapiens* and *Homo neanderthalensis* may suggests a genetic regulation of physical activity unique to *Homo sapiens*.

As noted earlier, evolution can occur through selection pressure, mutation, or genetic drift. Albeit with the limited state of current knowledge, it appears that genomic variants that are correlated with physical activity levels play a role in a wide variety of biological mechanisms (see Chapters 5, 6, 8, and 9), each with low effect sizes (i.e., physical activity levels between individuals with different alleles are not largely different). Thus, due to the few physical activity-related

SNPs that have hypothesized selective sweeps (4 of 104) and/or large effect sizes (0 of 104), in conjunction with the small community populations that existed 478–542 kya, it is likely that genetic drift is the major evolutionary process responsible for the genetic mechanisms that control physical activity in humans. If it is the case that the majority of physical activity regulators do not significantly influence reproductive viability in humans, especially in modern society (41), the lack of a mutation in genetic sequences associated with physical activity which do not kill or lower the host's reproductive fitness (also known as stabilizing selection) could explain why it appears the genetic mechanisms are highly diverse across species. Because of the lack of large effect sizes for the physical activity-related genomic variants, we hypothesize that the genes containing the identified SNPs have a different primary function and only affect physical activity indirectly. Supporting this hypothesis is a recent paper by Xu and Garland (65) where they compared the genomic structure of four mouse lines which have been independently bred for high physical activity since 1993. Xu and Garland surprisingly found that the genomic structure associated with physical activity in these independent lines were largely different and thus, these independent lines had evolved differing genomic approaches to increasing physical activity levels. Applied to the current question, it is possible that humans have evolved a variety of genetic mechanisms that control physical activity and the mechanisms that have evolved depend somewhat on the population and the environmental exposures of the population. Given the known population differences arising in the current large-scale genomic mapping efforts such as the International HapMap Consortium (2), it would not be surprising to discover multiple genetic mechanisms control physical activity.

Conclusion

The literature is very clear that physical activity is critical to health; however, physical activity levels continue to be low in most human populations. While genetics have been clearly shown to be an important factor in determining physical activity level, the exact genetic mechanisms that regulate physical activity are still elusive. We have continued to explore how the physical activity genetic regulating mechanisms may have evolved in the hope of informing future mechanistic investigations. We provide Figure 7.3 as a summary of potential evolutionary processes and factors that may have been involved in the development of genetic mechanisms that regulate physical activity, building from the foundation of the pyramid toward the current-day physical activity regulation. From the existing literature, it is unlikely that EE was a selection pressure that drove the evolution of physical activity genetic regulation. However, given the inverse relationship between food availability and physical activity, the hypothesized food availability selection pressure that helped evolve homeostatic control of daily EE may have also been involved in the evolution of physical activity regulation mechanisms. Since pre-technology farming populations generally exhibit much higher daily levels of physical activity duration than either Western or hunter-gatherer populations, this suggests that longer durations of daily activity coupled with lower intensities may have played a role in the development of the genetic physical activity regulating mechanisms. Attractive recent theories grounded in neuroeconomic theory regarding "dopamine thrift" suggest potential mechanisms through which longer duration/lower activity intensities and food availability pressures could have affected genetic control mechanisms. Juxtaposed against these theories are our calculations of 478–542 kya as the estimated age of the few protein-coding human genomic variants that are currently associated with physical activity. This time frame is much older than the onset of agriculture in human populations, arguing against a role for agriculture in the development of these protein-coding genomic variants. However, while extremely tentative, dating of one of the nonprotein-coding

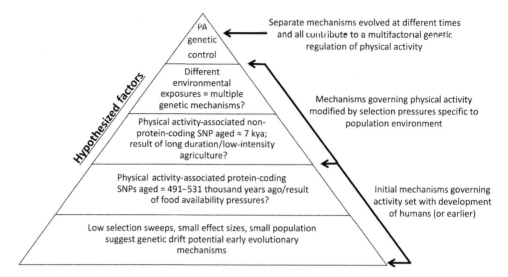

Figure 7.3 Summary of potential evolutionary processes that developed genetic control of physical activity. We propose that the foundational physical activity (PA) genetic regulatory mechanisms (base of the pyramid) were evolved early in the development of *Homo erectus* through genetic drift mechanisms. Later evolution of physical activity regulation (moving up the pyramid) was in response to selection pressure (e.g., finding food), leading to the current mechanisms that regulate physical activity. ★These extrapolations are based on current data and subject to change with an increase in aging data available.

SNPs associated with physical activity put the age of development of that variant near the onset of widespread agriculture. Thus, given the available data, we would propose that the foundational evolutionary process that *initially* resulted in genetic mechanisms that control physical activity was genetic drift (Figure 7.3), as opposed to either selection or mutation. We further propose that these initial genetic drift-induced mechanisms were altered in particular populations by differing environmental pressures (e.g., food availability, demands of agriculture) at differing times (Figure 7.3), resulting in a variety of genetic solutions to physical activity. Thus, in conclusion, we hypothesize that the genetic control of physical activity in humans may include a combination of mechanisms that arose in different time periods.

We acknowledge that many of our conclusions are based on extrapolations from extremely limited data sets. However, this type of investigation is critical in working toward an understanding of the biological and environmental factors that shaped humans' physical activity-regulating mechanisms. As such, our investigations present a framework by which future genomic-associated information can be further used to refine insights into the responsible physical activity-regulating mechanisms as well as the appropriateness of specific animal models.

Acknowledgments: This work was supported by funding from the Omar Smith Endowment at Texas A&M University.

References

1. **Abbo S, Lev–Yadun S** and **Gopher A.** Plant domestication and crop evolution in the near east: On events and processes. *Crit Rev Plant Sci* 31: 241–257, 2012.
2. **Altshuler DM, Gibbs RA, Peltonen L, Altshuler DM, Gibbs RA, Peltonen L, Dermitzakis E, Schaffner SF, Yu F, Peltonen L, Dermitzakis E, Bonnen PE, Altshuler DM, Gibbs RA,**

de Bakker PI, Deloukas P, Gabriel SB, Gwilliam R, Hunt S, Inouye M, Jia X, Palotie A, Parkin M, Whittaker P, Yu F, Chang K, Hawes A, Lewis LR, Ren Y, Wheeler D, Gibbs RA, Muzny DM, Barnes C, Darvishi K, Hurles M, Korn JM, Kristiansson K, Lee C, McCarrol SA, Nemesh J, Dermitzakis E, Keinan A, Montgomery SB, Pollack S, Price AL, Soranzo N, Bonnen PE, Gibbs RA, Gonzaga-Jauregui C, Keinan A, Price AL, Yu F, Anttila V, Brodeur W, Daly MJ, Leslie S, McVean G, Moutsianas L, Nguyen H, Schaffner SF, Zhang Q, Ghori MJ, McGinnis R, McLaren W, Pollack S, Price AL, Schaffner SF, Takeuchi F, Grossman SR, Shlyakhter I, Hostetter EB, Sabeti PC, Adebamowo CA, Foster MW, Gordon DR, Licinio J, Manca MC, Marshall PA, Matsuda I, Ngare D, Wang VO, Reddy D, Rotimi CN, Royal CD, Sharp RR, Zeng C, Brooks LD and McEwen JE. Integrating common and rare genetic variation in diverse human populations. *Nature* 467: 52–58, 2010.

3. **Arlettaz R, Christe P** and **Schaub M.** Food availability as a major driver in the evolution of life-history strategies of sibling species. *Ecol Evol* 7: 4163–4172, 2017.

4. **Beeler JA.** Thorndike's law 2.0: Dopamine and the regulation of thrift. *Front Neurosci* 6: 116, 2012.

5. **Beeler JA, Frazier CR** and **Zhuang X.** Dopaminergic enhancement of local food-seeking is under global homeostatic control. *Eur J Neurosci* 35: 146–159, 2012.

6. **Beeler JA, McCutcheon JE, Cao ZF, Murakami M, Alexander E, Roitman MF** and **Zhuang X.** Taste uncoupled from nutrition fails to sustain the reinforcing properties of food. *Eur J Neurosci* 36: 2533–2546, 2012.

7. **Beeler JA** and **Mourra D.** To do or not to do: Dopamine, affordability and the economics of opportunity. *Front Integr Neurosci* 12: 6, 2018.

8. **Benton MJ** and **Donoghue PC.** Paleontological evidence to date the tree of life. *Mol Biol Evol* 24: 26–53, 2007.

9. **Bjursell M, Gerdin AK, Lelliott CJ, Egecioglu E, Elmgren A, Törnell J, Oscarsson J** and **Bohlooly- Y M.** Acutely reduced locomotor activity is a major contributor to Western diet-induced obesity in mice. *Am J Physiol Endocrinol Metab* 294: E251–E260, 2008.

10. **Bouchard C, Rankinen T, Chagnon YC, Rice T, Pérusse L, Gagnon J, Borecki I, An P, Leon AS, Skinner JS, Wilmore JH, Province M** and **Rao DC.** Genomic scan for maximal oxygen uptake and its response to training in the HERITAGE Family Study. *J Appl Physiol (1985)* 88: 551–559, 2000.

11. **Bramble DM** and **Lieberman DE.** Endurance running and the evolution of Homo. *Nature* 432: 345–352, 2004.

12. **Brown CR, Brown MB, Roche EA, O'Brien VA** and **Page CE.** Fluctuating survival selection explains variation in avian group size. *Proc Natl Acad Sci U S A* 113: 5113–5118, 2016.

13. **Bruneau M, Walsh S, Selinsky E, Ash G, Angelopoulos TJ, Clarkson P, Gordon P, Moyna N, Visich P, Zoeller R, Thompson P, Gordish-Dressman H, Hoffman E, Devaney J** and **Pescatello LS.** A genetic variant in IL-15Rα correlates with physical activity among European-American adults. *Mol Genet Genomic Med* 6: 401–408, 2018.

14. **Casper RC.** The "drive for activity" and "restlessness" in anorexia nervosa: Potential pathways. *J Affect Disord* 92: 99–107, 2006.

15. **Chase PG, Dibble HL, Lindly J, Clark G** and **Guy L.** On the emergence of modern humans. *Current Anthropology* 31: 58–66, 1990.

16. **Comuzzie AG, Cole SA, Laston SL, Voruganti VS, Haack K, Gibbs RA** and **Butte NF.** Novel genetic loci identified for the pathophysiology of childhood obesity in the Hispanic population. *PLoS One* 7: e51954, 2012.

17. **Courtney SM** and **Massett MP.** Identification of exercise capacity QTL using association mapping in inbred mice. *Physiol Genomics* 44: 948–955, 2012.

18. **Darwin C.** The preservation of favoured races in the struggle for life. In: *On the Origin of Species by Means of Natural Section.* London: J. Murray, 1859, Chapt. 14.

19. **De Moor MH, Liu YJ, Boomsma DI, Li J, Hamilton JJ, Hottenga JJ, Levy S, Liu XG, Pei YF, Posthuma D, Recker RR, Sullivan PF, Wang L, Willemsen G, Yan H, DeGeus EJ** and **Deng HW.** Genome-wide association study of exercise behavior in Dutch and American adults. *Med Sci Sports Exerc* 41: 1887–1895, 2009.

20. **Ferguson DP, Dangott LJ, Schmitt EE, Vellers HL** and **Lightfoot JT.** Differential skeletal muscle proteome of high- and low-active mice. *J Appl Physiol* 116: 1057–1067, 2014.

21. **Ferguson DP, Dangott LJ, Vellers HL, Schmitt EE** and **Lightfoot JT.** Differential protein expression in the nucleus accumbens of high and low active mice. *Behav Brain Res* 291: 283–288, 2015.

22. **Fu W, O'Connor TD, Jun G, Kang HM, Abecasis G, Leal SM, Gabriel S, Rieder MJ, Altshuler D, Shendure J, Nickerson DA, Bamshad MJ, NHLBI ESP** and **Akey JM.** Analysis of 6,515 exomes reveals the recent origin of most human protein-coding variants. *Nature* 493: 216–220, 2013.

23. **Funkat A, Massa CM, Jovanovska V, Proietto J** and **Andrikopoulos S.** Metabolic adaptations of three inbred strains of mice (C57BL/6, DBA/2, and 129T2) in response to a high-fat diet. *J Nutr* 134: 3264–3269, 2004.

24. **Garland T, Jr, Dickerman A, Janis C** and **Jones J.** Phylogenetic analysis of covariance by computer simulation. *Syst Biol* 42: 265–292, 1993.

25. **Garland T, Jr** and **Kelly SA.** Phenotypic plasticity and experimental evolution. *J Exp Biol* 209: 2344–2361, 2006.

26. **Gielen M, Westerterp-Plantenga MS, Bouwman FG, Joosen AM, Vlietinck R, Derom C, Zeegers MP, Mariman EC** and **Westerterp KR.** Heritability and genetic etiology of habitual physical activity: A twin study with objective measures. *Genes Nutr* 9: 415, 2014.

27. **Goodrick CL, Ingram DK, Reynolds MA, Freeman JR** and **Cider NL.** Effects of intermittent feeding upon growth, activity, and lifespan in rats allowed voluntary exercise. *Exp Aging Res* 9: 203–209, 1983.

28. **Green RE, Krause J, Briggs AW, Maricic T, Stenzel U, Kircher M, Patterson N, Li H, Zhai W, Fritz MH, Hansen NF, Durand EY, Malaspinas AS, Jensen JD, Marques-Bonet T, Alkan C, Prüfer K, Meyer M, Burbano HA, Good JM, Schultz R, Aximu-Petri A, Butthof A, Höber B, Höffner B, Siegemund M, Weihmann A, Nusbaum C, Lander ES, Russ C, Novod N, Affourtit J, Egholm M, Verna C, Rudan P, Brajkovic D, Kucan Ž, Gušic I, Doronichev VB, Golovanova LV, Lalueza-Fox C, de la Rasilla M, Fortea J, Rosas A, Schmitz RW, Johnson PLF, Eichler EE, Falush D, Birney E, Mullikin JC, Slatkin M, Nielsen R, Kelso J, Lachmann M, Reich D** and **Pääbo S.** A draft sequence of the Neandertal genome. *Science* 328: 710–722, 2010.

29. **Hawks J, Wang ET, Cochran GM, Harpending HC** and **Moyzis RK.** Recent acceleration of human adaptive evolution. *Proc Natl Acad Sci U S A* 104: 20753–20758, 2007.

30. **Hedges SB, Dudley J** and **Kumar S.** TimeTree: a public knowledge-base of divergence times among organisms. *Bioinformatics* 22: 2971–2972, 2006.

31. **Kleiber M.** Body size and metabolic rate. *Physiol Rev* 27: 511–541, 1947.

32. **Klimentidis YC, Raichlen DA, Bea J, Garcia DO, Mandarino LJ, Alexander GE, Chen Z** and **Going SB.** Genome-wide association study of habitual physical activity in over 277,000 UK Biobank participants identifies multiple variants including CADM2 and APOE. *Int J Obesity* 42: 1161–1176, 2018.

33. **Kuhlwilm M, Gronau I, Hubisz MJ, de Filippo C, Prado-Martinez J, Kircher M, Fu Q, Burbano HA, Lalueza-Fox C, de la Rasilla M, Rosas A, Rudan P, Brajkovic D, Kucan Ž, Gušic I, Marques-Bonet T, Andrés AM, Viola B, Pääbo S, Meyer M, Siepel A** and **Castellano S.** Ancient gene flow from early modern humans into Eastern Neanderthals. *Nature* 530: 429–433, 2016.

34. **Lamb KL** and **Brodie DA.** Leisure-time physical activity as an estimate of physical fitness: A validation study. *J Clin Epidemiol* 44: 41–52, 1991.

35. **Lee RB.** *The Dobe Ju/'hoansi* (3rd ed.). Belmont, CA: Wadsworth Publishing, 2003.

36. **Lerman I, Harrison BC, Freeman K, Hewett TE, Allen DL, Robbins J** and **Leinwand LA.** Genetic variability in forced and voluntary endurance exercise performance in seven inbred mouse strains. *J Appl Physiol* 92: 2245–2255, 2002.

37. **Levine JA, McCrady SK, Lanningham-Foster LM, Kane PH, Foster RC** and **Manohar CU.** The role of free-living daily walking in human weight gain and obesity. *Diabetes* 57: 548–554, 2008.

38. **Lightfoot JT, Leamy LJ, Pomp D, Turner MJ, Fodor AA, Knab AM, Bowen RS, Ferguson DP, Moore-Harrison T** and **Hamilton A.** Strain screen and haplotype association mapping of wheel running in inbred mouse strains. *J Appl Physiol* 109: 623–634, 2010.

39. **Lightfoot JT, Bamman MM** and **Booth FW.** Translation goes both ways: The power of reverse translation from human trials into animal models. *Transl J Am Coll Sports Med* 2: 1–3, 2017.

40. **Lightfoot JT, Turner MJ, Pomp D, Kleeberger SR** and **Leamy LJ.** Quantitative trait loci (QTL) for physical activity traits in mice. *Physiol Genomics* 32: 401–408, 2008.

41. **Lightfoot JT.** Why control activity? Evolutionary selection pressures affecting the development of physical activity genetic and biological regulation. *Biomed Res Int* 2013: 821678, 2013.

42. **Lightfoot JT, De Geus EJC, Booth FW, Bray MS, den Hoed M, Kaprio J, Kelly SA, Pomp D, Saul MC, Thomis MA, Garland T** and **Bouchard C.** Biological/genetic regulation of physical activity level: Consensus from GenBioPAC. *Med Sci Sports Exerc In Press*: 2018.
43. **Lightfoot JT, Turner MJ, Knab AK, Jedlicka AE, Oshimura T, Marzec J, Gladwell W, Leamy LJ** and **Kleeberger SR.** Quantitative trait loci associated with maximal exercise endurance in mice. *J Appl Physiol (1985)* 103: 105–110, 2007.
44. **Lin X, Chan KK, Huang YT, Luo X, Liang L, Wilson J, Correa A, Levy D** and **Liu S.** Genetic determinants for leisure-time physical activity. *Med Sci Sports Exerc* 50: 1620–1628, 2018.
45. **Mäestu J, Lätt E, Rääsk T, Sak K, Laas K, Jürimäe J** and **Jürimäe T.** Ace I/D polymorphism is associated with habitual physical activity in pubertal boys. *J Physiol Sci* 63: 427–434, 2013.
46. **Maslow AH.** A theory of human motivation. *Psychol Rev* 50: 370–396, 1943.
47. **Meijer JH** and **Robbers Y.** Wheel running in the wild. *Proc Roy Soc B* 281: 20140210, 2014.
48. **Nitecki MH** and **Nitecki DV**. *Origins of Anatomically Modern Humans.* New York: Springer, 1994.
49. **Pontzer H.** Constrained total energy expenditure and the evolutionary biology of energy balance. *Exerc Sport Sci Rev* 43: 110–116, 2015.
50. **Pontzer H.** The crown joules: Energetics, ecology, and evolution in humans and other primates. *Evol Anthropol* 26: 12–24, 2017.
51. **Pontzer H, Brown MH, Raichlen DA, Dunsworth H, Hare B, Walker K, Luke A, Dugas LR, Durazo-Arvizu R, Schoeller D, Plange-Rhule J, Bovet P, Forrester TE, Lambert EV, Thompson ME, Shumaker RW** and **Ross SR.** Metabolic acceleration and the evolution of human brain size and life history. *Nature* 533: 390–392, 2016.
52. **Pontzer H, Durazo-Arvizu R, Dugas LR, Plange-Rhule J, Bovet P, Forrester TE, Lambert EV, Cooper RS, Schoeller DA** and **Luke A.** Constrained total energy expenditure and metabolic adaptation to physical activity in adult humans. *Curr Biol* 26: 410–417, 2016.
53. **Pontzer H, Raichlen DA, Wood BM, Mabulla AZ, Racette SB** and **Marlowe FW.** Hunter-gatherer energetics and human obesity. *PLoS One* 7: e40503, 2012.
54. **Powell R.** The future of human evolution. *Brit J Phil Sci* 63: 145–175, 2012.
55. **Rendeiro C, Masnik AM, Mun JG, Du K, Clark D, Dilger RN, Dilger AC** and **Rhodes JS.** Fructose decreases physical activity and increases body fat without affecting hippocampal neurogenesis and learning relative to an isocaloric glucose diet. *Sci Rep* 5: 9589, 2015.
56. **Rico-Sanz J, Rankinen T, Rice T, Leon AS, Skinner JS, Wilmore JH, Rao DC** and **Bouchard C.** Quantitative trait loci for maximal exercise capacity phenotypes and their responces to training in the HERITAGE Family Study. *Physiol Genomics* 16: 256–260, 2004.
57. **Schmidt SL, Harmon KA, Sharp TA, Kealey EH** and **Bessesen DH.** The effects of overfeeding on spontaneous physical activity in obesity prone and obesity resistant humans. *Obesity (Silver Spring)* 20: 2186–2193, 2012.
58. **Smith FH, Falsetti AB** and **Donnelly SM.** Modern human origins. *Am J Phys Anthrop* 32: 35–68, 1989.
59. **Stephens DW** and **Krebs JW**. *Foraging Theory.* Princeton, NJ: Princeton University Press, 1986.
60. **Theobald DL.** A formal test of the theory of universal common ancestry. *Nature* 465: 219–222, 2010.
61. **Vellers HL, Letsinger AC, Walker NR, Granados JZ** and **Lightfoot JT.** High fat high sugar diet reduces voluntary wheel running in mice independent of sex hormone involvement. *Front Physiol* 8: 628, 2017.
62. **Washburn SL** and **Lancaster CS.** The evolution of hunting. In: *Man The Hunter*, edited by Lee RB and Irven D. Chicago, IL: Aldine Publishing Company, 1968, p. 293–303.
63. **Westerterp KR** and **Speakman JR.** Physical activity energy expenditure has not declined since the 1980s and matches energy expenditures of wild mammals. *Int J Obesity* 32: 1256–1263, 2008.
64. **Wilkinson AV, Gabriel KP, Wang J, Bondy ML, Dong Q, Wu X, Shete S** and **Spitz MR.** Sensation-seeking genes and physical activity in youth. *Genes Brain Behav* 12: 181–188, 2013.
65. **Xu S** and **Garland T**, Jr. A mixed model approach to genome-wide association studies for selection signatures, with application to mice bred for voluntary exercise behavior. *Genetics* 207: 785–799, 2017.
66. **Yamada Y, Colman RJ, Kemnitz JW, Baum ST, Anderson RM, Weindruch R** and **Schoeller DA.** Long-term calorie restriction decreases metabolic cost of movement and prevents decrease of physical activity during aging in rhesus monkeys. *Exp Gerontol* 48: 1226–1235, 2013.

8

NEUROGENETICS OF MOTIVATION FOR PHYSICAL ACTIVITY

Justin S. Rhodes

Introduction

Movement is energetically costly, yet many animals travel vast distances as part of their normal life history. From a Darwinian evolutionary perspective, this would be unexpected unless it provided some fitness advantage for survival or reproductive success. Movement is often necessary to find food, shelter, or mates. Therefore, it is generally assumed that gene frequencies have been shaped by natural selection to support varying levels of physical activity depending on the local ecological conditions. At least two components are necessary for an individual to perform a voluntary behavior of any kind: they must be physically capable of performing the behavior and they must be motivated to do it. Both processes involve biological traits that are moldable by evolution and which, in part, shape genetic variation in physical activity levels. Physical constraints such as aerobic capacity (the maximal amount of oxygen an organism can consume during maximal physical exertion), muscle mass or composition, bone symmetry, and many others limit the ability of animals to move quickly or travel long distances (30). Hence, if ecological conditions demand that the animal displays challenging physical acts at the limit of their physical capability to survive and reproduce, then that will lead to the evolution of increased capacity for these exercise physiological features, to the extent that they are heritable.

While physical capability sets the upper limit for what an animal can possibly accomplish, animals typically choose not to perform at their limit. A substantial portion of variation in physical activity levels is expected to arise from differences in motivation for physical exertion (79). The exercise physiological features that animals are genetically endowed with (including the full extent of phenotypic plasticity) are usually far in excess of what the animal requires on a daily basis or even within a lifetime. Consider sedentary humans compared to marathon runners: the big difference is motivation not muscles (or capability). While it is certainly true that individuals are constrained by the exercise physiological capacities they are endowed with, and there are real biological differences between good and average marathon runners, the point is that most people possess the physical capability of training their bodies to accomplish a marathon, but they choose not to. On an evolutionary time scale, the principle that motivation contributes to behavioral variation applies equally well. Consider the long-standing idea that behavior evolves first, before specialized morphological and physiological adaptations arise (7, 43). There are many interesting examples of this phenomenon in currently living species such as marine iguanas in the Galapagos which basically are the same as mainland iguanas except for their behavior of swimming in the ocean (20). They have no special scales, webbed feet, or fins which other marine reptiles possess for swimming, because they haven't existed on earth long enough in the marine environment for these morphological features to evolve. However, one organ that probably has evolved slightly already is the iguana's brain that leads them to want to enter the marine environment and swim to obtain their food. This supports the "behavior evolves first" idea that the evolution of motivational systems in the brain precedes morphological adaptations in the periphery.

The "behavior evolves first" idea is also supported by direct experimental evidence. Over the last 25 years, Theodore Garland's group has conducted a replicated artificial selection experiment for increased voluntary wheel running in house mice (88, 94). If you look at the timeline of the discoveries, overall results suggest that the big changes initially were in neurological traits related to motivation (77–80), and then later changes in exercise physiological traits such as muscle phenotypes (41), aerobic capacity (76), and bone symmetry (31) became more evident. The interpretation is that in initial generations, variation in running was mostly attributed to differences in motivation to run, i.e., the reason why one mouse ran 5 km per day and another 1 km per day was not because of any differences in physical capability between the mice but rather because of differences in their intrinsic motivation for running. Several generations of selection increased motivation to a local maximum during which time variation in exercise physiological features became more and more significant contributors to the individual variation. As a result, changes in exercise physiological traits became more apparent in later generations. Taken together, these data strongly support the notion that motivation for physical activity can evolve, and is an important component of individual and species-level differences in activity levels. These data further imply that if the goal is to find genetic factors involved in the evolution of physical activity levels, then understanding how genes influence motivation to engage in the behavior is of paramount importance.

The purpose of this chapter is to provide an updated review on what is known about genetic variation underlying motivation for physical activity levels across individuals and species. The material is relevant in the broad sense, for understanding how behavior evolves, but also important in the narrower sense for human health. Arguably the single most important factor that has contributed to the decline of health in Western society is our increasingly sedentary lifestyle, which contributes to metabolic syndrome (28), obesity (65), diabetes (42), heart disease (67), stroke (55), and cancer (63). Not only is physical activity crucial for maintaining physical health, but evidence accumulated over the past 30 years has established that there are profound benefits of exercise on mental health as well (21, 39). Exercise is a useful strategy for coping with stress (37), treating depression (89), preventing relapse in drugs abuse (11), and delaying cognitive aging (16). Randomized human clinical trials have established that walking quickly for 40 minutes a day, three times a week for 6 months results in changes in brain functional and anatomical measures which support the pro-cognitive outcomes (24). An enormous literature in rodent models has established profound effects of exercise on brain anatomy, chemistry, and physiology providing mechanistic support for pro-cognitive outcomes (as reviewed in 18, 19, 97). One of the highlights of this literature is the landmark discovery that several weeks of voluntary wheel running increases the formation of entire new neurons in the dentate gyrus, a region of the brain crucial for learning and memory (96). Taken together, what this means for medicine is that we already know how to prevent the bulk of our health problems in a pretty broad sweeping way, and we usually have the physical capability to do it, yet we generally lack the motivation. Therefore, understanding genetic pathways which increase motivation for physical activity could have broad implications for preventative medicine.

The natural reward circuit as a molding block for evolution of behavior

The natural reward circuit is defined as a collection of interconnected brain regions involved in the perception of pleasure. In the 1950s, Olds and Milner conducted experiments with rats placed in operant boxes in which a lever could be pressed by the rat on a voluntary basis that would deliver mild electric shocks to various parts of the brain through differential placement of the electrode (69). They discovered that the rats would learn to self-administer shocks when the electrode was placed in numerous places throughout the brain. However, when they placed the electrode in certain regions, results were particularly striking. If the electrode was placed anywhere along the medial forebrain bundle, the axonal projections from the ventral tegmental area to the nucleus accumbens, or passing through the lateral hypothalamus, the rats would display an extraordinary motivation for the shock to the point of pressing so often as to forgo eating, drinking, and sleeping (Figure 8.1) (69). It is interesting to note from the original work that rats self-administered shocks to many different regions throughout the brain, suggesting the existence of an extended reward circuit that includes most of the brain (64, 100). This is consistent with the idea that a lot of real estate in the brain is involved in the perception of reward, and that a fundamental function of the brain, the organ which shapes behavior, is reward processing, in a manner that informs decision-making.

If one extends the idea of the stimulating electrode to extrinsic stimuli which are naturally capable of electrically activating the same circuit (albeit at a physiological level, and much less intensely than the electrode), then one way to coerce animals to behave a certain way is to make the behavior result in the electrical activation of the reward circuit and thereby perception of reward. In other words, if genes regulated the development of neural circuits in the brain in such a way that high levels of physical activity were perceived as rewarding because they activated the reward circuit and served as a positive reinforcer, then individuals would choose to display heightened activity. Therefore, the next logical question to ask is how physical activity stimulates

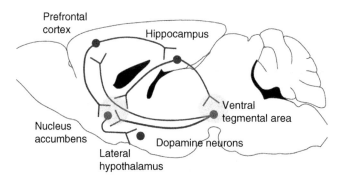

Figure 8.1   The natural reward circuit. A simplified illustration of interactions between the hippocampus and the natural reward circuit in the rodent brain. Forceful movement activates the hippocampus in proportion to the intensity or effort. The ventral midbrain and the nucleus accumbens, core nodes of the natural reward circuit, receive input from the hippocampus (32, 51). The highlighted areas indicate places where the neurophysiology may differ between individuals highly motivated for activity as compared to those less motivated. If the hippocampal input results in stronger activation of the ascending limb of the reward circuit through dopamine innervation of the nucleus accumbens, and prefrontal cortex, and subsequent activation of the lateral hypothalamus, physical activity would be reinforced. The precise cellular and molecular signatures and underlying sequence variants responsible for motivating physical activity as distinguished from other natural or artificial rewards (such as drugs of abuse) are not known and are currently actively being investigated.

the natural reward circuit, and what the difference is between the reward circuit of an animal that is unmotivated for physical activity versus an animal that is highly motivated for physical activity and which seeks out physical activity despite its high energetic costs and generation of fatigue. Here we come to a point where it starts getting complicated, because the old view that it will be one molecule or even a few has proven false (23). The reality is more likely a story about billions of neurons interacting with each other and with glial cells, with complex chemical signaling pathways involving hundreds if not thousands of molecules. These signaling pathways transmit information from one cell to the next, but there are numerous receptors and neurochemicals implicated at any one synapse. Realistically, it is a combination of multiple mixes that influence reward processing and that distinguish physical activity reward from other natural rewards or drugs of abuse.

Beyond dopamine

Dopamine has historically been considered the substrate for reward, and there is abundant evidence in the literature supporting this idea (91, 103). For example, dopamine levels increase in extracellular spaces in the nucleus accumbens in response to inherently rewarding stimuli such as sweet flavor (61), orgasms (72), and drugs of abuse (102). Moreover, the dopamine release depends critically on the perceived rewarding value of the stimuli which can change depending on the circumstances. In one study, rats were fed either a diet deficient or replete with salt, and then administered a saline solution directly into the mouth and extracellular dopamine in the nucleus accumbens was measured using carbon fiber voltammetry methods. This showed that the saline solution elicited a dopamine response only when the rats were deprived of salt, not when the diet contained sufficient salt. Moreover, the dopamine response was severely reduced in the salt-deprived rats if the salt taste receptors were pharmacologically blocked (17). In addition, the same group in a different study found clear evidence, as others have, that a bitter solution that elicits an aversive taste reaction reduces dopamine release (62). Taken together these data suggest that dopamine release in response to a stimulus is context dependent and matches the perceived rewarding value of the stimulus, rather than a direct response to the perception of the stimulus itself. Furthermore, these data constitute strong recent evidence in support of the dopamine reward hypothesis, demonstrating that stimuli that are perceived as rewarding increase dopamine in the nucleus accumbens (103).

On the other hand, serious questions have been raised about the validity of the hypothesis that dopamine is a substrate for reward as opposed to a more general role for dopamine as a salience detector, or in learning (5, 87). First, dopamine-deficient mice appear to find sweet flavor rewarding, and display the normal preference for sweet solutions, suggesting dopamine is not necessary for reward (14). More recent studies have established that dopamine-deficient mice can also perceive opioid reward (40). Second, stress and pain have also been found to increase dopamine in the nucleus accumbens, suggesting dopamine release is not specific to reward (1, 48, 85). In light of the conflicting evidence, it has been suggested that dopamine is released into the nucleus accumbens in response to an emotionally important event but does not distinguish between aversive and rewarding qualities, at least at this level of biological organization (nucleus accumbens dopamine as a whole) (85, 87). The large literature suggesting a role for dopamine in regulating neuronal plasticity, and especially reinforcement learning, supports this idea (4, 73, 86, 90, 101).

In light of the fact that physical activity involves rewarding and aversive emotional reactions, and that dopamine also functions in voluntary control of movement through the nigrostriatal pathway (35, 58), it is not surprising that the dopamine signaling pathway has been implicated in genetics of increased physical activity in several model systems now (10, 27, 53, 60, 79, 81, 83, 84, 99). However, the simple hypothesis that the difference would be in the amount of dopamine released or in the number of receptors has turned out to be false. For example, in the replicated selective breeding experiment for increased voluntary wheel running referenced previously, we discovered that the high-runner mice responded completely differently to drugs which block the dopamine reuptake transporter protein (77, 78). Similarly in a selective breeding experiment for increased and decreased voluntary wheel running in rats, the lines responded differently to a dopamine reuptake transporter blocker (10). The main cellular mechanism of action attributed to the psychoactive effects of the drugs which were used, cocaine, methylphenidate (Ritalin), and GBR 12909, was thought to be through increased dopamine in extracellular spaces. These drugs decreased wheel running in high-runner mice in a dose-dependent fashion whereas they had no effect or the opposite effect, and increased wheel running, in control mice (77, 78). The results demonstrated that some feature of the dopamine system had been altered by selection, but follow-up experiments found no differences in dopamine levels, or dopamine turnover in the nucleus accumbens (unpublished observations). Dopamine levels appear to have decreased in the dorsal raphe, the region of the brain containing the greatest density of serotonin neuron cell bodies, and DOPAC, which is a metabolite of dopamine, appears to have been reduced in the substantia nigra (98). Further, genes for two dopamine receptors displayed 20% increased expression in the hippocampus of the high-runner mice (9), but dopamine has diverse roles in different brain regions and the direct implications of these results for reward processing remain unclear. Additional experiments found no differences in dopamine receptors, or transporters in the nucleus accumbens or frontal cortical brain regions (unpublished data) using radiolabeled ligand binding assays established by Aaron Janowsky (45, 46). As described and characterized so well by the Nobel Prize laureate, Paul Greengard, dopamine receptors are only at the tip of an iceberg in terms of activing an entire intracellular signaling cascade involving many enzymes, interacting proteins, and molecular complexes (33). Any one of these could be altered at the genetic level to cause a change in the dopamine signal in response to a stimulus such as physical activity. Furthermore, dopamine neurons interact with neurons of many other types, so changes in other neurotransmitter systems could influence dopamine function through these interactions. Other neurotransmitter systems implicated in reward processing and motivation for physical activity include serotonin (38, 88, 98), glutamate (34, 92), gamma aminobutyric acid (GABA) (54), opioids (8, 71), and cannabinoids (22, 49, 50, 59, 74, 75, 93, 95). Each of these systems comes with their own degree of complexity in terms of signaling molecules downstream of receptors. Some of these receptors can be on presynaptic terminals and postsynaptic terminals to elicit a diverse array of effects on the reward circuit. Taken together, this paints a complex picture, and one that is only meaningful if considered at a systems level. The dopamine signaling system is clearly involved in the motivation for physical activity, but the specific molecular underpinnings are only beginning to become realized, and the answer is not one or two molecules, but the way in which systems-level gene expression is coordinated through development of a nervous system and alterations in chromatin structure in a cell type-specific manner (88).

Specificity of reward circuitry for promoting physical activity remains elusive

Unfortunately, determining the reward circuitry that promotes physical activity is an area in its infancy with little progress. Our understanding of how circuits in the brain are involved in motivation for specific behaviors is still remarkably rudimentary. Only a few reports illustrate specificity in the neural physiology underlying the perception of different types of rewards. Regina Carelli has done work showing that specific neurons in the nucleus accumbens are activated in response to sugar but are not activated in response to cocaine reward (13, 15). Other studies, attempting to find differential patterns of brain activation associated with expecting a food reward versus cocaine, have been only moderately successful in finding differential patterns of brain activation (106), and even then it is difficult to know whether these differences can be attributed to the magnitude of the perceived reward rather than the reward type. Even finding differential patterns of brain activation in response to aversive stimuli versus a reward is difficult as the majority of the brain activation response appears to reflect relative emotional potency rather than valence (47). In other words, when a subject is presented with a stimulus that is either very rewarding or very aversive, many of the same brain regions become activated. One possible explanation is that the majority of the brain response is a reflection of attention or arousal to the stimulus or learning about the stimulus so it can be approached or avoided in the future, and the learning, attention, and arousal are consistent between the two valences.

While some relevant regions and molecules have been identified for many different types of rewards, the question of specificity remains a major issue. When specificity is explicitly evaluated, often it is not found (29, 47, 68, 106). Therefore, how the different regions and molecules that have been identified mix differently to create different versions of motivation, particularly when it is directed at one or another reward such as a drug or exercise, the understanding becomes increasingly cloudy. The regions including the limbic system (amygdala, hippocampus, frontal cortex), natural reward circuit (ventral tegmental area to nucleus accumbens), and hypothalamus are activated for all sorts of natural and artificial rewards as well as for aversive stimuli such as in response to pain and stress. This variety of activation triggers suggest that in order to find specificity one will have to look at a more detailed aspect of the physiology, such as examining specific neurons and their firing rates similar to the work by Carelli mentioned briefly above. It appears that no one has tried to determine whether neurons can be found that are selectively sensitive to physical activity reward over other rewards. This area of investigation, finding the specificity of motivation for different types of natural rewards, will be important before we can really understand the motivation for physical activity at a neurobiological level.

An important clue about how the reward circuit may be modified to specifically promote one behavior over another comes not from studies exploring motivation for physical activity but rather from studies exploring motivation for pair-bonding behavior in voles. The leading hypothesis is that the evolution of monogamy in voles involves genetic changes in the promotor regions of genes which affect the way oxytocin and arginine vasopressin receptors are distributed and expressed on different nodes of the reward circuit (105). So, the idea is that the reward circuit itself remains unchanged (e.g., in terms of dopamine, opioids, cannabinoids, medial forebrain bundle, etc.). However, whenever two voles come into contact with each other, the peptides oxytocin in females and arginine vasopressin in males are released. The receptors for these two peptides in the brain are situated in such a way that they cause a differential level of electrical activation of the reward circuit and perception of reward. For example, monogamous female Prairie voles have more oxytocin receptors in the nucleus accumbens than polygynous female Montane voles (44, 82, 105). In males, the arginine vasopressin V1a receptor is concentrated in regions of the reward circuit in Prairie voles as compared to Montane voles (57, 104, 105). Moreover, individual differences in affiliative behavior in Prairie voles are associated with differential expression of the peptide receptors in the nodes of the natural reward circuit in expected ways based on their behavior (3, 36). Incredibly, the genetic regulatory mechanism for this differential spatial distribution and expression of the V1a receptors has been fairly well worked out in the voles, and appears to involve tandem repeated DNA sequences in the pro-motor region (57). Although the tandem repeat sequences cannot underlie variation in mon-ogamy/polygyny in *Microtus* voles more generally because many polygynous voles also have the repeated sequences (26), strong, direct molecular evidence supports the hypothesis that at least the Prairie vole variant of the promotor and resulting change in neuroanatomical distri-bution and expression of arginine vasopressin V1a receptors facilitates pair bonding. Both mice and meadow voles, which are polygynous species, can be coerced into displaying affiliative behavior if the appropriate neurons are engineered to express the Prairie vole variant of the V1a receptor (57, 104). Moreover, recent evidence demonstrates that this differential distribu-tion of receptors may increase the synchronicity of electrical activation between two key nodes of the reward circuit, the nucleus accumbens and prefrontal cortex, when the voles come in contact with each other (2). The degree of future affiliative behavior is greatly predicted by a measure of coherence between the electrical rhythms in each reward region during initial con-tact. Taken together, the vole work suggests that the evolution of a voluntary behavior results from changes in the way signaling systems involved in the behavior interact with the different nodes of the reward circuit. More specifically, the circuit appears to have to function in such a way that it facilitates coherence between different regions of the reward circuit at the time when the animals are performing the behavior. To the best of our knowledge, no study has explored coherence in electrical activation of the different nodes of the reward circuit during high levels of physical activity. It is possible that the evolution of increased motivation for physical activity required a change in the physiology of the circuit in such a way that coherence occurs between prefrontal cortex and nucleus accumbens during exhaustive physical exercise.

Physical activity activates the hippocampus, but the functional significance remains a mystery

Although no study has examined coherence between nodes of the reward circuit during phys-ical activity as was performed in the vole affiliative study, several studies have examined neuronal activation of different regions of the brain during physical activity. As it turns out, the region most activated from voluntary wheel-running behavior and forced treadmill running is the hippocampus (80). This is somewhat unexpected because the hippocampus is more known for its role in learning and memory than movement. However, a large literature has established that the hippocampal formation is instantaneously engaged at the onset and duration of strenuous physical movements, displaying a rhythmic synchronous activity of large numbers of neurons, which is proportional to the speed (or force) of the movement and persists for as long as phys-ical activity persists (6, 12, 56).

In addition to the literature establishing activation of the hippocampus in proportion to the intensity of physical activity, the hippocampus has an extensive literature for its role in motiv-ation, and it is often included as a peripheral reward region well interconnected with the central nodes of the reward circuit such as the ventral midbrain, nucleus accumbens, and prefrontal cortex (Figure 8.1) (70). It is possible that the physical activity-related electrical activation of the hippocampus stimulates the reward circuit to a greater degree in mice that are highly motivated for physical activity, though this would require additional testing to confirm. Finding sequence variants which affect the resulting development and function of hippocampus–reward circuit interactions could be a fruitful avenue for future research on the neurogenetics of motivation for physical activity.

Genetic regulatory mechanisms for increasing motivation for physical activity

It was thought that science would eventually find genetic differences in dopamine receptors and transporters in cocaine addiction, opioid receptors for heroin addiction, GABA and glutamate for alcoholism, and cannabinoid receptors for marijuana. However, results from human genetics over the past 20 years suggest instead that the heritability of drug addiction is highly overlapping with personality traits such as novelty seeking, and usually not specific to any one type of reward (52). Furthermore, the contribution of single candidate genes such as a dopamine receptor to a complex trait accounts for only a tiny fraction of the heritability, if any at all (66). Therefore, it is exceedingly unlikely that an approach that examines single candidate genes such as dopamine receptors will make headway into understanding the genetic mechanisms which regulate motivation for physical activity, at least with any degree of specificity distinguishing it from other rewards (25).

As described previously, genetic changes that lead to the development and function of a reward circuit that reinforces physical activity is a more realistic mechanism (25, 81, 88). Systems genetic analysis of gene expression changes in the striatum (both dorsal and ventral nucleus accumbens, main dopamine innervation region) of the high-runner mice implicated a network of genes that affect chromatin and/or transcriptional states (88). Chromatin can exist in multiple functional states, either in a condensed state that prohibits gene expression or a relaxed state that facilitates gene expression. Thus, sequence variants that affect chromatin structure could explain gene expression patterns in crucial regions of the reward circuit which could affect the way the cells respond to physical activity. Specifically, for the evolution of voluntary wheel running a structural polymorphism in the SMARCA4 protein is suggested to cause differential interaction with the BAZ1A protein, altering the distribution of the H1F0 histone subunit protein and thereby creating a chromatin state conducive for increased expression of the serotonin receptor and an orphan G protein-coupled receptor. Future work is needed to rigorously test this hypothesis by assessing the chromatin state through direct measurement.

Conclusions

In conclusion, heritable variation in motivation for physical activity is hypothesized to result from differences in the way neural signals involved in regulating the intensity of the physical activity interact with the natural reward circuit. Therefore, genetics of motivation for increased physical activity likely involve genetic programs for building a nervous system in which the act of intense physical activity produces a strong reward signal that leads to reinforcement of the behavior, and subsequent drive for the activity. We propose that a crucial location for the occurrence of neurological differences is at the interface between the hippocampus and various nodes of the reward circuit (Figure 8.1, shaded regions). This is because the hippocampus becomes electrically activated like no other region in the brain in proportion to exercise intensity. If the brain were wired in such a way that physical activity-induced neuronal activation stimulated the reward circuit, that would lead to reinforcement. However, the precise molecules and developmental trajectories that result in a brain predisposed for high or low motivation for physical activity are far from known. Models such as long-term selective breeding experiments for increased voluntary wheel running in mice and rats provide promising avenues for research and discovery in this area. Finding neurogenetic pathways that increase motivation for physical activity has broad implications for evolution of behavior. It also has important applications in preventative medicine. The health benefits of exercise are profound on all dimensions. Getting people to exercise is the hard part. Understanding the pathways which increase intrinsic drive for physical activity therefore holds the key to prolonged health and prosperity in the 21st century.

References

1. **Abercrombie ED, Keefe KA, DiFrischia DS,** and **Zigmond MJ.** Differential effect of stress on in vivo dopamine release in striatum, nucleus accumbens, and medial frontal cortex. *Journal of neurochemistry* 52: 1655–1658, 1989.

2. **Amadei EA, Johnson ZV, Kwon YJ, Shpiner AC, Saravanan V, Mays WD, Ryan SJ, Walum H, Rainnie DG,** and **Young LJ.** Dynamic corticostriatal activity biases social bonding in monogamous female prairie voles. *Nature* 546: 297, 2017.

3. **Barrett CE, Keebaugh AC, Ahern TH, Bass CE, Terwilliger EF,** and **Young LJ.** Variation in vasopressin receptor (Avpr1a) expression creates diversity in behaviors related to monogamy in prairie voles. *Hormones and behavior* 63: 518–526, 2013.

4. **Beeler JA** and **Mourra D.** To do or not to do: Dopamine, affordability and the economics of opportunity. *Frontiers in integrative neuroscience* 12: 6, 2018.

5. **Berridge KC** and **Robinson TE.** What is the role of dopamine in reward: Hedonic impact, reward learning, or incentive salience? *Brain research reviews* 28: 309–369, 1998.

6. **Bland BH** and **Oddie SD.** Theta band oscillation and synchrony in the hippocampal formation and associated structures: the case for its role in sensorimotor integration. *Behavioural brain research* 127: 119–136, 2001.

7. **Blomberg SP, Garland** Jr T, and **Ives AR.** Testing for phylogenetic signal in comparative data: Behavioral traits are more labile. *Evolution* 57: 717–745, 2003.

8. **Boecker H, Sprenger T, Spilker ME, Henriksen G, Koppenhoefer M, Wagner KJ, Valet M, Berthele A,** and **Tolle TR.** The runner's high: Opioidergic mechanisms in the human brain. *Cerebral cortex* 18: 2523–2531, 2008.

9. **Bronikowski A, Rhodes J, Garland** Jr T, **Prolla T, Awad T,** and **Gammie S.** The evolution of gene expression in mouse hippocampus in response to selective breeding for increased locomotor activity. *Evolution* 58: 2079–2086, 2004.

10. **Brown JD, Green CL, Arthur IM, Booth FW,** and **Miller DK.** Cocaine-induced locomotor activity in rats selectively bred for low and high voluntary running behavior. *Psychopharmacology* 232: 673–681, 2015.

11. **Brown RA, Abrantes AM, Read JP, Marcus BH, Jakicic J, Strong DR, Oakley JR, Ramsey SE, Kahler CW,** and **Stuart GL.** A pilot study of aerobic exercise as an adjunctive treatment for drug dependence. *Mental health and physical activity* 3: 27–34, 2010.

12. **Buzsaki G.** Theta oscillations in the hippocampus. *Neuron* 33: 325–340, 2002.

13. **Cameron CM, Wightman RM,** and **Carelli RM.** Dynamics of rapid dopamine release in the nucleus accumbens during goal-directed behaviors for cocaine versus natural rewards. *Neuropharmacology* 86: 319–328, 2014.

14. **Cannon CM** and **Palmiter RD.** Reward without dopamine. *Journal of neuroscience* 23: 10827–10831, 2003.

15. **Carelli RM, Ijames SG,** and **Crumling AJ.** Evidence that separate neural circuits in the nucleus accumbens encode cocaine versus "natural" (water and food) reward. *Journal of neuroscience* 20: 4255–4266, 2000.

16. **Colcombe S** and **Kramer AF.** Fitness effects on the cognitive function of older adults: A meta-analytic study. *Psychological science* 14: 125–130, 2003.

17. **Cone JJ, Fortin SM, McHenry JA, Stuber GD, McCutcheon JE,** and **Roitman MF.** Physiological state gates acquisition and expression of mesolimbic reward prediction signals. *Proceedings of the National Academy of Sciences* 113: 1943–1948, 2016.

18. **Cotman CW** and **Berchtold NC.** Exercise: A behavioral intervention to enhance brain health and plasticity. *Trends in neurosciences* 25: 295–301, 2002.

19. **Cotman CW, Berchtold NC,** and **Christie L-A.** Exercise builds brain health: Key roles of growth factor cascades and inflammation. *Trends in neurosciences* 30: 464–472, 2007.

20. **Dawson WR, Bartholomew GA,** and **Bennett AF.** A reappraisal of the aquatic specializations of the Galapagos marine iguana (Amblyrhynchus cristatus). *Evolution* 31: 891–897, 1977.

21. **Dishman RK, Berthoud HR, Booth FW, Cotman CW, Edgerton VR, Fleshner MR, Gandevia SC, Gomez-Pinilla F, Greenwood BN,** and **Hillman CH.** Neurobiology of exercise. *Obesity* 14: 345–356, 2006.

22. **Dubreucq S, Koehl M, Abrous DN, Marsicano G,** and **Chaouloff F.** CB1 receptor deficiency decreases wheel-running activity: Consequences on emotional behaviours and hippocampal neurogenesis. *Experimental neurology* 224: 106–113, 2010.

23. **Eichler EE, Flint J, Gibson G, Kong A, Leal SM, Moore JH,** and **Nadeau JH.** Missing heritability and strategies for finding the underlying causes of complex disease. *Nature reviews genetics* 11: 446, 2010.

24. **Erickson KI, Voss MW, Prakash RS, Basak C, Szabo A, Chaddock L, Kim JS, Heo S, Alves H,** and **White SM.** Exercise training increases size of hippocampus and improves memory. *Proceedings of the National Academy of Sciences* 108: 3017–3022, 2011.

25. **Ferguson DP, Dangott LJ, Vellers HL, Schmitt EE,** and **Lightfoot JT.** Differential protein expression in the nucleus accumbens of high and low active mice. *Behavioural brain research* 291: 283–288, 2015.

26. **Fink S, Excoffier L,** and **Heckel G.** Mammalian monogamy is not controlled by a single gene. *Proceedings of the National Academy of Sciences* 103: 10956–10960, 2006.

27. **Foley TE, Greenwood BN, Day HE, Koch LG, Britton SL,** and **Fleshner M.** Elevated central monoamine receptor mRNA in rats bred for high endurance capacity: Implications for central fatigue. *Behavioural brain research* 174: 132–142, 2006.

28. **Frugé AD, Byrd SH, Fountain BJ, Cossman JS, Schilling MW,** and **Gerard P.** Increased physical activity may be more protective for metabolic syndrome than reduced caloric intake. An analysis of estimated energy balance in US adults: 2007–2010 NHANES. *Nutrition, metabolism and cardiovascular diseases* 25: 535–540, 2015.

29. **Garavan H, Pankiewicz J, Bloom A, Cho J-K, Sperry L, Ross TJ, Salmeron BJ, Risinger R, Kelley D,** and **Stein EA.** Cue-induced cocaine craving: neuroanatomical specificity for drug users and drug stimuli. *American journal of psychiatry* 157: 1789–1798, 2000.

30. **Garland Jr T** and **Carter P.** Evolutionary physiology. *Annual review of physiology* 56: 579–621, 1994.

31. **Garland Jr T** and **Freeman PW.** Selective breeding for high endurance running increases hindlimb symmetry. *Evolution* 59: 1851–1854, 2005.

32. **Gasbarri A, Packard MG, Campana E,** and **Pacitti C.** Anterograde and retrograde tracing of projections from the ventral tegmental area to the hippocampal formation in the rat. *Brain research bulletin* 33: 445–452, 1994.

33. **Greengard P, Allen PB,** and **Nairn AC.** Beyond the dopamine receptor. *Neuron* 23: 435–447, 1999.

34. **Grigsby KB, Kovarik CM, Rottinghaus GE,** and **Booth FW.** High and low nightly running behavior associates with nucleus accumbens N-Methyl-d-aspartate receptor (NMDAR) NR1 subunit expression and NMDAR functional differences. *Neuroscience letters* 671: 50–55, 2018.

35. **Groves PM.** A theory of the functional organization of the neostriatum and the neostriatal control of voluntary movement. *Brain research reviews* 5: 109–132, 1983.

36. **Hammock EA** and **Young LJ.** Microsatellite instability generates diversity in brain and sociobehavioral traits. *Science* 308: 1630–1634, 2005.

37. **Harris AH, Cronkite R,** and **Moos R.** Physical activity, exercise coping, and depression in a 10-year cohort study of depressed patients. *Journal of affective disorders* 93: 79–85, 2006.

38. **Hayes DJ** and **Greenshaw AJ.** 5-HT receptors and reward-related behaviour: a review. *Neuroscience & biobehavioral reviews* 35: 1419–1449, 2011.

39. **Hillman CH, Erickson KI,** and **Kramer AF.** Be smart, exercise your heart: exercise effects on brain and cognition. *Nature reviews neuroscience* 9: 58, 2008.

40. **Hnasko TS, Sotak BN,** and **Palmiter RD.** Morphine reward in dopamine-deficient mice. *Nature* 438: 854, 2005.

41. **Houle-Leroy P, Guderley H, Swallow JG,** and **Garland Jr T.** Artificial selection for high activity favors mighty mini-muscles in house mice. *American journal of physiology – regulatory, integrative and comparative physiology* 284: R433–R443, 2003.

42. **Hu FB, Sigal RJ, Rich-Edwards JW, Colditz GA, Solomon CG, Willett WC, Speizer FE,** and **Manson JE.** Walking compared with vigorous physical activity and risk of type 2 diabetes in women: a prospective study. *JAMA* 282: 1433–1439, 1999.

43. **Huey RB, Hertz PE,** and **Sinervo B.** Behavioral drive versus behavioral inertia in evolution: A null model approach. *The American naturalist* 161: 357–366, 2003.

44. **Insel TR** and **Shapiro LE.** Oxytocin receptor distribution reflects social organization in monogamous and polygamous voles. *Proceedings of the National Academy of Sciences* 89: 5981–5985, 1992.

45. **Janowsky A, Mah C, Johnson RA, Cunningham CL, Phillips TJ, Crabbe JC, Eshleman AJ,** and **Belknap JK.** Mapping genes that regulate density of dopamine transporters and correlated behaviors in recombinant inbred mice. *Journal of pharmacology and experimental therapeutics* 298: 634–643, 2001.

46. **Janowsky A, Neve KA, Kinzie JM, Taylor B, de Paulis T,** and **Belknap JK.** Extrastriatal dopamine D2 receptors: distribution, pharmacological characterization and region-specific regulation by clozapine. *Journal of pharmacology and experimental therapeutics* 261: 1282–1290, 1992.

47. **Johnson ZV, Revis AA, Burdick MA,** and **Rhodes JS.** A similar pattern of neuronal Fos activation in 10 brain regions following exposure to reward-or aversion-associated contextual cues in mice. *Physiology & behavior* 99: 412–418, 2010.

48. **Kalivas PW** and **Duffy P.** Selective activation of dopamine transmission in the shell of the nucleus accumbens by stress. *Brain research* 675: 325–328, 1995.

49. **Keeney BK, Meek TH, Middleton KM, Holness LF,** and **Garland** Jr **T.** Sex differences in cannabinoid receptor-1 (CB1) pharmacology in mice selectively bred for high voluntary wheel-running behavior. *Pharmacology biochemistry and behavior* 101: 528–537, 2012.

50. **Keeney BK, Raichlen DA, Meek TH, Wijeratne RS, Middleton KM, Gerdeman GL,** and **Garland** Jr **T.** Differential response to a selective cannabinoid receptor antagonist (SR141716: rimonabant) in female mice from lines selectively bred for high voluntary wheel-running behaviour. *Behavioural pharmacology* 19: 812–820, 2008.

51. **Kelley A** and **Domesick V.** The distribution of the projection from the hippocampal formation to the nucleus accumbens in the rat: An anterograde and retrograde-horseradish peroxidase study. *Neuroscience* 7: 2321–2335, 1982.

52. **Kendler KS, Jacobson KC, Prescott CA,** and **Neale MC.** Specificity of genetic and environmental risk factors for use and abuse/dependence of cannabis, cocaine, hallucinogens, sedatives, stimulants, and opiates in male twins. *American Journal of Psychiatry* 160: 687–695, 2003.

53. **Knab AM** and **Lightfoot JT.** Does the difference between physically active and couch potato lie in the dopamine system? *International journal of biological sciences* 6: 133, 2010.

54. **Koob GF.** Drugs of abuse: Anatomy, pharmacology and function of reward pathways. *Trends in pharmacological sciences* 13: 177–184, 1992.

55. **Kyu HH, Bachman VF, Alexander LT, Mumford JE, Afshin A, Estep K, Veerman JL, Delwiche K, Iannarone ML,** and **Moyer ML.** Physical activity and risk of breast cancer, colon cancer, diabetes, ischemic heart disease, and ischemic stroke events: Systematic review and dose-response meta-analysis for the Global Burden of Disease Study 2013. *BMJ* 354: i3857, 2016.

56. **Li JY, Kuo TB, Hsieh IT,** and **Yang CC.** Changes in hippocampal theta rhythm and their correlations with speed during different phases of voluntary wheel running in rats. *Neuroscience* 213: 54–61, 2012.

57. **Lim MM, Wang Z, Olazábal DE, Ren X, Terwilliger EF,** and **Young LJ.** Enhanced partner preference in a promiscuous species by manipulating the expression of a single gene. *Nature* 429: 754, 2004.

58. **Lotharius J** and **Brundin P.** Pathogenesis of Parkinson's disease: Dopamine, vesicles and α-synuclein. *Nature reviews neuroscience* 3: 932, 2002.

59. **Lupica CR, Riegel AC,** and **Hoffman AF.** Marijuana and cannabinoid regulation of brain reward circuits. *British journal of pharmacology* 143: 227–234, 2004.

60. **Mathes WF, Nehrenberg DL, Gordon R, Hua K, Garland Jr T,** and **Pomp D.** Dopaminergic dysregulation in mice selectively bred for excessive exercise or obesity. *Behavioural brain research* 210: 155–163, 2010.

61. **McCutcheon JE, Beeler JA,** and **Roitman MF.** Sucrose-predictive cues evoke greater phasic dopamine release than saccharin-predictive cues. *Synapse* 66: 346–351, 2012.

62. **Mccutcheon JE, Ebner SR, Loriaux AL,** and **Roitman MF.** Encoding of aversion by dopamine and the nucleus accumbens. *Frontiers in neuroscience* 6: 137, 2012.

63. **Michaud DS, Giovannucci E, Willett WC, Colditz GA, Stampfer MJ,** and **Fuchs CS.** Physical activity, obesity, height, and the risk of pancreatic cancer. *JAMA* 286: 921–929, 2001.

64. **Milner PM.** Brain-stimulation reward: a review. *Canadian journal of psychology/Revue canadienne de psychologie* 45: 1, 1991.

65. **Mokdad AH, Ford ES, Bowman BA, Dietz WH, Vinicor F, Bales VS,** and **Marks JS.** Prevalence of obesity, diabetes, and obesity-related health risk factors, 2001. *JAMA* 289: 76–79, 2003.

66. **Munafo M, Matheson I,** and **Flint J.** Association of the DRD2 gene Taq1A polymorphism and alcoholism: A meta-analysis of case–control studies and evidence of publication bias. *Molecular psychiatry* 12: 454, 2007.

67. **Myers J, McAuley P, Lavie CJ, Despres J-P, Arena R,** and **Kokkinos P.** Physical activity and cardiorespiratory fitness as major markers of cardiovascular risk: Their independent and interwoven importance to health status. *Progress in cardiovascular diseases* 57: 306–314, 2015.

68. **Noori HR, Linan AC,** and **Spanagel R.** Largely overlapping neuronal substrates of reactivity to drug, gambling, food and sexual cues: A comprehensive meta-analysis. *European neuropsychopharmacology* 26: 1419–1430, 2016.

69. **Olds J** and **Milner P.** Positive reinforcement produced by electrical stimulation of septal area and other regions of rat brain. *Journal of comparative and physiological psychology* 47: 419, 1954.

70. **Otmakhova N, Duzel E, Deutch AY,** and **Lisman J.** The hippocampal-VTA loop: the role of novelty and motivation in controlling the entry of information into long-term memory. In: *Intrinsically motivated learning in natural and artificial systems.* New York: Springer, 2013, p. 235–254.

71. **Peciña S.** Opioid reward "liking" and "wanting" in the nucleus accumbens. *Physiology & behavior* 94: 675–680, 2008.

72. **Pfaus J, Damsma G, Nomikos GG, Wenkstern D, Blaha C, Phillips A,** and **Fibiger H.** Sexual behavior enhances central dopamine transmission in the male rat. *Brain research* 530: 345–348, 1990.

73. **Pignatelli M** and **Bonci A.** Role of dopamine neurons in reward and aversion: A synaptic plasticity perspective. *Neuron* 86: 1145–1157, 2015.

74. **Raichlen DA, Foster AD, Gerdeman GL, Seillier A,** and **Giuffrida A.** Wired to run: Exercise-induced endocannabinoid signaling in humans and cursorial mammals with implications for the "runner's high". *Journal of experimental biology* 215: 1331–1336, 2012.

75. **Raichlen DA, Foster AD, Seillier A, Giuffrida A,** and **Gerdeman GL.** Exercise-induced endocannabinoid signaling is modulated by intensity. *European journal of applied physiology* 113: 869–875, 2013.

76. **Rezende EL, Garland T, Chappell MA, Malisch JL,** and **Gomes FR.** Maximum aerobic performance in lines of Mus selected for high wheel-running activity: Effects of selection, oxygen availability and the mini-muscle phenotype. *Journal of experimental biology* 209: 115–127, 2006.

77. **Rhodes J** and **Garland T.** Differential sensitivity to acute administration of Ritalin, apormorphine, SCH 23390, but not raclopride in mice selectively bred for hyperactive wheel-running behavior. *Psychopharmacology* 167: 242–250, 2003.

78. **Rhodes J, Hosack G, Girard I, Kelley A, Mitchell G,** and **Garland T.** Differential sensitivity to acute administration of cocaine, GBR 12909, and fluoxetine in mice selectively bred for hyperactive wheel-running behavior. *Psychopharmacology* 158: 120–131, 2001.

79. **Rhodes JS, Gammie SC,** and **Garland Jr T.** Neurobiology of mice selected for high voluntary wheel-running activity. *Integrative and comparative biology* 45: 438–455, 2005.

80. **Rhodes JS, Garland Jr T,** and **Gammie SC.** Patterns of brain activity associated with variation in voluntary wheel-running behavior. *Behavioral neuroscience* 117: 1243, 2003.

81. **Roberts MD, Gilpin L, Parker KE, Childs TE, Will MJ,** and **Booth FW.** Dopamine D1 receptor modulation in nucleus accumbens lowers voluntary wheel running in rats bred to run high distances. *Physiology & behavior* 105: 661–668, 2012.

82. **Ross HE, Freeman SM, Spiegel LL, Ren X, Terwilliger EF,** and **Young LJ.** Variation in oxytocin receptor density in the nucleus accumbens has differential effects on affiliative behaviors in monogamous and polygamous voles. *Journal of neuroscience* 29: 1312–1318, 2009.

83. **Ruegsegger GN** and **Booth FW.** Running from disease: molecular mechanisms associating dopamine and leptin signaling in the brain with physical inactivity, obesity, and type 2 diabetes. *Frontiers in endocrinology* 8: 109, 2017.

84. **Ruegsegger GN, Brown JD, Kovarik MC, Miller DK,** and **Booth FW.** Mu-opioid receptor inhibition decreases voluntary wheel running in a dopamine-dependent manner in rats bred for high voluntary running. *Neuroscience* 339: 525–537, 2016.

85. **Salamone JD.** The involvement of nucleus accumbens dopamine in appetitive and aversive motivation. *Behavioural brain research* 61: 117–133, 1994.

86. **Salamone JD** and **Correa M.** The mysterious motivational functions of mesolimbic dopamine. *Neuron* 76: 470–485, 2012.

87. **Salamone JD, Correa M, Mingote SM,** and **Weber SM.** Beyond the reward hypothesis: alternative functions of nucleus accumbens dopamine. *Current opinion in pharmacology* 5: 34–41, 2005.

88. **Saul M, Majdak P, Perez S, Reilly M, Garland T**, and **Rhodes JS.** High motivation for exercise is associated with altered chromatin regulators of monoamine receptor gene expression in the striatum of selectively bred mice. *Genes, brain and behavior* 16: 328–341, 2017.

89. **Schuch FB, Vancampfort D, Richards J, Rosenbaum S, Ward PB**, and **Stubbs B.** Exercise as a treatment for depression: a meta-analysis adjusting for publication bias. *Journal of psychiatric research* 77: 42–51, 2016.

90. **Schultz W.** Dopamine reward prediction-error signalling: a two-component response. *Nature reviews neuroscience* 17: 183, 2016.

91. **Schultz W, Dayan P**, and **Montague PR.** A neural substrate of prediction and reward. *Science* 275: 1593–1599, 1997.

92. **Smith-Roe SL** and **Kelley AE.** Coincident activation of NMDA and dopamine D1Receptors within the nucleus accumbens core is required for appetitive instrumental learning. *Journal of neuroscience* 20: 7737–7742, 2000.

93. **Sparling P, Giuffrida A, Piomelli D, Rosskopf L**, and **Dietrich A.** Exercise activates the endocannabinoid system. *Neuroreport* 14: 2209–2211, 2003.

94. **Swallow JG, Carter PA**, and **Garland T.** Artificial selection for increased wheel-running behavior in house mice. *Behavior genetics* 28: 227–237, 1998.

95. **Thompson Z, Argueta D, Garland Jr T**, and **DiPatrizio N.** Circulating levels of endocannabinoids respond acutely to voluntary exercise, are altered in mice selectively bred for high voluntary wheel running, and differ between the sexes. *Physiology & behavior* 170: 141–150, 2017.

96. **Van Praag H, Kempermann G**, and **Gage FH.** Running increases cell proliferation and neurogenesis in the adult mouse dentate gyrus. *Nature neuroscience* 2: 266, 1999.

97. **Voss MW, Nagamatsu LS, Liu-Ambrose T**, and **Kramer AF.** Exercise, brain, and cognition across the life span. *Journal of applied physiology* 111: 1505–1513, 2011.

98. **Waters RP, Pringle R, Forster G, Renner K, Malisch J, Garland Jr T**, and **Swallow J.** Selection for increased voluntary wheel-running affects behavior and brain monoamines in mice. *Brain research* 1508: 9–22, 2013.

99. **Waters RP, Renner K, Pringle R, Summers CH, Britton S, Koch L**, and **Swallow J.** Selection for aerobic capacity affects corticosterone, monoamines and wheel-running activity. *Physiology & behavior* 93: 1044–1054, 2008.

100. **Wise RA.** Addictive drugs and brain stimulation reward. *Annual review of neuroscience* 19: 319–340, 1996.

101. **Wise RA.** Dopamine, learning and motivation. *Nature reviews neuroscience* 5: 483, 2004.

102. **Wise RA.** Neurobiology of addiction. *Current opinion in neurobiology* 6: 243–251, 1996.

103. **Wise RA** and **Rompre P-P.** Brain dopamine and reward. *Annual review of psychology* 40: 191–225, 1989.

104. **Young LJ, Nilsen R, Waymire KG, MacGregor GR**, and **Insel TR.** Increased affiliative response to vasopressin in mice expressing the V 1a receptor from a monogamous vole. *Nature* 400: 766, 1999.

105. **Young LJ** and **Wang Z.** The neurobiology of pair bonding. *Nature neuroscience* 7: 1048, 2004.

106. **Zombeck JA, Chen G-T, Johnson ZV, Rosenberg DM, Craig AB**, and **Rhodes JS.** Neuroanatomical specificity of conditioned responses to cocaine versus food in mice. *Physiology & behavior* 93: 637–650, 2008.

9

PERIPHERAL MECHANISMS ARISING FROM GENETICS THAT REGULATE ACTIVITY

David P. Ferguson

Introduction

Behavior traits, such as physical activity, are generally accepted to be a result of environmental and genetic/biological factors. A large amount of literature (7, 18, 19, 38, 39, 43, 45, 47, 50, 52–56) has examined the environmental influence on physical activity. While the literature has focused on factors such as culture, peer influence, and the "built environment" (i.e., access to sidewalks) (5, 54, 56), it has been shown that the main factors contributing to the control of voluntary physical activity are genetic and biological influences (27). Voluntary physical activity is an important trait to study because it has been positively correlated with decreases in cardiovascular disease, obesity, type 2 diabetes, and some types of cancer (27). With only 3.5% of adults meeting the recommended physical activity guidelines (51), physical inactivity is the second actual leading cause of death (~250,000 cases/year) in the US with an estimated $507 billion a year in healthcare costs (34). Thus, the identification of biological mechanisms that regulate voluntary physical activity could improve the quality of life of individuals and potentially reduce healthcare costs.

As described in Chapter 5, the use of animal models is a reliable approach to examine genetic mechanisms of physical activity and has several benefits over the human model. Specifically, mice can be bred to limit heterozygosity of the population, environmental factors can be controlled by the investigator, and the short lifespan of the animal provides the opportunity to measure physical activity across multiple generations (27). Inbred mice are produced using at least 20 consecutive generations of parent × offspring or sister × brother mating, allowing for mice to be genetically homozygous at all loci (30). Thus, the use of inbred mice allows for the rigorous control of heterozygosity of the genome as well as control of the environment allowing for investigation into the genetic regulation of physical activity. Furthermore, the mouse is an excellent model of the human genome given that there is approximately 75% homology between the mouse and human genome (8). While there is some discrepancy in homology between mice and humans, this difference appears to be a result of differences in noncoding regions of the genome (8). Thus, the demonstrated human–mouse genomic homology increases the probability that results from genetic studies using the mouse model can be directly translated to humans.

To evaluate voluntary physical activity in the mouse model, several methods have been utilized. The most frequently used methods in the literature have been wheel running, home cage activity, and/or maze activity. However, it has been suggested that studies using home cage activity and/or maze activity evaluate both physical activity level and fear/anxiety level (26). Therefore, in the mouse model, the method most often used to assess voluntary physical activity level is wheel running (31). Wheel running as a measure of physical activity has a similar physiological response as does partaking in physical activity by humans, such as self-selection of intensity, heart rate response, and neurological changes. Specifically it has been shown that humans self-select an average running intensity of 70% (12). Interestingly it has been shown that mice self-select a wheel running intensity of 65–70% (28). The self-selection of physical activity level results in similar cardiovascular and neurological adaptations between mice and humans. Adlam et al. (2) showed that during acute wheel running there was a significant increase in heart rate and blood pressure, with 5 weeks of wheel running resulting in a decreased resting heart rate and blood pressure (1). Similarly, it has been well established that regular bouts of moderate intensity exercise (60–70% of maximum heart rate) in humans result in a decrease of resting heart rate and systolic blood pressure over time (36). Additionally, mouse wheel running and human physical activity engagement result in similar neurological responses. Dishman et al. (10) characterized the norepinephrine, 5-hydroxytryptamine, dopamine, and gamma aminobutyric acid responses to wheel running and showed that there was an increase in norepinephrine and dopamine following mouse wheel running which led the authors to conclude that physical activity had a protective effect on brain monoamine depletion and thus an antidepressant affect (10). The human literature has documented similar findings of antidepressant effects following bouts of physical activity (11). However, due to the nature of the study, brain monoamines could not be directly measured in humans (10) for comparison to the mouse model. Given the similarities between human and mouse physiological parameters during voluntary exercise and voluntary wheel running, the use of the mouse wheel running model appears to be appropriate to determine the regulation of physical activity level and further allows the use of genetic linkage, transcriptome, and proteome analyses.

The physiological site of activity regulation is an evolving question, with current literature suggesting that multiple genes and environmental factors influence one's physical activity level (29). It has been proposed by Kelly et al. that the genetic control of voluntary physical activity is a result of both central drive and peripheral capability (22). Central drive is the result of mechanisms in the brain that influence the "want" to be active while the "capability" to be active is a result of peripheral factors that reduce pain/fatigue allowing for more sustained physical activity level (35). While Chapter 8 focuses on potential central pathways that influence physical activity, the remainder of this chapter focuses on peripheral factors that can be genetically controlled to regulate physical activity.

Peripheral factors affecting the capability to be physically activity

There is limited literature addressing the role of potential peripheral "capability to be active" factors in regulating physical activity. The available studies in this area have focused on skeletal muscle with potential peripheral factors that may be associated with physical activity regulation being components of substrate utilization and skeletal muscle contraction. Both these factors influence fatigue resistance, which interestingly is also affected by the dopaminergic systems and/or endocannabinoid systems (located centrally) (24, 25). Given that both the dopaminergic and endocannabinoid systems are involved with pain perception and since pain associated with activity has been correlated to skeletal muscle fatigue (16), it is possible that the fatigability

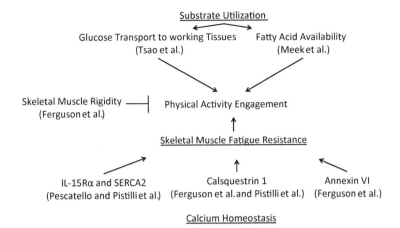

Figure 9.1 Schematic indicating the key processes involved with the peripheral regulation of physical activity along with associated journal citations. Specifically, substrate utilization and calcium homeostasis are the primary determinants to physical activity engagement. An increase in glucose transport and increasing fatty acid ability will increase physical activity. Optimal calcium homeostasis is achieved by an increase in annexin VI, calsequestrin 1, and the expression of the *IL-15αAA* and the associated increase in SERCA2. These calcium regulatory factors influence skeletal muscle fatigue resistance which will regulate skeletal muscle fatigue resistance. Lastly, an increase in proteins associated with skeletal muscle rigidity will decrease physical activity engagement.

of skeletal muscle – a peripheral factor influencing capability – could also influence physical activity level. Regardless of where these effects are exerted, there are at least two pathways through which peripheral factors may influence physical activity (Figure 9.1).

Inherent mechanisms by which skeletal muscle can regulate physical activity may include mechanisms associated with metabolism, contraction, and calcium flux (Figure 9.1). Specifically, the ability to transport glucose and fatty acids to the working tissue may increase physical activity levels. Furthermore, improved calcium homeostasis via IL-15Rα, annexin VI, and calsequestrin 1 may reduce skeletal muscle fatigue allowing for increased physical activity. Lastly, it should be noted that there is a unique set of proteins that increase skeletal muscle rigidity and their overexpression – as seen in low-active animals (14) – that may lead to a decrease in physical activity levels.

Substrate utilization may influence physical activity

Tsao et al. showed that an overexpression of glucose transport 4 (*Glut4*) in skeletal muscle led to a fourfold increase in wheel running as compared to control animals (57). The methodology used by Tsao et al. utilized an overexpression of *Glut4* in muscle and heart tissue of the 129/SV mouse strain (48) by splicing the MLCl promoter upstream of the *Glut4* gene. The authors observed a 45% increase in food intake and a fourfold increase in wheel running as compared to the control mice (~1 km ran for control mice and ~4 km ran for *Glut4* overexpressed mice) (57). The authors hypothesized that glucose transport was the rate-limiting step in skeletal muscle glucose uptake and therefore, an increase in glucose transporters could increase glucose uptake allowing for an increased physical activity response (57).

In addition to *Glut4*, there have been several studies that have shown nutritional factors may alter physical activity through alteration of substrate utilization. Researchers from the Garland lab have shown that mice bred for high activity for over 60 generations – mice whose activity had plateaued at approximately generation 25 – when treated with a high fat diet, significantly increased their daily wheel running by 160% (33). To date, this is the only treatment that Garland's research group has used that has increased the physical activity level of their high-active mice (32). Therefore, the authors suggested that treatment with a high-fat diet allowed for increased fat utilization as a primary fuel source, allowing for an increased capability resulting in a higher physical activity level in these mice whose activity had previously plateaued (33).

Skeletal muscle force of contraction and muscle fatigue may influence physical activity

During muscle contraction, the axon terminal of a motor neuron releases a neurotransmitter into the synaptic cleft. The neurotransmitters bind to receptors on the sarcolemma, which transmit an action potential to the transverse tubule (T tubule) of the sarcolemma. Once the action potential reaches the T tubule, there is a release of calcium (Ca^{2+}) from the sarcoplasmic reticulum (SR). Ca^{2+} binds to troponin C which causes a conformational change in tropomyosin, thereby exposing actin binding sites allowing for binding of the myosin head (41) and subsequent skeletal muscle contraction (41). Taking a broad view of skeletal muscle contraction, it is possible that biological factors that influence force production or fatigue at the motor neuron or fiber level could influence physical activity level. In fact, in 2015 Pistilli et al. showed that by knocking out IL-15Rα there was a shift in skeletal muscle fibers (with no change in the motor unit) to a fatigue-resistant phenotype, which also led to a 6.3-fold increase in wheel running (40). The authors concluded that the fatigue resistance, and increased physical activity, was due to an improved calcium homeostasis. Specifically, knocking out IL-15Rα altered the expression of key calcium regulating proteins, SERCA2 and calsequestrin 1, which prevented fatigue. The authors hypothesized that by preventing skeletal muscle fatigue, the muscle could maintain repeated bouts of contraction and therefore increase wheel running. Supporting this hypothesis is promising new research from the Pescatello lab that has demonstrated that men who are chronically active have the *IL-15Rα* 1775AA genotype as opposed to the *IL-15Rα* 1775CC genotype (6), confirming that the expression of *IL-15Rα* can influence physical activity levels in humans.

In 2014, we were the first to use the two-dimensional differential in gel electrophoresis (2D-DIGE) method to elucidate peripheral candidate proteins that were associated with physical activity regulation (14). The proteins that were differentially expressed between high- and low-active animals were primarily associated with metabolism, skeletal muscle structure, and calcium regulation. Using previous quantitative trait loci (QTL) mapping results, we selected key proteins of interest based on their expression in the 2D-DIGE results and if the protein's genetic code existed in a QTL region previously identified as being involved in the biological regulation of physical activity (14). With these criteria, annexin 6 and calsequestrin 1 were two highly likely candidate proteins involved in the peripheral regulation of physical activity.

The annexin family of proteins, which consists of 17 different proteins in animals, is involved primarily in Ca^{2+} homeostasis (46). Annexins are expressed in all tissues and share structural and functional similarities with other members of the annexin family, with the exception of annexin VI which contains a repeat sequence resulting in eight domains as opposed to the standard four (21). The combination of the similarities in structure and the expression in various tissues has led to difficulty in identifying the functions of individual members of the annexin family (13). In fact, functions of annexin VI have been hypothesized to include inhibition of blood coagulation, inhibition of protein kinase C, intracellular trafficking of endosomal vesicles, regulation of voltage-gated calcium cannels, structural modification of actin, and organization of lipid components of cell membranes (9, 13, 46). The function of annexin VI in muscle is still ambiguous partly because the role of annexin VI varies depending on the type of muscle. What is known is that annexin VI binds acidic phospholipids of membranes in a Ca^{2+}-dependent manner (3). Thus, the more calcium that is present, the more binding there is of annexin VI to lipid membranes.

The function of annexin VI in skeletal muscle is less studied as compared to cardiac and smooth muscle. Initially it was shown by Diaz-Munoz et al. that annexin VI bound calcium channels allowing for an increase in Ca^{2+} release (9). Additionally, Hazarika et al. demonstrated that in skeletal muscle annexin VI is associated with the SR and that during the initial phase of muscle contraction with the release of Ca^{2+} from channels of the sarcolemma, annexin VI binds to the T tubule and propagates the further release of Ca^{2+} (17). Thus, Hazarika et al. (17) proposed that annexin VI acts to stimulate more Ca^{2+} release from the SR, hence increasing force of contraction (17).

Another regulator of calcium homeostasis in skeletal muscle involved in regulation of physical activity based on proteomic overexpression is calsequestrin 1 (Casq1). Unlike annexin VI, Casq1 has been widely investigated for its function in skeletal muscle (4, 44). Casq1 is a Ca^{2+} buffer that helps to regulate the release of and reuptake of Ca^{2+} in skeletal muscle (42). Casq1 has a highly acidic C-terminal tail with a high binding affinity for Ca^{2+}. As Ca^{2+} binds to Casq1, a conformational change in the structure occurs allowing for a further increase in Ca^{2+} binding (4). It was initially thought that Casq1's only function was to remove Ca^{2+} from the myoplasm following muscle contraction; however, recent evidence has shown that Casq1 functions in the release of Ca^{2+} from the ryanodine receptor (RyR) (42). It has been suggested that Casq1 acts on the RyR to inhibit Ca^{2+} release through triadin and junctin (4). As a result of these functions, Casq1 acts as a Ca^{2+} sensor ensuring that Ca^{2+} levels are appropriately maintained in the muscle cell.

There have been several studies that evaluated Casq1 expression following regular bouts of exercise (20, 23, 37, 49). The studies by Jiao et al. (20) and Sugizaki et al. (49) were conducted in cardiac tissue and showed that with an increase in endurance training there was an increase in Casq1 protein expression, suggesting that Casq1 may play a role in the increased endurance. Kinnunen and Manttari (23) examined Casq1 protein expression in various skeletal muscle tissues following endurance or sprint training in a mouse model. Interestingly, the authors observed that depending on the muscle fiber composition and the type of training, there was a differential expression of Casq1 (23). Specifically, with endurance training there was a decrease in Casq1 in the soleus (slow-twitch fiber) while there was an increase in Casq1 in the extensor digitorum longus (EDL, fast twitch fiber) (23). Following sprint training, Casq1 was increased in the gastrocnemius (mixed muscle fiber) and the EDL, with no change in the soleus (23). The authors noted that in fast-twitch fiber muscle the Ca^{2+} storage capacity is three to four times higher and the release of and uptake of Ca^{2+} is more efficient compared to slow-twitch fibers (23). Thus, the authors propose that modulation of Casq1 following training allows for skeletal muscle to have increased capability to engage in the trained activity (23).

In summary, by showing that high-active animals have mechanisms that alter calcium homeostasis – increased expression of Anxn6 and Casq1 – our 2D-DIGE analysis (14) support Pistilli's earlier work (40) that showed through modification of *IL-15α* there was an alteration in calcium homeostasis in muscle which influenced physical activity level.

Adding to the complexity in the understanding of the peripheral regulation of physical activity is that low-active mice expressed their own unique protein signature in our 2D-DIGE results (14). This finding contradicted our original hypothesis which was that physical activity level was determined by a unique set of proteins and if an individual expressed more of those proteins they would be more active. Compared to the high-active mice, low-active mice had a reduction in glycolysis enzymes which we hypothesized slowed glycolysis and limited the generation of acetyl-CoA with a resultant slowing of the Krebs's cycle. Also, we observed an upregulation in electron transport chain enzymes in the low-active mice which might serve as compensation for the slowing of glycolysis and the Krebs's cycle, thus leading to no change in metabolism or physical activity (14). Additionally, the low-active mice had an increased expression in structural proteins of skeletal muscle (radixin, vinculin, vimentin, and the tubulins) that have been shown to increase rigidity and impair force production during skeletal muscle contraction. This overexpression of these structural proteins and potential increase in rigidity could increase fatigue and potentially impair physical activity engagement (14).

Combined, the above referenced studies encompassing both targeted and proteomic approaches, have provided tentative evidence that substrate utilization and skeletal muscle contractile performance may be primary peripheral factors that directly affect the capability to be active. However, these conclusions have been primarily based on correlative results highlighting the need for cause–effect research designs to provide mechanisms of activity regulation.

Confirming candidate genes' involvement in physical activity

An issue in many targeted genetics studies is the difficulty in providing cause–effect relationships between targeted genes/proteins and the phenotype being studied. In order to confirm the peripheral factors that influence physical activity, we utilized Vivo-Morpholinos to transiently silence annexin 6 and calsequestrin 1 genes in high-active mice. Vivo-Morpholinos are oligonucleotides bound to a morpholino ring that will bind to the target mRNA and block translation (15). The benefit of using Vivo-Morpholinos is that their use allows for partial silencing which is transient (15); thus we were able to knockdown annexin 6 and calsequestrin 1 in the high-active C57L/J mice to the levels of the C3H/HeJ low-active mice for 1 week. In effect, we were able to transiently convert the skeletal muscle of high-active mice to the phenotype of low-active mice (in regard to annexin 6 and calsequestrin 1) in order to quantitatively assess their role in physical activity regulation (15).

As shown in Figure 9.2, after baseline exposure to running wheels, mice treated with the annexin VI Vivo-Morpholino or the calsequestrin 1 Vivo-Morpholino had a 40% decrease in daily wheel running as compared to the control mice which received a Vivo-Morpholino that did not block the translation of any proteins. Once treatment with Vivo-Morpholinos ceased and the Vivo-Morpholinos were metabolized (~1 week), wheel running returned to control levels (14). From this data, we concluded that knocking down annexin VI and calsequestrin 1 to the level of a low-active mouse impaired the skeletal muscles' ability to maintain calcium homeostasis, resulting in an increased rate of fatigue which ultimately led to a decrease in wheel running.

While these results are exciting, this work could be greatly expanded. Specifically, since we only assessed wheel running as a measure of physical activity, there are a variety of further experiments that could be completed to further illustrate the balance between central (see Chapter 8) and peripheral factors regulating physical activity especially with the advancement of digital monitoring of home cages. For example, since the central drive to be active was not altered during Vivo-Morpholino treatments (14), quantifying the number of times a mouse gets on (and off) the running wheel would be an interesting approach to determine if the transiently silenced mice compensated for their reduced physical activity by engaging with the wheel more

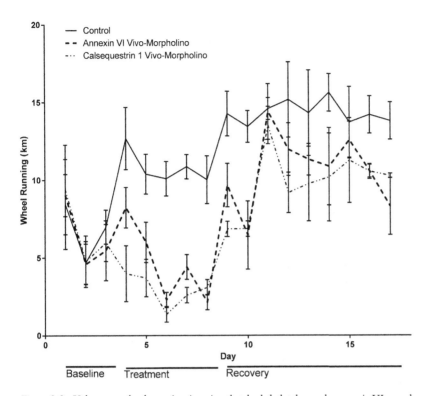

Figure 9.2 Voluntary wheel running in mice that had skeletal muscle annexin VI or calsequestrin 1 transiently knocked down by Vivo-Morpholinos. Wheel running was reduced when both annexin VI and calsequestrin was reduced and recovered once the Vivo-Morpholino was metabolized. Values are expressed as means ± standard deviations.

than the control mice. In short, the use of technologies such as Vivo-Morpholinos will allow other investigators to further delineate peripheral factors regulating physical activity.

Summary

The literature shows there are inherent mechanisms by which skeletal muscle can regulate physical activity with mechanisms associated with metabolism, contraction, and calcium flux (Figure 9.1). Specifically, the ability to transport glucose and fatty acids to the working tissue will increase physical activity levels. Furthermore, improved calcium homeostasis via IL-15Rα, annexin VI, and calsequestrin 1 will reduce skeletal muscle fatigue allowing for increased physical activity. Lastly, it should be noted that there is a unique set of proteins that increase skeletal muscle rigidity and their overexpression – as seen in low-active animals – may lead to a decrease in physical activity levels.

References

1. **Adlam D** and **Channon KM.** Radial artery graft string sign due to lumen obliteration by neointima: Insight from optical coherence tomography. *JACC Cardiovasc Interv* 4: 586–587, 2011.
2. **Adlam D, De Bono JP, Danson EJ, Zhang MH, Casadei B, Paterson DJ,** and **Channon KM.** Telemetric analysis of haemodynamic regulation during voluntary exercise training in mouse models. *Exp Physiol* 96: 1118–1128, 2011.

3. **Babiychuk EB** and **Draeger A.** Annexins in cell membrane dynamics. Ca(2+)-regulated association of lipid microdomains. *J Cell Biol* 150. 1113 1124, 2000.

4. **Beard NA**, **Wei L**, and **Dulhunty AF.** Ca(2+) signaling in striated muscle: The elusive roles of triadin, junctin, and calsequestrin. *Eur Biophys J* 39: 27–36, 2009.

5. **Ben-Joseph E**, **Lee JS**, **Cromley EK**, **Laden F**, and **Troped PJ.** Virtual and actual: Relative accuracy of on-site and web-based instruments in auditing the environment for physical activity. *Health Place* 19: 138–150, 2013.

6. **Bruneau M**, Jr., **Walsh S**, **Selinsky E**, **Ash G**, **Angelopoulos TJ**, **Clarkson P**, **Gordon P**, **Moyna N**, **Visich P**, **Zoeller R**, **Thompson P**, **Gordish-Dressman H**, **Hoffman E**, **Devaney J**, and **Pescatello LS.** A genetic variant in IL-15Ralpha correlates with physical activity among European-American adults. *Mol Genet Genomic Med*, 6: 401–408, 2018.

7. **Cheng Y**, **Macera CA**, **Davis DR**, **Ainsworth BE**, **Troped PJ**, and **Blair SN.** Physical activity and self-reported, physician-diagnosed osteoarthritis: Is physical activity a risk factor? *J Clin Epidemiol* 53: 315–322, 2000.

8. **Church DM**, **Goodstadt L**, **Hillier LW**, **Zody MC**, **Goldstein S**, **She X**, **Bult CJ**, **Agarwala R**, **Cherry JL**, **DiCuccio M**, **Hlavina W**, **Kapustin Y**, **Meric P**, **Maglott D**, **Birtle Z**, **Marques AC**, **Graves T**, **Zhou S**, **Teague B**, **Potamousis K**, **Churas C**, **Place M**, **Herschleb J**, **Runnheim R**, **Forrest D**, **Amos-Landgraf J**, **Schwartz DC**, **Cheng Z**, **Lindblad-Toh K**, **Eichler EE**, **Ponting CP**, and **Mouse Genome Sequencing Consortium.** Lineage-specific biology revealed by a finished genome assembly of the mouse. *PLoS Biol* 7: e1000112, 2009.

9. **Diaz-Munoz M**, **Hamilton SL**, **Kaetzel MA**, **Hazarika P**, and **Dedman JR**. Modulation of Ca2+ release channel activity from sarcoplasmic reticulum by annexin VI (67-kDa calcimedin). *J Biol Chem* 265: 15894–15899, 1990.

10. **Dishman RK**, **Renner KJ**, **Youngstedt SD**, **Reigle TG**, **Bunnell BN**, **Burke KA**, **Yoo HS**, **Mougey EH**, and **Meyerhoff JL.** Activity wheel running reduces escape latency and alters brain monoamine levels after footshock. *Brain Res Bull* 42: 399–406, 1997.

11. **Eikelboom R.** Human parallel to voluntary wheel running: Exercise. *Anim Behav* 57: F11–F12, 1999.

12. **Ekkekakis P**, **Hall EE**, and **Petruzzello SJ.** Variation and homogeneity in affective responses to physical activity of varying intensities: An alternative perspective on dose-response based on evolutionary considerations. *J Sports Sci* 23: 477–500, 2005.

13. **Enrich C**, **Rentero C**, **de Muga SV**, **Reverter M**, **Mulay V**, **Wood P**, **Koese M**, and **Grewal T.** Annexin A6-linking Ca(2+) signaling with cholesterol transport. *Biochim Biophys Acta* 1813: 935–947, 2011.

14. **Ferguson DP**, **Dangott LJ**, **Schmitt EE**, **Vellers HL**, and **Lightfoot JT**. Differential skeletal muscle proteome of high- and low-active mice. *J Appl Physiol (1985)* 116: 1057–1067, 2014.

15. **Ferguson DP**, **Schmitt EE**, and **Lightfoot JT.** Vivo-morpholinos induced transient knockdown of physical activity related proteins. *PloS One* 8: e61472, 2013.

16. **Ge HY**, **Nie H**, **Graven-Nielsen T**, **Danneskiold-Samsoe B**, and **Arendt-Nielsen L.** Descending pain modulation and its interaction with peripheral sensitization following sustained isometric muscle contraction in fibromyalgia. *Eur J Pain* 16: 196–203, 2012.

17. **Hazarika P**, **Kaetzel MA**, **Sheldon A**, **Karin NJ**, **Fleischer S**, **Nelson TE**, and **Dedman JR.** Annexin VI is associated with calcium-sequestering organelles. *J Cell Biochem* 46: 78–85, 1991.

18. **Heath GW** and **Troped PJ.** The role of the built environment in shaping the health behaviors of physical activity and healthy eating for cardiovascular health. *Future Cardiol* 8: 677–679, 2012.

19. **James P**, **Troped PJ**, **Hart JE**, **Joshu CE**, **Colditz GA**, **Brownson RC**, **Ewing R**, and **Laden F.** Urban sprawl, physical activity, and body mass index: Nurses' Health Study and Nurses' Health Study II. *Am J Public Health* 103: 369–375, 2013.

20. **Jiao Q**, **Bai Y**, **Akaike T**, **Takeshima H**, **Ishikawa Y**, and **Minamisawa S.** Sarcalumenin is essential for maintaining cardiac function during endurance exercise training. *Am J Physiol Heart Circ Physiol* 297: H576–582, 2009.

21. **Kaetzel MA** and **Dedman JR.** Annexin VI regulation of cardiac function. *Biochem Biophys Res Commun* 322: 1171–1177, 2004.

22. **Kelly SA**, **Nehrenberg DL**, **Peirce JL**, **Hua K**, **Steffy BM**, **Wiltshire T**, **Pardo-Manuel de Villena F**, **Garland T**, Jr., and **Pomp D.** Genetic architecture of voluntary exercise in an advanced intercross line of mice. *Physiological genomics* 42: 190–200, 2010.

23. **Kinnunen S** and **Manttari S.** Specific effects of endurance and spring training on protein expression of calsequestrin and SERCA in mouse skeletal muscle. *J Muscle Res Cell Motil* 33: 123–130, 2012.

24. **Knab AM, Bowen RS, Hamilton AT, Gulledge AA**, and **Lightfoot JT.** Altered dopaminergic profiles: Implications for the regulation of voluntary physical activity. *Behav Brain Res* 204: 147–152, 2009.

25. **Knab AM, Bowen RS, Hamilton AT**, and **Lightfoot JT.** Pharmacological manipulation of the dopaminergic system affects wheel-running activity in differentially active mice. *J Biol Regul Homeost Agents* 26: 119–129, 2012.

26. **Knab AM** and **Lightfoot JT.** Does the difference between physically active and couch potato lie in the dopamine system? *Int J Biol Sci* 6: 133–150, 2010.

27. **Lightfoot JT.** Current understanding of the genetic basis for physical activity. *J Nutr* 141: 526–530, 2011.

28. **Lightfoot JT.** Why control activity? Evolutionary selection pressures affecting the development of physical activity genetic and biological regulation. *Biomed Res Int* 2013: 821678, 2013.

29. **Lightfoot JT, EJC DEG, Booth FW, Bray MS, M DENH, Kaprio J, Kelly SA, Pomp D, Saul MC, Thomis MA, Garland T**, Jr, and **Bouchard C.** Biological/genetic regulation of physical activity level: Consensus from GenBioPAC. *Med Sci Sports Exerc* 50: 863–873, 2018.

30. **Lightfoot JT, Leamy L, Pomp D, Turner MJ, Fodor AA, Knab A, Bowen RS, Ferguson D, Moore-Harrison T**, and **Hamilton A**. Strain screen and haplotype association mapping of wheel running in inbred mouse strains. *J Appl Physiol (1985)* 109: 623–634, 2010.

31. **Lightfoot JT, Leamy L, Pomp D, Turner MJ, Fodor AA, Knab A, Bowen RS, Ferguson D, Moore-Harrison T**, and **Hamilton A.** Strain screen and haplotype association mapping of wheel running in inbred mouse strains. *J Appl Physiol* 109: 623–634, 2010.

32. **Meek TH, Dlugosz EM, Vu KT**, and **Garland T**, Jr. Effects of leptin treatment and Western diet on wheel running in selectively bred high runner mice. *Physiol Behav* 106: 252–258, 2012.

33. **Meek TH, Eisenmann JC**, and **Garland T**, Jr. Western diet increases wheel running in mice selectively bred for high voluntary wheel running. *Int J Obes (Lond)* 34: 960–969, 2010.

34. **Mokdad AH, Marks JS, Stroup DF**, and **Gerberding JL**. Actual causes of death in the United States, 2000. *JAMA* 291: 1238–1245, 2004.

35. **Moore-Harrison T** and **Lightfoot JT.** Driven to be inactive? The genetics of physical activity. *Prog Mol Biol Transl Sci* 94: 271–290, 2010.

36. **Morey SS.** ACSM revises guidelines for exercise to maintain fitness. *Am Fam Physician* 59: 473, 1999.

37. **Myllymaki T, Rusko H, Syvaoja H, Juuti T, Kinnunen ML**, and **Kyrolainen H**. Effects of exercise intensity and duration on nocturnal heart rate variability and sleep quality. *Eur J Appl Physiol* 112: 801–809, 2012.

38. **Orstad SL, McDonough MH, Klenosky DB, Mattson M**, and **Troped PJ.** The observed and perceived neighborhood environment and physical activity among urban-dwelling adults: The moderating role of depressive symptoms. *Soc Sci Med* 190: 57–66, 2017.

39. **Peterson KE, Dubowitz T, Stoddard AM, Troped PJ, Sorensen G**, and **Emmons KM**. Social context of physical activity and weight status in working-class populations. *J Phys Act Health* 4: 381–396, 2007.

40. **Pistilli EE, Bogdanovich S, Garton F, Yang N, Gulbin JP, Conner JD, Anderson BG, Quinn LS, North K, Ahima RS**, and **Khurana TS.** Loss of IL-15 receptor alpha alters the endurance, fatigability, and metabolic characteristics of mouse fast skeletal muscles. *J Clin Invest* 121: 3120–3132, 2011.

41. **Powers SK** and **Howley ET.** *Exercise Physiology. Theory and Application to Fitness and Performance.* New York: McGraw Hill, 2004.

42. **Protasi F, Paolini C, Canato M, Reggiani C**, and **Quarta M.** Lessons from calsequestrin-1 ablation in vivo: much more than a Ca(2+) buffer after all. *J Muscle Res Cell Motil* 32: 257–270, 2011.

43. **Rodriguez DA, Brown AL**, and **Troped PJ.** Portable global positioning units to complement accelerometry-based physical activity monitors. *Med Sci Sports Exerc* 37: S572–581, 2005.

44. **Rossi AE** and **Dirksen RT.** Sarcoplasmic reticulum: the dynamic calcium governor of muscle. *Muscle Nerve* 33: 715–731, 2006.

45. **Smith AL, Troped PJ, McDonough MH**, and **DeFreese JD.** Youth perceptions of how neighborhood physical environment and peers affect physical activity: a focus group study. *Int J Behav Nutr Phys Act* 12: 80, 2015.

46. **Song G, Harding SE, Duchen MR, Tunwell R, O'Gara P, Hawkins TE**, and **Moss SE**. Altered mechanical properties and intracellular calcium signaling in cardiomyocytes from annexin 6 null-mutant mice. *FASEB J* 16: 622–624, 2002.

47. **Starnes HA, Troped PJ, Klenosky DB**, and **Doehring AM.** Trails and physical activity: A review. *J Phys Act Health* 8: 1160–1174, 2011.

48. **Stenbit AE, Burcelin R, Katz EB, Tsao TS, Gautier N, Charron MJ,** and **Le Marchand-Brustel Y.** Diverse effects of Glut 4 ablation on glucose uptake and glycogen synthesis in red and white skeletal muscle. *J Clin Invest* 98: 629–634, 1996.

49. **Sugizaki MM, Leopoldo AP, Conde SJ, Campos DS, Damato R, Leopoldo AS, Nascimento AF, Oliveira Junior Sde A,** and **Cicogna AC.** Upregulation of mRNA myocardium calcium handling in rats submitted to exercise and food restriction. *Arq Bras Cardiol* 97: 46–52, 2011.

50. **Tamura K, Puett RC, Hart JE, Starnes HA, Laden F,** and **Troped PJ.** Spatial clustering of physical activity and obesity in relation to built environment factors among older women in three U.S. states. *BMC Public Health* 14: 1322, 2014.

51. **Troiano RP, Berrigan D, Dodd KW, Masse LC, Tilert T,** and **McDowell M.** Physical activity in the United States measured by accelerometer. *Med Sci Sports Exerc* 40: 181–188, 2008.

52. **Troped PJ** and **Saunders RP.** Gender differences in social influence on physical activity at different stages of exercise adoption. *Am J Health Promot* 13: 112–115, 1998.

53. **Troped PJ, Saunders RP, Pate RR, Reininger B,** and **Addy CL.** Correlates of recreational and transportation physical activity among adults in a New England community. *Prev Med* 37: 304–310, 2003.

54. **Troped PJ, Tamura K, Whitcomb HA,** and **Laden F.** Perceived built environment and physical activity in U.S. women by sprawl and region. *Am J Prev Med* 41: 473–479, 2011.

55. **Troped PJ, Wiecha JL, Fragala MS, Matthews CE, Finkelstein DM, Kim J,** and **Peterson KE.** Reliability and validity of YRBS physical activity items among middle school students. *Med Sci Sports Exerc* 39: 416–425, 2007.

56. **Troped PJ, Wilson JS, Matthews CE, Cromley EK,** and **Melly SJ.** The built environment and location-based physical activity. *Am J Prev Med* 38: 429–438, 2010.

57. **Tsao TS, Li J, Chang KS, Stenbit AE, Galuska D, Anderson JE, Zierath JR, McCarter RJ,** and **Charron MJ.** Metabolic adaptations in skeletal muscle overexpressing GLUT4: Effects on muscle and physical activity. *FASEB J* 15: 958–969, 2001.

10

TOXICANT AND DIETARY EXPOSURES AS UNIQUE ENVIRONMENTAL FACTORS THAT AFFECT THE GENETIC REGULATION OF ACTIVITY

Emily E. Schmitt and Heather L. Vellers

Introduction

As indicated in previous chapters, genetic background plays a crucial role in determining an individual's daily physical activity patterns; however, genetics is not the only factor driving physical activity. Like other behavioral phenotypes, physical activity is a complex behavior and is driven by various physiological variables not only influenced by genetics, but also, combined effects of genetics and environmental factors. When considering environmental influences on physical activity, the general thought is that common environmental factors, an example of which is our 'built environment" or presence and ease of access to sidewalks, parks, trails, and recreational facilities, is an important factor in determining individual activity engagement. This thought, however, has yet to be supported by evidence in adults where physical activity has been measured objectively (13, 18, 49). Thus, ease of access to a gym or parks does not necessarily prompt an increase in physical activity among individuals. Less commonly considered are unique environmental factors that affect physical activity, defined as all individual-specific experiences (see Chapter 6). Such factors have been calculated to account for 8–52% of the observed interindividual variation in daily activity patterns (33, 62, 66, 71). The precise unique environmental factors that directly influence an individual's physical activity are beginning to be studied, with work isolating factors including specific types of environmental chemicals and diet demonstrating a significant and detrimental effect of these factors on physical activity patterns. In this chapter, the purpose is to discuss two unique environmental influencers of the genetic regulation of activity and potential mechanisms (32) through which each are hypothesized to regulate activity.

How might unique environmental factors influence an individual's drive to be active?

Prior to genetics being considered a regulator of physical activity, work from the early 1920s and 1930s suggested that daily activity was controlled through biological mechanisms (58, 74). Wang, Richter, and colleagues (58, 65, 74) investigated the relationship between the female reproductive cycle and wheel-running behavior in rodents. In 1923, Wang et al. (74) reported a cyclical relationship between content inside the vagina of female rats and activity levels, and noted female mice were most active when they were in "heat" (74). Shortly thereafter, Slonaker (65) followed up on Wang's findings and concluded physical activity in females was driven by "copulation and successful stimulation of the cervis uteri," or what we presently refer to as the estrous cycle (65). In males, a role of the reproductive system on physical activity regulation was also apparent, when in 1925, Hoskins (30) demonstrated through castrating male rats that daily wheel running was significantly reduced and remained significantly lower than their control counterparts throughout their lifetime. Taken together, these initial studies were among the first to suggest a strong relationship between physical activity and the estrous cycle in females and between physical activity and testicular function in males.

Since these early studies, multiple other studies have shown a strong influence of sex hormones in regulating physical activity. For example, Gorzek et al. (25) found female ovariectomized mice displayed significant reductions in wheel-running activity by up to 80%, while physiological replacement of estrogen increased activity in these mice to approximately 54% of baseline. Additionally, Bowen and colleagues (9) found that removal of sex hormones resulted in approximately 90% decreases in the daily distances ran in male and female mice, while exogenous replacement of these hormones resulted in varying levels (35–110%) of recovered baseline activity. Further, Bowen, et al.'s (9) results revealed specific influences of each hormone on activity patterns, where recovered amounts of distance and duration ran were primarily influenced by testosterone administration while the recovery of speed was primarily influenced by 17β-estradiol.

While many studies have shown that sex hormones regulate physical activity, the mechanisms through which sex hormones work are somewhat unclear. Roy and Wade (59) examined the effect of nonaromatizable (dihydrotestosterone proprionate) and aromatizable (testosterone proprionate) androgen administration in male rats that underwent castration to determine whether the conversion of testosterone to estrogen through the aromatase complex was a pathway regulating male rat activity. The results showed the aromatizable form of testosterone had the greatest effect on physical activity, while the nonaromatizable form of testosterone had no effect on activity suggesting that activity regulation was dependent on testosterone conversion to estradiol via the aromatase complex (59). Conversely, more recent work by Bowen et al. (8), showed no effect on male mouse physical activity when the aromatase complex was inhibited through administration of reversible and irreversible aromatase pharmacological interventions, calling into question the applicability of Roy and Wade's results in a mouse model.

Lastly, in male mice only, Jardi et al. (31) investigated the role of testosterone, and identified a pathway through which testosterone elicits its effect on physical activity. These authors showed the free fraction of testosterone stimulated activity by acting on central (brain) dopaminergic pathways via the androgen receptor, and indirectly through the aromatase complex. Furthermore, using a muscle-specific androgen receptor knockout mouse model and then providing exogenous testosterone, the authors demonstrated that testosterone-induced increases in activity do not occur through muscle or peripheral mechanism(s) (31). Thus, in total, work demonstrates direct effects of testosterone and 17β-estradiol on physical activity regulation in male and female rodents (25, 31, 59). However, additional mechanistic work is needed in females to determine whether similar sex-dependent pathways as in males participate in physical activity regulation through these hormones. Additionally and perhaps most critically, the work by Jardi et al. (31) merged two separate bodies of literature involving the role sex hormones and dopamine play in regulating activity regulation with other studies previously linking wheel-running behavior in mice to genomic-dependent dopaminergic pathways (38, 39). Thus, the specific dopaminergic pathways stimulated by sex hormones and resulting physical activity may be dependent on genetic background, especially in the dopaminergic pathways (see Chapter 8).

As previously mentioned, unique environmental factors have been suggested to play significant direct roles in regulating physical activity. One potential pathway through which unique environmental factors may influence physical activity is via alteration in sex hormone levels given that alterations in sex hormone levels can have dramatic effects on physical activity levels. Thus, the remaining sections of this chapter will discuss specific, unique environmental factors that have been suggested to have direct effects on sex hormones, and thus, may indirectly affect physical activity.

Endocrine-disrupting chemicals

The harmful consequences of endocrine-disrupting chemicals (EDCs) on human health have been widely studied over the past few decades and growing evidence has supported that man-made chemicals contribute to adverse health effects on humans and wildlife (3). Not only do EDCs lead to harmful developmental, reproductive, neurological, and immune effects through the alteration of endocrine systems, they also cost the US healthcare system hundreds of billions of dollars (3). EDCs are defined as man-made synthetic substances that alter an organism's internal milieu which presents a risk of death, disease, or birth defect through absorption, ingestion, and inhalation (23). EDCs are found in, but not limited to, metals, plastics, personal care products, pesticides, pharmaceutical drugs, and industrial chemicals. Endocrine disruptors affect hormone response by mimicking hormones and binding agonistically or antagonistically to hormone receptors. EDCs may turn off, turn on, or modify hormonal signals, which affects normal functioning of tissues and organs (14). For example, EDCs can mimic estrogens, androgens, and thyroid hormones by competitively binding to the appropriate receptor and potentially producing over- or understimulation of these receptors (5). Exposures to EDCs are more dangerous if exposure occurs during "critical periods" of life when organisms are still developing and are more sensitive to hormonal disruption (23). The developing brain relies strongly on proper functioning hormones and disruption in hormone receptor function can lead to altered neural development of the brain (reviewed in 56). Specifically, it has recently been shown that EDCs can have a profound effect on early life brain development due to nervous system alterations in the hypothalamus–pituitary–thyroid gland axis (reviewed in 34). These alterations of the brain's connectivity and development have further been elucidated when mice exposed to low doses of a single EDC resulted in disruptions in midbrain dopaminergic nuclei of mice, where physical activity is thought to be regulated (67). Given that sex hormones regulate physical activity and that EDCs have a profound effect on hormone activity, it is possible that ECDs can cause lower physical activity levels through sex hormone disruption as illustrated in Figure 10.1.

While there are literally thousands of EDCs, there are some common EDCs that alter regulation of physical activity including bisphenol A (BPA), several different categories of phthalates, and a common fungicide, vinclozolin. BPA is a chemical produced in large quantities and is primarily used in production of plastics, PVC, and epoxy resins. BPA has been studied in a variety of *in vivo* and *in vitro* models, is estrogenic, and has been found to have significant adverse effects on mammary gland development in female mice (47) and sperm counts in males (42). Phthalates or phthalate esters are considered EDCs (35) and encompass a large group of compounds that share similar chemical structures. Common phthalates include diethylhexyl phthalate (DEHP), dibutyl phthalate (DBP), butyl benzyl phthalate (BBP), di-isononyl phthalate (DINP, DiBP, DIDP), and dipentyl phthalate (DPP); all have been shown to have adverse effects on human health primarily as antiandrogenic compounds (37, 55). Phthalate compounds have

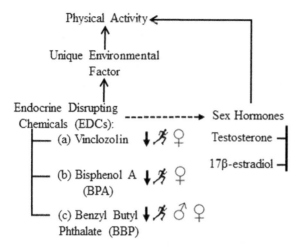

Figure 10.1 Schematic outlining the unique environmental factor of endocrine-disrupting chemicals (EDCs) and the effect on physical activity regulation. Research has shown that EDCs influence sex hormones, but the mechanisms through which the EDCs act to control activity are not fully understood (indicated by the dotted line). a) Vinclozolin exposure decreases activity in females. b) BPA exposure decreases physical activity in females. c) BBP exposure decreases physical activity in males and females.

been in the environment since the 1930s and are often found in plastics (most concerning in toys for infants) (35), and personal care products, such as perfumes, lubricants, aerosols, and nail polish products (75). Food is also a major source of phthalate exposure, specifically DEHP, with humans having diets high in meat and dairy showing a twofold increases in DEHP exposure (64). Finally, vinclozolin is a common fungicide used to control diseases in crops and has been characterized as an endocrine disruptor (antiandrogenic) and is a possible human carcinogen with exposure causing disease and abnormalities for up to four generations after exposure (2), with significant major morphological alterations observed in exposed male rats (27). In short, EDCs are ubiquitous in our environment with exposure ranging from personal care products to food packaging and processing. Disruption in hormone levels from EDC exposure can cause a variety of physiological problems that vary in severity and differ by sex, yet few studies have examined the direct relationship between EDC exposure and physical activity.

Endocrine disruptors' effect on physical activity

Given that sex hormone levels alter physical activity and EDC exposure alters sex hormone physiology, it is possible that EDCs affect physical activity level through their effects on sex hormones. The number of studies considering EDC influences on activity is few, with only three studies tackling the question of the effect of EDCs on physical activity (Table 10.1). The available studies have used animal models as they allow investigators to directly assess exposure to EDCs and resulting activity levels.

One of the earliest studies to investigate if a toxicant led to changes in activity levels was from Flynn et al. (21) who studied the fungicide vinclozolin. In 2001, Flynn et al. (21) showed that female rats, but not male rats, exposed to long-term dietary vinclozolin both pre- and postnatally had alterations in locomotor activity compared to control animals. The researchers fed pregnant rats soy-free diets containing vinclozolin (approximately 0, 0.8, 12, and 60 mg/kg/day for an adult) beginning on gestational day 7, and the diets were continuously fed to the

Table 10.1 Summary of studies demonstrating effects of endocrine-disrupting chemicals (EDCs) on physical activity in rodents

EDC	Study	Species	Species characteristics	Study design	Effect of EDC on physical activity
Vinclozolin	Flynn et al. (21)	Rat	Sprague Dawley male and female rats	2 weeks prior to mating, females were shifted from standard diet to irradiated soy-free diet. The vinclozolin-dosed diets began on gestation day 7 and continued through weaning on day 22. Weaned pups continued their respective diet until sacrifice on day 77. Resulting pups were randomly assigned to behavioral measures ranging from wheel-running activity to play behavior	In the high-dosed vinclozolin group, females (but not males) demonstrated decreased running-wheel activity
Bisphenol A (BPA)	Johnson et al. (32)	Mouse	Founder outbred adult California mice	2 weeks prior to mating, females were assigned to a diet group (control or BPA) and maintained their respective diets throughout gestation and lactation. Weaned males and females were then placed on the control diet for the remainder of the study	BPA-exposed females (but not males) were significantly less active than control counterparts as indicated by calorimetry measurements (cage activity), but no differences in voluntary wheel running were examined in either sex
Benzyl butyl phthalate (BBP)	Schmitt et al. (62)	Mouse	C57BL/6J inbred mice	Pregnant damns were exposed to BBP via oral gavage on days 9–16 of gestation. Resulting male and female pups were weaned and analyzed for the study	Male and female pups that were exposed to BBP prenatally showed significant decreases in voluntary wheel running compared to controls

offspring until sacrifice on postnatal day 77. It was found that females in the high-dose group were significantly less active than control animals, while treated males did not show significant alterations in wheel activity (21). Given that vinclozolin is antiandrogenic, Flynn et al.'s (21) results suggest that the decreased activity due to vinclozolin exposure was due to alterations in the androgenic system.

Johnson et al. (32) examined the effect of the antiestrogenic toxicant BPA on physical activity in founder outbred adult California mice (32). Two weeks before breeding, virgin female mice were randomly assigned to different diets and remained on the same diets throughout gestation and lactation. Diet #1 was a low-phytoestrogen diet supplemented with corn oil, diet #2 was the same as the first diet with 50 mg of BPA/kg feed weight, and diet #3 was the same phyto-estrogen diet supplemented with 0.1 parts per billion of ethinyl estradiol. Importantly, the authors found BPA-exposed females were significantly less active, as evident by several indirect calorim-etry measurements. In males, no significant differences were observed. Thus, while these results suggest that BPA exposure can affect physical activity, there are indications that males and females may be differentially affected due to differential mechanisms of physical activity regulation.

Schmitt and colleagues (62) found prenatal exposure to the antiandrogenic phthalate BBP resulted in decreased anogenital distances (indicates puberty development in male mice) and delayed vaginal openings (indicates puberty development in female mice). Additionally, serum testosterone concentrations were significantly lower in prenatally exposed male mice when measured during adolescent and adult years, indicating a lasting effect of *in utero* exposure to BBP on sex hormone function throughout life. In females, a similar decrease in testosterone and significant reductions in estrogen concentrations were found in prenatally exposed adults when compared to controls. Concurrent with these observations, wheel-running activity from 8 to 20 weeks of age in the BBP-exposed offspring was decreased (on average) by 20% in male and 15% in female mice compared to control counterparts. This study was the first to suggest maternal endocrine disruption can cause an altered hormone response, with a corresponding decreased activity throughout early adulthood in all offspring. Overall, these results suggest *in utero* exposure to a common antiandrogenic EDC can reduce sex hormone concentrations and physical activity in mice, regardless of sex (62).

To date, only three studies exist that directly assessed the impact of prenatal exposure of EDCs on physical activity in offspring (see Table 10.1). The results of these three studies con-firm that environmental toxicants can decrease physical activity and need to be considered as a possible factor causing physical inactivity. In addition, it appears that EDC effects on physical activity are mediated through sex hormone systems, and males and females appear to be differ-entially affected, perhaps indicating different mechanisms of action between sexes. Finally, even though the link has been made between the biological pathway interacting with the unique environment to control physical activity, it is also important to recognize that the dopaminergic system could play a factor as well (see Chapter 8). In a comprehensive review on neurotoxicity of EDCs, Masuo and Ishido (48) suggest that EDCs disrupt the development of the central dopamine system neurons in the brain by affecting monoaminergic neurons in the central ner-vous system. These neural effects of EDCs may play a role in causing the behavioral alterations observed when EDC effects on activity are study and are certainly a potential avenue for further investigation.

Effects of diet on physical activity regulation

Like EDCs, dietary intake is another unique environmental influence that potentially affects pathways of physical activity regulation. Observations that diet directly alters an individual's physical activity patterns dates back to studies in the early 1800s (52, 73) – as reviewed by Casper (12) – that documented "heightened physical activity" as a hallmark behavioral characteristic in individuals diagnosed with anorexia nervosa (AN; an eating disorder characterized by varying degrees of caloric deprivation and malnourishment). Casper (12) highlighted that heightened levels of activity (e.g., "restlessness" and "increased drive" to move), were typically found only after following a period of self-starvation. From this, Casper hypothesized that the caloric restriction related to AN led to increased physical activity, as opposed to the prevailing belief that increased physical activity led to AN. While Casper addressed the hypocaloric-induced hyperactivity response phenomenon as it relates to a diseased condition, this response falls in line with the theory that human locomotor activity has evolved partially to a selective pressure of food availability (discussed in 44). Briefly, throughout evolution, a foraging mechanism (e.g., foraging gene) is hypothesized to have been stimulated by food availability, where low food availability led to increased locomotor activity in search for food, while food abundance inhibited, or simply did not trigger this mechanism. In the current state of extremely high food abundance and availability in Western societies, it brings to question whether this shift of increased food availability has contributed to the low daily activity levels among US residents (69). Research specifically addressing the effect of dietary patterns on physical activity is in its infancy, however, evidence from both caloric restriction or overfeeding demonstrate links between feeding and physical activity. For the purposes of this chapter, this section will focus on evidence linking caloric restriction with increased activity with associated pathways through which this response occurs and evidence from work that has begun investigating the effect of caloric excess on activity.

Caloric restriction

The caloric restriction-induced increases in physical activity have been linked to various neurochemicals central to the brain, including leptin (4, 16, 26, 72), serotonin (28), and dopamine (36). The adipose tissue-derived hormone leptin, is one of the most widely known and investigated mechanisms associated with dietary restriction and increased activity (4, 19, 26, 29, 43, 72). The secretion of leptin is correlated with fat mass, where leptin secretion is increased with increases in fat mass, and decreased with decreases in fat mass (1). The involvement of leptin in diet and activity regulation has been tested through leptin administration in AN patients and activity-based anorexia (ABA) rodent models, where increased leptin reduced hyperactive responses (17, 43). A study by Verhagen et al. (72) demonstrated that low levels of leptin associated with increased wheel running was mediated through the ventral tegmental area of the brain, and speculated that the suppressed leptin levels induced an increased firing rate of the dopaminergic neurons. Interestingly, the dopaminergic neurons contain highly expressed leptin receptors (20), and may provide one mechanism through which leptin participates in caloric restriction-induced hyperactivity.

While plasma leptin has been suggested as a key player between caloric restriction and hyperactivity, such work is correlational and has not been directly tested. Some evidence suggests the hypocaloric-induced increases in physical activity are independent of leptin levels (28, 54). For example, one study by Morton et al. (54) demonstrated a hypocaloric-induced increased activity response independent of leptin, through fasting (fasted for 24 hours) wild-type and *ob/ob* (leptin-deficient) mice. Fasting in the leptin-deficient mice led to significant increases in both ambulatory and wheel-running activity. Hillebrand et al. (28) furthered this work by evaluating the effect of the atypical antipsychotic drug, olanzapine (Zyprexa), on wheel running in an ABA rat model, as well as measuring physical activity in a cohort of AN patients who were classified as "hyperactive" upon hospital admittance. Olanzapine is a thienobenzodiazepine compound, which has a high affinity for $5-HT_{2A/AC}$ receptors, histamine (H_1) receptors, adrenergic (α_1 receptors), and a moderate affinity for dopamine (D_1–D_4) receptors (10, 11, 53, 63). In Hillebrand, et al.'s study (28), olanzapine was found to inhibit the heightened wheel running in ABA rats as well as the hyperactive responses in patients with AN. However, olanzapine inhibited the hyperactive responses without altering plasma leptin levels suggesting that other nonleptin mechanisms were involved in the hyperactive responses. Hillebrand et al. (28) hypothesized that hypocaloric hyperactivity was mediated through serotonin activation (5-$HT_{2A/AC}$ receptors), histamine receptors, and/or dopamine given the high–moderate affinity of olanzapine on these systems. In rats, Klenotich et al. (36) expanded upon this thought by selectively blocking $5-HT_{2A/AC}$ receptors and dopamine receptors (DR) DR_2 and DR_3, and found that selective antagonism of DR_2 and DR_3 reduced ABA, whereas antagonism of $5-HT_{2A/AC}$ did not. Therefore, this study concluded that the D_2 and D_3 receptors were mechanisms through which olanzapine reduced activity in ABA rats. As noted previously, earlier work has established the dopaminergic system as a potential regulator of physical activity where biological (31) and genetic predisposition (38) link to influence physical activity. While the dopaminergic system presents one pathway through which caloric restriction could increase physical activity, it would be interesting to further investigate how caloric restriction, as a unique environmental factor, interacts with other biological/genetic factors to then influence physical activity.

Overfeeding

Compared to literature describing links between caloric restriction and increased activity, less work (Table 10.2) has described the effect of caloric excess on activity, especially in terms of potential mechanism(s) mediating how this response might occur. Of the studies in Table 10.2, only one has directly investigated a link between chronic overfeeding and physical activity. Similar to EDCs, chronic overfeeding has been observed to alter sex hormones levels and functions (7). In males, a direct effect of chronic overfeeding on sex hormones is known (7), where, in general, androgen levels are decreased and estrogens are increased. In females, however, direct ties between chronic overfeeding and sex hormone levels are unclear. For example, overfeeding-induced metabolic diseases in women (e.g., polycystic ovarian syndrome, type 2 diabetes, and obesity) show an opposing effect of chronic overfeeding on sex hormone levels as compared to men: increased androgens and decreases in estrogens (15). Given that it is established that sex hormones regulate activity, and that overfeeding potentially alters sex hormones (7), we hypothesized that alterations in sex hormones after chronic overfeeding were significant mediators of a reduced wheel-running activity in mice (71). With the chronic overfeeding of a high-fat, high-sugar diet, there was a significant reduction in acute wheel-running activity in males (~70%) and females (~57%) (71). However, this decreased activity did not appear to be mediated through alterations in sex hormones given that sex hormone levels between control and intervention animals did not differ and exogenous supplementation of sex hormones in overfed animals did not alter physical activity. Thus, chronic overfeeding decreased daily activity, but apparently through a mechanism(s) not involving sex hormones.

Another possible mediator of overfeeding-induced reductions in physical activity is the dopaminergic system, which as noted above, has been linked to hypocaloric-induced increases in physical activity through D_2 and D_3 receptors (36). The dopaminergic system was previously linked to genetic differences in wheel-running activity (38), has direct effects on physical activity via sex hormones (31), and is directly affected by overfeeding (68). Briefly, dopamine, as a neurotransmitter, functions via neural circuits to regulate pleasure, and through its production, reinforces

Table 10.2 Summary of studies demonstrating direct and indirect links between overfeeding and reduced activity in humans and rodents

Diet type	Study	Species	Subject characteristics	Study design	Effect of diet on physical activity
Excess calories	Levine et al. (41)	Human	22 healthy men and women, lean and obese sedentary individuals aged 39 ± 8 years	Weight maintenance feeding occurred during the first 10 experimental days, and baseline locomotor activity was also assessed during this time. These measurements were repeated again after 8 weeks of being overfed by 1000 kcal/day	Overfeeding reduced free-living walking to a similar degree in lean and obese subjects (~1.5 miles/day)
Excess calories	Schmidt et al. (61)	Human	55 healthy men and women aged 25–35 years classified as either obesity resistant (OR) or obesity prone (OP) defined by body mass index of 16.9–25.5 kg/m² and 19.6–30.6 kg/m², respectively	Spontaneous physical activity was measured using a physical activity monitoring system, either in a controlled eucaloric condition or during 3 days of overfeeding (1.4 × basal energy) and for the subsequent 3 days (ad libitum recovery period)	3 days following overfeeding, OP subjects significantly decreased the amount of time they spent walking (−2.0% of time), whereas OR subjects maintained their walking (+0.2%)
"Very high-fat diet"	Funkat et al. (24)	Mice	C57BL/6, DBA/2, and 129T2 aged 14 weeks	Mice were fed either a control or a high-fat (60% fat) diet for 6 weeks. During week 6, voluntary wheel-running activity was assessed for 7 days and readings were taken on days 5–7, then averaged, and expressed as cycles/day	129T2 mice fed either diet exhibited less voluntary activity compared with both C57BL/6 and DBA/2 mice. The high-fat diet decreased voluntary activity in both C57BL/6 and DBA/2 mice, but there was no further decrease in activity in the 129T2 mice

(continued)

Table 10.2 (Cont.)

Diet type	Study	Species	Subject characteristics	Study design	Effect of diet on physical activity
"Westernized diet"	Meek et al. (51)	Mice	Male selectively bred high-runner (HR) mouse line, and corresponding control (C) line aged 12 weeks	From 3 to 12 weeks of age, mice received either a standard chow diet or Western diet and wheel-running activity was assessed	Western diet initially caused increased caloric intake in both HR and C mice, but this effect was reversed during the last 4 weeks of the study. Western diet had little or no effect on wheel running in C mice, but increased revolutions per day by as much as 75% in HR mice, mainly through increased time spent running
"High fructose diet"	Rendeiro et al. (57)	Mice	Male C57BL/6J mice aged 14 weeks	Mice received either a diet containing fructose or glucose at 18% for 77 days. Wheel-running activity was assessed on days 76 and 77	Mice given the fructose diet traveled significantly less (~20% less) in comparison to animals fed the glucose diet
High–fat/high–sugar diet	Vellers et al. (71)	Mice	Male and female C57BL/6J mice aged 12 weeks	At 3 weeks of age, mice were assigned to either a control (CFD) or high-fat/high-sugar (HFHS) diet for 9–11 weeks. Acute wheel-running activity was assessed for 3 days at 12 weeks of age	HFHS diet decreased acute wheel-running activity in male (~70%) and female mice (~57%)
"Westernized diet"	Bjursell et al. (6)	Mice	Male C57Bl/6J mice aged 8 weeks	Mice were given Westernized diet or chow diet for 21 days. At weeks 3 and 7, mice were switched to the opposing diet and locomotor activity was analyzed for 24 hours	Mice that switched from chow to Westernized diet had significant reductions in locomotor activity after only 3–5 hours following the diet switch

rewarding behaviors. In mice, overfeeding via a high-fat diet suppresses dopamine production, with this suppression shown in areas of the brain known to house mechanisms regulating physical activity (e.g., striatum/nucleus accumbens) (60). Hence, it is possible that suppression of dopamine production, specific to dopamine receptors in areas of brain associated with activity regulation, could partially explain why motivation to be physically active decreases because of overfeeding. In this context, it is also important to consider genetic predisposition, where different physical activity phenotypes are influenced by divergent dopamine signaling pathways (high-active strain=dopamine 1-like receptor; low-active strain=dopamine reuptake) (38). Thus, it is possible that there is a potential interactive effect between overfeeding-induced alterations to dopamine signaling and a subsequent influence on physical activity. Even though it remains unknown whether the dopaminergic system links chronic overfeeding and reduced activity, the separate literature on overfeeding and physical activity and direct associations with dopaminergic pathways suggests there could be a possible link between overfeeding and dopaminergic control of physical activity.

When exploring potential mechanisms of an overfeeding-induced reduction in physical activity, another factor that is frequently suggested is body weight. Some work suggests that weight alone may influence physical activity primarily because the increased energy cost of movement with increased body weight correlates with declines in physical activity (e.g., 40, 70). However, this correlation does not arise in all cases, as has been demonstrated in numerous other studies (e.g., 21, 45, 46, 71). An important concept to bear in mind is that with overfeeding-induced increased body weight comes a myriad of other physiological and body composition changes. Thus, studies simply demonstrating a correlation with increased body weight and lowered activity cannot rule out other potential factors linking overfeeding with decreased physical activity. As noted above, other work that has assessed the influence of weight on activity primarily in mouse models has repeatedly shown an insignificant relationship between weight and activity (22, 45, 46, 71). Most recently, work by Friend et al. (22), ruled out an effect of body weight on activity, when restoration of DR_2 binding of the basal ganglia that was altered by the diet, recovered baseline activity in spite of no change in body weight. While the current understanding of whether body weight directly influences activity is limited to the mouse model, the available evidence suggests that weight is not an independent factor inhibiting physical activity. As such, body weight, among the host of other chronic overfeeding-induced body composition and physiological changes, must be further investigated to delineate which factor(s) are involved in pathways causing decreased physical activity.

While overfeeding in most studies has been shown (and associated) with reduced physical activity, there is evidence showing that genetic predisposition for specific physical phenotypes can interact with dietary intake and influence differential activity responses. Specifically, Meek et al. (51) utilized a specialized "Western diet" (42% fat) and found this diet actually increased wheel-running activity in mice selectively bred for high running-wheel activity when compared to a selected control line. The authors postulated the high-fat diet stimulated further increases in the already high-running activity-selected mouse line because these mice normally expended their available energy stores daily. The authors hypothesized that the extra fat in the Western diet provided an additional fuel source for these high-active mice (51). Meek et al. (50) further demonstrated the Western diet-induced increased wheel running in the high-active mouse line was linked to leptin sensitivity. When the authors gave leptin to the high-active mice that were on the standard diet, their activity levels increased and were similar to those animals on the Western diet (50). Lastly, another study by Funkat et al. (24), provided the specialized "very high-fat" diet to three different inbred mouse strains (C57BL/6, DBA/2, and 129T2), and found compared to baseline activity, wheel-running activity was significantly reduced in strains characterized with moderate activity (C57BL/6 and DBA/2; 46), while unchanged in

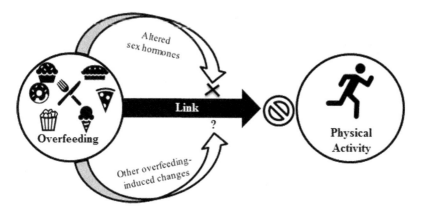

Figure 10.2 The effect of chronic overfeeding on physical activity regulation and potential mechanisms. Indirect evidence in humans (41, 61), and in mice (71) show chronic overfeeding inhibits physical activity. Of these studies, Vellers et al. (71) tested whether the primary sex hormones in males (testosterone) and females (17β-estradiol) were mechanisms linking chronic overfeeding with reduced physical activity; however, the findings demonstrated chronic overfeeding reduces activity independent of sex hormone involvement as depicted in the diagram.

a low-active strain (129T2) (45). Overall, the two studies by Meek et al. and Funkat et al. (24, 51) show a gene by "unique" environment interaction, where calorically dense diets appear to enhance physical activity in mice with a genetic predisposition to be highly active, with a decrease in activity in mice that do not have the selectively bred highly active genome. If extended to humans, these findings would likely suggest that only elite athletes would have enhanced physical activity with overfeeding and all other humans (i.e., majority of the population) would incur an inhibited physical activity level with overfeeding.

In summary, the collective evidence discussed in this section clearly presents an effect of diet on physical activity regulation. As depicted in Figure 10.2, the sex hormones are the only factors that have been directly assessed as potential mediators between overfeeding and reduced activity. Though work indicates sex hormones do not regulate diet-induced changes in activity, there are a myriad of other chronic overfeeding-induced changes that warrant future investigations (e.g., dopaminergic system). Despite the lack of clarity regarding how these mechanism(s) are linked, the knowledge that diet influences whether an individual is active or sedentary has substantial applications for exercise physiologists seeking to find modifiable factors to encourage regular daily physical activity in their clients. Therefore, as basic research continues to investigate mechanistic links between diet modifications and physical activity regulation, applied research is also needed to determine appropriate individual-based diets that effectively alter regular daily physical activity in clinical and healthy populations.

Conclusion and future directions

Interactions between genetics and the environment determine regulation of physical activity, with environmental influences, such as EDCs and diet, being modifiers of an individual's phenotype to be physically active or not. That there are known agents, such as diet and EDCs, which disrupt biological and/or genetic factors regulating an individual's drive to be active is a relatively new concept. To date, the focus on such environmental agents has primarily been on how each independently contributes to chronic diseases including cardiovascular and metabolic diseases with only a few studies considering how they alter human behaviors such as physical activity. Existing literature supports that the environment can play a unique role in regulating physical activity mechanisms; however, the mechanistic pathways through which activity is regulated are not fully delineated or understood. Additionally, the combined effects of exposure to poor diet and endocrine disruptors are unknown, but we would hypothesize that they would likely cause an even greater inhibition of physical activity. Therefore, as scientists, exercise physiologists, and other healthcare providers seek ways to promote increased daily physical activity, reducing environmental exposures and altering diet should be integral components to consider as interventions to increase physical activity.

References

1. **Ahima RS**, and **Flier JS**. Adipose tissue as an endocrine organ. *Trends in Endocrinology & Metabolism* 11: 327–332, 2000.
2. **Anway MD, Leathers C**, and **Skinner MK**. Endocrine disruptor vinclozolin induced epigenetic transgenerational adult-onset disease. *Endocrinology* 147: 5515–5523, 2006.
3. **Attina TM, Hauser R, Sathyanarayana S, Hunt PA, Bourguignon J-P, Myers JP, DiGangi J, Zoeller RT**, and **Trasande L**. Exposure to endocrine-disrupting chemicals in the USA: A population-based disease burden and cost analysis. *The Lancet Diabetes & Endocrinology* 4: 996–1003, 2016.
4. **Baranowska B, Baranowska-Bik A, Bik W**, and **Martynska L**. The role of leptin and orexins in the dysfunction of hypothalamo-pituitary-gonadal regulation and in the mechanism of hyperactivity in patients with anorexia nervosa. *Neuro Endocrinology Letters* 29: 37–40, 2008.
5. **Bigsby R, Chapin RE, Daston GP, Davis BJ, Gorski J, Gray LE, Howdeshell KL, Zoeller RT**, and **vom Saal FS**. Evaluating the effects of endocrine disruptors on endocrine function during development. *Environmental Health Perspectives* 107 Suppl. 4: 613–618, 1999.
6. **Bjursell M, Gerdin A-K, Lelliott CJ, Egecioglu E, Elmgren A, Törnell J, Oscarsson J**, and **Bohlooly-Y M**. Acutely reduced locomotor activity is a major contributor to western diet-induced obesity in mice. *American Journal of Physiology – Endocrinology and Metabolism* 294: E251–E260, 2008.
7. **Bouchard C, Tchernof A**, and **Tremblay A**. Predictors of body composition and body energy changes in response to chronic overfeeding. *International Journal of Obesity* 38: 236–242, 2014.
8. **Bowen RS, Ferguson DP**, and **Lightfoot JT**. Effects of aromatase inhibition on the physical activity levels of male mice. *Journal of Steroids & Hormonal Science* 1: 1, 2011.
9. **Bowen RS, Knab AM, Hamilton AT, McCall JR, Moore-Harrison TL**, and **Lightfoot JT**. Effects of supraphysiological doses of sex steroids on wheel running activity in mice. *Journal of Steroids & Hormonal Science* 3: 110, 2012.
10. **Bymaster FP, Hemrick-Luecke SK, Perry K**, and **Fuller R**. Neurochemical evidence for antagonism by olanzapine of dopamine, serotonin, α1-adrenergic and muscarinic receptors in vivo in rats. *Psychopharmacology* 124: 87–94, 1996.
11. **Bymaster FP, Rasmussen K, Calligaro DO, Nelson DL, DeLapp NW, Wong DT**, and **Moore NA**. In vitro and in vivo biochemistry of olanzapine: A novel, atypical antipsychotic drug. *The Journal of Clinical Psychiatry* 58: 1,478–436, 1997.
12. **Casper RC**. The "drive for activity" and "restlessness" in anorexia nervosa: Potential pathways. *Journal of Affective Disorders* 92: 99–107, 2006.
13. **Creatore MI, Glazier RH, Moineddin R, Fazli GS, Johns A, Gozdyra P, Matheson FI, Kaufman-Shriqui V, Rosella LC**, and **Manuel DG**. Association of neighborhood walkability with change in overweight, obesity, and diabetes. *JAMA* 315: 2211–2220, 2016.
14. **Diamanti-Kandarakis E, Bourguignon JP, Giudice LC, Hauser R, Prins GS, Soto AM, Zoeller RT**, and **Gore AC**. Endocrine-disrupting chemicals: An endocrine society scientific statement. *Endocrine Reviews* 30: 293–342, 2009.
15. **Escobar-Morreale HF, Álvarez-Blasco F, Botella-Carretero JI**, and **Luque-Ramírez M**. The striking similarities in the metabolic associations of female androgen excess and male androgen deficiency. *Human Reproduction* 2014.
16. **Exner C, Hebebrand J, Remschmidt H, Wewetzer C, Ziegler A, Herpertz S, Schweiger U, Blum W, Preibisch G**, and **Heldmaier G**. Leptin suppresses semi-starvation induced hyperactivity in rats: Implications for anorexia nervosa. *Molecular Psychiatry* 5: 476–481, 2000.

17. **Farooqi IS, Jebb SA, Langmack G, Lawrence E, Cheetham CH, Prentice AM, Hughes IA, McCamish MA,** and **O'Rahilly S.** Effects of recombinant leptin therapy in a child with congenital leptin deficiency. *New England Journal of Medicine* 341: 879–884, 1999.

18. **Ferdinand A, Bisakha S, Rahurkar S, Engler S,** and **Menachemi N.** The relationship between built environments and physical activity: A systematic review. *American Journal of Public Health* 102: e7-e13, 2012.

19. **Fernandes Maria Fernanda A, Matthys D, Hryhorczuk C, Sharma S, Mogra S, Alquier T,** and **Fulton S.** Leptin suppresses the rewarding effects of running via stat3 signaling in dopamine neurons. *Cell Metabolism* 22: 741–749, 2015.

20. **Figlewicz D, Evans S, Murphy J, Hoen M,** and **Baskin D.** Expression of receptors for insulin and leptin in the ventral tegmental area/substantia nigra (Vta/Sn) of the rat. *Brain Research* 964: 107–115, 2003.

21. **Flynn KM, Delclos KB, Newbold RR,** and **Ferguson SA.** Behavioral responses of rats exposed to long-term dietary vinclozolin. *Journal of Agricultural and Food Chemistry* 49: 1658–1665, 2001.

22. **Friend DM, Devarakonda K, O'Neal TJ, Skirzewski M, Papazoglou I, Kaplan AR, Liow J-S, Guo J, Rane SG,** and **Rubinstein M.** Basal ganglia dysfunction contributes to physical inactivity in obesity. *Cell Metabolism* 25: 312–321, 2017.

23. **Frye CA, Bo E, Calamandrei G, Calza L, Dessi-Fulgheri F, Fernandez M, Fusani L, Kah O, Kajta M, Le Page Y, Patisaul HB, Venerosi A, Wojtowicz AK,** and **Panzica GC.** Endocrine disrupters: A review of some sources, effects, and mechanisms of actions on behaviour and neuroendocrine systems. *Journal of Neuroendocrinology* 24: 144–159, 2012.

24. **Funkat A, Massa CM, Jovanovska V, Proietto J,** and **Andrikopoulos S.** Metabolic adaptations of three inbred strains of mice (C57bl/6, Dba/2, and 129t2) in response to a high-fat diet. *The Journal of Nutrition* 134: 3264–3269, 2004.

25. **Gorzek JF, Hendrickson KC, Forstner JP, Rixen JL, Moran AL,** and **Lowe DA.** Estradiol and tamoxifen reverse ovariectomy-induced physical inactivity in mice. *Medicine and Science in Sports and Exercise* 39: 248–256, 2007.

26. **Hebebrand J, Exner C, Hebebrand K, Holtkamp C, Casper R, Remschmidt H, Herpertz-Dahlmann B,** and **Klingenspor M.** Hyperactivity in patients with anorexia nervosa and in semistarved rats: evidence for a pivotal role of hypoleptinemia. *Physiology & Behavior* 79: 25–37, 2003.

27. **Hellwig J, van Ravenzwaay B, Mayer M,** and **Gembardt C.** Pre- and post-natal oral toxicity of vinclozolin in Wistar and Long-Evans rats. *Regulatory Toxicology and Pharmacology* 32: 42–50, 2000.

28. **Hillebrand JJ, van Elburg AA, Kas MJ, van Engeland H,** and **Adan RA.** Olanzapine reduces physical activity in rats exposed to activity-based anorexia: Possible implications for treatment of anorexia nervosa? *Biological Psychiatry* 58: 651–657, 2005.

29. **Holtkamp K, Herpertz-Dahlmann B, Mika C, Heer M, Heussen N, Fichter M, Herpertz S, Senf W, Blum WF,** and **Schweiger U.** Elevated physical activity and low leptin levels co-occur in patients with anorexia nervosa. *The Journal of Clinical Endocrinology & Metabolism* 88: 5169–5174, 2003.

30. **Hoskins RG.** The effect of castration on voluntary activity. *American Journal of Physiology* 324–330, 1925.

31. **Jardí F, Laurent MR, Kim N, Khalil R, Bundel D, Eeckhaut A, Helleputte L, Deboel L, Dubois V,** and **Schollaert D.** Testosterone boosts physical activity in male mice via dopaminergic pathways. *Scientific Reports* 8: 957, 2018.

32. **Johnson SA, Painter MS, Javurek AB, Ellersieck MR, Wiedmeyer CE, Thyfault JP,** and **Rosenfeld CS.** Sex-dependent effects of developmental exposure to bisphenol A and ethinyl estradiol on metabolic parameters and voluntary physical activity. *Journal of Developmental Origins of Health and Disease* 6: 539–552, 2015.

33. **Joosen AM, Gielen M, Vlietinck R,** and **Westerterp KR.** Genetic analysis of physical activity in twins. *The American Journal of Clinical Nutrition* 82: 1253–1259, 2005.

34. **Kajta M,** and **Wojtowicz AK.** Impact of endocrine-disrupting chemicals on neural development and the onset of neurological disorders. *Pharmacological Reports* 65: 1632–1639, 2013.

35. **Kamrin MA.** Phthalate risks, phthalate regulation, and public health: A review. *Journal of Toxicology and Environmental Health* 12: 157–174, 2009.

36. **Klenotich SJ, Ho EV, McMurray MS, Server CH,** and **Dulawa SC.** Dopamine D2/3 receptor antagonism reduces activity-based anorexia. *Transl Psychiatry* 5: e613, 2015.

37. **Kluwe WM, Haseman JK, Douglas JF**, and **Huff JE**. The carcinogenicity of dietary di(2-ethylhexyl) phthalate (DEHP) in Fischer 344 Rats and B6c3f1 mice. *Journal of Toxicology and Environmental Health* 10: 797–815, 1982.

38. **Knab A, Bowen R, Hamilton A**, and **Lightfoot J**. Pharmacological manipulation of the dopaminergic system affects wheel-running activity in differentially active mice. *Journal of Biological Regulators and Homeostatic Agents* 26: 119, 2012.

39. **Knab AM, Bowen RS, Hamilton AT, Gulledge AA**, and **Lightfoot JT**. Altered dopaminergic profiles: Implications for the regulation of voluntary physical activity. *Behavioural Brain Research* 204: 147–152, 2009.

40. **LaRoche DP, Marques NR, Shumila HN, Logan CR, St Laurent R**, and **Gonçalves M**. Excess body weight and gait influence energy cost of walking in older adults. *Medicine and Science in Sports and Exercise* 47: 1017, 2015.

41. **Levine JA, McCrady SK, Lanningham-Foster LM, Kane PH, Foster RC**, and **Manohar CU**. The role of free-living daily walking in human weight gain and obesity. *Diabetes* 57: 548–554, 2008.

42. **Li DK, Zhou Z, Miao M, He Y, Wang J, Ferber J, Herrinton LJ, Gao E**, and **Yuan W**. Urine bisphenol-A (BPA) level in relation to semen quality. *Fertility and Sterility* 95: 625–630.e621–624, 2011.

43. **Licinio J, Caglayan S, Ozata M, Yildiz BO, de Miranda PB, O'Kirwan F, Whitby R, Liang L, Cohen P**, and **Bhasin S**. Phenotypic effects of leptin replacement on morbid obesity, diabetes mellitus, hypogonadism, and behavior in leptin-deficient adults. *Proceedings of the National Academy of Sciences of the United States of America* 101: 4531–4536, 2004.

44. **Lightfoot JT**. Why control activity? Evolutionary selection pressures affecting the development of physical activity genetic and biological regulation. *BioMed Research International* 2013: 821678, 2013.

45. **Lightfoot JT, Leamy L, Pomp D, Turner MJ, Fodor AA, Knab A, Bowen RS, Ferguson D, Moore-Harrison T**, and **Hamilton A**. Strain screen and haplotype association mapping of wheel running in inbred mouse strains. *Journal of Applied Physiology* 109: 623–634, 2010.

46. **Lightfoot JT, Turner MJ, Daves M, Vordermark A**, and **Kleeberger SR**. Genetic influence on daily wheel running activity level. *Physiological Genomics* 19: 270–276, 2004.

47. **Markey CM, Luque EH, Munoz De Toro M, Sonnenschein C**, and **Soto AM**. In utero exposure to bisphenol A alters the development and tissue organization of the mouse mammary gland. *Biology of Reproduction* 65: 1215–1223, 2001.

48. **Masuo Y**, and **Ishido M**. Neurotoxicity of endocrine disruptors: Possible involvement in brain development and neurodegeneration. *Journal of Toxicology and Environmental Health, Part B* 14: 346–369, 2011.

49. **McGrath LJ, Hopkins WG**, and **Hinckson EA**. Associations of objectively measured built-environment attributes with youth moderate–vigorous physical activity: A systematic review and meta-analysis. *Sports Medicine* 45: 841–865, 2015.

50. **Meek TH, Dlugosz EM, Vu KT**, and **Garland** Jr T. Effects of leptin treatment and western diet on wheel running in selectively bred high runner mice. *Physiology & Behavior* 106: 252–258, 2012.

51. **Meek TH, Eisenmann JC**, and **Garland T**. Western diet increases wheel running in mice selectively bred for high voluntary wheel running. *International Journal of Obesity* 34: 960–969, 2010.

52. **Meyer BC**, and **Weinroth LA**. Observations on psychological aspects of anorexia nervosa: Report of a case. *Psychosomatic Medicine* 19: 389–398, 1957.

53. **Moore N**. Olanzapine: Preclinical pharmacology and recent findings. *The British Journal of Psychiatry* 41–44, 1998.

54. **Morton GJ, Kaiyala KJ, Fisher JD, Ogimoto K, Schwartz MW**, and **Wisse BE**. Identification of a physiological role for leptin in the regulation of ambulatory activity and wheel running in mice. *American Journal of Physiology – Endocrinology and Metabolism* 300: E392–E401, 2011.

55. **Parks LG, Ostby JS, Lambright CR, Abbott BD, Klinefelter GR, Barlow NJ**, and **Gray LE**, Jr. The plasticizer diethylhexyl phthalate induces malformations by decreasing fetal testosterone synthesis during sexual differentiation in the male rat. *Toxicological Sciences* 58: 339–349, 2000.

56. **Pinson A, Bourguignon JP**, and **Parent AS**. Exposure to endocrine disrupting chemicals and neurodevelopmental alterations. *Andrology* 4: 706–722, 2016.

57. **Rendeiro C, Masnik AM, Mun JG, Du K, Clark D, Dilger RN, Dilger AC**, and **Rhodes JS**. Fructose decreases physical activity and increases body fat without affecting hippocampal neurogenesis and learning relative to an isocaloric glucose diet. *Scientific Reports* 5: 2015.

58. **Richter CP**. A behavioristic study of the activity of the rat. *Comparative Psychology Monographs* 1922.

59. **Roy EJ** and **Wade GN**. Role of estrogens in androgen-induced spontaneous activity in male rats. *Journal of Comparative Physiological Psychology* 89: 573–579, 1975.

60. **Salamone JD**. Complex motor and sensorimotor functions of striatal and accumbens dopamine: Involvement in instrumental behavior processes. *Psychopharmacology (Berlin)* 107: 160–174, 1992.

61. **Schmidt SL, Harmon KA, Sharp TA, Kealey EH**, and **Bessesen DH**. The effects of overfeeding on spontaneous physical activity in obesity prone and obesity resistant humans. *Obesity* 20: 2186–2193, 2012.

62. **Schmitt EE, Vellers HL, Porter WW**, and **Lightfoot JT**. Environmental endocrine disruptor affects voluntary physical activity in mice. *Medicine and Science in Sports and Exercise* 48: 1251–1258, 2016.

63. **Schotte A, Janssen P, Gommeren W, Luyten W, Van Gompel P, Lesage A, De Loore K**, and **Leysen J**. Risperidone compared with new and reference antipsychotic drugs: in vitro and in vivo receptor binding. *Psychopharmacology* 124: 57–73, 1996.

64. **Serrano SE, Braun J, Trasande L, Dills R**, and **Sathyanarayana S**. Phthalates and diet: A review of the food monitoring and epidemiology data. *Environmental Health* 13: 43, 2014.

65. **Slonaker JR**. The effect of pubescence, oestruation and menopause on the voluntary activity in the albino rat. *American Journal of Physiology* 362–394, 1925.

66. **Stubbe JH, Boomsma DI, Vink JM, Cornes BK, Martin NG, Skytthe A, Kyvik KO, Rose RJ, Kujala UM**, and **Kaprio J**. Genetic influences on exercise participation in 37,051 twin pairs from seven countries. *PloS One* 1: e22, 2006.

67. **Tanida T, Warita K, Ishihara K, Fukui S, Mitsuhashi T, Sugawara T, Tabuchi Y, Nanmori T, Qi WM, Inamoto T, Yokoyama T, Kitagawa H**, and **Hoshi N**. Fetal and neonatal exposure to three typical environmental chemicals with different mechanisms of action: Mixed exposure to phenol, phthalate, and dioxin cancels the effects of sole exposure on mouse midbrain dopaminergic nuclei. Toxicology Letters 189: 40–47, 2009.

68. **Tellez LA, Medina S, Han W, Ferreira JG, Licona-Limon P, Ren X, Lam TT, Schwartz GJ**, and **de Araujo IE**. A gut lipid messenger links excess dietary fat to dopamine deficiency. *Science* 341: 800–802, 2013.

69. **Troiano RP, Berrigan D, Dodd KW, Mâsse LC, Tilert T**, and **McDowell M**. Physical activity in the United States measured by accelerometer. *Medicine and Science in Sports and Exercise* 40: 181, 2008.

70. **Tucker JM, Tucker LA, LeCheminant J**, and **Bailey B**. Obesity increases risk of declining physical activity over time in women: A prospective cohort Study. *Obesity* 21: E715–E720, 2013.

71. **Vellers HL, Letsinger AC, Walker NR, Granados JZ**, and **Lightfoot JT**. High fat high sugar diet reduces voluntary wheel running in mice independent of sex hormone involvement. *Frontiers in Physiology* 8: 2017.

72. **Verhagen LA, Luijendijk MC**, and **Adan RA**. Leptin reduces hyperactivity in an animal model for anorexia nervosa via the ventral tegmental area. *European Neuropsychopharmacology* 21: 274–281, 2011.

73. **Waller JV, Kaufman RM**, and **Deutsch F**. Anorexia nervosa: A psychosomatic entity. *Psychosomatic Medicine* 2: 3–16, 1940.

74. **Wang GH**. The relationship between spontaneous activity and oestrous cycle in the rat. *Comparative Psychology Monographs* 2: 1–27, 1923.

75. **Witorsch RJ**, and **Thomas JA**. Personal care products and endocrine disruption: A critical review of the literature. *Critical Reviews in Toxicology* 40 Suppl 3: 1–30, 2010.

SECTION 3

Systems genetics of exercise endurance and trainability

The previous section explored the systems genetics underlying the trait of physical activity, and its component parts. This (and the following) section will further explore genetic and molecular mechanisms driving variation in traits associated with performance – first for endurance-related tasks (Section 3) and then for strength-related tasks (Section 4). For each of the sections, we have experts provide some background context and primers associated with the key traits that underlie performance. Each author was tasked particularly to review traits at baseline (untrained state) and following acute and chronic exercise training – which highlights the similarities and differences between basic human variation and variation in the response to training. As you will have noted from the first part of the book, there is a lot yet to be learned in sport and exercise systems genetics, so our authors also highlight gaps in our knowledge and provide directions for future potential studies.

Chapter 11 starts off Section 3 with Dr. David Raichlen and colleagues providing a fantastic overview of human evolution related to the endurance trait. As many readers will have exercise science backgrounds, having the perspective on the endurance trait from an evolutionary perspective is unique and quite fascinating. Given that endurance and endurance-related traits are complex, Drs. Quindry and Roberts provide a primer in Chapter 12, reviewing the physiological traits that comprise the complex "endurance" phenotype and discuss underlying molecular drivers of these traits. In Chapters 13 (Dr. Michael Massett and colleagues) and 14 (Drs. Jacob Barber and Mark Sarzynski), our experts discuss the heritability of endurance-related phenotypes that have been gleaned so far from animal (Chapter 13) and human (Chapter 14) research models. Specific genetic contributions to cardiorespiratory fitness are then discussed by Dr. Reuben Howden and colleagues in Chapter 15. Given that mitochondria play such a crucial role in energy production, Dr. Mark Tarnopolsky reviews mitochondrial biology in Chapter 16, and discusses the unique aspects that mitochondrial genetics contribute to endurance-related traits, and to overall health and disease. While each chapter in Sections 3 and 4 will explore multiple pathways and genes, there are a few genetic variations that have been extensively studied in relation to sport and exercise-related traits. One of these variations is the common insertion/deletion variation in the angiotensin-converting enzyme (*ACE*) gene, which is reviewed by Dr. Linda Pescatello and colleagues in Chapter 17.

Together, the chapters in Section 3 provide a comprehensive review of traits underlying endurance and endurance-related traits both at baseline and following training, highlight gaps in our current knowledge, and provide a solid foundation for future work to complete the systems models.

11

THE EVOLUTION OF THE HUMAN ENDURANCE PHENOTYPE

David A. Raichlen, James T. Webber, and Herman Pontzer

Humans are exceptional endurance athletes. Compared to other quadrupedal mammals, our ability to engage in anaerobic activity such as sprinting is highly constrained. However, humans compare favorably to other species in athletic performance at moderate aerobic intensities (6, 7, 39). Understanding the evolutionary history of our endurance capabilities, along with adaptations that support human aerobic activity, may provide a foundation for exploring the underlying systems genetics of endurance sports and aerobic exercise.

In a sense, detailing the genetics of human performance is an evolutionary exploration, and here we discuss the evidence for how and why human endurance adaptations, and their underlying genetic associations, evolved. By doing so, we suggest human evolutionary physiology can play a key role in studies of exercise, health, and performance. In addition, as described in more detail below, a systems genetics approach is needed to fully understand the evolution of the endurance phenotype. Since many endurance adaptations in humans are confined to soft tissue, which does not fossilize, we must reconstruct our evolutionary history using comparative physiology. Genomic and genetic approaches can help us detail the specific changes, and timing of these changes, that have led humans to become the endurance primate. Thus, an evolutionary approach to human exercise physiology can both aid, and benefit from, genetic and genomic studies of exercise performance.

To build an evolutionary framework for exercise physiology, we review data from a combination of methodological approaches including analyses of the human fossil record, comparative physiology of humans and nonhuman primates, and studies of humans living more traditional lifestyles (e.g., hunter-gatherers). By drawing on data from these approaches, we will develop a model of the human endurance phenotype, a timeline for how and when it evolved, and a blueprint for how to use this evolutionary framework in future work.

Defining the endurance phenotype

Aerobic activities are those which can be sustained entirely by oxygen-based metabolism. The rate of oxygen consumption during an activity, called VO_2, is often used as a measure of energy for aerobic activities. Activity costs tend to increase with body size, and so to account for differences in body size, energy expenditure during an activity is often expressed as metabolic equivalents (METs), the ratio of activity energy expenditure to basal metabolic rate

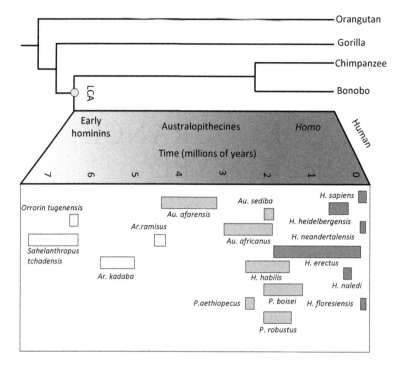

Figure 11.1 Phylogeny of Hominidae. This figure shows the relationships between extant great apes including modern humans and bipedal human ancestors. Individual hominin species (ancestors of modern humans following the divergence from living chimpanzees and bonobos) are shown along with their known dates of existence. Hominin species are shaded by their major grouping (early hominins, australopithecines, *Homo*).

(BMR; the rate of energy expenditure while completely at rest and fasted in a thermoneutral environment) (15). Thus, energy expenditure during sleep is 1 MET. The metabolic ceiling for aerobic activities – VO$_2$max, the maximum rate of oxygen consumption – is approximately 20 METs (54) for trained human athletes and is considerably lower (~5–10 METs) for untrained or elderly individuals (63). Walking at 5 km per hour is an approximately 3 MET activity, while running at 10 km per hour (~10 minutes per mile) is an approximately 10 MET activity (35).

We can define the human endurance phenotype by traits that improve our ability to sustain moderate to vigorous physical activity (MVPA; aerobic intensities between 3 and 10 METs) for periods greater than 20 minutes (see Chapter 12 in this volume for more detailed discussion of the human endurance phenotype). While endurance activities in traditional human societies often include endeavors other than walking and running (e.g., digging to extract wild tubers for food) (32), locomotion has been the focus of most research into the evolution of the human endurance phenotype (6, 7). For example, in humans, running distances greater than about 5 km requires sustained aerobic energy expenditure and is considered an endurance activity (26). Among extant primates, humans are the only taxon that regularly engages in endurance locomotor activities, suggesting selection for the endurance phenotype occurred sometime after the divergence of the human lineage from nonhuman apes (6) (Figure 11.1). Tracking an evolutionary increase in endurance capabilities allows us to identify the specific pressures that generated humans' unique athletic abilities.

Here, we focus on the evolution of locomotor-related traits that we can track through human evolution (i.e., in fossil taxa or through comparative physiology), dividing these traits into three adaptive categories. 1) locomotor energetics, 2) force resistance/stabilization required of high locomotor speeds, and 3) endurance (the ability to sustain locomotion over long distances). In defining the endurance phenotype this way, we are careful not to conflate adaptations that reduce energy costs of locomotion with traits that enhance endurance (see 39 for review and discussion). To fully understand how natural selection led to human endurance performance, we start by comparing human aerobic capabilities with those of our closest living relatives, and then discuss the underlying traits that explain taxonomic differences.

Comparative approach: Physical activity in extant apes and humans

Comparative biology offers a valuable methodological approach to examine evolutionary physiology in living taxa. By comparing performance or morphology in humans and our closest living relatives, the great apes (Figure 11.1), we can better understand how, and potentially when, major changes in evolutionary physiology occurred. We last shared a common ancestor with the genus *Pan* (living chimpanzees and bonobos) sometime between 6 and 8 million years ago. Any differences in endurance capabilities between humans and the *Pan* lineage should reflect either selection for increased endurance along the human lineage, or selection for decreased endurance along the chimpanzee and bonobo lineage. Thus, we can model changes in physical activity patterns across human evolutionary history by examining morphology and behavior in these taxa.

Field studies have tracked daily movement patterns in each of the three genera of great apes, providing a window into activity patterns of our last common ancestor with chimpanzees (see Figure 11.2). Studies of chimpanzees in the wild suggest they travel between 2 and 5 km per day on the ground, complemented by about 100 m/day of vertical climbing (1, 39, 41, 45). Although fewer data exist, bonobos seem to travel less than chimpanzees, with daily travel distances averaging 1.4 km/day (3). For the other great apes, movement is significantly shorter, with gorillas averaging 0.4–2.6 km/day (66), and orangutans averaging about 1 km/day (11, 18, 56). Even less is known about the aerobic intensities of physical activity patterns in the great apes. Data collected on walking velocities in chimpanzees suggest that most of their daily travel occurs at low intensities (2). For example, average walking speeds for males (1.94 km/hour) and

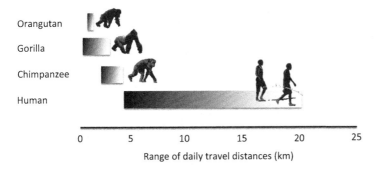

Orangutan

Gorilla

Chimpanzee

Human

0	5	10	15	20	25

Range of daily travel distances (km)

Figure 11.2 Range of daily walking distances for great apes. Human daily walking distances are longer than any of the other great apes, suggesting the need for skeletal and physiological adaptations supporting aerobic endurance. Estimates of walking distances for each species are taken from the literature. See text for further details and references.

females (2.20 km/hour) correspond to low aerobic intensities in humans walking at comparable speeds (<3 METs) (15). Interspecific differences in BMR and locomotor costs complicate this comparison of aerobic intensities in humans and chimpanzees, however given slow speeds used in the wild, it is unlikely chimpanzees engage in moderate intensity activity for any sustained period of time. Thus, despite limited data, the current evidence suggests living great apes engage in short daily travel at relatively slow speeds.

Comparing great ape activity to modern humans is complicated by changes in human lifestyles in industrialized societies that greatly reduce physical activity. However, there are extant human populations living lifestyles similar in some ways to those of our recent ancestors (e.g., hunter-gatherer populations), and we can use these groups as windows into physical activity patterns in the past. While the great apes seem to live relatively sedentary lifestyles, humans living in small-scale societies are highly active for large portions of their day (13, 46). For example, detailed recent studies of physical activity patterns in the Hadza, a hunting and gathering population living in northern Tanzania, suggest that high activity levels are common across the lifespan (30, 43, 44, 51). Hadza adults travel between 6 and 12 km/day; however, there is a high degree of variance, and adult males are known to travel over 20 km in a single day during hunting forays (43). In other hunter-gatherer populations, daily travel distances average 9.5–14.1 km per day across a wide range of diverse habitats (i.e., rain forests and open savannahs) (21, 31).

While intensities used during daily foraging vary considerably, we recently showed that Hadza adults spend about 75 minutes per day in moderate to vigorous aerobic intensities (i.e., > 3 METs). Although similarly detailed data are not available for other hunting and gathering groups, estimates of physical activity in these lifestyles are generally high, with foraging populations regularly engaging in more MVPA each day than people in industrialized societies perform in 1 week (13, 51). However, despite long periods of time spent in MVPA, living hunter-gatherers rarely engage in highly vigorous activity (52). Intensities that are similar to those experienced during long-distance running (10–14 METs) are performed for less than 10 minutes per day in Hadza hunter-gatherers. During hunting in other groups (i.e.!Kung, Ache), individuals walk at moderate to high speeds for long distances (~3 METs), punctuated only by short sprints to capture prey (14, 20; see also Chapter 12), suggesting that across hunter-gatherers, moderate aerobic intensities dominate their physical activities.

Thus, compared to great apes, human hunter-gatherers travel longer distances, and do so at higher intensity levels, however most of this movement occurs in the moderate range of aerobic intensities (3–6 METs). If living hunter-gatherers provide a window into activity levels in our earlier ancestors, the endurance phenotype for humans should be associated with adaptations that improve both endurance and sustained moderate intensity locomotion compared to morphology seen in the great apes.

Morphological approach: Analyses of the human fossil record

The previous discussion of comparative activity patterns suggests a fundamental difference between nonhuman ape-like lifestyles, and the human hunting and gathering lifestyle. A key element of reconstructing the evolution of human endurance activity is detailing how and when lifestyles in human ancestors shifted from more ape-like to more human-like, and specifically when hunting and gathering became the dominant human subsistence strategy. Combining data from human fossils with paleoecological data, we can reconstruct how and why hominin lifestyles underwent changes that altered physical activity patterns compared to our last common ancestor with the chimpanzee lineage. For the purposes of reconstructing changes in activity levels and endurance capabilities, we suggest the hominin record can be divided roughly into three key groups (see Figure 11.1): 1) the earliest hominins, 2) the genus *Australopithecus*, and 3) the genus *Homo*.

Ecological pressures and changing lifestyles in human evolution

Reconstructions of locomotion and behavior in the earliest hominins generally suggest that, although they walked bipedally, in many respects they more closely resemble nonhuman great apes in activity patterns and behavior (37). Because of this similarity, we generally assume the last common ancestor of humans and *Pan* (chimpanzees and bonobos) was more *Pan*-like (37). Further, as discussed above, all of the living apes share rather limited travel distances and speeds, suggesting a low-endurance phenotype was common among Miocene apes from which the human lineage emerged. Thus, changes in endurance capabilities along the human lineage are likely due to selection for increased time spent in moderate to vigorous aerobic intensities in hominins, rather than a decrease in endurance capabilities in the chimpanzee/bonobo lineage.

There is little known about the endurance capabilities of the earliest hominins, *Sahelanthropus tchadensis*, *Orrorin tugenensis*, and *Ardipithecus*. However, the retention of a grasping foot and other ape-like elements of the locomotor skeleton suggest the endurance capabilities of early hominins were no better than those of living apes. Indeed, the adoption of a bipedal (two-legged) walking gait in early hominins may have diminished endurance capabilities, at least initially, by removing the forelimbs from their role in supporting body weight and thus requiring more work from the hindlimb muscles (39).

The next major group of hominins, members of the genus *Australopithecus* (as well as the closely related *Paranthropus* group), show changes in the locomotor skeleton that suggest improved energy economy during walking (see 'Skeletal adaptations to high-speed, long-distance locomotion'). However, the *Australopithecus* postcranial skeleton contains a mix of traits that resemble both modern humans and living apes, including skeletal features of the upper limb and shoulder that suggest continued use of arboreal resources (12, 62, 65). Australopithecines have craniodental adaptations that likely supported omnivorous diets comprised primarily of fruits, and therefore a reliance on resources found mainly in forested habitats. During this time period, the earth's climate began a cooling trend that led to increasingly open, less heavily forested habitats (52). For a taxon that was reliant on forest-based resources for food, these habitat changes likely required increased daily walking distances, providing a selection pressure for increased energy economy. However, there is little evidence that *Australopithecus* species shifted to a meat-based diet, which would have necessitated a hunting and gathering lifestyle associated with high aerobic endurance requirements.

Beginning around 2.0 million years ago, with the early evolution of the genus *Homo*, there is a marked change in behavior that suggests hunting and gathering became an integral part of the hominin lifestyle. At this time, members of the genus *Homo* increased their reliance on meat, with evidence that there was some form of systematic hunting or power scavenging (stealing carcasses from primary hunters), since fossil prey animals found at sites with stone tools suggest our ancestors were gaining access to large sources of meat (9). As part of the development of the hunting and gathering lifestyle, ancestral hominins became central place foragers, which required a return to a home base following foraging bouts (30). Central place foraging allows for food sharing in a lifestyle dominated by variance in procurement across individuals, however, long-distance foraging bouts necessitate higher speeds so that individuals can return to the central place. Thus, we suggest the endurance phenotype is best understood as a suite of adaptations to movement at high speeds over long distances associated with this emergence of hunting and gathering in the genus *Homo*.

Skeletal adaptations to high-speed, long-distance locomotion

Reconstructing lifestyle transitions, and how they impacted endurance capabilities during human evolution, relies on analyses and interpretations of fossil skeletons. Although there remains a lively debate over how best to reconstruct the evolutionary links between skeletal morphology and locomotor performance, we believe there is an emerging consensus that the ecological and lifestyle changes described above led to changes in the hominin musculoskeletal system that supported a major transition in physical activity. In the following subsection, we detail these morphological changes as they relate to three key aspects of the endurance pheno-type: 1) energetics, 2) force resistance/stabilization, and 3) endurance.

Skeletal adaptations for energy economy

Several skeletal features suggest changes from the earliest hominins to the origins of the genus *Homo* are associated with selection to improve locomotor economy following the early evolution of bipedalism. The earliest hominins, including *Sahelanthropus tchadensis*, *Orrorin tugenensis*, and *Ardipithecus*, likely walked with energy economy more similar to those of living great apes, and substantially higher energy costs than living humans (39, 57). These reconstructions are based mainly on the functional morphology of the pelvis and hindlimb which suggests short limbs combined with more flexed limb postures (19), leading to large volumes of muscle activated to support the body during each step.

   However, beginning with the evolution of *Australopithecus*, we see changes to the lower limb that indicate an improvement in locomotor economy. For example, the lower limbs of australopiths are significantly longer than those of other great apes and earlier hominins (39). Long limbs reduce energy costs by smoothing the path of the center of mass during walking, minimizing the amount of muscle volume needed per step, and reducing the number of steps taken per unit distance (38–40, 42). In addition, australopiths had pelvic anatomy consistent with full extension of the hip during locomotion, which would have greatly reduced energy costs of walking compared with the crouched postures of chimpanzees (10, 19, 57). This increased hip and knee extension in australopiths is confirmed by recent analyses of the fossil footprints from Laetoli, Tanzania showing that, by at least 3.66 million years ago, australopiths walked with mechanics generally similar to modern humans (49, 50). Given the inverse correlation between limb length and energy costs of locomotion at both walking and running speeds, and the reduced costs associated with an extended hip posture, selection for improved locomotor economy was likely acting by 3–4 million years ago. Thus, improved energy economy during walking in australopiths may have laid the foundation for long-distance foraging bouts in early hunting and gathering members of the genus *Homo*.

Skeletal adaptations for high forces

While improved energy economy was beneficial at both low and high speeds of movement, higher walking and running speeds bring other challenges. Specifically, higher speed movement increases forces acting on the musculoskeletal system (8, 25, 28) and we should expect to see adaptations to force resistance in fossil taxa moving at high speeds. In addition, high forces, especially at initial ground contact, generate large pitching moments at both the waist and neck, and if these are not resisted in some way, high-speed motion would lead to potentially dangerous instability.

Beginning with *Homo erectus*, hominin postcranial evolution is dominated by adaptations for force resistance and stabilization mechanisms. Early members of the genus *Homo* have increased lower limb joint surface areas, which are linked to resisting higher loading environments (16, 53). In comparisons with earlier hominins such as *Australopithecus afarensis* and *A. africanus*, after taking into account differences in body size, *H. erectus* has increased femoral head and tibial plateau breadth, and decreased humeral relative to femoral diaphyseal bone strength compared with earlier hominins (16, 52). These changes in joint articular surface size in the lower limb, combined with a shift in patterns of diaphyseal strength in the upper and lower limb bones, suggests that *H. erectus* was likely managing higher lower limb loads during locomotion.

Higher loads due to increased ground reaction forces often lead to pitching moments in both the trunk and head in bipeds, which would require associated adaptations to maintain stability (27). *H. erectus* and modern humans show changes in two areas associated with maintaining stability during bipedal locomotion. First, pitching moments at the trunk are counteracted by activation of the gluteus maximus muscle (27, 61). Modern humans have an enlarged gluteus maximus with an increased attachment area on the superior portion of the iliac blade compared with other great apes (27). Evidence from the fossil record suggests this change in muscular morphology likely occurred with the evolution of *H. erectus*, based on comparisons of attachment site morphology on the pelvis (27).

In addition to managing trunk pitch, head pitch in response to increased ground reaction forces may cause disruptions to the visual system that can be dangerous when moving at high speeds on a complex landscape (58). To manage high-pitch velocities, the vestibulo-ocular system must respond to head movements and adjust eye position to allow the maintenance of vision (59, 60). Across mammals, increasing the radius of the semicircular canals is often considered an adaptation to high head velocities, minimizing the potential for saturation of the vestibulo-ocular system (59, 60). Spoor et al. (59, 60) have shown that *H. erectus* and modern humans have increased diameters of the posterior and anterior semicircular canals compared with australopiths and other great apes.

Combined, a change in lower limb joint surface areas, a shift towards stronger lower limb compared with upper limb long bones, increased gluteus maximus size, and enlarged semicircular canals suggest that *H. erectus* was adapted to a locomotor environment that included increased loads potentially over long periods of time. These increased loads are likely linked to increased walking and running speeds consistent with requirements of a hunting and gathering lifestyle. Thus, by the evolution of the genus *Homo*, we see skeletal adaptations that are linked to an increased reliance on higher aerobic intensity foraging behaviors.

Physiological adaptations for endurance

Evidence presented above suggests the human locomotor phenotype includes adaptations for higher loads during locomotion, which likely come with increased velocity, and reduced locomotor economy, and could be advantageous for moving over long distances. While these skeletal adaptations reflect the potential for a behavioral transition towards increased endurance, the main elements that make up the endurance phenotype lie in soft tissue that does not preserve in the fossil record (39). Using comparative biology, we can assess differences in endurance traits that do not fossilize; however, a detailed exploration of the evolution of the endurance phenotype requires analysis of how the underlying genetics of these traits shifted over time.

A key element of endurance is muscle fiber type distribution that impacts both mitochondrial density and fatigue resistance (5, 33, 34). Recent work shows that human lower limb muscles are biased towards myosin heavy chain (MHC) type I fibers, whereas chimpanzees and other primates have more mixed lower limb muscle fiber distributions. MHC I fibers have a higher density of mitochondria, relying less on glycolysis, and therefore muscle glycogen, allowing for an increase in the number of contractions possible prior to onset of fatigue (55). In addition, humans have greater hindlimb muscle mass compared to chimpanzees (36, 39, 64), which would increase muscle endurance given the greater density of mitochondria predicted for muscles with a larger percentage of type I fibers.

Fiber-type distributions are at least partially a product of underlying genetics. For example, the alpha-actinin-3 (*ACTN3*) gene is linked with fiber-type distribution, and individuals possessing the 577X allele have a significantly higher density of type I fibers compared with individuals possessing the 577R allele (67). In fact, elite endurance athletes include a higher proportion of individuals homozygous for the 577X allele compared with nonathletes and power-oriented athletes (68). MacArthur et al. (29) show that this endurance-linked mutation likely arose between 40,000 and 60,000 years ago, during the evolution of modern *H. sapiens*, suggesting increased selection pressures for improved endurance in populations of our own species. Examinations of the underlying genetics behind these muscle variables may provide further evidence of adaptive changes earlier in human evolution.

In addition to muscular traits that improve human endurance, humans also possess thermoregulatory adaptations that some suggest evolved to facilitate endurance activities in environments that would generate high heat stress (e.g., African savanna (23), but see (4) for an alternative view). For example, while all Old World monkeys and apes sweat, humans have a much higher percentage of eccrine subcutaneous sweat glands, and have much higher sweat rates than other primates, including apes (7, 23). Combined with a loss of dense fur, these adaptations would allow for enhanced thermoregulatory capabilities in hot environments during endurance activities. A recent study demonstrated that the density of eccrine sweat glands is under partial genetic control, through the engrailed-1 (*En1*) gene, which may provide a novel basis for exploring the evolution of human thermoregulatory capabilities (17).

While analyses of ancestral anatomy detail a shift in lifestyle that likely required enhanced endurance, soft tissue evidence of changing endurance capabilities does not fossilize. It is likely that changes in mitochondrial density, muscle fiber-type distributions, and thermoregulatory abilities shifted with the evolution of the genus *Homo*. Future work in comparative genetics and genomics can help evolutionary biologists clarify the timing of these adaptive changes in endurance, and will help fill in gaps in the story of the evolution of the human endurance phenotype.

An evolutionary framework for the endurance phenotype

Our review of evidence for changes in locomotion and endurance during human evolution suggests that a major transition occurred beginning around 2 million years ago. At this time, with the earth's climate changing, and associated increases in grasslands and decreases in forest cover in east and south Africa, ancestral humans adopted a hunting and gathering lifestyle. From comparative studies of living humans and great apes, we showed that this lifestyle change would have involved an increase in travel distance and locomotor intensity (predominantly moderate intensity physical activity). The hominin fossil record provides evidence for selection acting on the locomotor skeleton to support this type of behavioral change. While selection for improved locomotor economy seems to have occurred prior to the adoption of hunting and gathering (i.e., in *Australopithecus*), the evolution of the genus *Homo* is linked with adaptations to resist high locomotor forces and maintain stability at higher locomotor speeds. Because adaptations for endurance do not fossilize, it is difficult to know with certainty when traits associated with aerobic capacity evolved; however, a plausible hypothesis is that an increase in the density of slow-twitch muscle fibers in the lower limb, and an associated increase in mitochondrial density, was selected during the evolution of the genus *Homo*.

Evolutionary exercise physiology and human health

Based on this proposed evolutionary shift towards increased endurance activities, we can explore the importance of an evolutionary framework for understanding the genetic links between exercise (or lack thereof) and disease. Fundamental to this discussion is the understanding that selection acted on human physiology to enhance reproductive success, rather than to improve health (e.g., 24). Thus, any health-enhancing effects of exercise that are associated with our evolutionary history are linked to the reproductive fitness benefits of engaging in aerobic activity.

Recently, Lieberman (24) and Raichlen and Alexander (46) detailed models for evolutionary exercise physiology that suggest physiological systems evolved to respond plastically to exercise stress. When faced with increased demands, systems from our musculoskeletal system to our cardiovascular system and even our brains, respond by increasing capacity to adapt to new stress. When exercise demands are removed, an energy-saving mechanism is initiated that leads to system atrophy, reducing the energy costs of tissue maintenance. Given our reliance on physical activity and endurance behaviors to gain access to food, our physiological systems do not function well with capacity reductions, often leading to negative health outcomes.

Well-known examples of these exercise-induced capacity adaptations include increased peripheral capillary density, increased heart mass, and increased cardiac stroke volume in individuals engaged in aerobic exercise (46). Bone mineral density is increased through exercise, especially at young ages, which can lead to a higher overall peak bone mass and reduced risk of developing osteoporosis later in life (22). In addition, reductions in activity are associated with loss of muscle mass and strength (sarcopenia) (22).

Finally, endurance exercise has beneficial effects on the brain, with reduced age-related atrophy and increased functional connectivity at young ages (46–48). In fact, it is possible that evolutionary changes in endurance behaviors may have altered brain aging early on during the adoption of hunting and gathering (47). At this time, nearly 2 million years ago, human ancestors were all homozygous for apolipoprotein E (*APOE*) ε4, an allele that carries increased risk of cardiovascular disease and Alzheimer's disease. However, individuals who exercise experience large risk reductions for each of these diseases. Raichlen and Alexander (47) argue that the adoption of increased endurance-related activities may have allowed for an increase in the human lifespan in the context of genetic constraints such as *APOE-ε4*.

This evolutionary approach to exercise physiology helps us understand how and why our physiological systems respond to exercise. As a foundation for future studies, understanding the role of intensity and exercise duration on capacity changes in physiology may help us better determine optimal exercise patterns for maintaining the health of physiological systems. In addition, knowledge of ancestral genotypes, and their interactions with physical activity, may provide new avenues for examining precision exercise studies from an evolutionary perspective.

Conclusions: What can genetics bring to the evolutionary story and vice versa?

Here, we have argued that human evolution was driven, in many ways, by a shift from a relatively sedentary lifestyle to an increase in endurance activities likely tied to a changing climate and the associated adoption of a hunting and gathering lifestyle. Adaptations that appear during the evolution of *H. erectus*, beginning about 2 million years ago, suggest major changes in the endurance capabilities of these human ancestors that persist in modern *H. sapiens*. Thus, we owe our modern endurance athletic capabilities to key transitions during human evolution.

While the human fossil record provides clues to the evolution of the human endurance phenotype, a better understanding of the genetic and epigenetic underpinnings of the endurance phenotype will not only help improve health and athletic performance, but will enhance our understanding of human evolution. Thus, we suggest that analyses of human performance genetics can both benefit from an evolutionary approach and can improve our understanding of human evolutionary history. For example, testing the hypothesis that increased mitochondrial density evolved with the adoption of hunting and gathering in the genus *Homo* could benefit from a directed effort to examine the history of genes associated with muscle fiber type and mitochondrial density. A better understanding of the evolution of genes contributing to the endurance phenotype, and especially the timing and geographical variation of their evolutionary history, will help us more clearly identify the selection pressures that led to human endurance capabilities. By combining data from the fossil record with a systems genetic approach to human exercise performance, we can, perhaps, use an evolutionary framework to improve sports performance and health.

References

1. **Amsler SJ**. Energetic costs of territorial boundary patrols by wild chimpanzees. *Am J Primatol* 72: 93–103, 2010.
2. **Bates LA** and **Byrne RW**. Sex differences in the movement patterns of free-ranging chimpanzees (Pan troglodytes schweinfurthii): foraging and border checking. *Behav Ecol Sociobiol* 64: 247–255, 2009.
3. **Beaune D, Bretagnolle F, Bollache L, Hohmann G, Surbeck M, Bourson C,** and **Fruth B**. The Bonobo–Dialium positive interactions: seed dispersal mutualism. *Am J Primatol* 75: 394–403, 2013.
4. **Best A** and **Kamilar JM**. The evolution of eccrine sweat glands in human and nonhuman primates. *J Hum Evol* 117: 33–43, 2018.
5. **Bozek K, Wei Y, Yan Z, Liu X, Xiong J, Sugimoto M, Tomita M, Pääbo S, Pieszek R,** and **Sherwood CC**. Exceptional evolutionary divergence of human muscle and brain metabolomes parallels human cognitive and physical uniqueness. *PLoS Biol* 12: e1001871, 2014.
6. **Bramble DM** and **Lieberman DE**. Endurance running and the evolution of Homo. *Nature* 432: 345–352, 2004.
7. **Carrier DR**. The energetic paradox of human running and hominid evolution. *Curr Anthropol* 25: 483–495, 1984.
8. **Daoud AI, Geissler GJ, Wang F, Saretsky J, Daoud YA,** and **Lieberman DE**. Foot strike and injury rates in endurance runners: A retrospective study. *Med Sci Sports Exerc* 44: 1325–1334, 2012.
9. **Domínguez-Rodrigo M**. Hunting and scavenging by early humans: The state of the debate. *J World Prehist* 16: 1–54, 2002.
10. **Foster AD, Raichlen DA,** and **Pontzer H**. Muscle force production during bent-knee, bent-hip walking in humans. *J Hum Evol* 65: 294–302, 2013.
11. **Galdikas BM**. Orangutan diet, range, and activity at Tanjung Puting, Central Borneo. *Int J Primatol* 9: 1–35, 1988.
12. **Green DJ** and **Alemseged Z**. Australopithecus afarensis scapular ontogeny, function, and the role of climbing in human evolution. *Science* 338: 514–517, 2012.

13. **Gurven M**, **Jaeggi AV**, **Kaplan H**, and **Cummings D**. Physical activity and modernization among Bolivian Amerindians. *PLoS One* 8: e55679, 2013.
14. **Hill K** and **Hurtado AM**. Hunter-gatherers of the New World. *Am Sci* 77: 436–443, 1989.
15. **Jette M**, **Sidney K**, and **Blümchen G**. Metabolic equivalents (METS) in exercise testing, exercise prescription, and evaluation of functional capacity. *Clin Cardiol* 13: 555–565, 1990.
16. **Jungers WL**. Lucy's limbs: skeletal allometry and locomotion in Australopithecus afarensis. *Nature* 297: 676–678, 1982.
17. **Kamberov YG**, **Karlsson EK**, **Kamberova GL**, **Lieberman DE**, **Sabeti PC**, **Morgan BA**, and **Tabin CJ**. A genetic basis of variation in eccrine sweat gland and hair follicle density. *Proc Natl Acad Sci U S A* 112: 9932–9937, 2015.
18. **Knott C**, **Beaudrot L**, **Snaith T**, **White S**, **Tschauner H**, and **Planansky G**. Female-female competition in Bornean orangutans. *Int J Primatol* 29: 975–997, 2008.
19. **Kozma EE**, **Webb NM**, **Harcourt-Smith WEH**, **Raichlen DA**, **D'Aout K**, **Brown MH**, **Firestone E**, **Ross SR**, **Aerts P**, and **Pontzer H**. Hip extensor mechanics and the evolution of walking and climbing capabilities in humans, apes, and fossil hominins. *Proc Natl Acad Sci U S A* 115: 4134–4139, 2018.
20. **Lee RB**. Kung Bushmen subsistence: An input-output analysis. In: *Contributions to Anthropology: Ecological Essays*, edited by **Damas D**. Ottowa: National Museums of Canada, 1969, p. 73–94.
21. **Leonard WR** and **Robertson ML**. Comparative primate energetics and hominid evolution. *Am J Phys Anthropol* 102: 265–281, 1997.
22. **Lieberman D**. *The Story of the Human body: Evolution, Health, and Disease*. New York: Vintage, 2014.
23. **Lieberman DE**. Human locomotion and heat loss: An evolutionary perspective. *Compr Physiol* 5: 99–117, 2015.
24. **Lieberman DE**. Is exercise really medicine? An evolutionary perspective. *Curr Sports Med Rep* 14: 313–319, 2015.
25. **Lieberman DE**. What we can learn about running from barefoot running: An evolutionary medical perspective. *Exerc Sport Sci Rev* 40: 63–72, 2012.
26. **Lieberman DE** and **Bramble DM**. The evolution of marathon running. *Sports Med* 37: 288–290, 2007.
27. **Lieberman DE**, **Raichlen DA**, **Pontzer H**, **Bramble DM**, and **Cutright-Smith E**. The human gluteus maximus and its role in running. *J Exp Biol* 209: 2143–2155, 2006.
28. **Lieberman DE**, **Venkadesan M**, **Werbel WA**, **Daoud AI**, **D'Andrea S**, **Davis IS**, **Mang'Eni RO**, and **Pitsiladis Y**. Foot strike patterns and collision forces in habitually barefoot versus shod runners. *Nature* 463: 531, 2010.
29. **MacArthur DG**, **Seto JT**, **Raftery JM**, **Quinlan KG**, **Huttley GA**, **Hook JW**, **Lemckert FA**, **Kee AJ**, **Edwards MR**, and **Berman Y**. Loss of ACTN3 gene function alters mouse muscle metabolism and shows evidence of positive selection in humans. *Nat Genet* 39: 1261, 2007.
30. **Marlowe F**. *The Hadza: Hunter-Gatherers of Tanzania*. Berkeley, CA: University of California Press, 2010.
31. **Marlowe FW**. Hunter-gatherers and human evolution. *Evol Anthropol* 14: 54–67, 2005.
32. **Marlowe FW** and **Berbesque JC**. Tubers as fallback foods and their impact on Hadza hunter-gatherers. *Am J Phys Anthropol* 140: 751–758, 2009.
33. **Myatt JP**, **Schilling N**, and **Thorpe SK**. Distribution patterns of fibre types in the triceps surae muscle group of chimpanzees and orangutans. *J Anat* 218: 402–412, 2011.
34. **O'Neill MC**, **Umberger BR**, **Holowka NB**, **Larson SG**, and **Reiser PJ**. Chimpanzee super strength and human skeletal muscle evolution. *Proc Natl Acad Sci U S A* 114: 7343–7734, 2017.
35. **Office of Disease Prevention and Health Promotion**. Appendix 1. Translating scientific evidence about total amount and intensity of physical activity into guidelines. 2018. www.health.gov/paguidelines/guidelines/appendix1.aspx.
36. **Payne RC**, **Crompton RH**, **Isler K**, **Savage R**, **Vereecke EE**, **Günther MM**, **Thorpe S**, and **D'Août K**. Morphological analysis of the hindlimb in apes and humans. I. Muscle architecture. *J Anat* 208: 709–724, 2006.
37. **Pilbeam DT** and **Lieberman DE**. Reconstructing the last common ancestor of chimpanzees and humans. In: *Chimpanzees and Human Evolution*, edited by Muller MN, Wrangham RW, and Pilbeam DT. Cambridge, MA: The Belknap Press of Harvard University Press, 2017, p. 22–141.
38. **Pontzer H**. Ecological energetics in early Homo. *Curr Anthropol* 53: S346–S358, 2012.
39. **Pontzer H**. Economy and endurance in human evolution. *Curr Biol* 27: R613–R621, 2017.

40. **Pontzer H**. Effective limb length and the scaling of locomotor cost in terrestrial animals. *J Exp Biol* 210: 1752–1761, 2007.

41. **Pontzer H**. Locomotor ecology and evolution in chimpanzees and humans. In: *Chimpanzees and Human Evolution*, edited by Muller MN, Wrangham RW, and Pilbeam DT. Cambridge, MA: The Belknap Press of Harvard University Press, 2017, p. 259–285.

42. **Pontzer H**. Predicting the energy cost of terrestrial locomotion: A test of the LiMb model in humans and quadrupeds. *J Exp Biol* 210: 484–494, 2007.

43. **Pontzer H, Raichlen DA, Wood BM, Emery Thompson M, Racette SB, Mabulla AZ**, and **Marlowe FW**. Energy expenditure and activity among Hadza hunter-gatherers. *Am J Hum Biol* 27: 628–637, 2015.

44. **Pontzer H, Raichlen DA, Wood BM, Mabulla AZ, Racette SB**, and **Marlowe FW**. Hunter-gatherer energetics and human obesity. *PLoS One* 7: e40503, 2012.

45. **Pontzer H** and **Wrangham RW**. Climbing and the daily energy cost of locomotion in wild chimpanzees: implications for hominoid locomotor evolution. *J Hum Evol* 46: 315–333, 2004.

46. **Raichlen DA** and **Alexander GE**. Adaptive capacity: An evolutionary neuroscience model linking exercise, cognition, and brain health. *Trends Neurosci* 40: 408–421, 2017.

47. **Raichlen DA** and **Alexander GE**. Exercise, APOE genotype, and the evolution of the human life-span. *Trends Neurosci* 37: 247–255, 2014.

48. **Raichlen DA, Bharadwaj PK, Fitzhugh MC, Haws KA, Torre G-A, Trouard TP**, and **Alexander GE**. Differences in resting state functional connectivity between young adult endurance athletes and healthy controls. *Front Hum Neurosci* 10: 610, 2016.

49. **Raichlen DA** and **Gordon AD**. Interpretation of footprints from Site S confirms human-like bipedal biomechanics in Laetoli hominins. *J Hum Evol* 107: 134–138, 2017.

50. **Raichlen DA, Gordon AD, Harcourt-Smith WE, Foster AD**, and **Haas Jr WR**. Laetoli footprints preserve earliest direct evidence of human-like bipedal biomechanics. *PLoS One* 5: e9769, 2010.

51. **Raichlen DA, Pontzer H, Harris JA, Mabulla AZ, Marlowe FW, Josh Snodgrass J, Eick G, Colette Berbesque J, Sancilio A**, and **Wood BM**. Physical activity patterns and biomarkers of cardiovascular disease risk in hunter-gatherers. *Am J Hum Biol* 29: e22919, 2017.

52. **Rowan J** and **Reed KE**. The paleoclimatic record and Plio-Pleistocene paleoenvironments. In: *Handbook of Paleoanthropology*, edited by **Henke W** and **Tattersall I**. New York: Springer, 2015, p. 465–491.

53. **Ruff CB, Burgess ML, Ketcham RA**, and **Kappelman J**. Limb bone structural proportions and locomotor behavior in AL 288-1 ("Lucy"). *PLoS One* 11: e0166095, 2016.

54. **Scheadler CM** and **Devor ST**. VO2max measured with a self-selected work rate protocol on an automated treadmill. *Med Sci Sports Exerc* 47: 2158–2165, 2015.

55. **Schiaffino S** and **Reggiani C**. Fiber types in mammalian skeletal muscles. *Physiol Rev* 91: 1447–1531, 2011.

56. **Singleton I, Knott CD, Morrogh-Bernard HC, Wich SA**, and **van Schaik CP**. Ranging behaviour of orangutan females and social organization. In: *Orangutans: Geographic Variation in Behavioral Ecology and Conservation*, edited by **Wich SA, Utami Atmoko SS, Setia TM**, and **van Schaik CP**. Oxford: Oxford University Press, 2009, p. 205–213.

57. **Sockol MD, Raichlen DA**, and **Pontzer H**. Chimpanzee locomotor energetics and the origin of human bipedalism. *Proc Natl Acad Sci U S A* 104: 12265–12269, 2007.

58. **Spoor F, Garland T, Krovitz G, Ryan TM, Silcox MT**, and **Walker A**. The primate semicircular canal system and locomotion. *Proc Natl Acad Sci U S A* 104: 10808–10812, 2007.

59. **Spoor F, Hublin J-J, Braun M**, and **Zonneveld F**. The bony labyrinth of Neanderthals. *J Hum Evol* 44: 141–165, 2003.

60. **Spoor F, Wood B**, and **Zonneveld F**. Implications of early hominid labyrinthine morphology for evolution of human bipedal locomotion. *Nature* 369: 645, 1994.

61. **Stern JT**. Anatomical and functional specializations of the human gluteus maximus. *Am J Phys Anthropol* 36: 315–339, 1972.

62. **Stern JT**. Climbing to the top: A personal memoir of Australopithecus afarensis. *Evol Anthropol* 9: 113–133, 2000.

63. **Takeshima N, Kobayashi F, Watanabe T, Tanaka K, Tomita M**, and **Pollock ML**. Cardiorespiratory responses to cycling exercise in trained and untrained healthy elderly: With special reference to the lactate threshold. *Appl Human Sci* 15: 267–273, 2001.

64. **Thorpe SK, Crompton RH, Guenther MM, Ker RF,** and **McNeill Alexander R**. Dimensions and moment arms of the hind- and forelimb muscles of common chimpanzees (Pan troglodytes). *Am J Phys Anthropol* 110: 179–199, 1999.

65. **Ward CV**. Interpreting the posture and locomotion of Australopithecus afarensis: Where do we stand? *Am J Phys Anthropol* 119: 185–215, 2002.

66. **Yamagiwa J** and **Basabose AK**. Socioecological flexibility of gorillas and chimpanzees. In: *Primates and Cetaceans*, edited by **Yamagiwa J** and **Karczmarski L**. Tokyo: Springer, 2014, p. 43–74.

67. **Yang N, MacArthur DG, Gulbin JP, Hahn AG, Beggs AH, Easteal S,** and **North K**. ACTN3 genotype is associated with human elite athletic performance. *Am J Hum Genet* 73: 627–631, 2003.

12

ENDURANCE PHENOTYPE PRIMER

John C. Quindry and Michael D. Roberts

This chapter serves as a primer, summarizing individual physiological traits that contribute to overall endurance, endurance-related traits, and performance during endurance events. The chapter also summarizes basic molecular pathways that modify traits associated with endurance phenotypes and informs subsequent chapters on the genetic influences of these traits.

Introduction and evolutionary considerations of the endurance phenotype

Healthy humans have a remarkable capacity to engage in endurance activities. Genetic understanding of endurance capacity describes an emergent group of well-conserved traits which span an organizational hierarchy from subcellular to organismal. This primer is founded on classic understanding of human anthropometry, systems physiology, and tissue-level adaptations that inform endurance exercise capacity and adaptation. Descriptions of anthologized information are provided in brief, while more recently discovered roles of cell signaling mechanisms that ultimately underpin endurance capacity and adaptive responses will be covered in more detail. The reader is directed to Chapter 11 for additional details of endurance and evolution. For the sake of simplicity, human-, animal-, and cell culture-based investigations are woven into a common narrative which serves as a necessary background for subsequent understanding of the genetic foundations of endurance.

Within a given species, endurance exercise speed is size limited, and generally inverse to total body mass in terms of relative oxygen consumption (40, 42). However, when the importance of endurance supersedes speed, larger species and individuals are more often benefitted by: 1) increased metabolic flexibility favoring lipid utilization, and 2) fluid retention strategies that preserve cardiovascular dynamics, in addition to heat tolerance (42). Proportional expressions of these, and other, physiologic traits are often predictive of specialized endurance success across athletic competitions (e.g., 5 km, 40 km, 160 km runs) (78).

Acute physiologic adjustments to prolonged physical activity, and endurance adaptations, are largely independent of endurance performance capabilities (71). That is, prerequisite physiologic adjustments include acute alterations in cardiovascular work and blood flow redistribution, matched to accelerated ventilatory function and parsimonious access to macronutrients (9). It is important to remember, from an evolutionary perspective, that cellular "wisdom" self-regulates in the name of homeostatic preservation (14). Thus, endurance exercise adaptations are the cumulative effect of acute cellular stresses expressed across tissues and organ systems. Based on this rationale, the following sections briefly overview the most well-defined physiologic responses to acute and chronic endurance exercise. Subsequent sections detail cell signaling events responsible for endurance adaptations that underpin many of the physiologic outcomes described forthright.

Acute and chronic physiologic responses to endurance exercise

Metabolic flexibility

The endurance phenotype is characterized by metabolic flexibility. This point is ultimately underscored by natural selection of "thrifty" genes directed to promote energy storage and spare carbohydrate use (14). Given the importance of duration to endurance-type exercise, metabolic flexibility is perhaps best characterized by the ability to the support ATP regeneration via multiple macronutrient substrates in order to maintain steady-state workload demands. The topic of metabolic flexibility is immense and beyond the scope of this chapter, but the reader is directed to authoritative work on the topic (29). Suffice it to state that harnessing stored calories during exercise involves time-dependent macronutrient partitioning in a carbohydrate-sparing fashion (9). The topic is further nuanced in that the endurance phenotype responds to dietary manipulation and can favor a number of macronutrient-loading strategies including fat, carbohydrate, and ketones (9, 80).

Cardiorespiratory responses

Endurance exercise evokes prominent alterations to the integrated cardiorespiratory response. Elevated cardiac output is directly proportional to increased exercise intensity and reflects elevations in both heart rate and stroke volume (SV), with the latter exhibiting a plateau at intensities above moderate workloads (64). Of note, endurance-trained athletes possess significant increases in cardiac output for a given work intensity, primarily due to elevated SV (58). More recent investigations, aided by advanced *in vivo* imaging, indicate that SV may not plateau in elite distance runners as they exceed moderate intensity exercise (88). The respiratory system also supports endurance activities through ventilation–perfusion matching via increased tidal volume and respiratory rate. Most of the increased tidal volume comes from decreases in inspiratory reserve, a feature that is potentiated by muscular adaptations for inspiration with endurance training (37, 62).

Blood flow redistribution

During endurance exercise, blood flow is redistributed (vasodilation and constriction) to match tissue-level changes in bioenergetics demand, while simultaneously mitigating heat accumulation. Acute changes in blood flow ultimately influence oxygen consumption via the Fick principle (VO_2 = cardiac output − arteriovenous difference (a–vO_2)). Accordingly, cardiorespiratory responses require acute changes in blood flow and are accompanied by an increased a–vO_2 across a capillary bed (41). For a more in-depth discussion of this topic, the reader is directed to an authoritative review (42), but it is notable that blood flow adaptations to training are difficult to enumerate independent of the other physiologic systems (40, 78). While integrated blood flow responses to thermoregulation are included shortly, it is important to recognize that tissue-level adaptations for improved blood flow responses to endurance training are among the most well-described of the mechanisms detailed below.

Neuroendocrine influence on metabolic flexibility

Metabolic flexibility and carbohydrate-sparing during endurance exercise is facilitated, in part, by pairs of fast-acting hormones. Insulin and glucagon are central to fast-acting energy regulation, with the latter being responsible for carbohydrate and free fatty acid liberation during endurance exercise (16). Acute endurance exercise promotes energy availability through time-dependent glucagon release (77); a response that is blunted in trained individuals (19). Epinephrine (E) and norepinephrine (NE) further mediate the fast-acting hormonal influence on metabolic control, stimulating free fatty acid release and utilization simultaneous to carbohydrate-sparing effects. These are highly important time-dependent effects as E/NE levels rise gradually during endurance exercise. Not unlike glucagon, acute exercise-induced release of E/NE to a given moderate intensity workload is blunted in trained individuals (90). Collective attenuation of hormone release during exercise reveals an interesting feature about the endurance phenotype. Specifically, the immediate physiologic stress of long-duration muscular activity is better tolerated in exercise-trained individuals, a fact that speaks to innumerable tissue-level adaptations to be detailed shortly.

Thermoregulatory and blood volume perseveration

The aforementioned blood volume redistribution during endurance exercise is often complicated by the physiologic need to thermoregulate, and subsequently, counteract the resultant hypovolemia (58). Recent investigation of acute ultra-endurance physiology indicates SV will drift (first decreasing, then increasing) to moderate ongoing metabolic demands simultaneous to hypovolemia and thermoregulatory efforts (50). Long-term physiologic demands are also bolstered in the endurance phenotype through increased red blood cell content and increased hematocrit and red cell volume (55). Moreover, elevated exercise core temperatures potentiate the aforementioned hormonal responses to better control fuel utilization during endurance exercise (65). These adaptations are fundamental to improved thermoregulatory tolerance in endurance-trained individuals as compared to untrained individuals (58).

Section summary

From a comprehensive perspective, it is not surprising that the various aspects of organizational physiology which support endurance exercise are universally exhibited across the talent spectrum from mall walkers to Olympic marathon champions. Moreover, all physiologic aspects discussed herein are also subject to optimization via endurance training; a fact that is also independent of aerobic talent. Foundational understanding of these tissue- and cellular-level adaptations are described below.

Skeletal muscle and the myocardium: Responsiveness to endurance training

Endurance training promotes physiological adaptations in a variety of tissues. While describing an exhaustive list of tissue-level adaptations exceeds the scope of this chapter, selected thematic skeletal muscle and myocardial adaptations are described below. Following months of endurance training, well-documented skeletal muscle adaptations include: 1) increased mitochondrial expression of the tricarboxylic acid (TCA) cycle and fatty acid oxidation enzymes; 2) increased electron transport chain components (34); 3) expansion of mitochondrial volume via mitochondrial biogenesis (36), 4) majority transition of type IIX to IIA fibers, and limited transition of type II to type I fibers (~5–10%, quantified with histological myosin ATPase staining) (84); and 5) an approximately 20% increase in skeletal muscle capillary content via angiogenesis (44).

Ethical constraints dictate that parallel understanding of myocardial adaptations to endurance training are largely confined to data from animal studies. Notwithstanding, myocardial adaptations generally mimic skeletal muscle responses, including increased fatty acid oxidation enzymes (74), increased mitochondrial volume (79), and increased capillarization (12). Furthermore, landmark human-based studies report that months of endurance training increases maximal SV (21) as well as cardiac output during exercise by approximately 10% (22).

Whole-body adaptations resulting from skeletal muscle and myocardial adaptations

The novel introduction of endurance training, adhering to several months of American College of Sports Medicine prescriptive criteria, produces an approximately 15–30% increase in maximal oxygen consumption (VO_2max) (8). Subsequent scientific revelation introduced the idea that high-intensity interval training, involving interspersed intervals of supra-VO_2max running or cycling with inactive- or low-intensity recovery, elicits similar improvements in aerobic capacity. Notably, however, VO_2max adaptations to endurance training are heterogenic across the population. For instance, the HERITAGE Family Study revealed that 60 cycle training sessions over 20 weeks produced individual VO_2max increases ranging between no gain and a 100% increase (8). Application of heritability calculations to these data suggest approximately 50% of the VO_2max adaptations to endurance training are genetically predisposed, and this topic is the focus of a subsequent chapter (Chapter 14) on heritability and endurance capacity in humans (7). Genetic contributors aside, the majority of VO_2max adaptations to endurance training are cardiovascular in nature. Physiologically, this response is marked by increases in maximal stroke volume, as a primary influence on cardiac output, in addition to increased a–vO_2 difference (e.g., increases in muscle fiber capillary number and mitochondrial volume) (52).

Beyond increasing VO_2max, endurance training elevates lactate threshold (43), the work rate beyond which incremental increases in exercise intensity elicit a nonlinear increase in blood lactate concentration. Where untrained individuals experience lactate thresholds between 40% and 70% VO_2max, endurance-trained subjects exhibit a lactate threshold at or above 80% VO_2max (43). While the contributors to skeletal muscle fatigue involve accumulation of numerous metabolites and ions (e.g., inorganic phosphate, lactate, and potassium and hydrogen ions) as well as muscle glycogen depletion (28), lactate threshold is an important physiological parameter to consider, given that it is often more predicative of endurance performance than VO_2max (3). Numerous factors influence lactate threshold, including muscle fiber recruitment patterns, skeletal muscle oxidative capacity, the rate of O_2 delivery to muscle, glycolytic activation, and the ability to clear lactate (28). However, the aforementioned doubling of skeletal muscle oxidative capacity through increased mitochondrial function and volume, as well as capillary number, are the primary determinants of increased lactate threshold values with endurance training (43).

Endurance training may also increase exercise economy, or the workload performed at a given VO_2. While improvements in mechanical efficiency are well documented, the adaptive propensity is highly variable between individuals. In this regard, elite runners express a 30–40% difference in running economy (40). For example, athletes with a lower exercise economy ran approximately 16.5 km/hour at a VO_2 of 55 ml O_2/kg/min, whereas athletes with a higher exercise economy ran over 19.0 km/hour at this same VO_2. Genetic factors, muscle fiber type, fiber recruitment patterns during running, and external factors (e.g., wind resistance) likely contribute to heterogeneity in running economy. However, adaptation is also trainable, in that years of directed training produce 8–14% increases in the running economy of elite endurance athletes (40). While the nuanced mechanisms remain emergent, experts posit that a fast-to-slow conversion of myosin isoforms over long-term training periods may underpin adaptations in economy (40).

Molecular pathways that facilitate endurance training adaptations

Cellular-level adaptations to endurance training are widespread across skeletal muscle, myocardium, and numerous other tissues. Upon the introduction of sustained exercise, intracellular changes are acute and marked by a concert of biochemical alterations in metabolite levels, protein signaling, and gene expression patterns. Over a series of training bouts, these molecular events accumulate with tissue-level adaptations to produce the aforementioned increases in VO_2max, lactate threshold, and exercise economy. Collectively, these responses contribute to the genetics of cardiorespiratory fitness (detailed in Chapter 15), and are largely driven by mitochondrial adaptations (detailed in Chapter 16).

Given that exercise-responsive molecules orchestrate a plethora of signaling events and lead to extraordinary exercise adaptations, there is widespread interest in elucidating the interrelationships among these molecules. In this regard, recent advances in powerful 'omics'-based methods (e.g., metabolomics, phosphoproteomics, RNA sequencing) have been used to characterize metabolite, kinase, transcription factor, and RNA transcript profile changes following acute and chronic endurance training. For instance, RNA sequencing indicates that more than 3400 skeletal muscle mRNA transcripts are altered by 12 weeks of endurance training (47). While many altered transcripts associate with oxidative ATP production, 34 transcripts are previously unidentified targets within exercised muscle. Moreover, mass spectrometry-based phosphoproteomics demonstrate that approximately 15 minutes of high-intensity cycling exercise alters the phosphorylation status of more than 560 skeletal muscle proteins (32). Canonical protein signaling networks activated by endurance exercise include adenosine monophosphate-activated kinase (AMPK) and CaMK (as described below) in addition to a novel complement of muscle proteins subject to exercise-induced phosphorylation. Recent animal studies confirm that hundreds of myocardial proteins are acutely phosphorylated in response to treadmill running (31). Excitingly, the majority of these phospho-sites have not previously been associated with cardiac adaptive response to exercise.

Collectively, omics-based studies conceptualize two critical points: 1) thousands of molecules (e.g., kinases, transcription factors, mRNA transcripts, and epigenetic factors including miRNAs) coordinate to facilitate endurance exercise adaptations; and 2) the functional significance of molecular profiles in endurance exercised skeletal muscle, myocardia, and other tissues remain unknown. Indeed, understanding molecular pathways activated in exercised tissues is just emerging. A Common Fund Program from the National Institutes of Health (NIH), named the Molecular Transducers of Physical Activity Consortium (MoTrPAC), was a 2015 NIH initiative that identified a consortium to extensively investigate phosphoproteomic and transcriptomic alterations in endurance exercised skeletal muscle and other tissues. Ongoing efforts will continue to validate previously identified exercise-responsive molecules and identify new targets to better understand the molecular landscape that underpins endurance training adaptations. The following sections discuss the most well-characterized molecules and signaling pathways that promote endurance training adaptations at the cellular level to date. As noted above, one must appreciate the wealth of currently unidentified molecules and pathways that mediate endurance exercise adaptations, as will soon be revealed.

PGC-1α and VEGF

Peroxisome proliferator-activated receptor gamma coactivator 1 alpha (*PGC-1α*) and vascular endothelial growth factor (*VEGF*) are perhaps the two most well-studied molecular transcripts (and corresponding proteins) upregulated in response to endurance training in skeletal muscle and other tissues. Modern understanding dictates that PGC-1α is a "master regulator" of mitochondrial biogenesis (39). Specifically, the PGC-1α protein acts as a transcriptional coactivator and associates with nuclear transcription factors to up- or downregulate mRNA transcription rates of other target genes. PGC-1α, for example, regulates transcriptional activity of the peroxisome proliferator-activated receptor gamma (*PPARγ*) nuclear receptor gene. PGC-1α-induced increases in *PPARγ* DNA binding facilitates an upregulation of electron transport chain genes (66). PGC-1α also binds to and activates the nuclear respiratory factor-1 (*NRF1*) transcription factor in muscle cells, thereby upregulating genes that facilitate mitochondrial DNA replication (86). These findings are bolstered by numerous reports suggesting endurance training promotes mitochondrial biogenesis through the induction of PGC-1α protein expression following one or multiple bouts of training in animals (5) and humans alike (63). The effects of one exercise bout on *PGC-1α* mRNA and protein levels in human skeletal muscle are illustrated in Figure 12.1.

Compelling evidence indicates that increased *PGC-1α* mRNA is a foundational response to acute exercise, inasmuch as potent trigger for downstream adaptive responses. However, the role of PGC-1α is not an exclusive mediator for endurance exercise adaptations. As a case in point, global *Pgc-1α*-knockout mice express 17–44% lower mitochondrial content in skeletal and cardiac muscle as compared to wild-type mice. Despite this fact, skeletal muscle mitochondrial biogenesis still occurred in the knockout mice following 5 weeks of voluntary wheel running compared to untrained knockout mice (2) (Figure 12.2). Other observations indicate endurance exercise rapidly increases the mRNA expression of genes involved with skeletal muscle

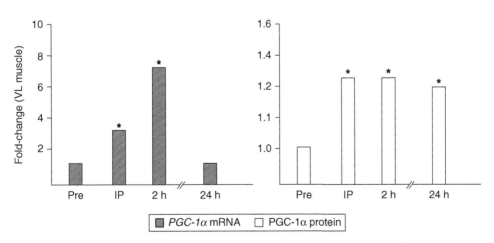

Figure 12.1 Figure demonstrating that *PGC-1α* mRNA increases in human vastus lateralis (VL) muscle up to 2 hours following exhaustive cycling at 65% VO_2max.
Source: Figure adapted from Mathai et al. (49).

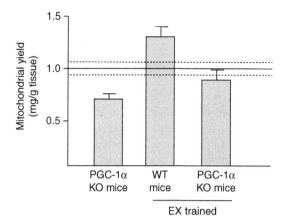

Figure 12.2 Recent data demonstrate in global *Pgc-1α* knockout (KO) mice that hindlimb muscle mitochondrial content is lower than wild-type controls. The solid and dashed lines represent the mean and variance measures of un-exercised wild-type (WT) mice. EX=exercise.

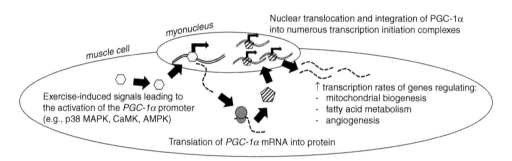

Figure 12.3 Endurance exercise rapidly activates multiple pathways (e.g., p38 MAPK pathway, CaMK pathway, and AMPK pathway) that subsequently activate the *PGC-1α* promoter and increases mRNA levels, and subsequent translation rates.

mitochondrial biogenesis via *Nrf1/2* transcription factor binding (e.g., cytochrome c and citrate synthase) prior to PGC-1α protein levels increasing after exercise (85). This important finding indicates exercise-induced mitochondrial biogenesis involves redundant stimuli that facilitate exercise-induced increases in mitochondrial content.

Beyond involvement with mitochondrial biogenesis, PGC-1α upregulates genes involved with skeletal muscle fatty acid metabolism (59), cardiac muscle mitochondrial function (4), and hepatic gluconeogenesis (53). Therefore, PGC-1α is a critical regulator of mitochondrial physiology and metabolic homeostasis in numerous tissues. Figure 12.3 summarizes exercise-induced *PGC-1α* mRNA and protein level upregulation of numerous metabolic processes.

Like PGC-1α, *VEGF* mRNA and protein expression responses to endurance exercise have been well-studied in various tissues. VEGF is a growth factor expressed in numerous cell types and secreted into the extracellular space. Once secreted, VEGF binds to cognate receptors (VEGFR1–3) on vascular endothelial cells initiating angiogenesis, or the formation of new capillaries (24). The VEGF family contains five proteins including VEGF-A, placenta growth factor, VEGF-B, VEGF-C, and VEGF-D (72). VEGF-A has been the most extensively studied form, and notably, numerous spliced *VEGF-A* mRNA variants (e.g., $VEGF_{165}$, $VEGF_{189}$, $VEGF_{206}$)

are translated into further differentiated VEGF-A isoforms. These VEGF isoforms possess altered receptor affinity binding (13), although the endurance exercise and training effects on mRNA isoform expression and spliced variants in different tissue types are not completely described.

VEGF mRNA and protein levels are elevated in rodent (6) and human skeletal muscle (67), as well as rodent myocardium (35) following acute and chronic endurance training. These cross-species data indicate VEGF is transcriptionally upregulated, rapidly translated, and secreted in order to initiate and maintain angiogenesis in multiple tissues exposed to acute and chronic exercise training scenarios. Advanced microscopy techniques have revealed, more mechanistically, that human skeletal myofibers rapidly produce and secrete VEGF protein containing vesicles into the extracellular space following extended duration cycling (33), and supports VEGF as fundamental to the endurance phenotype.

While a variety of factors activate the *VEGF* promoter, hypoxia is the most potent stimulator of *VEGF* mRNA expression. Classic investigations first revealed that lower muscle PO_2 levels during exercise rapidly activate the hypoxia-inducible factor 1α (HIF-1α) transcription factor which, in turn, binds to and activates the *VEGF* gene promoter (81). Alternately, findings from a study using the *Pgc-1α*-knockout mouse line, indicate that skeletal muscle AMPK activation by either prolonged endurance exercise, or pharmacological activation via 5-aminoimidazole-4-carboxamide-1-beta-D-ribofuranoside (AICAR), increases VEGF protein expression only in wild-type control mice (46). Moreover, in *Pgc-1α* knockout mice, basal VEGF protein levels are expressed at 60–80% of control mouse levels and the resulting capillary number is 20% lower than controls. Thus, skeletal muscle *VEGF* mRNA expression is also modulated through the AMPK-mediated activation of PGC-1α in a HIF-1α-independent manner. More importantly, these studies reinforce the notion that: 1) multiple molecules promote endurance exercise adaptations, and 2) PGC-1α and VEGF are two critical signaling molecules that facilitate physiological adaptations to endurance exercise with some degree of interdependence.

AMPK signaling

The 5′ AMP-activated protein kinase (AMPK) is a hetero-trimeric enzyme with a catalytic α subunit and regulatory β and γ subunits. Notably, the catalytic subunit catalyzes the phosphorylation of cytoplasmic and nuclear proteins as part of signal transduction and transcription factor activation. During exercise, AMPK is central to cellular energy sensing and homeostatic control in response to: 1) skeletal ATP turnover and increased AMP concentrations which bind to and activate AMPK (68), and 2) declining cellular glycogen levels which interact with AMPK β-subunit activity and reciprocal effects on subsequent glycogen level alterations (73).

Incumbent upon highly conserved metabolic regulators, AMPK is redundantly controlled independently of cellular bioenergetic status. For instance, stress-responsive molecules such as LKB1 and CaMKKβ phosphorylate and increase AMPK activity through interactions with the catalytic α-subunit AMPK at the Thr172 residue (68). Resultant AMPK activation increases cellular glucose uptake, facilitates fatty acid oxidation (54), promotes a decrease in anabolic processes (e.g., protein and glycogen synthesis) (68), increases mitochondrial biogenesis (89), and promotes fiber-type shift from type II glycolytic to oxidative fibers (69). Figure 12.4 summarizes the upstream activators and downstream physiological effects of AMPK activation.

Cross-species investigations indicate endurance exercise acutely increases phosphorylated AMPK levels and activity in skeletal muscle (15). Moreover, acute endurance exercise increases markers of AMPK activity in myocardium (17), aortic vessels (10), and pancreatic β-cells (11), reinforcing the concept that AMPK activation is evolutionarily conserved in metabolically active tissues in cross-species fashion. Emphasizing centrality to bioenergetics control, 4 weeks

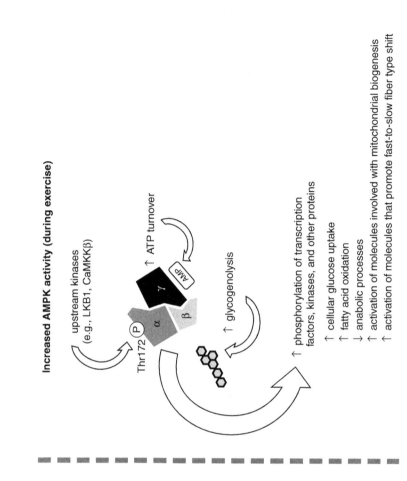

Low AMPK activity

catalytic subunit with
kinase domain

α

β

γ

regulatory
subunits

(cytoplasmic localization)

glycogen

Increased AMPK activity (during exercise)

upstream kinases
(e.g., LKB1, CaMKKβ)

Thr172 (P)

α

β

γ

AMP

↑ ATP turnover

↑ glycogenolysis

↑ phosphorylation of transcription
factors, kinases, and other proteins

↑ cellular glucose uptake
↑ fatty acid oxidation
↓ anabolic processes
↑ activation of molecules involved with mitochondrial biogenesis
↑ activation of molecules that promote fast-to-slow fiber type shift

Figure 12.4 Left: the unstimulated AMPK enzyme; right: increased AMPK activity (during exercise).

of AICAR administration in rodents induced a skeletal muscle gene expression profile that roughly paralleled endurance training. As such, treadmill running endurance was enhanced by 44% in treated animals (56). However, some skepticism remains as to the essentiality of AMPK activation facilitating endurance training adaptations in muscle. In this regard, basal mitochondrial markers were 20% lower in the gastrocnemius of AMPKα2-knockout mice versus wild-type controls, although wheel-running adaptations in knockout mice remained unmitigated in terms of oxidative capacity (38). Additionally, it has been reported mitochondrial biogenesis occurs in AMPKα2-knockout mice that undertake voluntary wheel running (69). These findings led both research groups to conclude that AMPK signaling may be most important for basal metabolic homeostasis, albeit redundant pathways or downstream substrates facilitate adaptations to more extreme bioenergetics challenges such as endurance training. In spite of seemingly disparate findings, the overwhelming body of evidence indicates that AMPK pathway activation is critically involved in promoting the oxidative phenotype in metabolically active tissues of exercised animals.

CaMKII–p38/MAPK

The calcium/calmodulin-dependent protein kinase II (CaMKII) enzyme facilitates endurance training adaptations in skeletal muscle. While multiple classes of CaMK enzymes exist, including CaMKI, CaMKII, and CaMKIV (75), only CaMKII isoforms are enriched in skeletal muscle (70). Skeletal muscle CaMKII activity is increased by rising cytosolic calcium concentrations during acute endurance exercise. This response results in increased calcium/calmodulin (Ca^{2+}/CaM) complexes and occurs in a species-independent fashion (70). In turn, Ca^{2+}/CaM binds to and activates CaMKII leading to autophosphorylation at the Thr287 residue as well as increased activity. Similar to AMPK, CaMKII phosphorylates cytoplasmic and nuclear proteins to promote signal transduction and transcription factor activation. For instance, CaMKII phosphorylates numerous proteins involved with transcriptional machinery formation in skeletal muscle (e.g., HDAC4, myogenin, SRF) and upregulates genes associated with an endurance phenotype (70). As a proof of concept, pharmacologic inhibition of CaMKII activity *in vitro* prevents calcium-induced increases in PGC-1α and mtTFA protein expression as well as mitochondrial biogenesis in L6 myotubes (61). A follow-up study confirmed these findings in isolated rat epitrochlearis muscle, further demonstrating that CaMKII phosphorylates p38 mitogen-activated protein kinase (MAPK) in order to facilitate PGC-1α protein expression and markers of mitochondrial biogenesis, and additional evidence exists suggesting CaMKII acutely phosphorylates p38/MAPK in skeletal muscle to promote an endurance phenotype (26).

CaMKII activation is also critical for increasing *GLUT4* gene expression through acetylating histones that flank the *GLUT4* promoter (60). This outcome is accomplished through CaMKII phosphorylating and inactivating the HDAC4 histone deacteylase enzyme. Calcium/calmodulin-sensitive CaMK kinase (CaMKK) is upstream of several CaMK enzymes, although it does not phosphorylate CaMKII (82). However, CaMKK phosphorylates AMPK at Thr172 and increases AMPK activity in order to increase GLUT4 and CD36 sarcolemmal localization as well as glucose and fatty acid uptake (1). Hence, increases in intracellular calcium during endurance exercise activate parallel signaling pathways (i.e., CaMKII and AMPK) which promote skeletal muscle mitochondrial biogenesis and nutrient uptake. Figure 12.5 summarizes the upstream activators and downstream physiological effects of CaMKII activation in skeletal muscle.

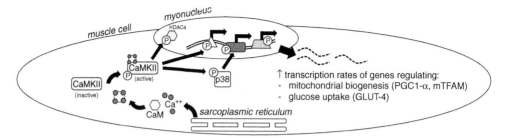

Figure 12.5 Calcium (Ca^{2+}) flux increases in the cytosol during endurance exercise.

SIRT1/3

Sirtuin (SIRT) proteins encompass seven (SITR1–7) deacetylase enzymes, although endurance exercise activates SIRT1 and SIRT3 through increased nuclear and mitochondrial nicotinamide adenine dinucleotide (NAD^+) concentrations (83). SIRT1 regulates mitochondrial biogenesis through deacetylating and increasing the integration of PGC-1α into nuclear transcriptional machinery (25). In muscle cells, SIRT1 overexpression increases PGC1α transcriptional activity and mitochondrial gene expression, promoting fatty acid oxidation (25). However, other studies report no reduction in mitochondrial function or number when SIRT1 protein or deacetylase activity is knocked out in myotubes or murine skeletal muscle (83). Conflicting data make it difficult to conclude whether endurance exercise-induced increases in nuclear NAD^+ and subsequent SIRT1-mediated PGC-1α deacetylation are required for mitochondrial adaptations.

The SIRT3 deacetylase enzyme is localized to mitochondria and enhances mitochondrial function like SIRT1. SIRT3 deacetylates and activates TCA cycle and β-oxidation enzymes (83), which during endurance exercise logically elevates NAD^+ concentrations, increasing fuel substrate oxidation rates. However, SIRT3 activation may attenuate mitochondrial biogenesis given that overexpression of SIRT3 in C2C12 myotubes depresses mitochondrial protein synthesis through the deacetylation of mitochondrial ribosomal protein L1 (87). Hence, during energy-deprived states (e.g., exercise or fasting), SIRT3 seemingly operates to upregulate the rate of mitochondrial fuel oxidation while shunting consumptive pathways such as mitochondrial biogenesis.

NRF2 signaling

Upregulation of antioxidant defense mechanisms is another noteworthy adaptation of endurance training in skeletal muscle and myocardial tissue. Nuclear respiratory factor 2 (NRF2) is the master regulator of antioxidant defense mechanisms of this response (57). In confirmation, endurance training increases NRF2 signaling across multiple tissues including skeletal muscle, myocardium, kidney, brain, liver, testes, and prostate (18). Multiple studies report acute treadmill bouts increase skeletal muscle and myocardium NRF2 protein levels as well as the expression of NRF2-dependent genes (e.g., *CAT*, *SOD2*, *HO-1*, *NQO1*, and glutathione synthesis genes) (18).

NRF2 is a member of the leucine zipper family of transcription factors. In basal, unstressed states, NRF2 localizes to the cytosol via association with KEAP1. Elevations in reactive oxygen species (ROS) during endurance exercise modify cysteine residues on KEAP1. This event promotes the dissociation of KEAP1 from NRF2, and allows NRF2 to translocate into the nucleus. Upon nuclear entry, NRF2 binds promoter regions of the genome containing antioxidant response elements altering expression of aforementioned endogenous antioxidant defenses and antiapoptotic regulators (e.g., Bcl-2) (76). Collectively, NRF2 activation through acute and chronic endurance training bolsters antioxidant defenses in numerous tissues and promotes mitochondrial homeostatic maintenance. Additionally, NRF2 nuclear localization and DNA binding post exercise contributes to mitochondrial biogenesis (85), further underscoring a critical role in endurance training adaptations.

eNOS and nitric oxide signaling

Nitric oxide (NO) is also fundamental to endurance training adaptations in skeletal muscle, myocardium, and vascular tissues. NO is produced endogenously via nitric oxide synthase (NOS) enzymes via L-arginine substrate utilization. The primary function of NO is to facilitate vasodilation through vascular smooth muscle relaxation (27). NOS isozymes are expressed in tissue-independent fashion (e.g., nNOS in nerve and skeletal muscle, iNOS in immune cells, and eNOS in endothelial nitric oxide) (51). Chronic endurance training increases skeletal muscle and myocardium NO levels (23). Phosphorylation of eNOS is observed post exercise, indicative of heightened activity in cardiac and skeletal muscle capillary beds (30).

Beyond vasodilation, NO also affects molecular signaling cascades in skeletal muscle and other tissues. For instance, eNOS knockout mice present impairments in basal mitochondrial function and a dysregulation in CamKII signaling (45). Moreover, NO influences *VEGF* mRNA and protein regulation in several exercised tissues (20). As yet another redundant factor in promoting mitochondrial biogenesis, NO directly activates skeletal muscle AMPK signaling, increasing *PGC-1α* mRNA and protein expression (48). Hence, elevation of NO during and following endurance exercise initiates signaling cascades which collectively increase mitochondrial number and function as well as angiogenesis.

Conclusion

One should appreciate the complex, tissue-wide, molecular signaling phenomena that occur in response to acute and chronic endurance training. Thematic of these outcomes, exercise adaptations operate through parallel or redundant signaling mechanisms including PGC-1α, VEGF, and AMPK. Foundational understanding of these and other molecules will give rise to new horizons in related mechanisms, yet to be elucidated through future omics-based endeavors and related loss of function in whole animal and cell culture models. Indeed, the interface between genetic responses to exercise will likely shed new light on classic understanding of endurance phenotypes and the underpinning physiologic responses necessary for long-duration exercise adaptations. Many of the most pressing scientific questions are already posed within this text.

References

1. **Abbott MJ**, **Edelman AM**, and **Turcotte LP**. CaMKK is an upstream signal of AMP-activated protein kinase in regulation of substrate metabolism in contracting skeletal muscle. *Am J Physiol Regul Integr Comp Physiol* 297: R1724–1732, 2009.
2. **Adhihetty PJ**, **Uguccioni G**, **Leick L**, **Hidalgo J**, **Pilegaard H**, and **Hood DA**. The role of PGC-1alpha on mitochondrial function and apoptotic susceptibility in muscle. *Am J Physiol Cell Physiol* 297: C217–225, 2009.
3. **Allen WK**, **Seals DR**, **Hurley BF**, **Ehsani AA**, and **Hagberg JM**. Lactate threshold and distance-running performance in young and older endurance athletes. *J Appl Physiol* 58: 1281–1284, 1985.

4. **Arany Z**, He H, Lin J, Hoyer K, Handschin C, Toka O, Ahmad F, Matsui T, Chin S, Wu PH, Rybkin, II, Shelton JM, Manieri M, Cinti S, Schoen FJ, **Bassel-Duby R**, Rosenzweig A, **Ingwall JS**, and **Spiegelman BM**. Transcriptional coactivator PGC-1 alpha controls the energy state and contractile function of cardiac muscle. *Cell Metab* 1: 259–271, 2005.

5. **Baar K, Wende AR**, Jones TE, Marison M, Nolte LA, Chen M, **Kelly DP**, and **Holloszy JO**. Adaptations of skeletal muscle to exercise: rapid increase in the transcriptional coactivator PGC-1. *FASEB J* 16: 1879–1886, 2002.

6. **Birot OJ**, Koulmann N, Peinnequin A, and **Bigard XA**. Exercise-induced expression of vascular endothelial growth factor mRNA in rat skeletal muscle is dependent on fibre type. *J Physiol* 552: 213–221, 2003.

7. **Bouchard C, Daw EW, Rice T, Perusse L, Gagnon J, Province MA, Leon AS, Rao DC, Skinner JS**, and **Wilmore JH**. Familial resemblance for VO2max in the sedentary state: the HERITAGE family study. *Med Sci Sports Exerc* 30: 252–258, 1998.

8. **Bouchard C,** and **Rankinen T**. Individual differences in response to regular physical activity. *Med Sci Sports Exerc* 33: S446–451, 2001.

9. **Burke LM**. Re-examining high-fat diets for sports performance: Did we call the "nail in the coffin" too soon? *Sports Med* 45 Suppl 1: S33–49, 2015.

10. **Cacicedo JM, Gauthier MS, Lebrasseur NK, Jasuja R, Ruderman NB**, and **Ido Y**. Acute exercise activates AMPK and eNOS in the mouse aorta. *Am J Physiol Heart Circ Physiol* 301: H1255–1265, 2011.

11. **Calegari VC, Zoppi CC, Rezende LF, Silveira LR, Carneiro EM**, and **Boschero AC**. Endurance training activates AMP-activated protein kinase, increases expression of uncoupling protein 2 and reduces insulin secretion from rat pancreatic islets. *J Endocrinol* 208: 257–264, 2011.

12. **Carlsson S, Ljungqvist A, Tornling G,** and **Unge G**. The myocardial capillary vasculature in repeated physical exercise. An experimental investigation in the rat. *Acta Pathol Microbiol Scand A* 86: 117–119, 1978.

13. **Cebe Suarez S, Pieren M, Cariolato L, Arn S, Hoffmann U, Bogucki A, Manlius C, Wood J**, and **Ballmer-Hofer K**. A VEGF-A splice variant defective for heparan sulfate and neuropilin-1 binding shows attenuated signaling through VEGFR-2. *Cell Mol Life Sci* 63: 2067–2077, 2006.

14. **Chakravarthy MV**, and **Booth FW**. Eating, exercise, and "thrifty" genotypes: Connecting the dots toward an evolutionary understanding of modern chronic diseases. *J Appl Physiol* 96: 3–10, 2004.

15. **Coffey VG, Zhong Z, Shield A, Canny BJ, Chibalin AV, Zierath JR**, and **Hawley JA**. Early signaling responses to divergent exercise stimuli in skeletal muscle from well-trained humans. *FASEB J* 20: 190–192, 2006.

16. **Coker RH**, and **Kjaer M**. Glucoregulation during exercise: The role of the neuroendocrine system. *Sports Med* 35: 575–583, 2005.

17. **Coven DL, Hu X, Cong L, Bergeron R, Shulman GI, Hardie DG**, and **Young LH**. Physiological role of AMP-activated protein kinase in the heart: Graded activation during exercise. *Am J Physiol* 285: E629–636, 2003.

18. **Done AJ**, and **Traustadottir T**. Nrf2 mediates redox adaptations to exercise. *Redox Biol* 10: 191–199, 2016.

19. **Drouin R, Lavoie C, Bourque J, Ducros F, Poisson D,** and **Chiasson JL**. Increased hepatic glucose production response to glucagon in trained subjects. *Am J Physiol* 274: E23–28, 1998.

20. **Dulak J, Jozkowicz A, Dembinska-Kiec A, Guevara I, Zdzienicka A, Zmudzinska-Grochot D, Florek I, Wojtowicz A, Szuba A,** and **Cooke JP**. Nitric oxide induces the synthesis of vascular endothelial growth factor by rat vascular smooth muscle cells. *Arterioscler Thromb Vasc Biol* 20: 659–666, 2000.

21. **Ehsani AA, Hagberg JM**, and **Hickson RC**. Rapid changes in left ventricular dimensions and mass in response to physical conditioning and deconditioning. *Am J Cardiol* 42: 52–56, 1978.

22. **Ekblom B, Astrand PO, Saltin B, Stenberg J**, and **Wallstrom B**. Effect of training on circulatory response to exercise. *J Appl Physiol* 24: 518–528, 1968.

23. **Gavin TP, Spector DA, Wagner H, Breen EC**, and **Wagner PD**. Nitric oxide synthase inhibition attenuates the skeletal muscle VEGF mRNA response to exercise. *J Appl Physiol (1985)* 88: 1192–1198, 2000.

24. **Gerhardt H, Golding M, Fruttiger M, Ruhrberg C, Lundkvist A, Abramsson A, Jeltsch M, Mitchell C, Alitalo K, Shima D**, and **Betsholtz C**. VEGF guides angiogenic sprouting utilizing endothelial tip cell filopodia. *J Cell Biol* 161: 1163–1177, 2003.

25. **Gerhart-Hines Z, Rodgers JT, Bare O, Lerin C, Kim SH, Mostoslavsky R, Alt FW, Wu Z,** and **Puigserver P.** Metabolic control of muscle mitochondrial function and fatty acid oxidation through SIRT1/PGC-1alpha. *EMBO J* 26: 1913–1923, 2007.

26. **Gibala MJ, McGee SL, Garnham AP, Howlett KF, Snow RJ,** and **Hargreaves M.** Brief intense interval exercise activates AMPK and p38 MAPK signaling and increases the expression of PGC-1alpha in human skeletal muscle. *J Appl Physiol (1985)* 106: 929–934, 2009.

27. **Gielen S, Sandri M, Erbs S,** and **Adams V.** Exercise-induced modulation of endothelial nitric oxide production. *Curr Pharm Biotechnol* 12: 1375–1384, 2011.

28. **Gladden LB.** Lactate metabolism: a new paradigm for the third millennium. *J Physiol* 558: 5–30, 2004.

29. **Goodpaster BH,** and **Sparks LM.** Metabolic flexibility in health and disease. *Cell Metab* 25: 1027–1036, 2017.

30. **Grijalva J, Hicks S, Zhao X, Medikayala S, Kaminski PM, Wolin MS,** and **Edwards JG.** Exercise training enhanced myocardial endothelial nitric oxide synthase (eNOS) function in diabetic Goto-Kakizaki (GK) rats. *Cardiovasc Diabetol* 7: 34, 2008.

31. **Guo H, Isserlin R, Emili A,** and **Burniston JG.** Exercise-responsive phosphoproteins in the heart. *J Mol Cell Cardiol* 111: 61–68, 2017.

32. **Hoffman NJ, Parker BL, Chaudhuri R, Fisher-Wellman KH, Kleinert M, Humphrey SJ, Yang P, Holliday M, Trefely S, Fazakerley DJ, Stockli J, Burchfield JG, Jensen TE, Jothi R, Kiens B, Wojtaszewski JF, Richter EA,** and **James DE.** Global phosphoproteomic analysis of human skeletal muscle reveals a network of exercise-regulated kinases and AMPK substrates. *Cell Metab* 22: 922–935, 2015.

33. **Hoier B, Prats C, Qvortrup K, Pilegaard H, Bangsbo J,** and **Hellsten Y.** Subcellular localization and mechanism of secretion of vascular endothelial growth factor in human skeletal muscle. *FASEB J* 27: 3496–3504, 2013.

34. **Holloszy JO.** Adaptation of skeletal muscle to endurance exercise. *Med Sci Sports* 7: 155–164, 1975.

35. **Iemitsu M, Maeda S, Jesmin S, Otsuki T,** and **Miyauchi T.** Exercise training improves aging-induced downregulation of VEGF angiogenic signaling cascade in hearts. *Am J Physiol Heart Circ Physiol* 291: H1290–1298, 2006.

36. **Irrcher I, Adhihetty PJ, Joseph AM, Ljubicic V,** and **Hood DA.** Regulation of mitochondrial biogenesis in muscle by endurance exercise. *Sports Med* 33: 783–793, 2003.

37. **Johnson BD, Aaron EA, Babcock MA,** and **Dempsey JA.** Respiratory muscle fatigue during exercise: Implications for performance. *Med Sci Sports Exerc* 28: 1129–1137, 1996.

38. **Jorgensen SB, Treebak JT, Viollet B, Schjerling P, Vaulont S, Wojtaszewski JF,** and **Richter EA.** Role of AMPKalpha2 in basal, training-, and AICAR-induced GLUT4, hexokinase II, and mitochondrial protein expression in mouse muscle. *Am J Physiol* 292: E331–339, 2007.

39. **Jornayvaz FR,** and **Shulman GI.** Regulation of mitochondrial biogenesis. *Essays Biochem* 47: 69–84, 2010.

40. **Joyner MJ.** Modeling: Optimal marathon performance on the basis of physiological factors. *J Appl Physiol (1985)* 70: 683–687, 1991.

41. **Joyner MJ.** Preclinical and clinical evaluation of autonomic function in humans. *J Physiol* 594: 4009–4013, 2016.

42. **Joyner MJ,** and **Casey DP.** Regulation of increased blood flow (hyperemia) to muscles during exercise: A hierarchy of competing physiological needs. *Physiol Rev* 95: 549–601, 2015.

43. **Joyner MJ,** and **Coyle EF.** Endurance exercise performance: The physiology of champions. *J Physiol* 586: 35–44, 2008.

44. **Klausen K, Andersen LB,** and **Pelle I.** Adaptive changes in work capacity, skeletal muscle capillarization and enzyme levels during training and detraining. *Acta Physiol Scand* 113: 9–16, 1981.

45. **Lee-Young RS, Ayala JE, Hunley CF, James FD, Bracy DP, Kang L,** and **Wasserman DH.** Endothelial nitric oxide synthase is central to skeletal muscle metabolic regulation and enzymatic signaling during exercise in vivo. *Am J Physiol Regul Integr Comp Physiol* 298: R1399–R1408, 2010.

46. **Leick L, Hellsten Y, Fentz J, Lyngby SS, Wojtaszewski JF, Hidalgo J,** and **Pilegaard H.** PGC-1alpha mediates exercise-induced skeletal muscle VEGF expression in mice. *Am J Physiol* 297: E92–103, 2009.

47. **Lindholm ME, Giacomello S, Werne Solnestam B, Fischer H, Huss M, Kjellqvist S,** and **Sundberg CJ.** The impact of endurance training on human skeletal muscle memory, global isoform expression and novel transcripts. *PLoS Genet* 12: e1006294, 2016.

48. **Lira VA, Brown DL, Lira AK, Kavazis AN, Soltow QA, Zeanah EH,** and **Criswell DS**. Nitric oxide and AMPK cooperatively regulate PGC-1 in skeletal muscle cells. *J Physiol* 588: 3551–3566, 2010.

49. **Mathai AS, Bonen A, Benton CR, Robinson DL,** and **Graham TE**. Rapid exercise-induced changes in PGC-1alpha mRNA and protein in human skeletal muscle. *J Appl Physiol (1985)* 105: 1098–1105, 2008.

50. **Mattsson CM, Stahlberg M, Larsen FJ, Braunschweig F,** and **Ekblom B**. Late cardiovascular drift observable during ultraendurance exercise. *Med Sci Sports Exerc* 43: 1162–1168, 2011.

51. **McAllister RM, Newcomer SC,** and **Laughlin MH**. Vascular nitric oxide: Effects of exercise training in animals. *Appl Physiol Nutr Metab* 33: 173–178, 2008.

52. **McGavock JM, Warburton DE, Taylor D, Welsh RC, Quinney HA,** and **Haykowsky MJ**. The effects of prolonged strenuous exercise on left ventricular function: A brief review. *Heart Lung* 31: 279–292, 2002.

53. **Meirhaeghe A, Crowley V, Lenaghan C, Lelliott C, Green K, Stewart A, Hart K, Schinner S, Sethi JK, Yeo G, Brand MD, Cortright RN, O'Rahilly S, Montague C,** and **Vidal-Puig AJ**. Characterization of the human, mouse and rat PGC1 beta (peroxisome-proliferator-activated receptor-gamma co-activator 1 beta) gene in vitro and in vivo. *Biochem J* 373: 155–165, 2003.

54. **Merrill GF, Kurth EJ, Hardie DG,** and **Winder WW**. AICA riboside increases AMP-activated protein kinase, fatty acid oxidation, and glucose uptake in rat muscle. *Am J Physiol* 273: E1107–1112, 1997.

55. **Montero D** and **Lundby C**. Red cell volume response to exercise training: Association with aging. *Scand J Med Sci Sports* 27: 674–683, 2017.

56. **Narkar VA, Downes M, Yu RT, Embler E, Wang YX, Banayo E, Mihaylova MM, Nelson MC, Zou Y, Juguilon H, Kang H, Shaw RJ,** and **Evans RM**. AMPK and PPARdelta agonists are exercise mimetics. *Cell* 134: 405–415, 2008.

57. **Nguyen T, Nioi P,** and **Pickett CB**. The Nrf2-antioxidant response element signaling pathway and its activation by oxidative stress. *J Biol Chem* 284: 13291–13295, 2009.

58. **Nielsen B, Hales JR, Strange S, Christensen NJ, Warberg J,** and **Saltin B**. Human circulatory and thermoregulatory adaptations with heat acclimation and exercise in a hot, dry environment. *J Physiol* 460: 467–485, 1993.

59. **Nikolic N, Rhedin M, Rustan AC, Storlien L, Thoresen GH,** and **Stromstedt M**. Overexpression of PGC-1alpha increases fatty acid oxidative capacity of human skeletal muscle cells. *Biochem Res Int* 2012: 714074, 2012.

60. **Ojuka EO, Goyaram V,** and **Smith JA**. The role of CaMKII in regulating GLUT4 expression in skeletal muscle. *Am J Physiol* 303: E322–331, 2012.

61. **Ojuka EO, Jones TE, Han DH, Chen M,** and **Holloszy JO**. Raising Ca2+ in L6 myotubes mimics effects of exercise on mitochondrial biogenesis in muscle. *FASEB J* 17: 675–681, 2003.

62. **Olafsson S** and **Hyatt RE**. Ventilatory mechanics and expiratory flow limitation during exercise in normal subjects. *J Clin Invest* 48: 564–573, 1969.

63. **Pilegaard H, Saltin B,** and **Neufer PD**. Exercise induces transient transcriptional activation of the PGC-1alpha gene in human skeletal muscle. *J Physiol* 546: 851–858, 2003.

64. **Poliner LR, Dehmer GJ, Lewis SE, Parkey RW, Blomqvist CG,** and **Willerson JT**. Left ventricular performance in normal subjects: A comparison of the responses to exercise in the upright and supine positions. *Circulation* 62: 528–534, 1980.

65. **Powers SK, Howley ET,** and **Cox R**. A differential catecholamine response during prolonged exercise and passive heating. *Med Sci Sports Exerc* 14: 435–439, 1982.

66. **Puigserver P, Wu Z, Park CW, Graves R, Wright M,** and **Spiegelman BM**. A cold-inducible coactivator of nuclear receptors linked to adaptive thermogenesis. *Cell* 92: 829–839, 1998.

67. **Richardson RS, Wagner H, Mudaliar SR, Henry R, Noyszewski EA,** and **Wagner PD**. Human VEGF gene expression in skeletal muscle: effect of acute normoxic and hypoxic exercise. *Am J Physiol* 277: H2247–H2252, 1999.

68. **Richter EA,** and **Ruderman NB**. AMPK and the biochemistry of exercise: implications for human health and disease. *Biochem J* 418: 261–275, 2009.

69. **Rockl KS, Hirshman MF, Brandauer J, Fujii N, Witters LA,** and **Goodyear LJ**. Skeletal muscle adaptation to exercise training: AMP-activated protein kinase mediates muscle fiber type shift. *Diabetes* 56: 2062–2069, 2007.

70. **Rose AJ, Frosig C, Kiens B, Wojtaszewski JF,** and **Richter EA**. Effect of endurance exercise training on Ca2+ calmodulin-dependent protein kinase II expression and signalling in skeletal muscle of humans. *J Physiol* 583: 785–795, 2007.

71. **San-Millan I,** and **Brooks GA**. Assessment of metabolic flexibility by means of measuring blood lactate, fat, and carbohydrate oxidation responses to exercise in professional endurance athletes and less-fit individuals *Sports Med* 48. 467–479, 2018.

72. **Shibuya M**. vascular endothelial growth factor (VEGF) and its receptor (VEGFR) signaling in angiogenesis: A crucial target for anti- and pro-angiogenic therapies. *Genes Cancer* 2: 1097–1105, 2011.

73. **Steinberg GR, Watt MJ, McGee SL, Chan S, Hargreaves M, Febbraio MA, Stapleton D,** and **Kemp BE**. Reduced glycogen availability is associated with increased AMPKalpha2 activity, nuclear AMPKalpha2 protein abundance, and GLUT4 mRNA expression in contracting human skeletal muscle. *Appl Physiol Nutr Metab* 31: 302–312, 2006.

74. **Stuewe SR, Gwirtz PA, Agarwal N,** and **Mallet RT**. Exercise training enhances glycolytic and oxidative enzymes in canine ventricular myocardium. *J Mol Cell Cardiol* 32: 903–913, 2000.

75. **Takemoto-Kimura S, Suzuki K, Horigane SI, Kamijo S, Inoue M, Sakamoto M, Fujii H,** and **Bito H**. Calmodulin kinases: Essential regulators in health and disease. *J Neurochem* 141: 808–818, 2017.

76. **Tebay LE, Robertson H, Durant ST, Vitale SR, Penning TM, Dinkova-Kostova AT,** and **Hayes JD**. Mechanisms of activation of the transcription factor Nrf2 by redox stressors, nutrient cues, and energy status and the pathways through which it attenuates degenerative disease. *Free Radic Biol Med* 88: 108–146, 2015.

77. **Trefts E, Williams AS,** and **Wasserman DH**. Exercise and the regulation of hepatic metabolism. *Prog Mol Biol Transl Sci* 135: 203–225, 2015.

78. **van der Zwaard S, van der Laarse WJ, Weide G, Bloemers FW, Hofmijster MJ, Levels K, Noordhof DA, de Koning JJ, de Ruiter CJ,** and **Jaspers RT**. Critical determinants of combined sprint and endurance performance: an integrative analysis from muscle fiber to the human body. *FASEB J* 32: 2110–2123, 2018.

79. **Vettor R, Valerio A, Ragni M, Trevellin E, Granzotto M, Olivieri M, Tedesco L, Ruocco C, Fossati A, Fabris R, Serra R, Carruba MO,** and **Nisoli E**. Exercise training boosts eNOS-dependent mitochondrial biogenesis in mouse heart: role in adaptation of glucose metabolism. *Am J Physiol* 306: E519–E528, 2014.

80. **Volek JS, Freidenreich DJ, Saenz C, Kunces LJ, Creighton BC, Bartley JM, Davitt PM, Munoz CX, Anderson JM, Maresh CM, Lee EC, Schuenke MD, Aerni G, Kraemer WJ,** and **Phinney SD**. Metabolic characteristics of keto-adapted ultra-endurance runners. *Metabolism* 65: 100–110, 2016.

81. **Wagner PD**. The critical role of VEGF in skeletal muscle angiogenesis and blood flow. *Biochem Soc Trans* 39: 1556–1559, 2011.

82. **Wayman GA, Tokumitsu H, Davare MA,** and **Soderling TR**. Analysis of CaM-kinase signaling in cells. *Cell Calcium* 50: 1–8, 2011.

83. **White AT** and **Schenk S**. NAD(+)/NADH and skeletal muscle mitochondrial adaptations to exercise. *Am J Physiol* 303: E308–E321, 2012.

84. **Wilson JM, Loenneke JP, Jo E, Wilson GJ, Zourdos MC,** and **Kim JS**. The effects of endurance, strength, and power training on muscle fiber type shifting. *J Strength Cond Res* 26: 1724–1729, 2012.

85. **Wright DC, Han DH, Garcia-Roves PM, Geiger PC, Jones TE,** and **Holloszy JO**. Exercise-induced mitochondrial biogenesis begins before the increase in muscle PGC-1α expression. *J Biol Chem* 282: 194–199, 2007.

86. **Wu Z, Puigserver P, Andersson U, Zhang C, Adelmant G, Mootha V, Troy A, Cinti S, Lowell B, Scarpulla RC,** and **Spiegelman BM**. Mechanisms controlling mitochondrial biogenesis and respiration through the thermogenic coactivator PGC-1. *Cell* 98: 115–124, 1999.

87. **Yang Y, Cimen H, Han MJ, Shi T, Deng JH, Koc H, Palacios OM, Montier L, Bai Y, Tong Q,** and **Koc EC**. NAD+-dependent deacetylase SIRT3 regulates mitochondrial protein synthesis by deacetylation of the ribosomal protein MRPL10. *J Biol Chem* 285: 7417–7429, 2010.

88. **Zhou B, Conlee RK, Jensen R, Fellingham GW, George JD,** and **Fisher AG**. Stroke volume does not plateau during graded exercise in elite male distance runners. *Med Sci Sports Exerc* 33: 1849–1854, 2001.

89. **Zong H, Ren JM, Young LH, Pypaert M, Mu J, Birnbaum MJ,** and **Shulman GI**. AMP kinase is required for mitochondrial biogenesis in skeletal muscle in response to chronic energy deprivation. *Proc Natl Acad Sci U S A* 99: 15983–15987, 2002.

90. **Zouhal H, Jacob C, Delamarche P,** and **Gratas-Delamarche A**. Catecholamines and the effects of exercise, training and gender. *Sports Med* 38: 401–423, 2008.

13

HERITABILITY OF ENDURANCE TRAITS FROM ANIMAL RESEARCH MODELS

Joshua J. Avila, Sean M. Courtney, and Michael P. Massett

Introduction

A variety of studies in humans indicate that genetics contribute significantly to individual variation in both baseline or intrinsic exercise capacity and the response to training, with heritability estimates of approximately 50% for each of these phenotypes (detailed in Chapter 14). Despite evidence of a genetic component influencing these phenotypes, the need for large sample sizes and variation in training paradigms have significantly limited replication of pertinent results in humans (22). Alternatively, three strategies have been employed to investigate the genetic basis of complex traits in rodent models: selective breeding, screening of multiple inbred strains for exercise phenotypes followed by quantitative trait loci (QTL) analyses, and candidate gene studies. Transgenic or knockout mice generated to alter expression level of genes known to be relevant to acute or chronic exercise typically exhibit marked changes in exercise performance or responses to training (11, 18, 20, 24, 45, 46). However, for the candidate gene approach to be fruitful, the gene must already be known to be involved in a pathway related to exercise or training responses (3). In contrast, other approaches can be used to identify the genetic basis for a complex trait with no *a priori* bias toward a particular gene, protein, tissue, or organ system. One such approach is selective breeding for endurance exercise capacity or the change in exercise capacity in response to training. Repeated selection on a specific exercise phenotype should enrich for alleles associated with the selected trait, resulting in divergent lines with markedly different phenotypes (10). The phenotypic variance attributed to additive genetic variance, or narrow-sense heritability, can be estimated in this selected population by regression, using phenotype values from parents and their offspring. Conversely, screening multiple inbred rodent strains for a specific phenotypic trait takes advantage of the natural genetic and phenotypic variation among strains. One benefit of using inbred rodents for analysis of complex traits is that strains inbred for at least 20 generations are essentially homozygous at all loci (55). Thus, under standardized environmental conditions, phenotypic differences observed among inbred strains are due predominantly to genetic variation. The proportion of phenotypic variation attributed to total genetic variation (i.e., broad-sense heritability) can then be estimated from these inbred strain populations. Two strains with differing phenotypes can be crossed and the offspring used for traditional linkage (i.e., QTL) analysis. Although several hundred second-generation offspring are typically used for linkage analysis, the power to detect QTL is dependent on multiple factors, including the magnitude of the phenotypic difference between the parental inbred strains and the QTL effect size (21). Alternatively, if a large number of inbred strains have been phenotyped, a genome-wide association study (GWAS) can be performed (6, 30, 59). For GWAS in mice, 30 or more inbred strains are generally sufficient to detect QTL of moderate effect, but the resolution and power are improved by utilizing a larger number of inbred strains (30, 59). Both linkage analysis and GWAS have been used to identify genomic regions and/or putative candidate genes for endurance exercise capacity or responses to training.

There are three commonly used paradigms for exercise training in rodents – swimming, voluntary wheel running, and "forced" wheel or treadmill running – and each has been used to study the genetic basis of exercise capacity and responses to training. Voluntary wheel running and treadmill running are known to induce adaptations in mice associated with endurance exercise training (2, 12, 15, 28, 43, 56, 60). However, there are inherent differences between the two paradigms (34) such that there is little correlation between treadmill running performance and voluntary wheel-running performance among mouse strains (36, 38, 39), suggesting the genetic factors influencing these two phenotypes are different. The genetic and environmental control of physical activity in rodents are discussed further in Chapters 5, 7, 8, 9, and 10 of this book.

This chapter will focus on treadmill running and swimming as a means to assess endurance exercise capacity and as an exercise paradigm to elicit responses to endurance training. The majority of these studies have utilized a graded exercise test to assess endurance exercise capacity reported as maximal time, distance, speed, or work. Changes in these variables, i.e., the difference between post-training exercise capacity and pretraining exercise capacity, represent the response to training. Human exercise studies suggest the genes influencing variation in pretraining or intrinsic endurance exercise capacity are different than those that determine the responses to training (7, 8, 54) (see Chapter 14). There is support for this from rodent-based studies as well (4, 33, 43, 44). Therefore, these phenotypes will be discussed individually in the subsequent sections.

Intrinsic endurance exercise capacity

Selected strains/artificial selection

Starting with a founder population of heterogeneous N:NIH rats, Koch and Britton developed a two-way artificial selection model of endurance running capacity based on maximal treadmill running performance (31). After 11 generations of selection, high-capacity runner (HCR) and low-capacity runner (LCR) selected lines differed by approximately 660 m (~4.5-fold) in treadmill running endurance (63). By generation 28, the difference increased to about 840 m (~8.3 fold) (52). In HCR, improved oxygen utilization was attributed to increased capillary density, higher oxygen extraction, and higher activity of oxidative metabolic enzymes (25, 26). Proteins involved in mitochondrial synthesis and function are also elevated in muscle from HCR rats (63). Thus, phenotypes associated with endurance exercise training cosegregated with the selected phenotype. Preliminary phenotypic and genetic analyses were conducted on F_1 and F_2 populations developed from parental LCR and HCR lines (52). The exercise phenotype in F_1 and F_2 generations was intermediate to the parental lines. Narrow-sense heritability calculated for maximal running distance based on parental through F_2 generation offspring was 60%. That is somewhat higher than heritability reported for running distance within the HCR and LCR lines (45%). Thus, the HCR/LCR lines are a viable model for QTL mapping and identification of genetic factors contributing to variation in endurance exercise capacity.

Inbred strain comparisons

Although not specifically selected for exercise capacity, strain differences in endurance exercise capacity measured by treadmill running and swimming have been reported for inbred mice and rats (5, 29, 36, 39, 58). In a survey of 11 inbred rat strains, the difference in endurance exercise performance measured by treadmill running is approximately 2.5-fold between the highest (DA/OlaHsd (DA)) and lowest (Copenhagen (COP)) performing strains (5). In mice, maximum treadmill running speed is approximately double in the highest (FVB/NJ (FVB)) versus lowest (C57BL/6J (B6)) performing strain (36, 58). Treadmill running distance during a maximal exercise test varied by 3.6-fold between ten inbred mouse strains (highest: BALB/cJ, lowest: A/J) (39). Based on differences in treadmill running performance among inbred strains of mice, broad-sense heritability estimates for endurance exercise capacity range from 31% to 73% (36, 39), whereas in rats heritability estimates range from 39% to 50% (5, 32). The large differences between inbred strains and high heritability provide evidence that endurance exercise capacity is significantly influenced by genetic background.

Genetic mapping

Although transgenic/knockout mouse approaches have identified some genes that influence exercise capacity, the data supporting putative candidate genes based on genome-wide approaches is lacking. Using traditional genome-wide linkage analysis, several QTL for endurance exercise capacity have been identified in rats (61) and mice (40, 42, 44). In the first study to identify QTL for aerobic running capacity in rats, Ways et al. utilized an F_2 population based on low-performing COP and high-performing DA strains for linkage analysis (61). Significant and suggestive QTL for aerobic running capacity were identified on rat chromosomes 16 (LOD 4.0) and 3 (LOD 2.2), respectively. To confirm these QTL, two congenic strains were developed by introgressing either a region of chromosome 3 or chromosome 16 from DA rats into the genetic background of COP rats (62). Exercise capacity was similar between chromosome 3 congenic and COP rats. Chromosome 16 congenic rats had significantly greater aerobic running capacity compared with COP rats, supporting the presence of a QTL for aerobic running capacity on this chromosome. The congenic region on chromosome 16 spans nearly the entire chromosome and requires additional fine-mapping to identify candidate genes for aerobic running capacity.

Lightfoot et al. (39) screened several strains of mice for endurance exercise performance using a graded treadmill test and identified DBA/2J and BALB/cJ as low- and high-performing strains, respectively. In a subsequent study, significant and suggestive QTL for maximal endurance exercise performance were identified on chromosomes X (LOD 2.26) and 8 (LOD 1.19), respectively, in F_2 mice derived from a cross between these strains (40). The confidence interval for the QTL on mouse chromosome 8 overlaps with the two running capacity QTL on rat chromosome 16 (the QTL regions on rat chromosome 16 are syntenic to regions of mouse chromosome 8) (61). This concordance between rats and mice supports the premise that a portion of the genetic regulation of endurance exercise capacity is conserved among species.

Similarly, Massett and Berk performed a strain screen using three inbred mouse strains and three F_1 hybrid strains (43). Significant differences in run time and work were identified among strains. The highest (FVB) and lowest (B6) performing strains were used to derive an intercross F_2 population (44). Significant QTL for pretraining endurance exercise capacity were identified on chromosomes 14 (LOD 3.72) and 19 (LOD 3.63) in a genome-wide linkage scan (Table 13.1). Suggestive QTL (LOD ≤3.4) were identified on chromosomes 1, 2, 3, and 8. Similarly, a reciprocal intercross-breeding scheme was used to generate F_2 mice from inbred 129S1/SvImJ (high-performing) and NZW/LacJ (low-performing) strains (42). A significant QTL was identified on chromosome 5 (LOD 4.26) in female mice only (Table 13.1). Suggestive QTL (LOD ≤3.0) were identified on chromosomes 6, 9, and 12. Subsequently, data from (FVB × B6)F_2 and (NZW × 129S1)F_2 populations were combined to increase the resolution of shared QTL and identify new QTL not identified in individual crosses. In the combined cross-analysis, a significant novel QTL for pretraining exercise time was identified on chromosome 12 (LOD 3.6) (Table 13.1). Results from this combined cross-analysis demonstrate that this approach can be useful in identifying novel QTL and reducing the confidence interval of previously identified QTL. The success of combining two mapping populations lends support for the use of larger and more diverse mapping populations to identify the genetic basis for exercise capacity.

To verify the presence of a QTL for endurance exercise capacity on chromosome 14, Courtney and Massett utilized a chromosome substitution strain (CSS) derived from A/J (A) and B6 inbred strains, denoted as B6.A14 (14). CSS mice are made by substituting a single chromosome from a donor inbred strain on the genetic background of a host inbred strain (recipient). Phenotypic differences between the recipient or background strain mice and CSS mice support the presence of a QTL on the substituted chromosome for the phenotype being measured. B6.A14 mice carry chromosome 14 from the low-performing A donor inbred strain on the genetic background of a host B6 inbred strain. Exercise capacity in B6.A14 mice is significantly lower than in B6 mice, suggesting the presence of a QTL on the substituted chromosome for exercise capacity. Subsequent linkage analysis in a (B6.A14 × B6)F_2 population identified a significant QTL for exercise time (LOD 2.28) and a suggestive QTL for work (LOD 2.19) in male mice. In contrast, no QTL was identified for exercise time, but a suggestive QTL for work (LOD 1.8) was identified in female (B6.A14 × B6)F_2 mice, suggesting that the genetic architecture underlying exercise capacity is different in males and females of these strains. Using a similar strategy, Kvedaras et al. measured exercise capacity in inbred B6 mice and mice from a CSS carrying A/J chromosome 10 on a B6 background (B6.A10) (35). Running distance was significantly lower in B6.A10 mice compared to inbred B6 indicating the presence of at least one QTL on chromosome 10. No sex differences were reported for this CSS. Collectively, these results support the presence of QTL for endurance exercise capacity on chromosomes 10 and 14 in A and B6 strains.

As an alternative to traditional linkage analyses, association mapping can be performed on phenotype data from a large number of inbred strains. To this end, endurance exercise capacity was measured in 34 strains of inbred mice (13). Exercise time in the highest performing strain (C58/J) was 2.7 times that of the lowest performing strain (A/J). These same strains showed a 16.5-fold difference in work performed. Subsequent genome-wide association mapping identified significant associations (P ≤1 × 10^{-6}) for exercise time on chromosomes 1, 2, 7, 11, and 13. The average confidence interval for the significant QTL was approximately 450 kb, which is markedly smaller than QTL identified by linkage analysis. The interval on chromosome 2 contains one gene, *Nfatc2*. This gene is associated with pathological cardiac hypertrophy (9), but has yet to be confirmed as a candidate gene for endurance exercise capacity. The genetic

Table 13.1 Significant quantitative trait loci (QTL) for intrinsic endurance exercise capacity

Study	Population	Phenotype	Chromosome	Peak, Mb	CI, Mb	Genes of interest
Lightfoot et al., 2007	(C × 2J)F$_2$	Time, min	8	74.8		–
			X	127.9		Hsh2d
Massett et al., 2009	(FVB × B6)F$_2$	Work, kg:m	14	7.5	0–73	Myh6, Myh7, Myoz1, Sgcg
			19	41.1	14–60	Ankrd2, Btaf1, Fxn, Plce1
Massett et al., 2015	(NZW × 129S1)F$_2$	Time, min	5	71.0	52–129	Atp2a2, Myl2, Nos1, Sgcb
	Combined cross	Time, min	12	105.6	89–110	Bdkrb2, Tdp1
			14	50.8	20–72	Myh6, Myh7, Myoz1, Sgcg
Courtney and Massett, 2012	Inbred strains	Time, min	1	180.7	178–181	Kif26b
			2	168.4	168.2–168.5	Nfatc2
			7	16.97	16.97–16.99	Sae1
			11	21.6	21–23	Mdh1
			11	24.5	24.5–25.6	–
			11	70.3	70.2–70.8	Chrne, Eno3
			13	58.95		Ntrk2
Ways et al., 2002	(COP × DA)F$_2$	Distance, m	8★	43.1	33–61	Sgcz, Slc25a4
			8★	18.0	14.5–25	Angpt2
			2★	25.2	25–49	Crat, Mymk
Ways et al., 2007	Congenic	Distance, m	8★		9–75	Irs2, Slc27a1
			14★		25–42	Slc18a3
Courtney and Massett, 2014	(B6.A14 × B6)F$_2$	Time, min	14	104.9	99–114	Ednrb
Kvedaras et al., 2017	B6.A10 CSS	Distance, m	10			–

Peak, position of QTL peak in megabases (Mb); CI, 95% confidence interval in Mb; (C × 2J)F$_2$, cross between BALB/cJ and DBA/2J strains; (FVB × B6)F$_2$, cross between FVB/NJ and C57BL/6J strains; (NZW × 129S1)F$_2$, cross between NZW/LacJ and 129S1/SvImJ strains; Combined cross, data combined from (FVB × B6)F$_2$ and (NZW × 129S1)F$_2$ populations; (COP × DA)F$_2$, cross between Copenhagen and DA rat strains; Congenic, COP.DA-(D16Rat12-D16Rat90)/Mco rat congenic strain; (B6.A14 × B6)F$_2$, cross between C57BL/6J-Chr14[A/J/NaJ] and C57BL/6J strains; B6.A10 CSS, C57BL/6J-Chr10[A/J/NaJ]; ★, Rat genome positions have been converted to approximate syntenic regions in mouse genome. All QTL peak positions and intervals were mapped to build 37.2 of the National Center for Biotechnology Information mouse genome. Genes of Interest, genes within region associated with exercise performance, or cardiac, and/or skeletal muscle structure/function; Hsh2d, hematopoietic SH2 domain containing; Myh6, myosin, heavy polypeptide 6, cardiac muscle, alpha; Myh7, myosin, heavy polypeptide 7, cardiac muscle, beta; Myoz1, myozenin 1; Sgcg, sarcoglycan, gamma (dystrophin–associated glycoprotein); Ankrd2, ankyrin repeat domain 2 (stretch responsive muscle); Btaf1, B-TFIID TATA-box binding protein associated factor 1; *Fxn*, frataxin; *Plce1*, phospholipase C, epsilon 1; *Atp2a2*, ATPase, Ca^{2+} transporting, cardiac muscle, slow twitch 2; *Myl2*, myosin, light polypeptide 2, regulatory, cardiac, slow; *Nos1*, nitric oxide synthase 1, neuronal; *Sgcb*, sarcoglycan, beta (dystrophin-associated glycoprotein); *Bdkrb2*, bradykinin receptor, beta 2; *Tdp1*, tyrosyl-DNA phosphodiesterase 1; *Kif26b*, kinesin family member 26B; *Nfactc2*, nuclear factor of activated T cells, cytoplasmic, calcineurin dependent 2; *Sae1*, SUMO1 activating enzyme subunit 1; *Mdh1*, malate dehydrogenase 1, NAD (soluble); *Chrne*, cholinergic receptor, nicotinic, epsilon polypeptide; *Eno3*, enolase 3, beta muscle; *Ntrk2*, neurotrophic tyrosine kinase, receptor, type; *Sgcz*, sarcoglycan zeta; *Slc25a4*, solute carrier family 25 (mitochondrial carrier, adenine nucleotide translocator), member 4; *Angpt2*, angiopoietin 2; *Crat*, carnitine acetyltransferase; *Mymk*, myomaker, myoblast fusion factor; *Irs2*, insulin receptor substrate 2; *Slc27a1*, solute carrier family 27 (fatty acid transporter), member 1; *Slc18a3*, solute carrier family 18 (vesicular monoamine), member 3; *Ednrb*, endothelin receptor type B.

marker *D20S857* was linked to the response to exercise training (change in VO_2max) in African Americans in the HERITAGE Family Study (54) and maps to a region on human chromosome 20. This region is syntenic with the putative QTL on mouse chromosome 2. Hence, association mapping using a large panel of inbred strains provides a higher-resolution approach to gene discovery for endurance exercise capacity and related traits.

Responses to exercise training

Selected strains/artificial selection

Similar to their approach for endurance exercise capacity, Koch et al. created a rat model of low and high responders to aerobic exercise training to investigate the genetic basis for the response to exercise training (33). They utilized heterogeneous N/NIH rats in a two-way artificial selection based on changes in maximal running distance to develop high-response trainer (HRT) and low-response trainer (LRT) lines. Rats trained 3 days per week for 8 weeks. The workload progressively increased each session, exposing all rats to the same absolute training stimulus. After 15 generations of selection, HRT improved their exercise capacity by about 223 m, whereas LRT exhibited a reduction in distance of about 65 m. Estimated narrow-sense heritability for the response to training at generation 15 was relatively low (10%) compared with pretraining (34%) and post-training (43%) exercise capacity. Additionally, the response to training was not dependent upon endurance exercise capacity as both groups had similar pretraining exercise capacity. This was also reflected in the low genetic correlation between endurance exercise capacity and change in distance (0.14), suggesting these phenotypes are determined by different genetic factors. Physiologically, LRT animals have a dysregulated metabolic profile characterized by insulin resistance, increased adipose mass, and decreased angiogenesis following exercise when compared to HRT (37). Thus, physiological adaptations to training appear to cosegregate with the change in distance in HRT and LRT lines. At this time, no genetic analysis utilizing the HRT and LRT lines has been published.

Inbred strain comparisons

Several studies have compared training responses across multiple inbred strains of mice or rats. All have consistently reported high-responding strains having training responses at least three to four times higher than the lowest responding strains (4, 33, 43). In ten inbred strains of rats, training responses differed by 3.9-fold following 8 weeks of treadmill training at the same absolute workload. Strain means ranged from −80 m (PVG) to +239 m (LEW), while individual responses ranged from −438 m to +754 m (33). Massett and Berk reported that responses to 4 weeks of exercise training at the same relative workload (~65% max) varied significantly across three inbred (BALB/cJ, C57BL/6J, FVB/NJ) and three F_1 hybrid (CB6F1/J, B6FF1, FB6F1) mouse strains (43). Among the inbred strains, the response to treadmill training was greatest in FVB/NJ and smallest in BALB/cJ mice. The C57BL/6J strain had a low response to training that was similar to BALB/cJ and significantly less than FVB/NJ. Responses in the hybrid strains varied relative to each other and relative to their respective parental strains. Mean responses in hybrids were greater than both parental strains (CB6F1/J), intermediate to their parents (FB6F1), or similar to the lower performing parental strain (B6FF1), implying that responses to training are complex, significantly influenced by genetic background, and potentially influenced by maternal inheritance (43). Using a swim training model, adaptations to 5 weeks of training were compared in six inbred strains of mice (29). The change in exercise capacity was not reported; however, there was an approximately 6.5-fold difference in exercise capacity after training between the highest (632 minutes) and lowest (97 minutes) performing strains. Similar to Massett and Berk, the BALB/cByJ as well as A/J were identified as low-responding strains. The C57BL/6J and DBA/2J were the highest responding strains in that study.

In a large strain screen, Avila et al. characterized the response to exercise training in 24 genetically diverse strains of inbred mice following 4 weeks of treadmill training (4). As expected, endurance exercise capacity was significantly different between strains when expressed as time (range: 21–42 minutes) and work performed (range: 0.42–3.89 kg:m). In response to training, changes in exercise capacity were significantly different between strains, ranging from −2.2 to +8.7 minutes. The change in exercise capacity expressed as work performed also varied from a decrease of 0.24 kg:m to an increase of 2.30 kg:m. Collectively, the surveys of inbred rat and mouse strains indicate that responses to training vary markedly among strains and are significantly influenced by genetic background.

Despite reporting similar ranges of responses among strains, the estimated genetic contribution to this variation is not consistent. Estimated heritability for responses to training in inbred rats was 13% (33). This value is similar to that observed in selected lines developed from heterogeneous N/NIH rats. In contrast, genetic background accounted for 37–58% of the variance in responses to training in inbred mice (4, 43). In (FVB × B6)F_2 mice estimated heritability for the change in work was 53% (44). The estimated contribution by genetic factors to training responses in mice is comparable to that reported for change in VO$_2$max following exercise training in humans (7, 23, 50). The differences between heritability estimates for responses to training in rats and mice can be partly attributed to differences in environmental variance. The training paradigms differed significantly between rat and mouse models (8 weeks vs. 4 weeks, absolute vs. relative intensity). Therefore, it is not unexpected that the contributions of environmental and genetic factors to phenotypic variance might differ. Furthermore, heritability estimates are population specific. Regardless, studies of training responses from rats and mice indicate that this response is a heritable trait with a significant genetic component.

Quantitative trait locus mapping

While the majority of linkage and association studies have focused on endurance exercise capacity (Table 13.1), a few studies have been conducted to identify the genetic basis for the response to training. An intercross breeding scheme between low-responding B6 and high-responding FVB strains was used to generate (FVB × B6)F$_2$ offspring for linkage analysis (44). After 4 weeks of treadmill training, changes in exercise capacity ranged from −1.67 to +4.55 kg:m. Suggestive QTL for the change in work were identified on chromosomes 11 (LOD 2.30) and 14 (LOD 2.25) (Table 13.2). In a subsequent study, a reciprocal intercross breeding strategy was used to generate an F$_2$ population from low-responding NZW and high-responding 129S1 strains (42). Training responses in (NZW × 129S1)F$_2$ mice were highly variable with a mean increase in exercise capacity of 1.5 ± 3.7 minutes (range: −10.1 to 12.4 minutes). Cross direction (female NZW × male 129S1 or female 129S1 × male NZW) did not significantly affect the response to training. Suggestive QTL for response to training were identified on chromosomes 1 (LOD 2.47) and 6 (LOD 2.73) (Table 13.2) with the QTL on chromosome 1 identified in female mice only.

Both linkage studies for exercise training responses incorporated relatively small populations of animals (<300 each). Therefore, a combined cross-analysis was performed utilizing both F$_2$ populations (42). Genome-wide linkage analysis yielded a significant QTL on chromosome 6 (LOD 3.7) for change in exercise time (Table 13.2). Several suggestive QTL (LOD <3.0) also were identified using this approach (Table 13.2). Although the confidence interval for the QTL on chromosome 6 was relatively large (71 Mb), these findings support the use of combining data from multiple crosses to identify QTL for responses to training not observed in smaller mapping populations.

Mouse–rat–human comparative genomics

For most of the animal studies discussed above, the QTL intervals for endurance exercise capacity and responses to training are relatively large. These large intervals contain hundreds of genes, many of which are not obviously associated with exercise capacity or training responses. One approach to prioritizing regions or genes for future investigation is to identify regions of chromosomal synteny across species for endurance exercise and training response QTL (17). For example, QTL for endurance exercise capacity and responses to training on mouse chromosome 14 are concordant with regions of the human genome identified in the HERITAGE Family Study linked to exercise capacity in the sedentary state and training-induced changes in maximal oxygen consumption (ΔVO_2max) (8, 42, 44, 54). Single nucleotide polymorphisms (SNPs) associated with training responses in humans also map to regions sytenic with QTL on chromosome 14 (53, 57). One of these SNPs, in the gene mitochondrial intermediate peptidase (*MIPEP*), was used to predict training responses in humans based on baseline gene expression in skeletal muscle (57). This collection of evidence suggests that mouse chromosome 14 should be considered for more detailed analyses of the genetic basis for endurance exercise capacity and responses to training.

Similarly, QTL intervals on chromosomes 6, 8, and 19 align with concordant QTL from other species. QTL for endurance exercise capacity in rats and mice overlap on chromosome 8 (40, 61). Several linkage markers for VO$_2$max in the sedentary state in humans (8, 54) also fall within these QTL intervals suggesting potential concordance among mouse, rat, and human QTL. On chromosome 19, QTL for endurance exercise capacity and responses to training identified in mice contain genes associated with training responses (*BTAF1*, *PIP5K1B*) (16, 57), and fitness (*ANKRD22*) (51) in humans. The significant QTL for responses to training in mice on chromosome 6 contains *Cpvl*, a carboxypeptidase gene. This transcript was included in a group of genomic predictors for responses to exercise training in humans (57). Collectively,

Table 13.2 Significant and suggestive quantitative trait loci (QTL) for responses to endurance exercise training

Study	Population	Phenotype	Chromosome	Peak, Mb	CI, Mb	Genes of interest
Massett et al., 2009	(FVB × B6)F₂	Change in work, kg:m	11	72.6	47–109	*Ace, Myh1, Myocd, Myh4, Slc2a4*
			14	69.8	0–122	*Myh6, Myh7, Myoz1, Sgcg*
Massett et al., 2015	(NZW × 129S1)F₂	Change in time, min	1	42.7	21–166	*Mstn, Myog Tnnt2*
			6	86.8	33–127	*Chrm2, Kcna5, Mtpn, Pparg*
	Combined cross	Change in time, min	6	58.2★	41–112	*Cav3, Dysf*
			8	95.3	82–117	*Mmp2, Rln3*
			11	42	33–113	*Ace, Myh1, Myocd, Myh4, Slc2a4*
			19	27.5	9–37	*Ankrd1, Anxa1, Btaf1, Fxn*

Peak, position of QTL peak in megabases (Mb); CI, 95% confidence interval in Mb; (FVB × B6) F₂, cross between FVB/NJ and C57BL/6J strains; (NZW × 129S1)F₂, cross between NZW/LacJ and 129S1/SvImJ strains; Combined cross, data combined from (FVB × B6)F₂ and (NZW × 129S1)F₂ populations; ★, indicates significant QTL. All QTL peak positions and intervals were mapped to build 37.2 of the National Center for Biotechnology Information mouse genome. Genes of Interest, genes within region associated with exercise performance, or cardiac, and/or skeletal muscle structure/function; *Ace,* angiotensin I converting enzyme (peptidyl-dipeptidase A) 1, *Myh1,* myosin, heavy polypeptide 1, skeletal muscle, adult; *Myh4,* myosin, heavy polypeptide 4, skeletal muscle; *Myocd,* myocardin; *Slc2a4,* solute carrier family 2 (facilitated glucose transporter), member 4; *Myh6,* myosin, heavy polypeptide 6, cardiac muscle, alpha; *Myh7,* myosin, heavy polypeptide 7, cardiac muscle, beta; *Myoz1,* myozenin 1; *Sgcg,* sarcoglycan, gamma (dystrophin-associated glycoprotein); *Mstn,* myostatin; *Myog,* myogenin; *Tnnt2,* troponin T2, cardiac; *Chrm2,* cholinergic receptor, muscarinic 2, cardiac; *Kcna5,* potassium voltage-gated channel, shaker-related subfamily, member 5; *Mtpn,* myotrophin; *Pparg,* peroxisome proliferator activated receptor gamma; *Cav3,* caveolin 3; *Dysf,* dysferlin; *Mmp2,* matrix metallopeptidase 2; *Rln3,* relaxin 3; *Ankrd1,* ankyrin repeat domain 1 (cardiac muscle); *Anxa1,* annexin A1; *Btaf1,* B-TFIID TATA-box binding protein associated factor 1.

these examples suggest that there is some concordance among mouse, rat, and human QTL for endurance exercise capacity and responses to training. However, the large confidence intervals from linkage analyses in rodents require some fine mapping to effectively utilize comparative mapping as an approach for candidate gene discovery.

Summary and future directions

Data from animal models confirm that endurance exercise capacity and responses to training are heritable traits and these traits are determined by multiple genetic factors. The high heritability estimates for endurance exercise capacity in inbred mice suggest that a high percentage of the variation in exercise capacity is determined by genetic factors. The heritability estimates for the response to training are lower, likely reflecting the greater influence of environmental factors and gene by environment interactions on the response to training. This complex nature of the responses to exercise training has made identifying genetic factors challenging. The two inbred line crosses yielded moderately significant QTL for responses to training. The combined cross-analyses strengthened the evidence for a QTL on chromosome 6, but the region is quite large. The wide variation in training responses in the inbred mouse strains tested thus far suggests that additional loci can be identified using the GWAS approach. Any overlap between the relatively small regions identified using this approach and previously identified QTL would strengthen the evidence that these regions contain putative candidate genes influencing responses to training.

Some of the difficulty in identifying genetic factors is related to the complex nature of the phenotype. To maximize the ability to detect genetic variants and identify candidate genes, several factors should be considered going forward. A well-defined phenotype is paramount to successful gene identification. The published exercise testing and training paradigms are quite variable (4, 19, 28, 33, 49). Therefore, some consideration should be given to better defining the measurement of exercise capacity in mice and the outcome variable (i.e., time, work, oxygen consumption) used to define it. Similarly, an appropriate training regimen eliciting maximal changes in exercise capacity, but capable of being utilized for large numbers of animals, needs to be identified. Additionally, assessment of the adaptations to training in mice should be expanded to better identify the appropriate target organ for gene and protein mapping studies. For example, functional changes in cardiac performance with endurance training have yet to be assessed in multiple strains of mice. Finally, inbred strain surveys have typically utilized animals of one sex (4, 13, 29, 36, 39, 43, 58). However, a few sex-specific QTL were identified in F_2 populations (14, 42), suggesting that the genetic architecture underlying these traits differs. Therefore, expanding our knowledge of the contribution of sex to these exercise phenotypes could facilitate discovery of the genetic networks underlying endurance exercise capacity and the responses to training.

To date, individual line crosses and GWAS approaches have been used identify genomic regions of interest. Although the line crosses have yielded some significant loci, the identified regions contain hundreds of genes. The GWAS approach applied to endurance exercise capacity identified several small regions containing only a few genes, but with 34 inbred strains was still somewhat underpowered (6, 30). The current data for training responses in inbred strains will likely yield similar results but are underpowered for identifying genetic factors influencing training responses. Future studies should focus on the GWAS approach, but also utilize the recently developed mouse and rat models designed to maximize genetic heterogeneity. Approximately 500 or less Diversity Outbred and/or Collaborative Cross mice have been used to identify QTL for physiological and behavioral traits (1, 41). A similar number might be sufficient for genetic analyses of endurance exercise capacity and/or training responses. Heterogeneous stock rats also could be used for higher resolution mapping; however, the number of animals required (>1000) could be prohibitive for exercise training studies (64). Conversely, examining smaller populations as a whole with meta-analytic approaches could circumvent the need for conducting such large training studies (27). Finally, combining genome-wide gene expression with genetic linkage or association mapping has successfully identified candidate genes for metabolic and disease-related traits (47, 48). Utilizing such a systems biology approach could expedite identification of candidate genes or proteins underlying the variation in endurance exercise capacity and the responses to training, and better define the genetic architecture underlying these complex phenotypes.

References

1. **Abu-Toamih Atamni HJ, Ziner Y, Mott R, Wolf L, Iraqi FA.** Glucose tolerance female-specific QTL mapped in collaborative cross mice. *Mamm Genome* 28: 20–30, 2017.

2. **Allen DL, Harrison BC, Maass A, Bell ML, Byrnes WC, Leinwand LA.** Cardiac and skeletal muscle adaptations to voluntary wheel running in the mouse. *J Appl Physiol* 90: 1900–1908, 2001.

3. **Andreux PA, Williams EG, Koutnikova H, Houtkooper RH, Champy M-F, Henry H, Schoonjans K, Williams RW, Auwerx J.** Systems genetics of metabolism: The use of the BXD murine reference panel for multiscalar integration of traits. *Cell* 150: 1287–1299, 2012.

4. **Avila JJ, Kim SK, Massett MP.** Differences in exercise capacity and responses to training in 24 inbred mouse strains. *Front Physiol* 8: 974, 2017.

5. **Barbato JC, Koch LG, Darvish A, Cicila GT, Metting PJ, Britton SL.** Spectrum of aerobic endurance running performance in eleven inbred strains of rats. *J Appl Physiol* 85: 530–536, 1998.

6. **Bennett BJ, Farber CR, Orozco L, Kang HM, Ghazalpour A, Siemers N, Neubauer M, Neuhaus I, Yordanova R, Guan B, Truong A, Yang W, He A, Kayne P, Gargalovic P, Kirchgessner T, Pan C, Castellani LW, Kostem E, Furlotte N, Drake TA, Eskin E, Lusis AJ.** A high-resolution association mapping panel for the dissection of complex traits in mice. *Genome Res* 20: 281–290, 2010.

7. **Bouchard C, An P, Rice T, Skinner JS, Wilmore JH, Gagnon J, Pérusse L, Leon AS, Rao DC.** Familial aggregation of VO(2max) response to exercise training: results from the HERITAGE Family Study. *J Appl Physiol* 87: 1003–1008, 1999.

8. **Bouchard C, Rankinen T, Chagnon YC, Rice T, Pérusse L, Gagnon J, Borecki I, An P, Leon AS, Skinner JS, Wilmore JH, Province M, Rao DC.** Genomic scan for maximal oxygen uptake and its response to training in the HERITAGE Family Study. *J Appl Physiol* 88: 551–559, 2000.

9. **Bourajjaj M, Armand A-S, da Costa Martins PA, Weijts B, van der Nagel R, Heeneman S, Wehrens XH, De Windt LJ.** NFATc2 is a necessary mediator of calcineurin-dependent cardiac hypertrophy and heart failure. *J Biol Chem* 283: 22295–22303, 2008.

10. **Britton SL, Koch LG.** Animal genetic models for complex traits of physical capacity. *Exerc Sport Sci Rev* 29: 7–14, 2001.

11. **Calvo JA, Daniels TG, Wang X, Paul A, Lin J, Spiegelman BM, Stevenson SC, Rangwala SM.** Muscle-specific expression of PPARgamma coactivator-1alpha improves exercise performance and increases peak oxygen uptake. *J Appl Physiol* 104: 1304–1312, 2008.

12. **Chow LS, Greenlund LJ, Asmann YW, Short KR, McCrady SK, Levine JA, Nair KS.** Impact of endurance training on murine spontaneous activity, muscle mitochondrial DNA abundance, gene transcripts, and function. *J Appl Physiol* 102: 1078–1089, 2007.

13. **Courtney SM, Massett MP.** Identification of exercise capacity QTL using association mapping in inbred mice. *Physiol Genomics* 44: 948–955, 2012.

14. **Courtney SM, Massett MP.** Effect of chromosome substitution on intrinsic exercise capacity in mice. *F1000Res* 3: 9, 2014.

15. **De Angelis K, Wichi RB, Jesus WRA, Moreira ED, Morris M, Krieger EM, Irigoyen MC.** Exercise training changes autonomic cardiovascular balance in mice. *J Appl Physiol* 96: 2174–2178, 2004.

16. **Dias RG, Silva MSM, Duarte NE, Bolani W, Alves CR, Junior JRL, da Silva JL, de Oliveira PA, Alves GB, de Oliveira EM, Rocha CS, Marsiglia JDC, Negrao CE, Krieger EM, Krieger JE, Pereira AC.** PBMCs express a transcriptome signature predictor of oxygen uptake responsiveness to endurance exercise training in men. *Physiol Genomics* 47: 13–23, 2015.

17. **DiPetrillo K, Wang X, Stylianou IM, Paigen B.** Bioinformatics toolbox for narrowing rodent quantitative trait loci. *Trends Genet* 21: 683–692, 2005.

18. **Fan W, Waizenegger W, Lin CS, Sorrentino V, He M-X, Wall CE, Li H, Liddle C, Yu RT, Atkins AR, Auwerx J, Downes M, Evans RM.** Pparδ promotes running endurance by preserving glucose. *Cell Metab* 25: 1186–1193.e4, 2017.

19. **Ferreira JCB, Rolim NPL, Bartholomeu JB, Gobatto CA, Kokubun E, Brum PC.** Maximal lactate steady state in running mice: effect of exercise training. *Clin Exp Pharmacol Physiol* 34: 760–765, 2007.

20. **Fewell JG, Osinska H, Klevitsky R, Ng W, Sfyris G, Bahrehmand F, Robbins J.** A treadmill exercise regimen for identifying cardiovascular phenotypes in transgenic mice. *Am J Physiol* 273: H1595–605, 1997.

21. **Flint J, Valdar W, Shifman S, Mott R.** Strategies for mapping and cloning quantitative trait genes in rodents. *Nat Rev Genet* 6: 271–286, 2005.

22. **Hagberg JM, Rankinen T, Loos RJF, Pérusse L, Roth SM, Wolfarth B, Bouchard C.** Advances in exercise, fitness, and performance genomics in 2010. *Med Sci Sports Exerc* 43: 743–752, 2011.

23. **Hamel P, Simoneau JA, Lortie G, Boulay MR, Bouchard C.** Heredity and muscle adaptation to endurance training. *Med Sci Sports Exerc* 18: 690–696, 1986.

24. **Haubold KW, Allen DL, Capetanaki Y, Leinwand LA.** Loss of desmin leads to impaired voluntary wheel running and treadmill exercise performance. *J Appl Physiol* 95: 1617–1622, 2003.

25. **Henderson KK, Wagner H, Favret F, Britton SL, Koch LG, Wagner PD, Gonzalez NC.** Determinants of maximal O(2) uptake in rats selectively bred for endurance running capacity. *J Appl Physiol* 93: 1265–1274, 2002.

26. **Howlett RA, Gonzalez NC, Wagner HE, Fu Z, Britton SL, Koch LG, Wagner PD.** Selected contribution: skeletal muscle capillarity and enzyme activity in rats selectively bred for running endurance. *J Appl Physiol* 94: 1682–1688, 2003.

27. **Kang EY, Han B, Furlotte N, Joo JWJ, Shih D, Davis RC, Lusis AJ, Eskin E.** Meta-analysis identifies gene-by-environment interactions as demonstrated in a study of 4,965 mice. *PLoS Genet* 10: e1004022, 2014.

28. **Kemi OJ, Loennechen JP, Wisløff U, Ellingsen Ø.** Intensity-controlled treadmill running in mice: cardiac and skeletal muscle hypertrophy. *J Appl Physiol* 93: 1301–1309, 2002.

29. **Kilikevicius A, Venckunas T, Zelniene R, Carroll AM, Lionikaite S, Ratkevicius A, Lionikas A.** Divergent physiological characteristics and responses to endurance training among inbred mouse strains. *Scand J Med Sci Sports* 23: 657–668, 2013.

30. **Kirby A, Kang HM, Wade CM, Cotsapas C, Kostem E, Han B, Furlotte N, Kang EY, Rivas M, Bogue MA, Frazer KA, Johnson FM, Beilharz EJ, Cox DR, Eskin E, Daly MJ.** Fine mapping in 94 inbred mouse strains using a high-density haplotype resource. *Genetics* 185: 1081–1095, 2010.

31. **Koch LG, Britton SL.** Artificial selection for intrinsic aerobic endurance running capacity in rats. *Physiol Genomics* 5: 45–52, 2001.

32. **Koch LG, Meredith TA, Fraker TD, Metting PJ, Britton SL.** Heritability of treadmill running endurance in rats. *Am J Physiol* 275: R1455–60, 1998.

33. **Koch LG, Pollott GE, Britton SL.** Selectively bred rat model system for low and high response to exercise training. *Physiol Genomics* 45: 606–614, 2013.

34. **Kregel KC, Allen DL, Booth FW, Fleshner MR, Henriksen EJ, Musch TI, O'Leary DS, Parks CM, Poole DC, Ra'anan AW, Sheriff DD.** *Resource Book for the Design of Animal Exercise Protocols.* Bethesda, MD: American Physiological Society, 2006.

35. **Kvedaras M, Minderis P, Fokin A, Ratkevicius A, Venckunas T, Lionikas A.** Forced running endurance is influenced by gene(s) on mouse chromosome 10. *Front Physiol* 8: 9, 2017.

36. **Lerman I, Harrison BC, Freeman K, Hewett TE, Allen DL, Robbins J, Leinwand LA.** Genetic variability in forced and voluntary endurance exercise performance in seven inbred mouse strains. *J Appl Physiol* 92: 2245–2255, 2002.

37. **Lessard SJ, Rivas DA, Alves-Wagner AB, Hirshman MF, Gallagher IJ, Constantin-Teodosiu D, Atkins R, Greenhaff PL, Qi NR, Gustafsson T, Fielding RA, Timmons JA, Britton SL, Koch LG, Goodyear LJ.** Resistance to aerobic exercise training causes metabolic dysfunction and reveals novel exercise-regulated signaling networks. *Diabetes* 62: 2717–2727, 2013.

38. **Lightfoot JT, Turner MJ, Daves M, Vordermark A, Kleeberger SR.** Genetic influence on daily wheel running activity level. *Physiol Genomics* 19: 270–276, 2004.

39. **Lightfoot JT, Turner MJ, Debate KA, Kleeberger SR.** Interstrain variation in murine aerobic capacity. *Med Sci Sports Exerc* 33: 2053–2057, 2001.

40. **Lightfoot JT, Turner MJ, Knab AK, Jedlicka AE, Oshimura T, Marzec J, Gladwell W, Leamy LJ, Kleeberger SR.** Quantitative trait loci associated with maximal exercise endurance in mice. *J Appl Physiol* 103: 105–110, 2007.

41. **Logan RW, Robledo RF, Recla JM, Philip VM, Bubier JA, Jay JJ, Harwood C, Wilcox T, Gatti DM, Bult CJ, Churchill GA, Chesler EJ.** High-precision genetic mapping of behavioral traits in the diversity outbred mouse population. *Genes Brain Behav* 12: 424–437, 2013.

42. **Massett MP, Avila JJ, Kim SK.** Exercise capacity and response to training quantitative trait loci in a NZW X 129S1 intercross and combined cross analysis of inbred mouse strains. *PLoS One* 10: e0145741, 2015.

43. **Massett MP, Berk BC.** Strain-dependent differences in responses to exercise training in inbred and hybrid mice. *Am J Physiol Regul Integr Comp Physiol* 288: R1006–13, 2005.

44. **Massett MP, Fan R, Berk BC.** Quantitative trait loci for exercise training responses in FVB/NJ and C57BL/6J mice. *Physiol Genomics* 40: 15–22, 2009.

45. **Momken I, Lechêne P, Ventura-Clapier R, Veksler V.** Voluntary physical activity alterations in endothelial nitric oxide synthase knockout mice. *Am J Physiol Heart Circ Physiol* 287: H914–H920, 2004.

46. **Nie Y, Sato Y, Wang C, Yue F, Kuang S, Gavin TP.** Impaired exercise tolerance, mitochondrial biogenesis, and muscle fiber maintenance in miR-133a-deficient mice. *FASEB J* 30: 3745–3758, 2016.

47. **Parker CC, Gopalakrishnan S, Carbonetto P, Gonzales NM, Leung E, Park YJ, Aryee E, Davis J, Blizard DA, Ackert-Bicknell CL, Lionikas A, Pritchard JK, Palmer AA.** Genome-wide association study of behavioral, physiological and gene expression traits in outbred CFW mice. *Nat Genet* 48: 919–926, 2016.

48. **Parks BW, Sallam T, Mehrabian M, Psychogios N, Hui ST, Norheim F, Castellani LW, Rau CD, Pan C, Phun J, Zhou Z, Yang W-P, Neuhaus I, Gargalovic PS, Kirchgessner TG, Graham M, Lee R, Tontonoz P, Gerszten RE, Hevener AL, Lusis AJ.** Genetic architecture of insulin resistance in the mouse. *Cell Metab* 21: 334–346, 2015.

49. **Petrosino JM, Heiss VJ, Maurya SK, Kalyanasundaram A, Periasamy M, LaFountain RA, Wilson JM, Simonetti OP, Ziouzenkova O.** Graded maximal exercise testing to assess mouse cardio-metabolic phenotypes. *PLoS One* 11: e0148010, 2016.

50. **Prud'homme D, Bouchard C, Leblanc C, Landry F, Fontaine E.** Sensitivity of maximal aerobic power to training is genotype-dependent. *Med Sci Sports Exerc* 16: 489–493, 1984.

51. **Rampersaud E, Nathanson L, Farmer J, Meshbane K, Belton RL, Dressen A, Cuccaro M, Musto A, Daunert S, Deo S, Hudson N, Vance JM, Seo D, Mendez A, Dykxhoorn DM, Pericak-Vance MA, Goldschmidt-Clermont PJ.** Genomic signatures of a global fitness index in a multi-ethnic cohort of women. *Ann Hum Genet* 77: 147–157, 2013.

52. **Ren Y-Y, Overmyer KA, Qi NR, Treutelaar MK, Heckenkamp L, Kalahar M, Koch LG, Britton SL, Burant CF, Li JZ.** Genetic analysis of a rat model of aerobic capacity and metabolic fitness. *PLoS One* 8: e77588, 2013.

53. **Rice TK, Sarzynski MA, Sung YJ, Argyropoulos G, Stütz AM, Teran-Garcia M, Rao DC, Bouchard C, Rankinen T.** Fine mapping of a QTL on chromosome 13 for submaximal exercise capacity training response: The HERITAGE Family Study. *Eur J Appl Physiol* 112: 2969–2978, 2012.

54. **Rico-Sanz J, Rankinen T, Rice T, Leon AS, Skinner JS, Wilmore JH, Rao DC, Bouchard C.** Quantitative trait loci for maximal exercise capacity phenotypes and their responses to training in the HERITAGE Family Study. *Physiol Genomics* 16: 256–260, 2004.

55. **Silver LM.** *Mouse Genetics: Concepts and Applications.* New York: Oxford University Press, 1995.

56. **Swallow JG, Garland T, Carter PA, Zhan WZ, Sieck GC.** Effects of voluntary activity and genetic selection on aerobic capacity in house mice (Mus domesticus). *J Appl Physiol* 84: 69–76, 1998.

57. **Timmons JA, Knudsen S, Rankinen T, Koch LG, Sarzynski M, Jensen T, Keller P, Scheele C, Vollaard NBJ, Nielsen S, Akerström T, MacDougald OA, Jansson E, Greenhaff PL, Tarnopolsky MA, van Loon LJC, Pedersen BK, Sundberg CJ, Wahlestedt C, Britton SL, Bouchard C.** Using molecular classification to predict gains in maximal aerobic capacity following endurance exercise training in humans. *J Appl Physiol* 108: 1487–1496, 2010.

58. **Totsuka Y, Nagao Y, Horii T, Yonekawa H, Imai H, Hatta H, Izaike Y, Tokunaga T, Atomi Y.** Physical performance and soleus muscle fiber composition in wild-derived and laboratory inbred mouse strains. *J Appl Physiol* 95: 720–727, 2003.

59. **Wang J, Liao G, Usuka J, Peltz G.** Computational genetics: from mouse to human? *Trends Genet* 21: 526–532, 2005.

60. **Waters RE, Rotevatn S, Li P, Annex BH, Yan Z.** Voluntary running induces fiber type-specific angiogenesis in mouse skeletal muscle. *Am J Physiol Cell Physiol* 287: C1342–C1348, 2004.

61. **Ways JA, Cicila GT, Garrett MR, Koch LG.** A genome scan for loci associated with aerobic running capacity in rats. *Genomics* 80: 13–20, 2002.

62. **Ways JA, Smith BM, Barbato JC, Ramdath RS, Pettee KM, DeRaedt SJ, Allison DC, Koch LG, Lee SJ, Cicila GT.** Congenic strains confirm aerobic running capacity quantitative trait loci on rat chromosome 16 and identify possible intermediate phenotypes. *Physiol Genomics* 29: 91–97, 2007.
63. **Wisløff U, Najjar SM, Ellingsen O, Haram PM, Swoap S, Al-Share Q, Fernström M, Rezaei K, Lee SJ, Koch LG, Britton SL.** Cardiovascular risk factors emerge after artificial selection for low aerobic capacity. *Science* 307: 418–420, 2005.
64. **Woods LCS, Mott R.** Heterogeneous stock populations for analysis of complex traits. *Methods Mol Biol* 1488: 31–44, 2017.

14

HERITABILITY OF ENDURANCE TRAITS FROM HUMAN RESEARCH MODELS

Jacob L. Barber and Mark A. Sarzynski

Chapter 13 summarized published work related to the heritability of endurance traits at baseline and in response to exercise training in animal models. This chapter will summarize published work that quantifies genetic contributions to endurance-related traits both in the intrinsic state (i.e., in the sedentary state at baseline) and following exercise training using traditional family and twin study approaches in humans. Please refer to Chapter 12 for a primer on the endurance phenotype.

Heritability of intrinsic levels of endurance traits

There are large interindividual differences in endurance-related phenotypes, which may be affected by age, sex, physical activity, and fitness levels (13). Additionally, numerous twin and family studies have provided evidence that endurance-related traits clearly aggregate in families and have a significant genetic component in the intrinsic state. Twin and family studies represent the ideal design to investigate the influences of genes and the environment on a trait given that family members not only share similar genetic profiles but are also exposed to similar environmental influences. The rationale is that the trait levels will be more similar for individuals having the same genes (monozygotic (MZ) twins) or sharing about 50% of their genes (dizygotic (DZ) twins, parent–offspring, siblings) compared to unrelated individuals (between twin pairs or families). From comparisons of intrapair differences between MZ and DZ twins, it is possible to separate the relative contribution of genotype and environment for any attribute by deriving a coefficient of heritability. Heritability is defined as the proportion of observed phenotypic variance in a population that is attributable to individual genetic differences. If MZ twins show more similarity for a given trait than DZ twins, this provides evidence of a significant genetic component of the trait, whereas if MZ and DZ twins exhibit equal similarity for a trait, it is likely the environment influences the trait more than genetic factors. Similarly, in family studies a pattern of significant correlations between parents and offspring and between siblings, but not between spouses, suggests that the familial resemblance is primarily due to genetic factors.

For example, a study of 42 brothers and 66 DZ and 106 MZ twins of both sexes found that the interclass correlations of absolute maximal oxygen uptake or VO_2max (l/min) were 0.57, 0.84, and 0.92 (all $P < 0.01$), respectively (12). The **HERITAGE** Family Study examined the

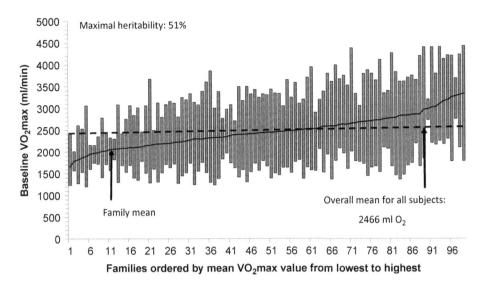

Figure 14.1 Mean baseline VO₂max across white families from the HERITAGE Family Study, with families ranked by family mean.

familial resemblance for VO₂max in 426 sedentary adults from 86 nuclear families. The authors found that intrinsic levels of VO₂max aggregate in families, as there was about 2.7 times more variance between different families than within families for adjusted VO₂max (9) (Figure 14.1). It can be seen in Figure 14.1 that some families in HERITAGE tended to have below-average VO₂max values, while others had above-average values.

Furthermore, the authors estimated that the genetic heritability of intrinsic VO₂max was 51% in HERITAGE (9). This heritability estimate is similar to the aforementioned study of 106 MZ twins and 66 DZ twins that found heritability estimates ranging from 38% to 47% for VO₂max (12). However, to date the calculated heritability estimates of VO₂max show wide variation across studies, with twin studies tending to report higher estimates (Table 14.1) (18, 24, 26, 33). A meta-analysis of seven twin and sibling studies in children to young adults (*N*=1088) found weighted heritability estimates of 59% and 72% for absolute (ml/min) and relative (ml/kg/min) VO₂max (33). In 2017, a systematic review and meta-analysis of twin and family studies was performed on the heritability of intrinsic VO₂max (24). Six twin studies and two family studies were included in the meta-analysis, which found that the weighted means of the heritability of absolute VO₂max and VO₂max adjusted for body weight and adjusted for fat-free mass were 0.68 (95% confidence interval (CI) 0.59–0.77), 0.56 (95% CI 0.47–0.65) (Figure 14.2), and 0.44 (95% CI 0.13–0.75), respectively (24). The authors found that estimation method, study type, and exercise mode did not significantly influence the heritability estimates of VO₂max, while the heritability estimates were significantly higher in studies comprised of only males (0.69; 95% CI 0.55–0.83) compared to studies including both males and females (0.49; 95% CI 0.42–0.56). Thus, sex differences appear to partially explain the heterogeneity in the heritability estimates of absolute and relative VO₂max. This could be the result of sex differences in body composition, as heritability estimates of absolute VO₂max tend to be higher compared to those adjusting for body weight or composition. Importantly, no study of only females has been performed to better address and compare sex differences in the heritability of VO₂max. Results

Table 14.1 Heritability estimates for endurance-related traits in the intrinsic/untrained state

Trait	Study design	Number of studies	Heritability	References
VO$_2$max	Nuclear families	6	0.20–0.52	18, 24, 26, 33
(adjusted for body weight)	Twins	8	0.38–0.93	
Submaximal aerobic	Nuclear families	4	0.00–0.74	5, 18, 24, 26, 33
performance	Twins	3	0.00–0.90	
(e.g., VO$_2$ at 50% or 80% of maximum)				

Study		Heritability (95% CI)	%Weight
Klissouras et al. 1971		0.93 (0.59, 1.28)	5.04
Bouchard et al. 1986		0.39 (0.21, 0.57)	11.53
Fagard et al. 1991		0.78 (0.53, 1.03)	8.14
Sundet et al. 1994		0.62 (0.57, 0.67)	22.37
Rodas et al. 1998		0.52 (0.09, 0.95)	3.49
Bouchard et al. 1998		0.52 (0.40, 0.64)	16.85
Foraita et al. 2015		0.42 (0.28, 0.56)	14.66
Schutte et al. 2016		0.55 (0.45, 0.65)	17.91
Overall (I^2 = 63.6%, P = 0.007)		**0.56 (0.47, 0.65)**	**100.00**

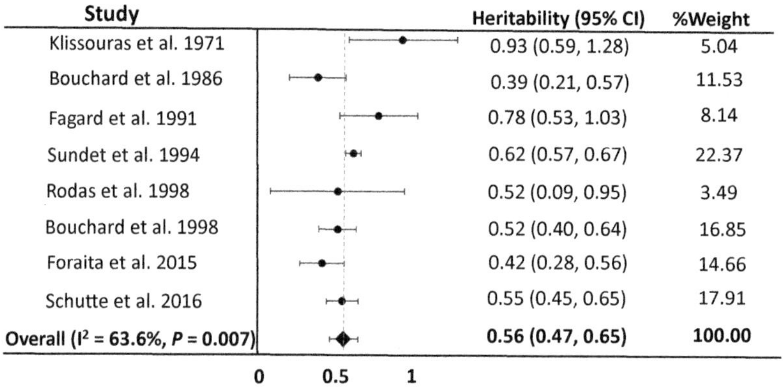

Figure 14.2 Meta-analysis of heritability estimates of intrinsic VO$_2$max adjusted by body weight.

from HERITAGE found the strongest familial correlations of intrinsic VO$_2$max between mothers and daughters and that the best heritability models incorporated maternal inheritance with the father's contribution being environmental (9). The authors estimated the maternal heritability of intrinsic VO$_2$max ranged from 29% to 36% and most likely represents the contribution of mitochondrial DNA, which is transmitted by the mother to the zygote with no contribution from the father. The strong maternal inheritance could also be mediated by *in utero* maternal epigenetic factors.

In addition to VO$_2$max, several other maximal and submaximal endurance-related traits have been shown to have significant genetic heritability levels as estimated from twin and family studies (Table 14.1) (5, 18, 24, 26, 33). In the study of 66 DZ twins and 106 MZ twins of both sexes, the range of heritability estimates for relative total work output during 90 minutes of maximal exercise, maximal oxygen pulse, and maximal ventilation were 0.66–0.70, 0.49–0.55, and 0.51–0.95, respectively (12). A study of 22 pairs of DZ and 31 pairs of MZ twins found that heritability estimates of submaximal endurance traits adjusted for body weight were high for low-power outputs and became nonsignificant at higher power outputs (15). The estimated heritability of VO$_2$ (ml/kg/min) at submaximal absolute intensities was 0.90 at 50 W, 0.78 at 75 W, 0.46 at 100 W, and 0.0 at 125 and 150 W, respectively (15). The estimated heritability of VO$_2$ at submaximal relative intensities was nonsignificant for VO$_2$ at a heart rate of 150 and 0.63 for VO$_2$ at a respiratory exchange ratio of 0.95 (20). Similarly, in HERITAGE the heritability

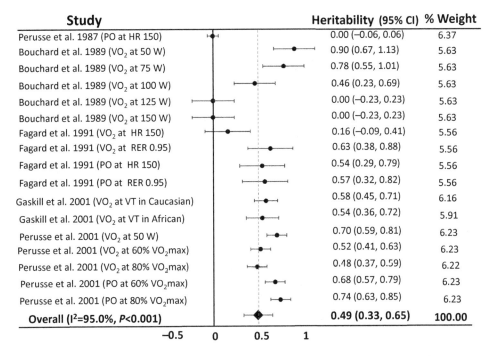

Study	Heritability (95% CI)	% Weight
Perusse et al. 1987 (PO at HR 150)	0.00 (−0.06, 0.06)	6.37
Bouchard et al. 1989 (VO$_2$ at 50 W)	0.90 (0.67, 1.13)	5.63
Bouchard et al. 1989 (VO$_2$ at 75 W)	0.78 (0.55, 1.01)	5.63
Bouchard et al. 1989 (VO$_2$ at 100 W)	0.46 (0.23, 0.69)	5.63
Bouchard et al. 1989 (VO$_2$ at 125 W)	0.00 (−0.23, 0.23)	5.63
Bouchard et al. 1989 (VO$_2$ at 150 W)	0.00 (−0.23, 0.23)	5.63
Fagard et al. 1991 (VO$_2$ at HR 150)	0.16 (−0.09, 0.41)	5.56
Fagard et al. 1991 (VO$_2$ at RER 0.95)	0.63 (0.38, 0.88)	5.56
Fagard et al. 1991 (PO at HR 150)	0.54 (0.29, 0.79)	5.56
Fagard et al. 1991 (PO at RER 0.95)	0.57 (0.32, 0.82)	5.56
Gaskill et al. 2001 (VO$_2$ at VT in Caucasian)	0.58 (0.45, 0.71)	6.16
Gaskill et al. 2001 (VO$_2$ at VT in African)	0.54 (0.36, 0.72)	5.91
Perusse et al. 2001 (VO$_2$ at 50 W)	0.70 (0.59, 0.81)	6.23
Perusse et al. 2001 (VO$_2$ at 60% VO$_2$max)	0.52 (0.41, 0.63)	6.23
Perusse et al. 2001 (VO$_2$ at 80% VO$_2$max)	0.48 (0.37, 0.59)	6.22
Perusse et al. 2001 (PO at 60% VO$_2$max)	0.68 (0.57, 0.79)	6.23
Perusse et al. 2001 (PO at 80% VO$_2$max)	0.74 (0.63, 0.85)	6.23
Overall (I^2=95.0%, P<0.001)	**0.49 (0.33, 0.65)**	**100.00**

−0.5   0   0.5   1

Figure 14.3 Meta-analysis of heritability estimates of submaximal endurance phenotypes in the untrained state.

estimates were 0.52 and 0.48 for VO$_2$ at 60% and 80% of VO$_2$max, respectively (27), while heritability estimates for VO$_2$ at ventilatory threshold were 0.58 for white and 0.54 for black individuals (21). The heritability estimates for submaximal endurance traits are summarized in the systematic review and meta-analysis by Miyamoto-Mikami et al. (24), which found a weighted mean heritability estimate of 0.49 (95% CI 0.33–0.65) for submaximal endurance traits (Figure 14.3).

Lastly, one twin study examined longitudinal changes in genetic influences of intrinsic endurance-related traits. Specifically, the heritability of maximal walking speed over 10 m and a 6-min walking endurance test were estimated in 63 MZ and 67 DZ pairs of older (63–75 years) twin sisters at baseline and 3 years later (25). The authors found that the heritability estimate of walking speed was similar at baseline (56%) and follow-up (60%), while heritability of walking endurance increased from baseline (40%) to follow-up (60%). Additional analyses showed the genetic influences at baseline and follow-up were highly correlated for both traits (r$_g$=0.71–0.72), suggesting expression of the same genetic factors at both time points. However, the results also suggest a small proportion of newly expressed genetic factors at follow-up for both traits (25). A study of older twins followed over 6 years found an increase in genetic variance of self-reported physical functioning (17). The authors postulate that these results conform to the genetic-evolutionary theories of aging that suggest genetic variability in the underlying traits for physical functioning tend to vary more at older ages due to changes in gene expression in different body systems or the weakening influence of beneficial genes that were strongly active in early life (17, 27).

Human variation in endurance training responses

Both animal and human studies provide strong evidence that there is a significant genetic component to endurance-related traits. Importantly, the genetic component is thought to affect both the intrinsic level of endurance in the untrained state and responsiveness to endurance training. In general, the heritability estimates tend to be lower for endurance response phenotypes as compared to intrinsic phenotypes. This section will briefly summarize important studies highlighting variation in endurance trait response to exercise training and the role of genetic factors in these responses.

The beneficial effects of endurance exercise training on several health outcomes and physical performance have been well documented (28). However, numerous studies have also shown large heterogeneity in the adaptation to exercise training (13). In the early 1980s, Dr. Claude Bouchard led a series of carefully controlled and standardized exercise training studies that showed the individual differences in training-induced changes in several endurance-related phenotypes were large, with the range between low and high responders reaching severalfold (6, 7, 10, 23, 34). The most extensive data on individual differences in trainability come from the HERITAGE Family Study, in which healthy but sedentary subjects followed a highly standardized, fully monitored and enforced, laboratory-based endurance-training program consisting of 60 exercise sessions over 20 weeks (204 families, 742 subjects) (11). In the entire HERITAGE cohort, the average increase in VO_2max was 384 ml/min with a standard deviation of 202 ml/min, while individual training responses varied from no change to increases of more than 1000 ml/min (8, 13). This heterogeneity in the response of VO_2max has been shown in several endurance training studies (31), as shown in Figure 14.4.

Interestingly, the marked interindividual differences in VO_2max responsiveness in HERITAGE was not accounted for by baseline VO_2max level, age, sex, or race. The HERITAGE Family Study is uniquely qualified to examine the contributions of these factors on responsiveness to standardized exercise training given its study design. Specifically, the HERITAGE cohort consisted of black and white families with both parents and three or more adult offspring that completed the same standardized and supervised endurance training program (11). Thus, analyses

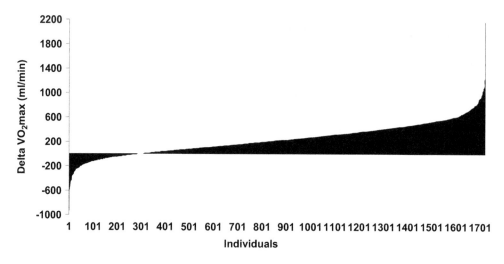

Figure 14.4 Heterogeneity of VO_2max response to endurance exercise training across 1724 participants from 8 studies and 14 different interventions.

in HERITAGE could examine the independent or combined effects of age (parents vs. offspring or continuous variable), sex, and race (black vs. white) on exercise responsiveness. For example, the same heterogeneity in response levels can be found in those who began the program with a low VO_2max and in those who were initially above the VO_2max median (13). A similar pattern of interindividual variation in training responses was observed for other endurance-related phenotypes in HERITAGE, including submaximal exercise stroke volume, cardiac output, heart rate, and blood pressure (15, 35, 36). These data demonstrate that interindividual variability in response to exercise training is common across diverse populations and exercise programs.

Heritability of the response of endurance traits to exercise training

Results from twin and family studies suggest that the marked interindividual differences in the trainability of phenotypes governing endurance performance is highly familial and genetically determined. Key twin and family studies examining these issues are summarized below.

Twin studies

A study of ten pairs of MZ twins subjected to 20 weeks of endurance training found a wide range of individual training gains in absolute VO_2max (0–41%), but the distribution of responses was not random among the twins. The intraclass correlation of VO_2max response (l/min) was 0.77, indicating that members of the same twin pair responded similarly to training, whereas there was almost eight times (F ratio=7.8) more variance between pairs of twins than within pairs for absolute VO_2max response (29). These results were replicated in two other studies of endurance training in MZ twins (16, 22), which showed intraclass correlations in response of VO_2max (l/min) of 0.44 and 0.65. Pooled results of the trainability of VO_2max in MZ twins from the three above-mentioned studies show there is about nine times more variance between genotypes than within genotypes in the response of VO_2max to standardized endurance training protocols (32). Similarly, pooled analysis of four twin studies (N=41 pairs) found the within-MZ pair correlation for relative VO_2max response to endurance training was 0.38 (95% CI 0.04–0.64) (37). A study of nine pairs of MZ twins aged 11–14 years that completed 6 months of endurance training used the between-pair variance to represent the heritability and found the heritability of relative VO_2max response to be 46% (19).

A significant intrapair resemblance of 0.60 for change in VO_2max was also observed in a study of seven male MZ twin pairs subjected to a negative energy balance protocol over a period of 3 months (14). The daily energy deficit was induced entirely by exercise training performed twice daily on a cycle ergometer, 9 out of 10 days, over a period of 93 days while subjects were kept on a constant daily energy and nutrient intake (14). In addition to VO_2max, there were significant within-pair resemblances in training response for submaximal exercise measures of VO_2 (r=0.87 and 0.76 at 50 and 150 W, respectively), respiratory quotient (r=0.86 and 0.87 at 100 and 150 W, respectively), and heart rate (r=0.70 and 0.63 at 50 and 150 W, respectively) (14). Lastly, two studies of MZ twins have also shown significant within-pair resemblance in training response for total power output during a 90-min maximal exercise test, with the ratio of between pairs to within pairs variances ranging from 5.5 to 11, and the intraclass coefficient for twin resemblance in response ranging from 0.69 to 0.83 (16, 22).

In summary, these studies showed that twin pairs are significantly more alike than unrelated individuals in their cardiorespiratory responses to standardized endurance training programs. Thus, a substantial genetic component exists in exercise training-induced changes in endurance-related phenotypes.

Family studies

To date, the only family study to examine the heritability of endurance-related phenotypes to exercise training is the HERITAGE Family Study. In HERITAGE, the increase in absolute VO_2max in 481 individuals from 99 two-generation families of Caucasian descent showed 2.5 times more variance between families than within families (8). Furthermore, under the most parsimonious model, the maximal heritability of absolute VO_2max response adjusted for age and sex was 47%. The authors found that adjusting for baseline VO_2max did not change the heritability estimate, indicating that the familial and genetic factors underlying intrinsic VO_2max and VO_2max response to training appear to be different. These findings are generally in agreement with those from pharmacological interventions. Combined analyses of genome-wide association study results from three trials of statin efficacy ($N=3928$) showed there was no overlap between the genetic variants associated with variation in the lipid levels of the cohort at baseline compared with those associated with the change in lipid levels (4). Thus, available evidence both from exercise and pharmacological interventions appear to show that the genetic factors influencing response to intervention differ from those affecting the intrinsic state of complex phenotypes.

In addition to VO_2max, significant familial aggregation and the heritability of training-induced changes in several other endurance-related phenotypes, including submaximal aerobic performance (27), resting and submaximal stroke volume, cardiac output, and heart rate were found in HERITAGE (1–3, 30). The response to exercise training of all measured submaximal endurance performance phenotypes showed significant familial resemblance in white families in HERITAGE, with maximal heritability values of 57% for ΔVO_2 at 50 W, 23% and 44% for ΔVO_2 at 60% and 80% of VO_2max, and 33% and 45% for ΔPower output at 60% and 80% of VO_2max (27). Analyses in HERITAGE also found a moderate familial component in the response of VO_2 at the ventilatory threshold to endurance exercise training in white subjects (heritability of 22%) and a larger component in black subjects (heritability of 51%) (21).

Submaximal exercise stroke volume and cardiac output were also characterized by a significant familial aggregation in response to endurance training in HERITAGE, as the between-family variation in adjusted stroke volume and cardiac output training responses at 50 W were 1.5 to 2.2 times greater than the within-family variation (2). In white families of HERITAGE, maximal heritability estimates were 29% and 38% for stroke volume and cardiac output training responses at 50 W, and 24% and 30% for the training-induced changes in stroke volume and cardiac output at 60% of VO_2max (12). In the entire HERITAGE cohort, there was 1.8 times more variance between families than within families for the response of submaximal heart rate (13), with maximal heritability estimates reaching 34% and 29% for heart rate training responses at 50 W and 60% of VO_2max, respectively, in white families (1).

Conclusion

Heterogeneity in the levels of complex traits is a normal biological phenomenon, which is not limited to the endurance-related phenotypes discussed in this chapter. It is ubiquitous and commonly observed in both the intrinsic (untrained) state and in response to training. Furthermore, interindividual differences in endurance traits are not randomly distributed, as they are characterized by significant familial aggregation. Significant heritability estimates have been reported for both intrinsic levels and training-induced changes in several endurance-related phenotypes, confirming that familial factors account for some of the interindividual variation in these phenotypes. Both twin and family studies show that individuals with the same genotype are more likely to have similar baseline levels of endurance traits, as well as respond more similarly to training than those with different genotypes. However, the evidence also suggests that there are *separate* genetic components affecting endurance-related phenotypes at baseline in the untrained state and in response to exercise training. Better understanding the genetic factors underlying interindividual differences in responsiveness to acute and regular exercise will allow for a better understanding of the biology of exercise response, as well as the potential to utilize genetic information in personalized exercise medicine.

References

1. **An P, Perusse L, Rankinen T, Borecki IB, Gagnon J, Leon AS, Skinner JS, Wilmore JH, Bouchard C**, and **Rao DC.** Familial aggregation of exercise heart rate and blood pressure in response to 20 weeks of endurance training: The HERITAGE family study. *Int J Sports Med* 24: 57–62, 2003.

2. **An P, Rice T, Gagnon J, Leon AS, Skinner JS, Bouchard C, Rao DC**, and **Wilmore JH.** Familial aggregation of stroke volume and cardiac output during submaximal exercise: The HERITAGE Family Study. *Int J Sports Med* 21: 566–572, 2000.

3. **An P, Rice T, Perusse L, Borecki IB, Gagnon J, Leon AS, Skinner JS, Wilmore JH, Bouchard C**, and **Rao DC.** Complex segregation analysis of blood pressure and heart rate measured before and after a 20-week endurance exercise training program: The HERITAGE Family Study. *Am J Hypertens* 13: 488–497, 2000.

4. **Barber MJ, Mangravite LM, Hyde CL, Chasman DI, Smith JD, McCarty CA, Li X, Wilke RA, Rieder MJ, Williams PT, Ridker PM, Chatterjee A, Rotter JI, Nickerson DA, Stephens M**, and **Krauss RM.** Genome-wide association of lipid-lowering response to statins in combined study populations. *PLoS One* 5: e9763, 2010.

5. **Beunen GP, Peeters MW**, and **Malina RM.** Twin studies in sports performance. In: *Genetic and Molecular Aspects of Sport Performance*, edited by Bouchard C and Hoffman EP. West Sussex, UK: Wiley-Blackwell, 2011, p. 101–109.

6. **Bouchard C.** Human adaptability may have a genetic basis. In: *Risk Reduction and Health Promotion: Proceedings of the 18th Annual Meeting of the Society of Prospective Medicine*, edited by Landry F. Ottawa: Canadian Public Health Association, 1983, p. 463–476.

7. **Bouchard C.** Individual differences in the response to regular exercise. *Int J Obes Relat Metab Disord* 19 Suppl 4: S5–8, 1995.

8. **Bouchard C, An P, Rice T, Skinner JS, Wilmore JH, Gagnon J, Perusse L, Leon AS**, and **Rao DC.** Familial aggregation of VO(2max) response to exercise training: Results from the HERITAGE Family Study. *J Appl Physiol* 87: 1003–1008, 1999.

9. **Bouchard C, Daw EW, Rice T, Perusse L, Gagnon J, Province MA, Leon AS, Rao DC, Skinner JS**, and **Wilmore JH.** Familial resemblance for VO2max in the sedentary state: The HERITAGE family study. *Med Sci Sports Exerc* 30: 252–258, 1998.

10. **Bouchard C, Dionne FT, Simoneau JA**, and **Boulay MR.** Genetics of aerobic and anaerobic performances. *Exerc Sport Sci Rev* 20: 27–58, 1992.

11. **Bouchard C, Leon AS, Rao DC, Skinner JS, Wilmore JH**, and **Gagnon J.** The HERITAGE family study. Aims, design, and measurement protocol. *Med Sci Sports Exerc* 27: 721–729, 1995.

12. **Bouchard C, Lesage R, Lortie G, Simoneau JA, Hamel P, Boulay MR, Perusse L, Theriault G**, and **Leblanc C.** Aerobic performance in brothers, dizygotic and monozygotic twins. *Med Sci Sports Exerc* 18: 639–646, 1986.

13. **Bouchard C**, and **Rankinen T.** Individual differences in response to regular physical activity. *Med Sci Sports Exerc* 33: S446–451, 2001.

14. **Bouchard C, Tremblay A, Despres JP, Theriault G, Nadeau A, Lupien PJ, Moorjani S, Prudhomme D**, and **Fournier G.** The response to exercise with constant energy intake in identical twins. *Obes Res* 2: 400–410, 1994.

15. **Bouchard C, Tremblay A, Nadeau A, Despres JP, Theriault G, Boulay MR, Lortie G, Leblanc C**, and **Fournier G.** Genetic effect in resting and exercise metabolic rates. *Metabolism* 38: 364–370, 1989.

16. **Boulay MR LG, Simoneau JA, Bouchard C.** Sensitivity of maximal aerobic power and capacity to anaerobic training is partly genotype dependent. In: *Sport and Human Genetics*, edited by Malina R., and Bouchard C. Champaign, IL: Human Kinetics, 1986, p. 173–181.

17. **Christensen K, Frederiksen H, Vaupel JW, and McGue M.** Age trajectories of genetic variance in physical functioning: A longitudinal study of Danish twins aged 70 years and older. *Behav Genet* 33: 125–136, 2003.

18. **Costa AM, Breitenfeld L, Silva AJ, Pereira A, Izquierdo M, and Marques MC.** Genetic inheritance effects on endurance and muscle strength: An update. *Sports Med* 42: 449–458, 2012.

19. **Danis A, Kyriazis Y, and Klissouras V.** The effect of training in male prepubertal and pubertal monozygotic twins. *Eur J Appl Physiol* 89: 309–318, 2003.

20. **Fagard R, Bielen E, and Amery A.** Heritability of aerobic power and anaerobic energy generation during exercise. *J Appl Physiol* 70: 357–362, 1991.

21. **Gaskill SE, Rice T, Bouchard C, Gagnon J, Rao DC, Skinner JS, Wilmore JH, and Leon AS.** Familial resemblance in ventilatory threshold: The HERITAGE Family Study. *Med Sci Sports Exerc* 33: 1832–1840, 2001.

22. **Hamel P, Simoneau JA, Lortie G, Boulay MR, and Bouchard C.** Heredity and muscle adaptation to endurance training. *Med Sci Sports Exerc* 18: 690–696, 1986.

23. **Lortie G, Simoneau JA, Hamel P, Boulay MR, Landry F, and Bouchard C.** Responses of maximal aerobic power and capacity to aerobic training. *Int J Sports Med* 5: 232–236, 1984.

24. **Miyamoto-Mikami E, Zempo H, Fuku N, Kikuchi N, Miyachi M, and Murakami H.** Heritability estimates of endurance-related phenotypes: A systematic review and meta-analysis. *Scand J Med Sci Sports* 28: 834–845, 2018.

25. **Ortega-Alonso A, Sipila S, Kujala UM, Kaprio J, and Rantanen T.** Longitudinal changes in genetic and environmental influences on older women's walking ability. *Scand J Med Sci Sports* 19: 669–677, 2009.

26. **Perusse L.** Role of genetic factors in sport performance: Evidence from family studies. In: *Genetic and Molecular Aspects of Sport Performance*, edited by Bouchard C and Hoffman EP. West Sussex, UK: Wiley-Blackwell, 2011, p. 90–100.

27. **Perusse L, Gagnon J, Province MA, Rao DC, Wilmore JH, Leon AS, Bouchard C, and Skinner JS.** Familial aggregation of submaximal aerobic performance in the HERITAGE Family study. *Med Sci Sports Exerc* 33: 597–604, 2001.

28. **Physical Activity Guidelines Advisory Committee.** *Physical Activity Guidelines Advisory Committee Report, 2008.* Washington, DC: Department of Health and Human Services, 2008.

29. **Prud'homme D, Bouchard C, Leblanc C, Landry F, and Fontaine E.** Sensitivity of maximal aerobic power to training is genotype-dependent. *Med Sci Sports Exerc* 16: 489–493, 1984.

30. **Rice T, An P, Gagnon J, Leon AS, Skinner JS, Wilmore JH, Bouchard C, and Rao DC.** Heritability of HR and BP response to exercise training in the HERITAGE Family Study. *Med Sci Sports Exerc* 34: 972–979, 2002.

31. **Ross LM, Church TS, Blair SN, Durstine JL, Hagberg JM, Martin CK, Rankinen T, Ross R, Bouchard C, and Sarzynski MA.** Prevalence of Vo2max low response across nine aerobic exercise interventions. *Med Sci Sports Exerc* 49: 838, 2017.

32. **Sarzynski MA, Rankinen T, and Bouchard C.** Twin and family studies of training responses. In: *Genetic and Molecular Aspects of Sport Performance*, edited by Bouchard C and Hoffman EP. West Sussex, UK: Wiley-Blackwell, 2011, p. 110–120.

33. **Schutte NM, Nederend I, Hudziak JJ, Bartels M, and de Geus EJ.** Twin-sibling study and meta-analysis on the heritability of maximal oxygen consumption. *Physiol Genomics* 48: 210–219, 2016.

34. **Simoneau JA, Lortie G, Boulay MR, Marcotte M, Thibault MC, and Bouchard C.** Inheritance of human skeletal muscle and anaerobic capacity adaptation to high-intensity intermittent training. *Int J Sports Med* 7: 167–171, 1986.

35. **Wilmore JH, Stanforth PR, Gagnon J, Rice T, Mandel S, Leon AS, Rao DC, Skinner JS, and Bouchard C.** Cardiac output and stroke volume changes with endurance training: The HERITAGE Family Study. *Med Sci Sports Exerc* 33: 99–106, 2001.

36. **Wilmore JH, Stanforth PR, Gagnon J, Rice T, Mandel S, Leon AS, Rao DC, Skinner JS, and Bouchard C.** Heart rate and blood pressure changes with endurance training: The HERITAGE Family Study. *Med Sci Sports Exerc* 33: 107–116, 2001.

37. **Zadro JR, Shirley D, Andrade TB, Scurrah KJ, Bauman A, and Ferreira PH.** The beneficial effects of physical activity: Is it down to your genes? A systematic review and meta-analysis of twin and family studies. *Sports Med Open* 3: 4, 2017.

15

GENETIC CONTRIBUTIONS TO CARDIORESPIRATORY FITNESS

Reuben Howden, Benjamin D.H. Gordon, and Ebony C. Gaillard

Introduction

In the animal kingdom, humans are impressive runners. While human sprint speed does not compare favorably with other animals (e.g., ~10 m/s for ~15 secs vs. 15–20 m/s for several minutes in horses), human capacity for endurance running is seldom rivaled (1). Cardiopulmonary function is a key feature of endurance running capacity and therefore the cardiopulmonary system was an important component in the genetic development (evolution) of *Homo*.

Cardiorespiratory fitness (CRF) is broadly defined as the capacity of circulatory and respiratory systems to deliver energy substrates and oxygen to muscles contributing to prolonged exercise. The principal components of CRF have been described beginning with the work of A.V. Hill and colleagues early in the 20th century (2). Low CRF is well established as an indicator of all-cause mortality risk (3, 4). Moreover, the health benefits of engaging in habitual exercise training that likely leads to improved CRF are well described (e.g., 5–8). Since CRF is determined mainly by cardiovascular and pulmonary capacity during exercise, this chapter will focus on these traits and their genetic underpinnings.

The standard measure for CRF is maximum capacity for oxygen consumption (VO_2max), which is a robust and reproducible measure with a reliability coefficient of at least 0.95 (9, 10). However, VO_2 max is defined by the Fick equation $Q \text{ Å} \sim A - VO_2$ difference, where Q is cardiac output (l/min) and $A-VO_2$ difference is the difference in oxygen content between arterial and venous blood, an index for cellular oxygen uptake. The Fick equation does not consider pulmonary function and is therefore a contradiction in terms as a measure of CRF (oxygen supply vs. oxygen uptake, i.e., exercising muscle does not uptake all oxygen supplied). Predicting cardiopulmonary fitness via VO_2max assessment has become an important determinant of not only the degree of adaptation to exercise training, but also mortality risk (11). The latter raises the question of whether a high CRF (via genetics or exercise training) is more or less important than simply engaging in physical activity regardless of its influence on CRF: genetics versus environment.

It has been argued that reaching a high level of performance (e.g., CRF) is solely dependent upon accumulating hours of so-called deliberate practice and is not limited by individual genotype (12, 13). Ericsson's model proposed that all individuals possess the necessary genetics to become expert performers. This suggests that any individual with sufficient determination could become competitive at the elite level, including sports performance, as long as they accumulate enough deliberate practice hours (the common figure suggested is 10,000 hours). However, it has been reported that athletes in sports where CRF is important can achieve elite status with considerably less "deliberate practice" than 10,000 hours (14, 15), suggesting a capacity for accelerated progression or responsiveness to training; ergo, a genetic component. In any case, the premise of Ericsson's "deliberate practice" model has been criticized in several reports, not least of all in a recent meta-analysis on deliberate practice and human performance in a number of categories, which found the deliberate practice only explained 18% of sports performance variability (16). This does not discount the critical importance of deliberate practice (training) to reach maximum possible individual performance. Indeed, failure of individuals to reach their maximum potential at a given activity has long been associated with a lack of commitment to practice or training (17). However, it does appear that a considerable proportion of human CRF levels are not explained by deliberate practice. Contributing factors to this large proportion of variability may include opportunity, environment, socioeconomic status, ethnic background, and sex, among others.

Interestingly, there is considerable variation between sedentary individuals in CRF, suggesting innate capacity (18). Evidence from twin human and inbred mouse (19) studies, as well as interindividual differences and sexual dimorphism (20), suggests genetic contributions to CRF and responses to exercise training (18, 21). These contributions are described in more detail in Chapters 13 and 14 of this book. To understand more about specific genes that may contribute to CRF, it is prudent to consider factors that determine or limit CRF and the genetics modifying those factors.

Cardiac function

Cardiac function is a major component of CRF and therefore is a key feature of the Fick equation describing VO_2. The job of the heart is to generate blood pressure and flow, moving deoxygenated blood through the pulmonary vasculature for gas exchange and then oxygenated, nutrient-rich blood through to the exchange vessels. Baseline cardiac function can provide insight into individual fitness levels. For example, lower resting heart rate (HR) suggests a larger stroke volume (SV) for a given cardiac output (Q). Variation in human HR carries approximately 50% heritability (22). However, in inbred mice, significant variation in resting HR, comprising a 296.4 bpm difference between 129/Svlm and Castaneous strains has been reported (23). Interestingly, there does not appear to be a relationship between untrained resting HR (23) and voluntary wheel running in inbred mice (24), suggesting that a low sedentary resting HR, usually associated with fitness, is not related to motivation for exercise. Strong evidence exists for resting HR being a heritable trait, with estimates ranging from approximately 51% to 65% (22, 25–28).

A higher maximum Q, within certain limits, results in higher CRF as determined by VO_2max (Fick equation). In the HERITAGE Family Study, heritability of SV and Q was approximately 40%, suggesting a moderate genetic influence on baseline cardiac function. Moreover, assessed at different submaximal exercise intensities (% VO_2max) heritability estimates for SV and Q were similar to baseline (41–46%) (29).

Variation in HR responses to exercise, before and after training, also suggest a genetic component to cardiac adaptation to exercise training. In HERITAGE, HRs at 50 W workload (HR50) were assessed before and after a 20-week endurance exercise training program (30). Interestingly, the mean training-induced reduction in HR50 was almost matched by the standard deviation. This variation in training responsiveness produced a heritability estimate of 34%, which may be important not only for exercise performance improvements, but also the degree to which mortality risk can be lowered. Previous reports have suggested that improvements in CRF are important in lowering mortality risk (11). Therefore, presumably the slope of the correlation between improved CRF and mortality risk may be influenced by genetics. However, this remains a controversial idea particularly in twin or rodent studies when habitual physical activity began in adulthood (31–33).

Cardiac function, QTL, and candidate genes

Limited work has been done to identify chromosomal regions (quantitative trait loci (QTL)) that associate with cardiac function. Inbred (30 strains) and recombinant inbred (29 AXB/BXA strains) mouse strain distributions for cardiac function were reported as continuous in quiescent mice (23). This suggests that cardiac phenotypes related to CRF such as resting HR are complex, meaning many genes are likely involved, which is not surprising. Others reported similar inbred strain distributions, although recorded resting HRs were generally higher, possibly due to using older mice and electrocardiographs (ECGs) were recorded in mice that were not quiescent (34). The conditions under which ECGs for cardiac function calculations are recorded is critical to consider since, for example, HR is highly sensitive to even minor stimuli (e.g., sound, smell, and vibration) detected by the research participant or animal which influences results. This is an important consideration, because although the genetic influences on inbred mouse HR responses to exercise have not been reported, there is evidence that genetic factors influencing cardiac function may differ when stress levels change (e.g., rest vs. exercise vs. training; see below).

QTL identified as associated with resting HR include mouse chromosomes 6 (23), 2, and 15 (35), rat chromosomes 2 (36), 3 (37) and 8 (38), and human chromosome 4 (39). However, these QTL are quite broad and therefore is it challenging to assess concordance between species. In any case, as stated previously, subtle differences in the precise conditions under which HRs were recorded and their influence on "resting" HR also make such a comparison difficult. Some of the previously identified HR QTL overlap with regions also reported to be associated with other cardiovascular phenotypes (e.g., blood pressure) (36), which should not be surprising, but does increase confidence in the importance of these chromosomal regions in cardiovascular regulation.

Proposed candidate genes within published QTL for resting HR include, but are not limited to, corticotropin-releasing factor receptor 2 and neuropeptide Y on mouse chromosome 6 (23), which have been associated with HR regulation elsewhere (40–42). Cholinergic receptor, nicotinic, polypeptide-α (*Chrna1*) on mouse chromosome 2 arising from a comparison between BALB/J and CBA/CaJ mice was identified as a candidate gene for resting HR (35). The influence of the parasympathetic nervous system on HR is well known and therefore, it is plausible that *Chrna1* could be important in HR regulation.

Studies reporting HR QTL are at least 10 years old and little has been done in terms of successful identification of genes within these QTL that have a functional influence on cardiovascular function. This is a problem well recognized especially for phenotypes that are influenced by many genes (complex traits) (43), but this may improve as the research tools needed to unravel the complexity of physiological phenomena continues to develop (44, 45).

Candidate genes associated with a complex and easily influenced phenotype such as HR are likely numerous. Cardiac function is influenced by multiple factors, including but not limited to peripheral neural inputs, central nervous system function, vascular function, and pulmonary function. The complexity of interactions within the cardiorespiratory system (46) makes genetic regulation very difficult to dissect. However, there has been progress in identifying candidates tor which there is evidence of an association between cardiac function and exercise (e.g., 47–51), which could be extrapolated to CRF. It is, however, beyond the scope of this chapter to discuss all reported genes associated with cardiac function or indeed CRF and therefore we discuss prominent examples only.

Aging is associated with reductions in cardiac function, but exercise training to improve CRF has been shown to attenuate this decline (52–54). The genetic influences on cardiac function adaptation to exercise training in the aged appear to be associated with an attenuation of the known switch in myosin heavy chain isoform from α to β and therefore lower sarcoplasmic reticulum Ca^{2+} ATPase activity (55, 56). This effect of exercise training was reported in aged rats and was controlled via an attenuated age-related decline in myocyte thyroid receptor (TR) protein expression (47), which has been associated with rat cardiac hypertrophy (57). A similar effect on TR protein expression was also reported after exercise training in post-myocardial infarction (58). Taken together, these studies suggest that exercise training induced improvements in cardiac function and therefore CRF may in part operate through changes in TR expression during aging or pathology.

An increase in left ventricular mass is a well-established adaptation to exercise training that improves CRF. Genes that have been reported as associated with left ventricular mass include, but are not limited to, angiotensin-converting enzyme (*ACE*; (59, 60, 61), peroxisome proliferator-activated receptor alpha (*PPARα*; 62), G-protein β3 subunit (*GNB3*; 63) and aldosterone synthase (*CYP11B2*; 64).

A polymorphism in the *ACE* gene (deletion/insertion) has received significant attention in association with ventricular hypertrophy with (59, 60) and without (61) hypertension. Moreover, associations between *ACE* polymorphisms and athletic ability have already been reviewed (65). It is well known that ACE plays a key role in vascular function by producing the vasoconstrictor angiotensin II and degrades vasodilator kinins (66). It is also well established that increases in sympathetic nerve activity during exercise lead to increased production of angiotensin II, which acts as a nonadrenergic vasoconstrictor contributing to blood flow redistribution supporting active muscle function. This role of angiotensin II in blood flow redistribution is a critical component to maximizing delivery of oxygen and nutrient-rich blood to active muscle during exercise and therefore CRF. Moreover, ACE has been associated with exercising muscle function, especially in sprinters (67), but it is beyond the scope of this chapter to discuss exercising muscle function in detail.

Calcineurin is a well-known component of calcium signaling, especially in myocardial hypertrophy (68). Indeed, calcineurin deficiency in mice was associated with lower cardiac mass (69). Moreover, calcineurin polymorphisms were reported to influence cardiac adaptations to cycle-ergometry training, assessed by postexercise HR responses. Other polymorphisms in the same gene are associated with resting HR, which is of well-established clinical significance (70).

Interestingly, there is evidence that genes influencing cardiac function at rest in untrained subjects are not necessarily important in cardiac adaptations induced by exercise training. For example, heme oxygenase 1 (*HMOX1*), which is involved in heme catabolism under conditions of oxidative stress and hypoxia among other stressors, has been shown to influence SV and Q at rest and in response to exercise. However, *HMOX1* was not associated with SV and Q adaptations induced by exercise training (71).

Differential genetic regulators of the same phenotypes have been shown previously. A QTL associated with baseline HR (chromosome 6) (23) was different from a QTL associated with HR responses to oxidative stress (chromosomes 3, 5, and 9) (72). This serves to illustrate the complexity of genetic influences on cardiac function, a major component of CRF.

Respiratory function

The respiratory system functions to move oxygen (O_2) from ambient air into blood and for excess carbon dioxide (CO_2) to be move from blood to ambient air (gas exchange), a critical component of CRF. Dalton's law of partial pressures describes the relative concentrations of gases in a mixture (e.g., blood gases) where the total pressure of a gas mixture is the sum of the partial pressures exerted by each gas within that mixture. For example, the partial pressure of oxygen (PO_2) in pulmonary capillary blood is lower than the PO_2 in alveolar space and therefore oxygen will move (diffuse) into the blood and bind to hemoglobin. Conversely, pulmonary capillary blood PCO_2 is higher than alveolar PCO_2, which drives movement of CO_2 from blood into alveolar space.

Factors effecting gas exchange between the alveoli and blood are described by Fick's law of diffusion where surface area for gas exchange, the distance gases must travel in order to move from one space to another, and the partial pressure difference between the two spaces principally effect diffusion in biological and nonbiological systems. This process is facilitated by the anatomy and physiology of the respiratory system, for example, the close proximity of pulmonary capillaries to alveoli reducing the distance gases must travel during diffusion or the density of the erythrocytes in pulmonary capillaries for oxygen to bind to thus helping to maintain gas concentration gradients in the right direction.

In addition to gas exchange governed by diffusion, intercostal and diaphragmatic muscle function are key components of pulmonary capacity. Moreover, oxygenation of blood is facilitated by the pulmonary and cardiovascular systems being regulated in concert. For example, pulmonary inspiration is accompanied by vagal nerve inhibition, increasing Q and pulmonary blood flow when pulmonary oxygen levels are highest.

Pulmonary function tests are used to measure pulmonary capacity in health and disease, and include measures of forced vital capacity (FVC), forced expiratory volume in 1 second (FEV_1), and forced expiratory flow at 25–75% FVC (FEF_{25-75}). Attenuation of age-related decline and improvement in respiratory function as well as exercise performance are all associated with habitual physical activity (73). Interestingly, the highest level of pulmonary function has been reported in elite athletes and although increases in diffusion capacity are possible for habitual exercisers, it appears unlikely that nonelite athletes will reach the pulmonary capacities of elite athletes. This suggests a genetic influence on pulmonary capacity.

Heritability of and QTL for pulmonary function

Early estimates of pulmonary function heritability between parents and offspring in FEV_1 and FEF_{25-75} were between 40% and 50% (74). In Swedish twins, heritability estimates for FVC and FEV_1 were reported as 48% and 67% respectively (75) (mean age ~65 years), which was similar to an earlier estimate for FEV_1 of 77% in American male twins between 42 and 56 years of age (76). Interestingly, Hubert et al. (1982) also reported that the variation in FVC was explained by pack-years of smoking, as well as genetically driven factors related to body size, demonstrating a gene–environment interaction. Heritability estimates for pulmonary function are quite consistent compared to cardiac phenotypes, perhaps because pulmonary function is less sensitive to acute environmental influences.

There are a limited number of studies regarding QTL analyses associated with pulmonary function. Part of the complication is the number of potential phenotypes of interest that are commonly used to assess different aspects of pulmonary function. Using minute ventilation, breathing frequency, and tidal volume to represent resting pulmonary function in a recombinant inbred mouse strain set (29 strains), no significant phenotypic differences or QTL were found (23). In human studies, a region on chromosome 6 was associated with FEV_1 and the FEV_1/FVC ratio (77). This suggests that if functional tests of pulmonary function are used to assess phenotypes, it is more likely that heritability estimates and pulmonary function QTL are identified. There is much work to be done regarding genetic influences of pulmonary function in relation to CRF.

Pulmonary function and genetics

One approach to increase oxygen-carrying capacity and therefore CRF is living at high altitude and training at low altitude. The premise of this strategy is to stimulate red blood cell production at high altitude while maintaining high-quality training at low altitude. Extensive study of the efficacy of "live high, train low" has revealed responders or nonresponders with regard to increased altitude-induced erythropoietin (EPO) stimulation (78). For example, altitude exposure-induced increases in packed cell volume was matched by an increase in VO_2max in responders only. The differential responsiveness to altitude-induced improvements in oxygen-carrying capacity between individuals suggests a genetic component.

Hypoxia-inducible factor 1α (HIF-1α) mediates EPO expression, in response to low ambient PO_2 at high altitude, resulting in an increase in red blood cell count, improved gas exchange, increasing oxygen-carrying capacity and CRF. As suggested earlier, results from reports on this topic have been inconsistent with increases (79, 80), no change (81, 82), or no response in red blood cell production despite increases in plasma EPO concentrations (83), although the length of time spent at altitude may also be an important factor in the interindividual differences in responses to hypoxia exposure (84).

Alveolar angiogenesis in response to exercise training improves pulmonary function and potentially CRF. The genetic influences on alveolar angiogenesis are quite well characterized and are mediated by VEGF and FGF (85). Increased vascularization of alveoli induced by exercise training could potentially improve pulmonary gas exchange and therefore CRF but it has not been demonstrated in humans yet. Conversely, some studies have had difficulty in demonstrating that alveolar capillaries specifically are capable of an angiogenic response during induced pulmonary hypertension, at least in rats (86, 87).

Hypoxia, pulmonary function, and genetics

The reduction in ambient PO_2 with height above sea level and therefore VO_2max means that altitude presents increasing limitations on pulmonary function (88) and CRF. At sea level, arterial PO_2 (PaO_2) remains close to resting levels even as exercise intensity increases because ambient PO_2 (101.3 kPa) is high enough for effective gas exchange (89, 90). However, as ambient PO_2 declines with increasing altitude, resting PaO_2 levels become progressively more difficult to achieve. Low PaO_2 at high altitude has been reported previously (91–94) making pulmonary gas exchange increasingly more difficult, particularly during exercise (e.g., mountaineering). In an attempt to maintain PaO_2, pulmonary function responses to reduced ambient PO_2 include increases in pulmonary ventilation (Ve). Pugh et al. (1964) demonstrated that a 2 l/min VO_2 at sea level resulted in a 40 l/min Ve. However, at 5800 m altitude, a Ve of about 180 l/min was required to achieve the same VO_2. At 7400 m altitude, the same VO_2 was not possible (95). Exceptionally low VO_2max levels are present at Mt. Everest's summit, estimated at less than 20 ml/min/kg compared to a typical sea-level VO_2max of 50–70 ml/kg/min (91, 95). Previous to the first "oxygenless" ascent to the summit of Mt. Everest by Messner and Habeler in 1978, studies conducted by Rodolfo Margaria and Joseph Barcroft suggested it was not possible for humans (96).

At the time of writing, only 208 people have been able to climb Mt. Everest without supplemental oxygen since 1978. This suggests a special ability possessed by a limited number of successful Mt. Everest climbers (>4800 people), which could have a genetic component, although this is poorly understood. Certainly, a high CRF is important for successful mountaineering, which is well known to possess a genetic influence (see earlier in this section) (97).

High-altitude versus sea-level dwellers

Several populations live at altitude and therefore hypobaric hypoxia. This provides an interesting opportunity to understand the resulting chronic adaptations. An estimated 140 million people reside at altitudes above 2500 m (98) and for thousands of years, several populations have inhabited altitudes exceeding 3000 m (99).

Nahua, Quechua, and Ayamara in the Andes, Ethiopians in Northern Africa, Sherpa, Tibetans, and Ladakhi on the Tibetan Plateau, and the Kyrgyz in the Asian Tien-Shan and Pamir mountains are examples of populations living in high-altitude regions (99, 100). Natural selection appears to have influenced survival and hence reproductive success in relation to pulmonary function in a hypobaric hypoxic environment and interestingly the adaptations are divergent between high-altitude dwellers in different regions. As an example, heritability estimates for resting ventilation, ventilator response to hypobaric hypoxia, hemoglobin concentration, and PaO_2 differed between Tibetan and Andean high-altitude populations (101, 102). Specifically, Tibetan populations had a higher resting ventilation (19.7 l/min; males) compared to Andean Aymara populations (13.4 l/min; males) despite lifelong adaptation at a similar altitude (101). However, the variation in resting ventilation measurements taken from the Tibetan populations was higher than the Andean population for both males and females, which could have contributed to the differences between the populations (101).

Other differences in pulmonary function between Tibetan and Andean populations include the hypoxic ventilator response (HVR), which is a standard test for ventilatory reactivity, where the Tibetan HVR was higher. Interestingly, HVR heritability was estimated at 13% higher in the Tibetan population (101), although the genetic mechanisms associated with the differences in pulmonary function between these populations are poorly understood.

Similar genetic variation between Tibetan and sea-level populations have been reported (103–106), which may be due to insufficient selection pressure for different HVRs in Tibet (107). However, HVRs in Andean populations were significantly different from both Tibetan and sea-level populations. The strategy of higher resting ventilation and HVR could be considered beneficial under conditions of low ambient PO_2 to ensure sufficient gas exchange and blood oxygenation. However, blood oxygen saturation was lower in the Tibetan, compared to the Andean populations (101). Although speculative, taken together, these studies do suggest that natural selection played a role in the success of these populations in their hypoxic environments, even though the phenotypic outcomes differed. However, one important consideration that must not be overlooked when discussing the impact of natural selection on gas exchange adaptations is whether there has been sufficient time for high-altitude dwellers to be affected by the process of natural selection or whether each individual born in to these populations have to adapt to ambient conditions after birth.

The Andean populations in question have resided at high altitude for approximately 11,000 years and Tibetan populations for twice as long. Using calculations for assessing the required length of time for adaptations to occur by natural selection (108), these time spans equate to approximately 550 and 1100 generations respectively, which should provide enough opportunity for sufficient meiotic events for significant adaptation by natural selection to improve gas exchange ability at high altitude. This suggests permanent genomic differences between these high-altitude dwellers and sea-level inhabitants.

Candidate genes for pulmonary function responses and adaptations to hypoxia

Although the genetic regulation of pulmonary responses to hypoxia is not well understood, a number of potential candidate genes have been identified. For example, HIF transcription factors are protective against hypoxic injury (109–111). During prolonged hypoxia, HIF increases EPO expression, increasing erythrocyte number (polycythemia) and improving blood oxygenation (112), although this response may take weeks of exposure to occur (95). HIF is involved in many other physiological and developmental processes which have been reviewed elsewhere (113), but this does highlight the genetic influences on hypoxia-induced responses and adaptations. Moreover, HIF has been implicated in the regulation of angiogenesis involving vascular endothelial growth factor and EPO in response to exercise training and therefore improved CRF (for review, see 114).

The proinflammatory cytokine tumor necrosis factor-α (TNF-α) production increases during hypoxia. This effect is especially important in lung disease patients, increasing pulmonary inflammation and reducing pulmonary function. However, the precise role of TNF-α, in addition to interleukin-1 (IL-1; both α and β) during hypoxia is not clear because it has been reported to attenuate *EPO* gene expression (115, 116), as well as increase *HIF-1* expression (117). Interestingly, TNF-α is associated with endothelial damage, which could be detrimental to CRF. However, chronic exercise training has been shown to attenuate TNF-α expression at least in heart failure patients (118), further illustrating the importance of habitual physical activity and improved CRF.

Summary

CRF can be defined by the capacity of the cardiorespiratory system to deliver oxygenated blood to muscles contributing to prolonged exercise. Physical activity designed to improve CRF is an important component of reducing health risks. This chapter provides a brief overview of the kinds of genetic influences on innate CRF, responsiveness to exercise training to improve CRF, and examples of candidate genes that may be involved.

Importantly, human evolution has involved running and therefore humans are endowed with numerous and complex genetic mechanisms associated with exercise capacity (i.e., running capacity improved survival). However, there is considerable between-individual variation in the extent to which genetics influence CRF and individual responsiveness to training. This suggests that some individuals possess a genetic advantage, not just in terms of athletic performance, but also in their capacity to reduce health risks by engaging in habitual physical activity. On the other hand, the accepted concept of larger CRF gains with exercise training in those with a low innate CRF may confer an advantage in terms of reductions in CRF-related health risks. It is not clear, however, if innate CRF is the crucial component to reduced health risk or engaging in habitual physical activity that results in improved CRF.

Both cardiovascular and pulmonary function are the key components of CRF and major genetic influences have been reported, including estimates of genetic contributions to interindividual differences, QTL analyses, and candidate gene proposals. In the future, it will be challenging to dissect the complexity of genetic influences on CRF because gene expression combinations are not consistent under differing environmental conditions (e.g., sea level vs. altitude (hypoxia). However, it may be possible to improve our understanding of these genetics mechanisms to design individualized training programs based on genotype, to maximize exercise training responsiveness and therefore the accompanying health benefits.

References

1. **Bramble**, **D.M.** and **D.E. Lieberman**, Endurance running and the evolution of Homo. *Nature*, 2004. 432(7015): p. 345–52.
2. **Hill**, **A.V.** and **H. Lupton**, Muscular exercise, lactic acid, and the supply and utilization of oxygen. *QJM*, 1923. 16(62): p. 135–71.
3. **Laukkanen**, **J.A.**, et al., The predictive value of cardiorespiratory fitness for cardiovascular events in men with various risk profiles: a prospective population-based cohort study. *Eur Heart J*, 2004. 25(16): p. 1428–37.
4. **Kodama**, **S.**, et al., Cardiorespiratory fitness as a quantitative predictor of all-cause mortality and cardiovascular events in healthy men and women: a meta-analysis. *JAMA*, 2009. 301(19): p. 2024–35.
5. **Myers**, **J.**, et al., Exercise capacity and mortality among men referred for exercise testing. *N Engl J Med*, 2002. 346(11): p. 793–801.
6. **Church**, **T.S.**, et al., Effects of different doses of physical activity on cardiorespiratory fitness among sedentary, overweight or obese postmenopausal women with elevated blood pressure: a randomized controlled trial. *JAMA*, 2007. 297(19): p. 2081–91.
7. **Kelley**, **G.A.** and **K.S. Kelley**, Efficacy of aerobic exercise on coronary heart disease risk factors. *Prev Cardiol*, 2008. 11(2): p. 71–5.
8. **Church**, **T.S.**, et al., Effects of aerobic and resistance training on hemoglobin A1c levels in patients with type 2 diabetes: a randomized controlled trial. *JAMA*, 2010. 304(20): p. 2253–62.
9. **Boulay**, **M.R.**, et al., A test of aerobic capacity: description and reliability. *Can J Appl Sport Sci*, 1984. 9(3): p. 122–6.
10. **Prud'Homme**, **D.**, et al., Reliability of assessments of ventilatory thresholds. *J Sports Sci*, 1984. 2(1): p. 13–24.
11. **Lee**, **D.C.**, et al., Mortality trends in the general population: the importance of cardiorespiratory fitness. *J Psychopharmacol*, 2010. 24(4 Suppl): p. 27–35.
12. **Ericsson**, **K.A.**, **R.T. Krampe**, and **S. Heizmann**, Can we create gifted people? *Ciba Found Symp*, 1993. 178: p. 222–31.
13. **Ericsson**, **K.A.**, Deliberate practice and acquisition of expert performance: a general overview. *Acad Emerg Med*, 2008. 15(11): p. 988–94.
14. **Gibbons**, **T.**, *The Path to Excellence: A Comprehensive View of Development of US Olympians Who Competed from 1984–1998*. Colorado Springs, CO: United States Olympic Committee, 2002.
15. **Baker**, **J.**, **J. Côté**, and **J. Deakin**, Expertise in ultra-endurance triathletes early sport involvement, training structure, and the theory of deliberate practice. *J Appl Sport Psychol*, 2005. 17(1): p. 64–78.
16. **Macnamara**, **B.N.**, **D.Z. Hambrick**, and **F.L. Oswald**, Deliberate practice and performance in music, games, sports, education, and professions: a meta-analysis. *Psychol Sci*, 2014. 25(8): p. 1608–18.
17. **Watson**, **J.B.**, *Behaviorism*, revised edn. New York: WW Norton & Company, 1930.
18. **Bouchard**, **C.** and **T. Rankinen**, Individual differences in response to regular physical activity. *Med Sci Sports Exerc*, 2001. 33(6 Suppl): p. S446–51.
19. **Swallow**, **J.G.**, et al., Effects of voluntary activity and genetic selection on aerobic capacity in house mice (Mus domesticus). *J Appl Physiol (1985)*, 1998. 84(1): p. 69–76.
20. **Pate**, **R.R.** and **A. Kriska**, Physiological basis of the sex difference in cardiorespiratory endurance. *Sports Med*, 1984. 1(2): p. 87–89.
21. **Prud'homme**, **D.**, et al., Sensitivity of maximal aerobic power to training is genotype-dependent. *Med Sci Sports Exerc*, 1984. 16(5): p. 489–93.
22. **Zhang**, **K.**, et al., Human heart rate: heritability of resting and stress values in twin pairs, and influence of genetic variation in the adrenergic pathway at a microribonucleic acid (microrna) motif in the 3'-UTR of cytochrome b561 [corrected]. *J Am Coll Cardiol*, 2014. 63(4): p. 358–68.
23. **Howden**, **R.**, et al., The genetic contribution to heart rate and heart rate variability in quiescent mice. *Am J Physiol Heart Circ Physiol*, 2008. 295(1): p. H59–68.

24. **Lightfoot, J.T.**, et al., Genetic influence on daily wheel running activity level. *Physiol Genomics*, 2004. 19(3): p. 270–6.

25. **Ditto, B.**, Familial influences on heart rate, blood pressure, and self-report anxiety responses to stress: results from 100 twin pairs. *Psychophysiology*, 1993. 30(6): p. 635–45.

26. **De Geus, E.J., D.I. Boomsma**, and **H. Snieder**, Genetic correlation of exercise with heart rate and respiratory sinus arrhythmia. *Med Sci Sports Exerc*, 2003. 35(8): p. 1287–95.

27. **Dalageorgou, C.**, et al., Heritability of QT interval: how much is explained by genes for resting heart rate? *J Cardiovasc Electrophysiol*, 2008. 19(4): p. 386–91.

28. **Wu, T., F.A. Treiber**, and **H. Snieder**, Genetic influence on blood pressure and underlying hemodynamics measured at rest and during stress. *Psychosom Med*, 2013. 75(4): p. 404–12.

29. **An, P.**, et al., Familial aggregation of stroke volume and cardiac output during submaximal exercise: the HERITAGE Family Study. *Int J Sports Med*, 2000. 21(8): p. 566–72.

30. **An, P.**, et al., Evidence of major genes for exercise heart rate and blood pressure at baseline and in response to 20 weeks of endurance training: the HERITAGE family study. *Int J Sports Med*, 2003. 24(7): p. 492–8.

31. **Edington, D.W., A.C. Cosmas**, and **W.B. McCafferty**, Exercise and longevity: evidence for a threshold age. *J Gerontol*, 1972. 27(3): p. 341–3.

32. **Goodrick, C.L.**, et al., Effects of intermittent feeding upon growth and life span in rats. *Gerontology*, 1982. 28(4): p. 233–41.

33. **Kujala, U.M., J. Kaprio**, and **M. Koskenvuo**, Modifiable risk factors as predictors of all-cause mortality: the roles of genetics and childhood environment. *Am J Epidemiol*, 2002. 156(11): p. 985–93.

34. **Xing, S.**, et al., Genetic influence on electrocardiogram time intervals and heart rate in aging mice. *Am J Physiol Heart Circ Physiol*, 2009. 296(6): p. H1907–13.

35. **Sugiyama, F.**, et al., QTL associated with blood pressure, heart rate, and heart weight in CBA/CaJ and BALB/cJ mice. *Physiol Genomics*, 2002. 10(1): p. 5–12.

36. **Alemayehu, A.**, et al., Reciprocal rat chromosome 2 congenic strains reveal contrasting blood pressure and heart rate QTL. *Physiol Genomics*, 2002. 10(3): p. 199–210.

37. **Kreutz, R.**, et al., Evidence for primary genetic determination of heart rate regulation: chromosomal mapping of a genetic locus in the rat. *Circulation*, 1997. 96(4): p. 1078–81.

38. **Silva, G.J.**, et al., Genetic mapping of a new heart rate QTL on chromosome 8 of spontaneously hypertensive rats. *BMC Med Genet*, 2007. 8: p. 17.

39. **Martin, L.J.**, et al., Major quantitative trait locus for resting heart rate maps to a region on chromosome 4. *Hypertension*, 2004. 43(5): p. 1146–51.

40. **Stiedl, O.** and **M. Meyer**, Cardiac dynamics in corticotropin-releasing factor receptor subtype-2 deficient mice. *Neuropeptides*, 2003. 37(1): p. 3–16.

41. **Tovote, P.**, et al., Central NPY receptor-mediated alteration of heart rate dynamics in mice during expression of fear conditioned to an auditory cue. *Regul Pept*, 2004. 120(1–3): p. 205–14.

42. **Warner, M.R.** and **M.N. Levy**, Neuropeptide Y as a putative modulator of the vagal effects on heart rate. *Circ Res*, 1989. 64(5): p. 882–9.

43. **Kleeberger, S.R.** and **D.A. Schwartz**, From quantitative trait locus to gene: a work in progress. *Am J Respir Crit Care Med*, 2005. 171(8): p. 804–5.

44. **Kloosterman, B.**, et al., From QTL to candidate gene: genetical genomics of simple and complex traits in potato using a pooling strategy. *BMC Genomics*, 2010. 11: p. 158.

45. **Drinkwater, N.R.** and **M.N. Gould**, The long path from QTL to gene. *PLoS Genet*, 2012. 8(9): p. e1002975.

46. **De Burgh Daly, M.**, Interactions between respiration and circulation, in: Cherniack NS, Widdicombe JG, eds. *Handbook of Physiology, Section 3: The Respiratory System, Vol II: Control of Breathing, Part 2*. Bethesda, MD: American Physiological Society; 1986, p. 529–94.

47. **Iemitsu, M.**, et al., Exercise training improves cardiac function-related gene levels through thyroid hormone receptor signaling in aged rats. *Am J Physiol Heart Circ Physiol*, 2004. 286(5): p. H1696–705.

48. **Jin, H.**, et al., Effects of exercise training on cardiac function, gene expression, and apoptosis in rats. *Am J Physiol Heart Circ Physiol*, 2000. 279(6): p. H2994–3002.

49. **Das, H.**, et al., Stem cell therapy with overexpressed VEGF and PDGF genes improves cardiac function in a rat infarct model. *PLoS One*, 2009. 4(10): p. e7325.

50. **Jamshidi, Y.**, et al., Peroxisome proliferator–activated receptor α gene regulates left ventricular growth in response to exercise and hypertension. *Circulation*, 2002. 105(8): p. 950–5.

51. **Boström, P.**, et al., C/EBPβ controls exercise-induced cardiac growth and protects against pathological cardiac remodeling. *Cell*, 2010. 143(7): p. 1072–1083.

52. **Levy, W.C.**, et al., Effect of endurance exercise training on heart rate variability at rest in healthy young and older men. *Am J Cardiol*, 1998. 82(10): p. 1236–1241.

53. **Li, Y.**, et al., Age-related differences in effect of exercise training on cardiac muscle function in rats. *Am J Physiol*, 1986. 251(1 Pt 2): p. H12–18.

54. **Wei, J.Y.**, et al., Chronic exercise training protects aged cardiac muscle against hypoxia. *J Clin Invest*, 1989. 83(3): p. 778–84.

55. **McNally, E.M.**, et al., Full-length rat alpha and beta cardiac myosin heavy chain sequences. Comparisons suggest a molecular basis for functional differences. *J Mol Biol*, 1989. 210(3): p. 665–71.

56. **Tate, C.A.**, et al., SERCA2a and mitochondrial cytochrome oxidase expression are increased in hearts of exercise-trained old rats. *Am J Physiol*, 1996. 271(1 Pt 2): p. H68–72.

57. **Kinugawa, K.**, et al., Regulation of thyroid hormone receptor isoforms in physiological and pathological cardiac hypertrophy. *Circ Res*, 2001. 89(7): p. 591–8.

58. **Xu, X.**, et al., Post-myocardial infarction exercise training beneficially regulates thyroid hormone receptor isoforms. *J Physiol Sci*, 2018. 68(6): p. 743–8.

59. **Schunkert, H.**, et al., Association between a deletion polymorphism of the angiotensin-converting-enzyme gene and left ventricular hypertrophy. *N Engl J Med*, 1994. 330(23): p. 1634–8.

60. **Celentano, A.**, et al., Cardiovascular risk factors, angiotensin-converting enzyme gene I/D polymorphism, and left ventricular mass in systemic hypertension. *Am J Cardiol*, 1999. 83(8): p. 1196–200.

61. **Kuznetsova, T.**, et al., Left ventricular mass in relation to genetic variation in angiotensin II receptors, renin system genes, and sodium excretion. *Circulation*, 2004. 110(17): p. 2644–50.

62. **Jamshidi, Y.**, et al., Peroxisome proliferator – activated receptor alpha gene regulates left ventricular growth in response to exercise and hypertension. *Circulation*, 2002. 105(8): p. 950–5.

63. **Poch, E.**, et al., Genetic variation of the gamma subunit of the epithelial Na+ channel and essential hypertension. Relationship with salt sensitivity. *Am J Hypertens*, 2000. 13(6 Pt 1): p. 648–53.

64. **Kupari, M.**, et al., Left ventricular size, mass, and function in relation to angiotensin-converting enzyme gene polymorphism in humans. *Am J Physiol*, 1994. 267(3 Pt 2): p. H1107–11.

65. **Puthucheary, Z.**, et al., The ACE gene and human performance: 12 years on. *Sports Med*, 2011. 41(6): p. 433–48.

66. **Coates, D.**, The angiotensin converting enzyme (ACE). *Int J Biochem Cell Biol*, 2003. 35(6): p. 769–73.

67. **Gunel, T.**, et al., Effect of angiotensin I-converting enzyme and alpha-actinin-3 gene polymorphisms on sport performance. *Mol Med Rep*, 2014. 9(4): p. 1422–6.

68. **Molkentin, J.D.**, et al., A calcineurin-dependent transcriptional pathway for cardiac hypertrophy. *Cell*, 1998. 93(2): p. 215–28.

69. **Bueno, O.F.**, et al., Impaired cardiac hypertrophic response in calcineurin Abeta-deficient mice. *Proc Natl Acad Sci U S A*, 2002. 99(7): p. 4586–91.

70. **He, Z.H.**, et al., Polymorphisms in the calcineurin genes are associated with the training responsiveness of cardiac phenotypes in Chinese young adults. *Eur J Appl Physiol*, 2010. 110(4): p. 761–7.

71. **He, Z.**, et al., Association between HMOX-1 genotype and cardiac function during exercise. *Appl Physiol Nutr Metab*, 2008. 33(3): p. 450–60.

72. **Howden, R.**, et al., Cardiac physiologic and genetic predictors of hyperoxia-induced acute lung injury in mice. *Am J Respir Cell Mol Biol*, 2012. 46(4): p. 470–8.

73. **American College of Sports** Medicine, et al., American College of Sports Medicine position stand. Exercise and physical activity for older adults. *Med Sci Sports Exerc*, 2009. 41(7): p. 1510–30.

74. **Lewitter, F.I.**, et al., Genetic and environmental determinants of level of pulmonary function. *Am J Epidemiol*, 1984. 120(4): p. 518–30.

75. **McClearn, G.E.**, et al., Genetic and environmental influences on pulmonary function in aging Swedish twins. *J Gerontol*, 1994. 49(6): p. 264–8.

76. **Hubert, H.B.**, et al., Genetic and environmental influences on pulmonary function in adult twins. *Am Rev Respir Dis*, 1982. 125(4): p. 409–15.

77. **Wilk, J.B.**, et al., Linkage and association with pulmonary function measures on chromosome 6q27 in the Framingham Heart Study. *Hum Mol Genet*, 2003. 12(21): p. 2745–51.

78. **Levine, B.D.** and **J. Stray-Gundersen**, Point: positive effects of intermittent hypoxia (live high:train low) on exercise performance are mediated primarily by augmented red cell volume. *J Appl Physiol (1985)*, 2005. 99(5): p. 2053–5.

79. **Wehrlin, J.P.**, et al., Live high-train low for 24 days increases hemoglobin mass and red cell volume in elite endurance athletes. *J Appl Physiol (1985)*, 2006. 100(6): p. 1938-45.

80. **Stray-Gundersen, J., R.F. Chapman**, and **B.D. Levine**, "Living high-training low" altitude training improves sea level performance in male and female elite runners. *J Appl Physiol (1985)*, 2001. 91(3): p. 1113–20.

81. **Ashenden, M.J.**, et al., "Live high, train low" does not change the total haemoglobin mass of male endurance athletes sleeping at a simulated altitude of 3000 m for 23 nights. *Eur J Appl Physiol Occup Physiol*, 1999. 80(5): p. 479–84.

82. **Ashenden, M.J.**, et al., Effects of a 12-day "live high, train low" camp on reticulocyte production and haemoglobin mass in elite female road cyclists. *Eur J Appl Physiol Occup Physiol*, 1999. 80(5): p. 472–8.

83. **Gore, C.J.**, et al., Increased serum erythropoietin but not red cell production after 4 wk of intermittent hypobaric hypoxia (4,000–5,500 m). *J Appl Physiol (1985)*, 2006. 101(5): p. 1386–93.

84. **Friedmann, B.**, et al., Individual variation in the reduction of heart rate and performance at lactate thresholds in acute normobaric hypoxia. *Int J Sports Med*, 2005. 26(7): p. 531–6.

85. **Lewis, B.S.**, et al., Angiogenesis by gene therapy: a new horizon for myocardial revascularization? *Cardiovasc Res*, 1997. 35(3): p. 490–7.

86. **Schraufnagel, D.E.**, Monocrotaline-induced angiogenesis. Differences in the bronchial and pulmonary vasculature. *Am J Pathol*, 1990. 137(5): p. 1083–90.

87. **Peao, M.N.**, et al., Neoformation of blood vessels in association with rat lung fibrosis induced by bleomycin. *Anat Rec*, 1994. 238(1): p. 57–67.

88. **West, J.B.**, Human physiology at extreme altitudes on Mount Everest. *Science*, 1984. 223(4638): p. 784–8.

89. **Powers, S.K.** and **E.T. Howley**, *Exercise Physiology: Theory and Application to Fitness and Performance.* New York: McGraw-Hill Humanities/Social Sciences/Languages, 2014.

90. **Scroop, G.C.** and **N.J. Shipp**, Exercise-induced hypoxemia: fact or fallacy? *Med Sci Sports Exerc*, 2010. 42(1): p. 120–6.

91. **West, J.B.**, et al., Maximal exercise at extreme altitudes on Mount Everest. *J Appl Physiol Respir Environ Exerc Physiol*, 1983. 55(3): p. 688–98.

92. **Peacock, A.J.** and **P.L. Jones**, Gas exchange at extreme altitude: results from the British 40th Anniversary Everest Expedition. *Eur Respir J*, 1997. 10(7): p. 1439–44.

93. **Grocott, M.P.**, et al., Arterial blood gases and oxygen content in climbers on Mount Everest. *N Engl J Med*, 2009. 360(2): p. 140–9.

94. **West, J.B.**, Arterial blood measurements in climbers on Mount Everest. *Lancet*, 2009. 373(9675): p. 1589–90.

95. **Pugh, L.G.**, et al., Muscular exercise at great altitudes. *J Appl Physiol*, 1964. 19: p. 431–40.

96. **Bailey, D.M.**, The last "oxygenless" ascent of Mt. Everest. *Br J Sports Med*, 2001. 35(5): p. 294–6.

97. **Burtscher, M., H. Gatterer**, and **A. Kleinsasser**, Cardiorespiratory fitness of high altitude mountaineers: the underestimated prerequisite. *High Alt Med Biol*, 2015. 16(2): p. 169–70.

98. **Moore, L.G., S. Niermeyer**, and **S. Zamudio**, Human adaptation to high altitude: regional and life-cycle perspectives. *Am J Phys Anthropol*, 1998. Suppl 27: p. 25–64.

99. **Stobdan, T., J. Karar**, and **M.A. Pasha**, High altitude adaptation: genetic perspectives. *High Alt Med Biol*, 2008. 9(2): p. 140–7.

100. **Shriver, M.D.**, et al., Finding the genes underlying adaptation to hypoxia using genomic scans for genetic adaptation and admixture mapping. *Adv Exp Med Biol*, 2006. 588: p. 89–100.

101. **Beall, C.M.**, et al., Ventilation and hypoxic ventilatory response of Tibetan and Aymara high altitude natives. *Am J Phys Anthropol*, 1997. 104(4): p. 427–47.

102. **Beall, C.M.**, et al., Quantitative genetic analysis of arterial oxygen saturation in Tibetan highlanders. *Hum Biol*, 1997. 69(5): p. 597–604.

103. **Kawakami, Y.**, et al., Relationship between hypoxic and hypercapnic ventilatory responses in man. *Jpn J Physiol*, 1981. 31(3): p. 357–68.

104. **Collins, D.D.**, et al., Hereditary aspects of decreased hypoxic response. *J Clin Invest*, 1978. 62(1): p. 105–10.

105. **Moore, G.C.**, et al., Respiratory failure associated with familial depression of ventilatory response to hypoxia and hypercapnia. *N Engl J Med*, 1976. 295(16): p. 861–5.

106. **Saunders, N.A., S.R. Leeder**, and **A.S. Rebuck**, Ventilatory response to carbon dioxide in young athletes: a family study. *Am Rev Respir Dis*, 1976. 113(4): p. 497–502.

107. **Beall, C.M.**, Tibetan and Andean contrasts in adaptation to high-altitude hypoxia. *Adv Exp Med Biol*, 2000. 475: p. 63–74.

108. **Aldenderfer, M.S.**, Moving up in the world: archaeologists seek to understand how and when people came to occupy the Andean and Tibetan plateaus. *Am Sci*, 2003. 91(6): p. 542–549.

109. **Smith, T.G., P.A. Robbins**, and **P.J. Ratcliffe**, The human side of hypoxia-inducible factor. *Br J Haematol*, 2008. 141(3): p. 325–34.

110. **Maxwell, P.H.**, Hypoxia-inducible factor as a physiological regulator. *Exp Physiol*, 2005. 90(6): p. 791–7.

111. **Yi, X.**, et al., Sequencing of 50 human exomes reveals adaptation to high altitude. *Science*, 2010. 329(5987): p. 75–78.

112. **West, J.B., American College of Physicians**, and **American Physiological Society**, The physiologic basis of high-altitude diseases. *Ann Intern Med*, 2004. 141(10): p. 789–800.

113. **Semenza, G.L.**, Hydroxylation of HIF-1: oxygen sensing at the molecular level. *Physiology (Bethesda)*, 2004. 19: p. 176–82.

114. **Ohno, H.**, et al., Effect of exercise on HIF-1 and VEGF signaling. *J Phys Fitness Sports Med*, 2012. 1(1): p. 5–16.

115. **Faquin, W.C., T.J. Schneider**, and **M.A. Goldberg**, Effect of inflammatory cytokines on hypoxia-induced erythropoietin production. *Blood*, 1992. 79(8): p. 1987–94.

116. **Jelkmann, W.**, et al., Monokines inhibiting erythropoietin production in human hepatoma cultures and in isolated perfused rat kidneys. *Life Sci*, 1992. 50(4): p. 301–8.

117. **Hellwig-Burgel, T.**, et al., Interleukin-1beta and tumor necrosis factor-alpha stimulate DNA binding of hypoxia-inducible factor-1. *Blood*, 1999. 94(5): p. 1561–7.

118. **Niebauer, J.**, et al., Exercise training in chronic heart failure: effects on pro-inflammatory markers. *Eur J Heart Fail*, 2005. 7(2): p. 189–93.

16

GENETIC CONTRIBUTIONS TO MITOCHONDRIAL TRAITS

Mark Tarnopolsky

Introduction

Given the importance of mitochondrial biogenesis to endurance exercise, the aim of this chapter is to evaluate the potential for variants in mitochondrial DNA (mtDNA), nuclear genes encoding mitochondrial proteins (NuGEMPs), or nuclear genes that control mitochondrial biogenesis to influence mitochondrial function/adaptations. It has long been known that increased mitochondrial mass and function are associated with endurance exercise training (33, 35). It is not surprising that maximal oxygen consumption at the whole body level (VO$_2$max) increases co-temporal with total mitochondrial mass (12, 53), and mitochondrial cristae density (64), given that complex IV of the mitochondrial respiratory chain is the terminal oxygen acceptor for cellular metabolism.

It is important to consider that mitochondria can respond to different stimuli by increasing the total mass and/or increasing the efficiency of individual mitochondria. In general, most studies use citrate synthase activity/protein, mitochondrial mRNA transcript abundance, voltage-dependent anion channel (VDAC) protein, mtDNA content, or mitochondrial volume density (electron microscopy) to measure total mitochondrial mass in response to endurance exercise training (52, 85, 96). A crude functional measure is the ratio of a respiratory chain enzyme activity (i.e., cytochrome *c* oxidase (COX))/total mitochondrial volume (i.e., citrate synthase); however, classical respirometry or high-resolution respirometry can be expressed relative to total mitochondrial or muscle mass and provides a mitochondrial functional metric (70). It is far beyond this chapter to review every paper evaluating the mitochondrial response to exercise; however, a general increase in mitochondrial mass is usually seen in response to training volume (12, 52, 53), with additional small increases in function (capacity/mitochondria) seen with higher-intensity interval-type training (for a review, see 7) or nitrates (42). The dramatic adaptability of skeletal muscle mitochondrial mass in response to stimuli can also be seen with hypodynamia, reducing mitochondrial mass by about 25% after only 2 weeks of leg immobilization (1).

Although it is generally accepted that increased red blood cell mass and stroke volume are the main determinants of exercise-induced increases in VO$_2$max (45), the importance of peripheral mitochondrial adaptations is reflected in the severe reduction of VO$_2$max in patients with mtDNA mutations (94), and impaired peripheral oxygen extraction (91). Consequently, exercise intolerance is a defining feature for many mitochondrial disorders that usually manifests during endurance type activities (93). A major component of this review will be exploring the potential for mtDNA, mitochondrial biogenesis-associated genes, or NuGEMP DNA variants to influence the increase in VO$_2$peak with endurance exercise training and/or peak endurance performance in top sport athletes. I will first provide a background of mitochondrial biology followed by an exploration of the genetic contributions to mitochondrial traits. Finally, I will suggest avenues for future research.

Mitochondrial biology

Origin and structure of mitochondria and mitochondrial DNA

Mitochondria are bilayer organelles that exist in nearly every mammalian cell, with the exception of mature red blood cells. They are thought to have origins as α-protobacteria that established a symbiotic relationship with a proto-eukaryotic cell approximately 1.5 billion years ago to create eukaryotic cells. With evolution, the majority of the genes encoding for mitochondrial proteins have been transferred to the nucleus, and these are referred to as NuGEMPs. As a reflection of their bacterial origin, mitochondria retain their own 16,569 bp intronless circular DNA (mtDNA) that undergoes polycistronic replication as opposed to gene-specific expression in nuclear DNA. mtDNA encodes for 37 gene products including 22 tRNAs, 2 rRNAs, and 13 protein subunits; yet a fully functional mitochondrion requires about 1300 gene products for proper structure and function with 1158 of these catalogued by the Broad Institute (MitoCarta; www.broadinstitute.org/scientific-community/science/programs/metabolic-disease-program/publications/mitocarta/mitocarta-in-0).

Why the few remaining mtDNA gene products are so conserved across the vertebrates and were not transferred to nuclear DNA control is unclear; however, it is postulated that they are highly hydrophobic and/or subtle differences in the genetic code between the genomes constrained transfer (20), and/or they are necessary to form the template core of the respiratory chain that functions as series circuit (personal communication, Doug Wallace, 2017). The NuGEMPs that are transcribed in the nucleus and translated in the cytosol are then imported into the mitochondria through a series of proteins that include the transporter of the outer mitochondrial membrane proteins (TOMM; i.e., TOMM20, TOMM70), the transporter of the inner mitochondrial membrane proteins (TIMM; i.e., TIMM23, TIMM22), and mitochondrial chaperones (i.e., hsp60, hsp72). Mutations in the TIMM8A protein can lead to a mitochondrial disorder with dystonia and deafness called the Mohr–Tranebjaerg syndrome (78).

Another unique aspect of mitochondrial genetics is that mtDNA is exclusively inherited through maternal transmission. This fact allowed for the tracking of *Homo sapiens* evolution from an ancestral mitochondrial Eve or matrilinear most recent common ancestor who was thought to have existed about 100,000–150,000 years ago in South Africa or Botswana (72), and allowed for tracking of human evolution out of Africa (15). In fact, any two humans can determine when they last shared a common mother by analyzing mtDNA sequence variants. Specific mtDNA sequences that define specific branches of human evolution are called haplogroups. The first mtDNA haplogroup that defined *Homo sapiens* is called L and the emergence of L0 defined the mitochondrial Eve (44, 77). Random mutations in mtDNA likely played a role in evolution, as reflected in the fact that haplogroups found in Siberia render the mitochondria more uncoupled and this leads to greater heat production that may have promoted survival in colder environments (81). Haplogroups also influence the penetrance of pathogenic mitochondrial DNA mutations (9). Given that mtDNA polymorphisms that define the haplogroups can

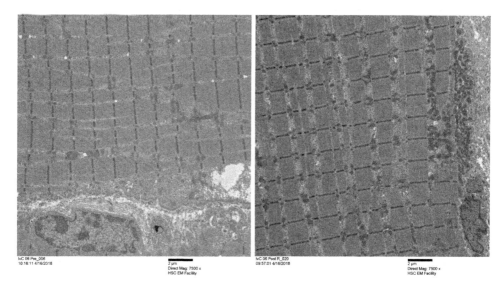

Figure 16.1 Mitochondrial ultrastructure. Transmission electron micrograph of mitochondria (25,000×) before (PRE) and after (POST) 2 months of endurance exercise training. IMF=intermyofibrillar mitochondria; SS=sub-sarcolemmal mitochondria; N=nucleus.

also lead to differences in coupled versus uncoupled mitochondrial respiration (39, 81), it is conceptually attractive to hypothesize that these polymorphisms may partially determine the evolution of the endurance trait (see Chapter 11). mtDNA also exhibits heteroplasmy within a cell and tissue with a varying proportion of two different mtDNA variants at the same nucleotide position. This is particularly important for pathogenic mutations where a higher proportion of a mutant versus wild-type mtDNA variant in skeletal muscle is associated with a greater deleterious effect on function (37).

Mitochondria have an outer membrane (OMM) and a highly convoluted inner membrane (IMM) that envelopes the matrix and interacts with the OMM through contact sites. Mitochondria are present in proportion to the energy needs of the tissue, with cardiac cells having up to 20%, and skeletal muscle about 4% mitochondrial volume density. Mitochondria are traditionally considered to be static cylindrical tube-like structures; however, mitochondria form complex dynamic networks within cells (48). Mitochondrial fusion and fission are important processes to allow for intercellular movement and optimal function (14, 58). This dynamic movement of mitochondria is likely important in mtDNA complementation, allowing for regional alterations in mitochondrial abundance in response to intracellular signals, and altering mitochondrial abundance in response to changes in need for energy. The importance of fusion and fission is reflected in that mutations within such genes (i.e., *OPA1*, *Mfn2*, and *DLP1*) result in neurological disease (27, 107). Mitochondria are distributed in sub-sarcolemmal and intermyofibrillar regions in skeletal muscle, with increased density after endurance exercise training (Figure 16.1).

Mitochondrial biogenesis and regulation

Mitochondrial biogenesis is the process of increasing mitochondrial mass in response to physiological stimuli such as growth or exercise. This is a complex process that involves mitochondrial fusion and fission and mtDNA replication. Even a cursory discussion of these processes is far beyond the scope of this focused chapter; however, it is important to discuss the basics of mtDNA replication and transcriptional control during exercise. Seminal work by Dr. Bruce Spiegelman's laboratory led to the identification of the "master regulator of mitochondrial biogenesis" called peroxisome proliferator-activated receptor gamma coactivator 1-alpha (PGC1α, gene=*PPARGC1A*) (74). PGC1α functions as a coactivator of nuclear transcription factors that upregulate NuGEMPs with histone-mediated transcription factor docking (73). It appears that PGC1α can also migrate to the mitochondria in response to physiological stimuli to function as an activator of mtDNA replication in conjunction with mitochondrial transcription factor A (Tfam) and sirtuin 1 (SIRT1) (5). Several splice variants have been discovered with evidence suggesting that the alternate promotor derived PGC1α4 mediates skeletal muscle hypertrophy (80). Others have found that both the truncated PGC1α4 and the canonical nontruncated PGC1α splice variants are activated by both acute resistance and endurance exercise and the adenosine monophosphate kinase (AMPK) activator, AICAR (103). There are several cellular signals that trigger mitochondrial biogenesis in response to acute exercise including oxidative stress, calcium transients/MAP kinase, and alterations in energy charge (i.e., increases in AMP) (11, 23, 36, 54). These alterations in cellular homeostasis activate several protein kinases that lead to transcription factor or coactivator activation.

AMPK is considered the main sensor of the exercise signal leading to mitochondrial biogenesis (36, 49, 67, 68). The protein is activated by phosphorylation in response to lower energy charge (higher AMP) during exercise and this leads to phosphorylation and/or nuclear translocation of downstream proteins and kinases that leads to an upregulation of mitochondrial biogenesis (i.e., PGC1α), activation of autophagy (i.e., ULK1), lipid oxidation (i.e., PPARα/δ), peroxisomal biogenesis, and antioxidant defences (10, 67). Important PGC1α-mediated transcription factors that upregulate NuGEMPs include *NRF1, NRF2, MEF2, PPARα/δ,* and *ERRα*. The newly transcribed NuGEMP mRNAs are exported to the cytosol for translation and import into the mitochondria. Oxidative stress can also be an activator of mitochondrial biogenesis through PGC1α activation (2, 4, 23), and calcium transients can also activate PGC1α through MAP kinase activation (11).

It is not clear how the exercise signal is transduced to the mitochondria to coordinately initiate mtDNA transcription but translocation of PGC1α to the mitochondria is a likely candidate (5). Given that mtDNA copy number increases with endurance exercise-mediated mitochondrial biogenesis, there must be mtDNA replication (i.e., making new copies of mtDNA). The replication of mtDNA requires many proteins and Tfam is important in mtDNA stability. Since mtDNA does not have true chromatin or histones, Tfam is thought to have a histone-like function in the mitochondria (40). Replication of mtDNA requires polymerase gamma 1 (POLG1) and POLG2. Mutations in the *POLG1* gene and to a lesser extent, *POLG2*, lead to a wide spectrum of disorders from fatal infantile hepatoencephalopathy to later-onset ataxia, neuropathy, and Parkinsonian features (63, 83). The DNA helicase *C10orf2* (twinkle) is required to unwind the highly coiled mtDNA prior to DNA replication. In contrast to the documentation of many dozens of pathogenic mutations in the *POLG1* gene (83), it may appear unusual that there are no known mutations responsible for human neurological disease in *PPARGC1A* (PGC1α gene) in spite of animal evidence for this possibility (90). The lack of demonstration of mutations in the *PPARGC1A* gene in patients with mitochondrial disease may be due to compensatory upregulation of *PGC1β* and *PRC* genes that are also involved in mitochondrial biogenesis coactivation (79, 88).

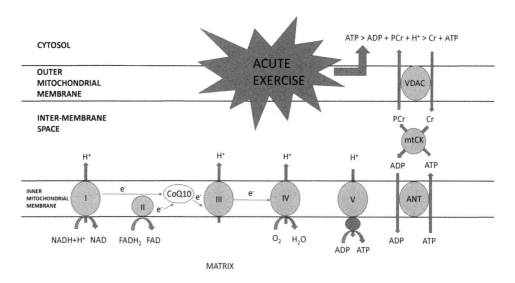

Figure 16.2 Mitochondrial respiratory chain. Carbohydrate, fat, and some amino acids can be oxidized and lead to the production of reduced co-factors, NADH+H$^+$ and FADH$_2$. These reduced cofactors are oxidized by linked multienzyme complexes embedded in the inner mitochondrial membrane (respiratory chain) with complex I and II gaining electrons from NADH+H$^+$ and FADH$_2$, respectively. The electrons are transferred to coenzyme Q10 which becomes reduced and the electrons are transferred to complex III (ubiquinol–cytochrome c reductase) and the electrons are then used to reduce cytochrome c. Cytochrome c is a mobile carrier protein that delivers its electrons to cytochrome c oxidase (COX, complex IV) and the electrons are used to reduce molecular oxygen to water. The potential energy from intermediary metabolism is used to pump protons (H$^+$) from the matrix of the mitochondria to the intermembrane space at complexes I, III, and IV. This causes an increase in proton concentration (lower pH) and this potential energy is captured as they flow through complex V back into the matrix to rephosphorylate ADP to ATP. ATP and ADP are translocated across the intermitochondrial membrane through the adenine nucleotide translocase (ANT) where through the catalytic activity of mitochondrial creatine kinase (mtCK), ATP is used to rephosphorylate creatine (Cr) to phosphocreatine (PCr). The phosphocreatine and creatine are exchanged across the outer mitochondrial membrane through the porin/voltage-dependent ion channel (VDAC) and the mitochondrial-derived phosphocreatine is then used to rephosphorylate ADP back to ATP in the cytosol (101).

Functions of mitochondria

The classical role of mitochondria is energy metabolism, where reducing equivalents from carbohydrate fat, and to some extent amino acids, can be used to generate ATP in the presence of oxygen (Figure 16.2). Mitochondria are also involved in a variety of other physiological and pathophysiologic processes including oxidative stress, inflammasome activation, telomere maintenance, and activation of apoptosis. Given that the respiratory chain depends on the flow of electrons, it is not surprising that unpaired electrons (free radicals) can be formed by the respiratory chain with complex I and III being traditionally considered as the main sites of free radical generation (100). Although an increase in oxidative stress is felt to be a component of neurodegenerative disorders and even aging (62), free radicals are thought to be signaling molecules in physiological adaptation and their suppression can attenuate exercise-induced mitochondrial adaptations (71) and attenuate adaptations to endurance exercise (29, 69, 76). Some of the negative effects of antioxidants could be through the inhibition of free radical-induced stimulation of AMPK, CaMKII (60), and PGC1α (23). In contrast, others have found no attenuation of exercise adaptations with antioxidants

(32, 104–106) or reported mixed results (61). Dysfunction of the mitochondria can lead to a release of danger-associated molecular pattern (DAMP) molecules such as mtDNA and formyl proteins that can activate an NLRP3-mediated increase in caspase-1 activation and the release of characteristic cytokines (IL-1β, IL-18) (86). Telomeres function to protect the ends of chromosomes and are a "replicometer" of aging. Telomere shortening is associated with mitochondrial dysfunction, partially through an increase in oxidative stress (82). Dysfunctional mitochondria can also release cytochrome c into the cytosol, activating caspase 9 that, in turn, activates caspases 3 and 7 to trigger ATP-dependent preprogrammed cell death (apoptosis).

Given the complexity of the mitochondrion, it is not surprising that there are many mtDNA and NuGEMP DNA mutations that can impair the ability to generate ATP (3, 34, 37, 99, 107). The emergence of mitochondrial medicine in the late 1980s focused on the identification of mtDNA mutations and characterization of many mitochondrial diseases by their impact upon the maximal enzyme activity (34, 99, 108). The majority of exercise physiology studies focusing on mitochondrial adaptation have also relied on the measurement of maximal enzyme activity (usually COX) as a reflection of the respiratory chain capacity with citrate synthase as a measure of total mitochondrial mass (12, 52, 85). Other proteins such as VDAC and measurements of mitochondrial DNA can also be used to measure the increase in total mitochondria in response to endurance exercise training. Of course, these assays determine the Vmax of the enzymes complexes in isolation, while newer techniques such as high-resolution respirometry allow for linked assays, especially in skinned muscle fibers versus isolated mitochondria (70).

Exercise adaptations and mtDNA variants

Mitochondrial disorders

The most dramatic influence of mtDNA variants upon exercise capacity are the deleterious effects of specific mutations (3, 93, 97). The most striking influence of a single mtDNA point mutation we have seen in the laboratory is the severe reduction of VO_2max in patients with the mitochondrial encephalomyopathy, lactic acidosis, and stroke-like episodes (MELAS) m.3271T>C and MELAS m.3243A>G transition variants of <10 ml/kg/min (97). Numerous publications have reported exercise intolerance, low aerobic capacity, and lifelong exercise intolerance in patients with a variety of mtDNA point mutations (18, 19, 37, 93, 95), with cytochrome b mutations being rather muscle symptom specific (3). Encouragingly, even with such a severe exercise intolerance, endurance exercise training can improve exercise capacity, VO_2max, and quality of life in mitochondrial disease patients through an increase in mitochondrial mass (38, 94).

Healthy individuals

There have been several summaries regarding the influence of mtDNA variants upon athletic performance (8, 25), and here I will highlight some of the main studies. A study of 114 healthy Spanish men found that those with haplogroup J had lower VO_2max as compared with non-J haplogroups (59). The lower VO_2max was thought to be related to the known lower oxidative stress (reactive oxygen species (ROS) production) and ATP generation efficiency of mitochondrial of haplogroup J (59). In another study, the enrichment of mtDNA haplogroup T (m.13368A) was less in elite male endurance athletes versus sedentary controls and thus, haplogroup T was considered a negative predictor of elite athletic performance (13). Finally, another Spanish study confirmed the lower VO_2max association with haplogroup J in 70 healthy sedentary men, but not in 50 aerobically trained men (50).

In contrast, is there evidence that specific mtDNA haplogroups (as defined by single or several transition or transversion variants) or single nucleotide mtDNA polymorphisms can positively influence mitochondrial traits? The first attempt to study the influence of mtDNA variants upon VO₂max or the adaptation to endurance training was by Dr. Claude Bouchard's group in 1991 and 1993 where polymerase chain reaction restriction fragment length polymorphism (PCR-RFLP) analysis found that men who carried unique patterns in two regions of the *ND5* mtDNA subunit and one region in the tRNA^{thr} gene had higher VO₂max levels at baseline, while those with an *ND2* restriction pattern had lower VO₂max levels at baseline (21, 22). After endurance exercise training, those with a *HincII* restriction pattern in *ND5* showed lower VO₂max responses (22). Another Spanish group looked at haplogroups that were enriched in elite male Caucasian endurance athletes and found that 15.7% of the elite endurance athletes were from haplogroup V, with fewer in the sedentary cohort (7.5%) (66). Another Spanish study looked at the mtDNA haplotype of 81 healthy men and found that those with J had lower VO₂max values than non-J, with H accounting for most of the difference (51). The finding of a lower VO₂max in haplogroup J was confirmed in 114 healthy male Spanish subjects. Interestingly, haplogroup H also showed higher oxidative damage versus J (50, 51). It would have been of interest to perform skeletal muscle electron microscopy and PGC1α analysis in the latter study to see if the association was mediated by ROS induction of mitochondrial biogenesis through a PGC1α-mediated mechanism.

A Japanese study evaluated the mtDNA sequence of 100 elite male endurance athletes and 672 controls and found that the endurance athletes showed a slight but significant enrichment of sub-haplogroups D4e2 and D4g (55). This same Japanese group studied 79 Olympic-level endurance/middle-distance athletes versus 672 controls and found an enrichment of 8.9% versus 3.7%, respectively for haplogroup G1 (57). They examined 100 elite male athletes in the first study and the 672 controls from the second study and found that the athletes had an enrichment of m.152C>T, m.514(CA)n (CA ≥5) and a poly-A stretch at m.568–573 (C ≥7) in the noncoding control region (56). Finally, a Korean study compared 75 endurance/middle-distance athletes to 265 nonathletic controls and found an enrichment for haplogroups M★ and N9 and a paucity of B compared to the control group (41).

Exercise adaptations, NuGEMP variants, and mitochondrial biogenesis genes

Mitochondrial disorders

As with mtDNA variants, there are several NuGEMP mutations associated with severe endurance exercise intolerance including *YARS2*, *ISCU*, *TMEM126B*, and *TRMT5* (43, 87). To my knowledge, there have not been reports of a significant relationship between nuclear-encoded subunits of the respiratory chain and VO₂max or endurance exercise adaptability. Given that the mitochondrial adaptations to endurance exercise are predominantly through changes in mitochondrial mass mediated by mitochondrial biogenesis and that mitochondrial biogenesis has PGC1α as a "master regulator," it is not surprising that most of the described genetic associations for mitochondrial traits are found in this gene and associated biogenesis genes.

Healthy individuals

A large study looked at maximal treadmill exercise duration in 3783 young, white and black men and women at baseline and again after a 20-year period (*N*=2335) (84). They found that a favorable single nucleotide polymorphism (SNP) in *PPARGC1A* (the PGC1α gene) and three other genes was associated with baseline treadmill performance in black individuals and specific SNPs in *PPARGC1A* (rs3774909) and *HIF1A* (rs1957757) were associated with baseline treadmill performance in white individuals. Four favorable SNPs in different genes (including *PPARGC1A*) were associated with less decline in treadmill performance after 20 years (84). Given the role of PGC1α as the master regulator of mitochondrial biogenesis (74), it is not surprising that the *PPARGC1A* gene came up on an unbiased gene discovery platform.

There is a common *PPARGC1A* SNP termed Gly482Ser (rs8192678) seen in about 35–50% of humans (28). It has been shown that humans with this specific SNP show an attenuated binding of PGC1α to MEF2 (109), and impaired *TFAM* expression (16). This SNP impairs skeletal muscle slow-twitch fiber-type transition following endurance exercise training (89). Not surprisingly the Gly482Ser SNP was slightly, but significantly, less prevalent in elite endurance athletes (29.1%) as compared to sedentary controls with a 2.5-fold lower VO_2max (40.0%) (47). Others have found a lower enrichment of homozygous 482Ser in elite Caucasian endurance athletes (46). Somewhat paradoxically, it has been shown that homozygosity for 482Ser (~11% of the population) has the greatest propensity to adapt to endurance exercise (28). Furthermore, ethnicity may play a role in these associations as a Japanese cohort found that homozygosity for 482Ser was associated with a higher lactate threshold with no influence on VO_2max (65), and there was no relationship between the Gly482Ser polymorphism and VO_2max adaptation to endurance training (65). Another study in Turkish elite endurance athletes found that Gly482 was more enriched in controls (60%) versus endurance athletes (38.3%) (98). Finally, a study in elite Chinese endurance athletes found no enrichment for any of 133 SNPs within 11 genes associated with PGC1α (*PPARGC1A, PPARGC1B, PPRC1, TFAM, TFB1M, TFB2M, NRF1, GABPA, GABPB1, ERRα,* and *SIRT1*) (30).

Independent associations between PPARα/δ SNPs have also been evaluated in the context of endurance capacity. PPARδ is encoded by the *PPARD* gene and this protein is involved in mitochondrial function and lipid oxidation. A large study evaluated the enrichment of three specific SNPs (rs2267668, rs2016520, and rs1053049) in the *PPARD* gene in 704 controls and 120 endurance athletes and found a significantly higher enrichment of the A/C/C haplotype in the controls (7.25%) versus the athletes (0.83%) (47). Another study found that the specific *PPARD* DNA variant (c.294T>C) associated with the rs2016520 SNP was not more enriched in top sport endurance athletes; however, the presence of homozygosity for *PPARGC1A* Gly482 *and PPARD* CC genotype was more prevalent in the athletes (24). PPARα is encoded for by the *PPARA* and has similar functions to PPARδ. One study found that a specific *PPARA* polymorphism G/G (rs4253778) was slightly more enriched (*P*=0.051) associated in 155 Israeli endurance athletes (*N*=155) versus controls (*N*=240), and they confirmed a lower enrichment of the *PPARGC1A* Gly482Ser SNP (47). Another study looked at a *PPARA* intron 7 variant (G>C; rs4253778) and found that G/G was enriched in endurance athletes (*N*=60) versus controls (*N*=110) (98).

Compared to single SNP analysis methods, a more complex analysis involves the potential interacting effects of multiple SNPs in genes involved in pathways related to aerobic capacity. As one can imagine, there are likely dozens to hundreds of potential SNPs in any given gene and hundreds of genes involved in aspects of aerobic capacity (cardiac output, capillary density, energy storage and mobilization, and mitochondrial biogenesis). Although one study found an enrichment of *PPARGC1A* Gly482 *and PPARD* CC in endurance athletes (24), when this group evaluated an "endurance genotype score" based upon the sum of these scores from six polymorphisms within the *PPARGC1A-NRF-TFAM* axis they found that *none* of the elite endurance athletes ($N=81$) had the ideal (100) genotype score; however, the score was higher (38.9%) for the athletes versus controls (30.6%) (26).

Conclusion

Given the complexities of biological systems (as highlighted by Dr. Bourchard's closing comments), and the fact that 1.5 billion years of mitochondrial evolution would have placed enormous selective pressure on achieving the most efficient mitochondria, it is not surprising that a given haplogroup/mtDNA variants does not *strongly* associate with VO_2max or the adaptive propensity for mitochondrial adaptation. When an enrichment of a haplogroup is reported to segregate with VO_2max or endurance adaptation, the relative difference between the athletes and controls or the responders and nonresponders can appear large by relative terms (up to 100% different); however, most studies show that the absolute enrichment and differences between the groups is in the 5–15% range. Consequently, mtDNA variants should not be used to encourage or dissuade an athlete from sport participation. Furthermore, even with severe mtDNA mutations that massively lower VO_2max, endurance exercise training can still lead to a significant increase in VO_2max, exercise performance, and quality of life (92).

A big issue when looking at mtDNA haplogroups is that within a given country the enrichment of the haplogroups will be somewhat homogenous based upon evolutionary migration patterns (i.e., the haplogroups in Korea and Japan will be very different than those in Spain). In addition, for strong statistical association studies even with common diseases (31), the sample size will need to be much larger and include many ethnicities as compared to the rather small and country/ethnicity-centric studies published to date. Another serious issue is that most of the studies exclusively used men and it is not appropriate to extrapolate the findings from men to women. The latter issue is particularly apparent given that women, likely through 17-β-estradiol, have lower oxidative stress; and a haplogroup such as H that likely works through higher ROS-inducing mitochondrial biogenesis would be less likely to associate in women.

By the same rationale of evolutionary pressure on mitochondrial efficiency, it would be surprising if NuGEMPs that encode for mitochondrial structural proteins would be strongly associated with mitochondrial adaptation. Even DNA variants in mitochondrial biogenesis proteins including PGC1α are not *strongly* associated with VO_2max or exercise capacity and these associations can be opposite depending upon the ethnicity. It is highly likely that the lack of a strong association between a SNP in any single gene and exercise performance or VO_2max is due to many factors, not the least of which is that the effect of any SNP is likely influenced by genetic factors such as a permissive haplotype, SNPs in biogenesis-associated genes, SNPs in mitochondrial structural genes, and SNPs in other related mitochondrial proteins such as membrane transporters, chaperones, nucleotide transporters, etc. The fact that about 30% of top sport endurance athletes have an "unfavorable" *PPARGC1A* SNP (24, 46) shows that these variants do not exert an overriding influence on endurance athletic performance. Finally, it is known that epigenetic influences (including gut microbiota) can strongly influence gene expression (6), even in the mitochondria (17), and these effects can hinder the ability to make genotype–phenotype correlations.

Another issue to consider in future studies is the influence of new technology upon the ability to discover genetic determinants of exercise capacity. For example, the first study that I am aware of that looked at mtDNA variants and endurance adaptations (21), used PCR-RFLP to look at a few mtDNA variants detected by the creation or removal of a restriction site; whereas, next-generation sequencing (NGS) can now provide up to 5000× reads of every base pair (16) of the mtDNA. Many of the genotype/phenotype association studies have used SNP-chip methods to look at specified SNPs, yet NGS-based whole-exome sequencing can provide an unbiased evaluation of all the nucleotides within the exons (~1% of all genomic material) of the entire genome (~22,000 genes). To explore the potential for variants in the intronic regions (~99% of all genomic material), it is now possible to use whole-genome sequencing. The latter method is particularly powerful when used in conjunction with RNA sequencing that can look at sequence variants in the transcribed exons and alternative splicing variants. Consequently, determining the contribution of DNA variants to exercise capacity will require large numbers of subjects and a combination of mtDNA sequencing, whole-genome sequencing, methylation arrays, and RNA sequencing in skeletal muscle. Initiatives such as the National Institutes of Health-sponsored Molecular Transducers of Physical Activity in Humans (www.commonfund. nih.gov/moleculartransducers/overview), and the Gene SMART Study (102), will likely provide important answers to many of the questions concerning genetic contributions to mitochondrial traits. To further illustrate the complexity of the issue, a large study (GAMES) with 1520 endurance athletes and 2760 controls from Australia, Ethiopia, Japan, Kenya, Poland, Russia, and Spain failed to find a marker or series of genetic markers that strongly segregated with the endurance phenotype (75).

Acknowledgements: Dr. Tarnopolsky's research in the area of exercise biochemistry and mitochondrial medicine is funded by the Canadian Institute for Health Research and kind donations from Dan Wright and family, Warren Lammert and family, and Giant Tiger Stores. Dr Lauren Skelly kindly provided the electron microscopy images in Figure 16.1.

References

1. **Abadi A, Glover EI, Isfort RJ, Raha S, Safdar A, Yasuda N, Kaczor JJ, Melov S, Hubbard A, Qu X, Phillips SM**, and **Tarnopolsky M.** Limb immobilization induces a coordinate down-regulation of mitochondrial and other metabolic pathways in men and women. *PLoS One* 4: e6518, 2009.
2. **Adamovich Y, Shlomai A, Tsvetkov P, Umansky KB, Reuven N, Estall JL, Spiegelman BM**, and **Shaul Y.** The protein level of PGC-1alpha, a key metabolic regulator, is controlled by NADH-NQO1. *Mol Cell Biol* 33: 2603–2613, 2013.
3. **Andreu AL, Hanna MG, Reichmann H, Bruno C, Penn AS, Tanji K, Pallotti F, Iwata S, Bonilla E, Lach B, Morgan-Hughes J**, and **DiMauro S.** Exercise intolerance due to mutations in the cytochrome b gene of mitochondrial DNA. *N Engl J Med* 341: 1037–1044, 1999.
4. **Aquilano K, Baldelli S, Pagliei B, Cannata SM, Rotilio G**, and **Ciriolo MR.** p53 orchestrates the PGC-1alpha-mediated antioxidant response upon mild redox and metabolic imbalance. *Antioxid Redox Signal* 18: 386–399, 2013.
5. **Aquilano K, Vigilanza P, Baldelli S, Pagliei B, Rotilio G**, and **Ciriolo MR.** Peroxisome proliferator-activated receptor gamma co-activator 1alpha (PGC-1alpha) and sirtuin 1 (SIRT1) reside in mitochondria: possible direct function in mitochondrial biogenesis. *J Biol Chem* 285: 21590–21599, 2010.
6. **Barres R, Osler ME, Yan J, Rune A, Fritz T, Caidahl K, Krook A**, and **Zierath JR.** Non-CpG methylation of the PGC-1alpha promoter through DNMT3B controls mitochondrial density. *Cell Metab* 10: 189–198, 2009.
7. **Bishop DJ, Granata C**, and **Eynon N.** Can we optimise the exercise training prescription to maximise improvements in mitochondria function and content? *Biochim Biophys Acta* 1840: 1266–1275, 2014.
8. **Bray MS, Hagberg JM, Perusse L, Rankinen T, Roth SM, Wolfarth B**, and **Bouchard C.** The human gene map for performance and health-related fitness phenotypes: the 2006–2007 update. *Med Sci Sports Exerc* 41: 35–73, 2009.
9. **Brown MD, Starikovskaya E, Derbeneva O, Hosseini S, Allen JC, Mikhailovskaya IE, Sukernik RI**, and **Wallace DC.** The role of mtDNA background in disease expression: a new primary LHON mutation associated with Western Eurasian haplogroup J. *Hum Genet* 110: 130–138, 2002.

10. **Bujak AL, Crane JD, Lally JS, Ford RJ, Kang SJ, Rebalka IA, Green AE, Kemp BE, Hawke TJ, Schertzer JD**, and **Steinberg GR.** AMPK activation of muscle autophagy prevents fasting induced hypoglycemia and myopathy during aging. *Cell Metab* 21: 883–890, 2015.

11. **Cao W, Daniel KW, Robidoux J, Puigserver P, Medvedev AV, Bai X, Floering LM, Spiegelman BM**, and **Collins S.** p38 mitogen-activated protein kinase is the central regulator of cyclic AMP-dependent transcription of the brown fat uncoupling protein 1 gene. *Mol Cell Biol* 24: 3057–3067, 2004.

12. **Carter SL, Rennie CD, Hamilton SJ**, and **Tarnopolsky.** Changes in skeletal muscle in males and females following endurance training. *Can J Physiol Pharmacol* 79: 386–392, 2001.

13. **Castro MG, Terrados N, Reguero JR, Alvarez V**, and **Coto E.** Mitochondrial haplogroup T is negatively associated with the status of elite endurance athlete. *Mitochondrion* 7: 354–357, 2007.

14. **Chen H, Vermulst M, Wang YE, Chomyn A, Prolla TA, McCaffery JM**, and **Chan DC.** Mitochondrial fusion is required for mtDNA stability in skeletal muscle and tolerance of mtDNA mutations. *Cell* 141: 280–289, 2010.

15. **Chen YS, Torroni A, Excoffier L, Santachiara-Benerecetti AS**, and **Wallace DC.** Analysis of mtDNA variation in African populations reveals the most ancient of all human continent-specific haplogroups. *Am J Hum Genet* 57: 133–149, 1995.

16. **Choi YS, Hong JM, Lim S, Ko KS**, and **Pak YK.** Impaired coactivator activity of the Gly482 variant of peroxisome proliferator-activated receptor gamma coactivator-1alpha (PGC-1alpha) on mitochondrial transcription factor A (Tfam) promoter. *Biochem Biophys Res Commun* 344: 708–712, 2006.

17. **Clark A** and **Mach N.** The crosstalk between the gut microbiota and mitochondria during exercise. *Front Physiol* 8: 319, 2017.

18. **Connolly BS, Feigenbaum AS, Robinson BH, Dipchand AI, Simon DK**, and **Tarnopolsky MA.** MELAS syndrome, cardiomyopathy, rhabdomyolysis, and autism associated with the A3260G mitochondrial DNA mutation. *Biochem Biophys Res Commun* 402: 443–447, 2010.

19. **Darin N, Hedberg-Oldfors C, Kroksmark AK, Moslemi AR, Kollberg G**, and **Oldfors A.** Benign mitochondrial myopathy with exercise intolerance in a large multigeneration family due to a homoplasmic m.3250T>C mutation in MTTL1. *Eur J Neurol* 24: 587–593, 2017.

20. **de Grey AD.** Forces maintaining organellar genomes: is any as strong as genetic code disparity or hydrophobicity? *Bioessays* 27: 436–446, 2005.

21. **Dionne FT, Turcotte L, Thibault MC, Boulay MR, Skinner JS**, and **Bouchard C.** Mitochondrial DNA sequence polymorphism, VO2max, and response to endurance training. *Med Sci Sports Exerc* 23: 177–185, 1991.

22. **Dionne FT, Turcotte L, Thibault MC, Boulay MR, Skinner JS**, and **Bouchard C.** Mitochondrial DNA sequence polymorphism, VO2max, and response to endurance training. *Med Sci Sports Exerc* 25: 766–774, 1993.

23. **Espinoza MB, Aedo JE, Zuloaga R, Valenzuela C, Molina A**, and **Valdes JA.** Cortisol induces reactive oxygen species through a membrane glucocorticoid receptor in rainbow trout myotubes. *J Cell Biochem* 118: 718–725, 2017.

24. **Eynon N, Meckel Y, Alves AJ, Yamin C, Sagiv M, Goldhammer E**, and **Sagiv M.** Is there an interaction between PPARD T294C and PPARGC1A Gly482Ser polymorphisms and human endurance performance? *Exp Physiol* 94: 1147–1152, 2009.

25. **Eynon N, Moran M, Birk R**, and **Lucia A.** The champions' mitochondria: is it genetically determined? A review on mitochondrial DNA and elite athletic performance. *Physiol Genomics* 43: 789–798, 2011.

26. **Eynon N, Ruiz JR, Meckel Y, Moran M**, and **Lucia A.** Mitochondrial biogenesis related endurance genotype score and sports performance in athletes. *Mitochondrion* 11: 64–69, 2011.

27. **Feely SM, Laura M, Siskind CE, Sottile S, Davis M, Gibbons VS, Reilly MM**, and **Shy ME.** MFN2 mutations cause severe phenotypes in most patients with CMT2A. *Neurology* 76: 1690–1696, 2011.

28. **Franks PW, Barroso I, Luan J, Ekelund U, Crowley VE, Brage S, Sandhu MS, Jakes RW, Middelberg RP, Harding AH, Schafer AJ, O'Rahilly S**, and **Wareham NJ.** PGC-1alpha genotype modifies the association of volitional energy expenditure with [OV0312]O2max. *Med Sci Sports Exerc* 35: 1998–2004, 2003.

29. **Gomez-Cabrera MC, Domenech E, Romagnoli M, Arduini A, Borras C, Pallardo FV, Sastre J**, and **Vina J.** Oral administration of vitamin C decreases muscle mitochondrial biogenesis and hampers training-induced adaptations in endurance performance. *Am J Clin Nutr* 87: 142–149, 2008.

30. **He ZH, Hu Y, Li YC, Gong LJ, Cieszczyk P, Maciejewska-Karlowska A, Leonska-Duniec A, Muniesa CA, Marin-Peiro M, Santiago C, Garatachea N, Eynon N,** and **Lucia A.** PGC-related gene variants and elite endurance athletic status in a Chinese cohort: a functional study. *Scand J Med Sci Sports* 25: 184–195, 2015.

31. **Herrnstadt C** and **Howell N.** An evolutionary perspective on pathogenic mtDNA mutations: haplogroup associations of clinical disorders. *Mitochondrion* 4: 791–798, 2004.

32. **Higashida K, Kim SH, Higuchi M, Holloszy JO,** and **Han DH.** Normal adaptations to exercise despite protection against oxidative stress. *Am J Physiol Endocrinol Metab* 301: E779–784, 2011.

33. **Holloszy JO, Oscai LB, Don IJ,** and **Mole PA.** Mitochondrial citric acid cycle and related enzymes: adaptive response to exercise. *Biochem Biophys Res Commun* 40: 1368–1373, 1970.

34. **Holt IJ, Harding AE,** and **Morgan-Hughes JA.** Deletions of muscle mitochondrial DNA in patients with mitochondrial myopathies. *Nature* 331: 717–719, 1988.

35. **Hoppeler H, Luthi P, Claassen H, Weibel ER,** and **Howald H.** The ultrastructure of the normal human skeletal muscle. A morphometric analysis on untrained men, women and well-trained orienteers. *Pflugers Arch* 344: 217–232, 1973.

36. **Jager S, Handschin C, St-Pierre J,** and **Spiegelman BM.** AMP-activated protein kinase (AMPK) action in skeletal muscle via direct phosphorylation of PGC-1alpha. *Proc Natl Acad Sci U S A* 104: 12017–12022, 2007.

37. **Jeppesen TD, Schwartz M, Frederiksen AL, Wibrand F, Olsen DB,** and **Vissing J.** Muscle phenotype and mutation load in 51 persons with the 3243A>G mitochondrial DNA mutation. *Arch Neurol* 63: 1701–1706, 2006.

38. **Jeppesen TD, Schwartz M, Olsen DB, Wibrand F, Krag T, Duno M, Hauerslev S,** and **Vissing J.** Aerobic training is safe and improves exercise capacity in patients with mitochondrial myopathy. *Brain* 129: 3402–3412, 2006.

39. **Ji F, Sharpley MS, Derbeneva O, Alves LS, Qian P, Wang Y, Chalkia D, Lvova M, Xu J, Yao W, Simon M, Platt J, Xu S, Angelin A, Davila A, Huang T, Wang PH, Chuang LM, Moore LG, Qian G,** and **Wallace DC.** Mitochondrial DNA variant associated with Leber hereditary optic neuropathy and high-altitude Tibetans. *Proc Natl Acad Sci U S A* 109: 7391–7396, 2012.

40. **Kanki T, Nakayama H, Sasaki N, Takio K, Alam TI, Hamasaki N,** and **Kang D.** Mitochondrial nucleoid and transcription factor A. *Ann NY Acad Sci* 1011: 61–68, 2004.

41. **Kim KC, Cho HI,** and **Kim W.** MtDNA haplogroups and elite Korean athlete status. *Int J Sports Med* 33: 76–80, 2012.

42. **Larsen FJ, Schiffer TA, Borniquel S, Sahlin K, Ekblom B, Lundberg JO,** and **Weitzberg E.** Dietary inorganic nitrate improves mitochondrial efficiency in humans. *Cell Metab* 13: 149–159, 2011.

43. **Legati A, Reyes A, Ceccatelli Berti C, Stehling O, Marchet S, Lamperti C, Ferrari A, Robinson AJ, Muhlenhoff U, Lill R, Zeviani M, Goffrini P,** and **Ghezzi D.** A novel de novo dominant mutation in ISCU associated with mitochondrial myopathy. *J Med Genet* 54: 815–824, 2017.

44. **Lewin R.** The unmasking of mitochondrial Eve. *Science* 238: 24–26, 1987.

45. **Lundby C, Montero D,** and **Joyner M.** Biology of VO2 max: looking under the physiology lamp. *Acta Physiol (Oxf)* 220: 218–228, 2017.

46. **Maciejewska A, Sawczuk M, Cieszczyk P, Mozhayskaya IA,** and **Ahmetov, II.** The PPARGC1A gene Gly482Ser in Polish and Russian athletes. *J Sports Sci* 30: 101–113, 2012.

47. **Maciejewska-Karlowska A, Hanson ED, Sawczuk M, Cieszczyk P,** and **Eynon N.** Genomic haplotype within the peroxisome proliferator-activated receptor delta (PPARD) gene is associated with elite athletic status. *Scand J Med Sci Sports* 24: e148–155, 2014.

48. **Mannella CA, Buttle K, Rath BK,** and **Marko M.** Electron microscopic tomography of rat-liver mitochondria and their interaction with the endoplasmic reticulum. *Biofactors* 8: 225–228, 1998.

49. **Marcinko K, Sikkema SR, Samaan MC, Kemp BE, Fullerton MD,** and **Steinberg GR.** High intensity interval training improves liver and adipose tissue insulin sensitivity. *Mol Metab* 4: 903–915, 2015.

50. **Marcuello A, Martinez-Redondo D, Dahmani Y, Casajus JA, Ruiz-Pesini E, Montoya J, Lopez-Perez MJ,** and **Diez-Sanchez C.** Human mitochondrial variants influence on oxygen consumption. *Mitochondrion* 9: 27–30, 2009.

51. **Martinez-Redondo D, Marcuello A, Casajus JA, Ara I, Dahmani Y, Montoya J, Ruiz-Pesini E, Lopez-Perez MJ,** and **Diez-Sanchez C.** Human mitochondrial haplogroup H: the highest VO2max consumer – is it a paradox? *Mitochondrion* 10: 102–107, 2010.

52. **McKenzie S, Phillips SM, Carter SL, Lowther S, Gibala MJ,** and **Tarnopolsky MA.** Endurance exercise training attenuates leucine oxidation and BCOAD activation during exercise in humans. *Am J Physiol Endocrinol Metab* 278: E580–587, 2000.

53. **Meinild Lundby AK, Jacobs RA, Gehrig S, de Leur J, Hauser M, Bonne TC, Fluck D, Dandanell S, Kirk N, Kaech A, Ziegler U, Larsen S,** and **Lundby C.** Exercise training increases skeletal muscle mitochondrial volume density by enlargement of existing mitochondria and not de novo biogenesis. *Acta Physiol (Oxf)* 222, 2018.

54. **Merry TL** and **Ristow M.** Nuclear factor erythroid-derived 2-like 2 (NFE2L2, Nrf2) mediates exercise-induced mitochondrial biogenesis and the anti-oxidant response in mice. *J Physiol* 594: 5195–5207, 2016.

55. **Mikami E, Fuku N, Kong QP, Takahashi H, Ohiwa N, Murakami H, Miyachi M, Higuchi M, Tanaka M, Pitsiladis YP,** and **Kawahara T.** Comprehensive analysis of common and rare mitochondrial DNA variants in elite Japanese athletes: a case-control study. *J Hum Genet* 58: 780–787, 2013.

56. **Mikami E, Fuku N, Takahashi H, Ohiwa N, Pitsiladis YP, Higuchi M, Kawahara T,** and **Tanaka M.** Polymorphisms in the control region of mitochondrial DNA associated with elite Japanese athlete status. *Scand J Med Sci Sports* 23: 593–599, 2013.

57. **Mikami E, Fuku N, Takahashi H, Ohiwa N, Scott RA, Pitsiladis YP, Higuchi M, Kawahara T,** and **Tanaka M.** Mitochondrial haplogroups associated with elite Japanese athlete status. *Br J Sports Med* 45: 1179–1183, 2011.

58. **Mishra P, Varuzhanyan G, Pham AH,** and **Chan DC.** Mitochondrial dynamics is a distinguishing feature of skeletal muscle fiber types and regulates organellar compartmentalization. *Cell Metab* 22: 1033–1044, 2015.

59. **Monaco C, Whitfield J, Jain SS, Spriet LL, Bonen A,** and **Holloway GP.** Activation of AMPKalpha2 is not required for mitochondrial FAT/CD36 accumulation during exercise. *PLoS One* 10: e0126122, 2015.

60. **Morales-Alamo D, Ponce-Gonzalez JG, Guadalupe-Grau A, Rodriguez-Garcia L, Santana A, Cusso R, Guerrero M, Dorado C, Guerra B,** and **Calbet JA.** Critical role for free radicals on sprint exercise-induced CaMKII and AMPKalpha phosphorylation in human skeletal muscle. *J Appl Physiol (1985)* 114: 566–577, 2013.

61. **Morrison D, Hughes J, Della Gatta PA, Mason S, Lamon S, Russell AP,** and **Wadley GD.** Vitamin C and E supplementation prevents some of the cellular adaptations to endurance-training in humans. *Free Radic Biol Med* 89: 852–862, 2015.

62. **Muhammad MH** and **Allam MM.** Resveratrol and/or exercise training counteract aging-associated decline of physical endurance in aged mice; targeting mitochondrial biogenesis and function. *J Physiol Sci*, 2017.

63. **Naviaux RK** and **Nguyen KV.** POLG mutations associated with Alpers' syndrome and mitochondrial DNA depletion. *Ann Neurol* 55: 706–712, 2004.

64. **Nielsen J, Gejl KD, Hey-Mogensen M, Holmberg HC, Suetta C, Krustrup P, Elemans CPH,** and **Ortenblad N.** Plasticity in mitochondrial cristae density allows metabolic capacity modulation in human skeletal muscle. *J Physiol* 595: 2839–2847, 2017.

65. **Nishida Y, Iyadomi M, Higaki Y, Tanaka H, Kondo Y, Otsubo H, Horita M, Hara M,** and **Tanaka K.** Association between the PPARGC1A polymorphism and aerobic capacity in Japanese middle-aged men. *Intern Med* 54: 359–366, 2015.

66. **Nogales-Gadea G, Pinos T, Ruiz JR, Marzo PF, Fiuza-Luces C, Lopez-Gallardo E, Ruiz-Pesini E, Martin MA, Arenas J, Moran M, Andreu AL,** and **Lucia A.** Are mitochondrial haplogroups associated with elite athletic status? A study on a Spanish cohort. *Mitochondrion* 11: 905–908, 2011.

67. **O'Neill HM, Holloway GP,** and **Steinberg GR.** AMPK regulation of fatty acid metabolism and mitochondrial biogenesis: implications for obesity. *Mol Cell Endocrinol* 366: 135–151, 2013.

68. **O'Neill HM, Maarbjerg SJ, Crane JD, Jeppesen J, Jorgensen SB, Schertzer JD, Shyroka O, Kiens B, van Denderen BJ, Tarnopolsky MA, Kemp BE, Richter EA,** and **Steinberg GR.** AMP-activated protein kinase (AMPK) beta1beta2 muscle null mice reveal an essential role for AMPK in maintaining mitochondrial content and glucose uptake during exercise. *Proc Natl Acad Sci U S A* 108: 16092–16097, 2011.

69. **Paulsen G, Cumming KT, Holden G, Hallen J, Ronnestad BR, Sveen O, Skaug A, Paur I, Bastani NE, Ostgaard HN, Buer C, Midttun M, Freuchen F, Wiig H, Ulseth ET, Garthe I, Blomhoff R, Benestad HB,** and **Raastad T.** Vitamin C and E supplementation hampers cellular

adaptation to endurance training in humans: a double-blind, randomised, controlled trial. *J Physiol* 592: 1887–1901, 2014.

70. **Picard M, Taivassalo T, Ritchie D, Wright KJ, Thomas MM, Romestaing C,** and **Hepple RT.** Mitochondrial structure and function are disrupted by standard isolation methods. *PLoS One* 6: e18317, 2011.

71. **Picklo MJ** and **Thyfault JP.** Vitamin E and vitamin C do not reduce insulin sensitivity but inhibit mitochondrial protein expression in exercising obese rats. *Appl Physiol Nutr Metab* 40: 343–352, 2015.

72. **Poznik GD, Henn BM, Yee MC, Sliwerska E, Euskirchen GM, Lin AA, Snyder M, Quintana-Murci L, Kidd JM, Underhill PA,** and **Bustamante CD.** Sequencing Y chromosomes resolves discrepancy in time to common ancestor of males versus females. *Science* 341: 562–565, 2013.

73. **Puigserver P, Adelmant G, Wu Z, Fan M, Xu J, O'Malley B,** and **Spiegelman BM.** Activation of PPAR gamma coactivator-1 through transcription factor docking. *Science* 286: 1368–1371, 1999.

74. **Puigserver P, Wu Z, Park CW, Graves R, Wright M,** and **Spiegelman BM.** A cold-inducible coactivator of nuclear receptors linked to adaptive thermogenesis. *Cell* 92: 829–839, 1998.

75. **Rankinen T, Fuku N, Wolfarth B, Wang G, Sarzynski MA, Alexeev DG, Ahmetov, II, Boulay MR, Cieszczyk P, Eynon N, Filipenko ML, Garton FC, Generozov EV, Govorun VM, Houweling PJ, Kawahara T, Kostryukova ES, Kulemin NA, Larin AK, Maciejewska-Karlowska A, Miyachi M, Muniesa CA, Murakami H, Ospanova EA, Padmanabhan S, Pavlenko AV, Pyankova ON, Santiago C, Sawczuk M, Scott RA, Uyba VV, Yvert T, Perusse L, Ghosh S, Rauramaa R, North KN, Lucia A, Pitsiladis Y,** and **Bouchard C.** No evidence of a common DNA variant profile specific to world class endurance athletes. *PLoS One* 11: e0147330, 2016.

76. **Ristow M, Zarse K, Oberbach A, Kloting N, Birringer M, Kiehntopf M, Stumvoll M, Kahn CR,** and **Bluher M.** Antioxidants prevent health-promoting effects of physical exercise in humans. *Proc Natl Acad Sci U S A* 106: 8665–8670, 2009.

77. **Rito T, Richards MB, Fernandes V, Alshamali F, Cerny V, Pereira L,** and **Soares P.** The first modern human dispersals across Africa. *PLoS One* 8: e80031, 2013.

78. **Roesch K, Curran SP, Tranebjaerg L,** and **Koehler CM.** Human deafness dystonia syndrome is caused by a defect in assembly of the DDP1/TIMM8a-TIMM13 complex. *Hum Mol Genet* 11: 477–486, 2002.

79. **Rowe GC, El-Khoury R, Patten IS, Rustin P,** and **Arany Z.** PGC-1alpha is dispensable for exercise-induced mitochondrial biogenesis in skeletal muscle. *PLoS One* 7: e41817, 2012.

80. **Ruas JL, White JP, Rao RR, Kleiner S, Brannan KT, Harrison BC, Greene NP, Wu J, Estall JL, Irving BA, Lanza IR, Rasbach KA, Okutsu M, Nair KS, Yan Z, Leinwand LA,** and **Spiegelman BM.** A PGC-1alpha isoform induced by resistance training regulates skeletal muscle hypertrophy. *Cell* 151: 1319–1331, 2012.

81. **Ruiz-Pesini E, Mishmar D, Brandon M, Procaccio V,** and **Wallace DC.** Effects of purifying and adaptive selection on regional variation in human mtDNA. *Science* 303: 223–226, 2004.

82. **Sahin E, Colla S, Liesa M, Moslehi J, Muller FL, Guo M, Cooper M, Kotton D, Fabian AJ, Walkey C, Maser RS, Tonon G, Foerster F, Xiong R, Wang YA, Shukla SA, Jaskelioff M, Martin ES, Heffernan TP, Protopopov A, Ivanova E, Mahoney JE, Kost-Alimova M, Perry SR, Bronson R, Liao R, Mulligan R, Shirihai OS, Chin L,** and **DePinho RA.** Telomere dysfunction induces metabolic and mitochondrial compromise. *Nature* 470: 359–365, 2011.

83. **Saneto RP** and **Naviaux RK.** Polymerase gamma disease through the ages. *Dev Disabil Res Rev* 16: 163–174, 2010.

84. **Sarzynski MA, Rankinen T, Sternfeld B, Grove ML, Fornage M, Jacobs DR,** Jr., **Sidney S,** and **Bouchard C.** Association of single-nucleotide polymorphisms from 17 candidate genes with baseline symptom-limited exercise test duration and decrease in duration over 20 years: the Coronary Artery Risk Development in Young Adults (CARDIA) fitness study. *Circ Cardiovasc Genet* 3: 531–538, 2010.

85. **Short KR, Vittone JL, Bigelow ML, Proctor DN, Rizza RA, Coenen-Schimke JM,** and **Nair KS.** Impact of aerobic exercise training on age-related changes in insulin sensitivity and muscle oxidative capacity. *Diabetes* 52: 1888–1896, 2003.

86. **Simmons JD, Lee YL, Mulekar S, Kuck JL, Brevard SB, Gonzalez RP, Gillespie MN,** and **Richards WO.** Elevated levels of plasma mitochondrial DNA DAMPs are linked to clinical outcome in severely injured human subjects. *Ann Surg* 258: 591–596, 2013.

87. Sommerville EW, Ng YS, Alston CL, Dallabona C, Gilberti M, He L, Knowles C, Chin SL, Schaefer AM, Falkous G, Murdoch D, Longman C, de Visser M, Bindoff LA, Rawles JM, Dean JCS, Petty RK, Farrugia ME, Haack TB, Prokisch H, McFarland R, Turnbull DM, Donnini C, Taylor RW, and Gorman GS. Clinical features, molecular heterogeneity, and prognostic implications in YARS2-related mitochondrial myopathy. *JAMA Neurol* 74: 686–694, 2017.

88. Srivastava S, Diaz F, Iommarini L, Aure K, Lombes A, and Moraes CT. PGC-1alpha/beta induced expression partially compensates for respiratory chain defects in cells from patients with mitochondrial disorders. *Hum Mol Genet* 18: 1805–1812, 2009.

89. Steinbacher P, Feichtinger RG, Kedenko L, Kedenko I, Reinhardt S, Schonauer AL, Leitner I, Sanger AM, Stoiber W, Kofler B, Forster H, Paulweber B, and Ring-Dimitriou S. The single nucleotide polymorphism Gly482Ser in the PGC-1alpha gene impairs exercise-induced slow-twitch muscle fibre transformation in humans. *PLoS One* 10: e0123881, 2015.

90. Szalardy L, Zadori D, Plangar I, Vecsei L, Weydt P, Ludolph AC, Klivenyi P, and Kovacs GG. Neuropathology of partial PGC-1alpha deficiency recapitulates features of mitochondrial encephalopathies but not of neurodegenerative diseases. *Neurodegener Dis* 12: 177–188, 2013.

91. Taivassalo T, Abbott A, Wyrick P, and Haller RG. Venous oxygen levels during aerobic forearm exercise: an index of impaired oxidative metabolism in mitochondrial myopathy. *Ann Neurol* 51: 38–44, 2002.

92. Taivassalo T, Gardner JL, Taylor RW, Schaefer AM, Newman J, Barron MJ, Haller RG, and Turnbull DM. Endurance training and detraining in mitochondrial myopathies due to single large-scale mtDNA deletions. *Brain* 129: 3391–3401, 2006.

93. Taivassalo T, Jensen TD, Kennaway N, DiMauro S, Vissing J, and Haller RG. The spectrum of exercise tolerance in mitochondrial myopathies: a study of 40 patients. *Brain* 126: 413–423, 2003.

94. Taivassalo T, Shoubridge EA, Chen J, Kennaway NG, DiMauro S, Arnold DL, and Haller RG. Aerobic conditioning in patients with mitochondrial myopathies: physiological, biochemical, and genetic effects. *Ann Neurol* 50: 133–141, 2001.

95. Tarnopolsky MA, Maguire J, Myint T, Applegarth D, and Robinson BH. Clinical, physiological, and histological features in a kindred with the T3271C melas mutation. *Muscle Nerve* 21: 25–33, 1998.

96. Tarnopolsky MA, Rennie CD, Robertshaw HA, Fedak-Tarnopolsky SN, Devries MC, and Hamadeh MJ. Influence of endurance exercise training and sex on intramyocellular lipid and mitochondrial ultrastructure, substrate use, and mitochondrial enzyme activity. *Am J Physiol Regul Integr Comp Physiol* 292: R1271–1278, 2007.

97. Tarnopolsky MA, Roy BD, and MacDonald JR. A randomized, controlled trial of creatine monohydrate in patients with mitochondrial cytopathies. *Muscle Nerve* 20: 1502–1509, 1997.

98. Tural E, Kara N, Agaoglu SA, Elbistan M, Tasmektepligil MY, and Imamoglu O. PPAR-alpha and PPARGC1A gene variants have strong effects on aerobic performance of Turkish elite endurance athletes. *Mol Biol Rep* 41: 5799–5804, 2014.

99. Wallace DC, Brown MD, and Lott MT. Mitochondrial DNA variation in human evolution and disease. *Gene* 238: 211–230, 1999.

100. Wong HS, Dighe PA, Mezera V, Monternier PA, and Brand MD. Production of superoxide and hydrogen peroxide from specific mitochondrial sites under different bioenergetic conditions. *J Biol Chem* 292: 16804–16809, 2017.

101. Wyss M, Smeitink J, Wevers RA, and Wallimann T. Mitochondrial creatine kinase: a key enzyme of aerobic energy metabolism. *Biochim Biophys Acta* 1102: 119–166, 1992.

102. Yan X, Eynon N, Papadimitriou ID, Kuang J, Munson F, Tirosh O, O'Keefe L, Griffiths LR, Ashton KJ, Byrne N, Pitsiladis YP, and Bishop DJ. The gene SMART study: method, study design, and preliminary findings. *BMC Genomics* 18: 821, 2017.

103. Ydfors M, Fischer H, Mascher H, Blomstrand E, Norrbom J, and Gustafsson T. The truncated splice variants, NT-PGC-1alpha and PGC-1alpha4, increase with both endurance and resistance exercise in human skeletal muscle. *Physiol Rep* 1: e00140, 2013.

104. Yfanti C, Akerstrom T, Nielsen S, Nielsen AR, Mounier R, Mortensen OH, Lykkesfeldt J, Rose AJ, Fischer CP, and Pedersen BK. Antioxidant supplementation does not alter endurance training adaptation. *Med Sci Sports Exerc* 42: 1388–1395, 2010.

105. Yfanti C, Fischer CP, Nielsen S, Akerstrom T, Nielsen AR, Veskoukis AS, Kouretas D, Lykkesfeldt J, Pilegaard H, and Pedersen BK. Role of vitamin C and E supplementation on IL-6 in response to training. *J Appl Physiol (1985)* 112: 990–1000, 2012.

106. **Yfanti C, Nielsen AR, Akerstrom T, Nielsen S, Rose AJ, Richter EA, Lykkesfeldt J, Fischer CP**, and **Pedersen BK.** Effect of antioxidant supplementation on insulin sensitivity in response to endurance exercise training. *Am J Physiol Endocrinol Metab* 300: E761–770, 2011.

107. **Yu-Wai-Man P, Trenell MI, Hollingsworth KG, Griffiths PG**, and **Chinnery PF.** OPA1 mutations impair mitochondrial function in both pure and complicated dominant optic atrophy. *Brain* 134: e164, 2011.

108. **Zeviani M** and **Antozzi C.** Defects of mitochondrial DNA. *Brain Pathol* 2: 121–132, 1992.

109. **Zhang SL, Lu WS, Yan L, Wu MC, Xu MT, Chen LH**, and **Cheng H.** Association between peroxisome proliferator-activated receptor-gamma coactivator-1alpha gene polymorphisms and type 2 diabetes in southern Chinese population: role of altered interaction with myocyte enhancer factor 2C. *Chin Med J (Engl)* 120: 1878–1885, 2007.

17

ANGIOTENSIN-CONVERTING ENZYME AND THE GENOMICS OF ENDURANCE PERFORMANCE

Linda S. Pescatello, Lauren M.L. Corso, Lucas P. Santos,
Jill Livingston, and Beth A. Taylor

Introduction

The preceding Chapters 15 and 16 focused on the overall genetic influence on cardiorespiratory fitness and mitochondrial function during physical performance, respectively. This chapter will focus specifically on the influence of the angiotensin-converting enzyme gene (*ACE*) on human physical performance that was first studied by Montgomery and colleagues in 1998 (39). *ACE* has now become the most investigated gene in relation to human physical performance (57). Our search in PubMed located 316 citations that involved *ACE* and all types of physical performance. The number of yearly citations in PubMed from 1998 to 2017 involving *ACE* and all types of physical performance is displayed in Figure 17.1. Please note the search terms for this search differed slightly from the search conducted for this chapter on *ACE* and endurance performance, as we wished to emphasize the extent to which *ACE* is cited in the exercise performance literature.

ACE (OMIM 106180) is located on the long arm of chromosome 17 band 17q23.3, has the genomic coordinates 17:63,477,060–63,498,379 (GRCh38/hg38:CM000679.2), is 21,319 bp long, and consists of 26 exons and 25 introns (25). The *ACE* gene has 22 transcripts (splice variants), is a member of three Ensembl protein families, and is associated with five phenotypes (http://grch37.ensembl.org/index.html). These phenotypes include diabetes mellitus, renal disease, Alzheimer's disease, cancer and tumor burden, and athletic performance. *ACE* encodes an enzyme (ACE) that is a peptidyldipeptide hydrolase belonging to the class of zinc metallopeptidase (11, 25, 51). ACE is involved in catalyzing the conversion of angiotensin I into a physiologically active peptide, angiotensin II. Angiotensin II is a potent vasopressor and aldosterone-stimulating peptide that regulates blood pressure (BP) and fluid–electrolyte balance and is also involved with muscle function (45, 57). ACE also inactivates bradykinin, a potent vasodilator. ACE plays a key regulatory role in the renin–angiotensin–aldosterone system (RAAS), as will be discussed later in this chapter.

Rigat et al. found that an insertion (I)/deletion (D) of an Alu repetitive element polymorphism in intron 16 of the *ACE* gene involving about 250 bp was strongly associated with circulating plasma ACE levels, with the mean plasma ACE level of DD genotype subjects about

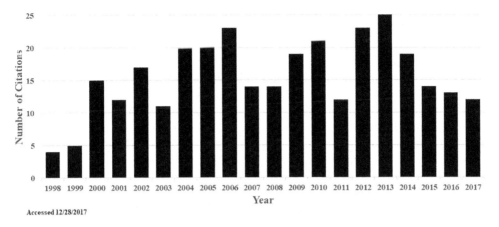

Accessed 12/28/2017

Figure 17.1 Angiotensin-converting enzyme gene (*ACE*) and physical performance number of citations per year in PubMed.

two times that of subjects with II genotype, with ID subjects having intermediate levels between the two homozygous genotypes (51, 52). This polymorphism is now called *ACE* rs4340, a structural variant (30), with the genomic coordinates ch17:63488531–63488532 (GRCh38/hg38). There are several dbSNP entries all tagging *ACE* rs4340 that include rs4343, rs4341, rs1799752 (named as present on 23andMe chips), rs4646994, and rs13447447. The structural variant *ACE* rs4340 has become the most investigated variant in ACE in relation to physical performance. Therefore, *ACE* rs4340 will be the focus of this chapter in relation to endurance exercise performance. In both common and scientific usage, endurance exercise has come to mean structured and planned physical activity using large muscle groups that could be continued for more than a few minutes that would be expected to maintain or improve cardiorespiratory fitness or endurance capacity (44). See Chapter 12 of this book for a primer on endurance exercise-related phenotypes.

The purpose of this chapter is to present a systematic review of *ACE* in relation to endurance exercise performance and other endurance exercise health-related outcomes as well as to provide a discussion on the systems through which *ACE* may affect endurance exercise performance. Specially, we will: 1) overview the systematic review methodology; 2) briefly discuss the regulation of the classical and nonclassical RAAS in relation to *ACE*, endurance exercise, and other endurance exercise health-related outcomes; 3) summarize the influence of *ACE* on endurance exercise performance and other endurance exercise health-related outcomes and the systems by which *ACE* may operate; and 4) conclude with take-home messages from this systematic review. As first originally postulated by Montgomery and colleagues (39), the working hypothesis of this chapter is that adults with the *ACE* I allele will exhibit superior endurance exercise performance compared with adults with the *ACE* D allele.

Systematic review methods

Trial selection process

A comprehensive Boolean search was run in PubMed (including Medline) and Scopus from earliest coverage to December 28, 2017 to locate all qualifying systematic reviews, meta-analyses, and primary level trials that examined the influence of *ACE* polymorphisms on endurance performance and/or endurance exercise health-related outcomes. The full search strategy for *ACE* and endurance performance and endurance performance health-related outcomes for potential qualifying trials was: ("exercise"[majr] OR exercise[ti] OR exercises[ti] OR exercising[ti] OR postexercise[ti] OR running[MeSH] OR running[ti] OR bicycling[MeSH] OR bicycling OR bicycle★ OR cycling[ti] OR treadmill★ OR ergometer OR "endurance training" OR "endurance exercise" OR "endurance athlete" OR "endurance athletes" OR "speed training" OR "circuit training" OR "training duration" OR "training frequency" OR "training intensity" OR "aerobic endurance" OR "aerobic training" OR "interval training" OR "combination training" OR "combined training" OR plyometric★ OR "HIIT" OR walking[MeSH] OR walking[ti] OR swimming OR swimmer★ OR hiker★ OR hiking OR mountaineer★ OR climber OR climbers OR climbing OR "military training" OR walking OR ironman OR triathlon★ OR triathlete★ OR marathon★ OR ultramarathon★ OR rowing OR rower★ OR skiing OR skier★ OR "endurance sport" OR "endurance sports" OR soccer OR football OR rugby OR hockey OR tennis OR basketball OR lacrosse OR athlete★ OR "endurance performance" OR "physical endurance" OR "physical performance" OR endurance[ti]) AND (Genetics[majr] OR genetics[ti] OR gene[ti] OR genes[ti] OR "genotype" OR "genotypes" OR chromosome[ti] OR chromosomes[ti] OR "SNP" OR "SNPS" OR allele OR alleles OR genotype★[ti] OR phenotype★[ti] OR genome[ti] OR polymorphism OR polymorphisms OR polymorphic OR "trait loci" OR "gene map" OR "autosomal gene" OR "trait locus" OR "trait loci" OR "candidate genes" OR "candidate gene" OR "quantitative trait loci" OR "mitochondrial genome" OR "nuclear genome" OR autosome★ OR microrna[ti] OR micrornas[ti] OR mirna[ti] OR mirnas[ti] OR loci[ti] OR "DNA" OR genetic★ OR "Insertion/deletion" OR "I/D" OR genetics[sh] OR "Physical Endurance/genetics"[MAJR]) AND (ace[ti] OR "angiotensin converting enzyme" OR "angiotensin converting enzymes" OR "angiotensin 1 converting enzyme" OR "angiotensin 2 converting enzyme" OR "Peptidyl-Dipeptidase A"[nm]) NOT ("ace inhibitor"[ti] OR "ace inhibitors"[ti] OR "angiotensin converting enzyme inhibitor"[ti] OR "angiotensin converting enzyme inhibitors"[ti] OR "Angiotensin-Converting Enzyme Inhibitors"[MeSH]).

At minimum, qualifying trials met the following criteria: 1) included adult samples ≥18 years that were generally healthy and free from chronic disease; 2) performed *ACE* genotyping; 3) disclosed the *Frequency Intensity, Time, and Type* or *FITT* of the endurance exercise intervention; 4) reported a measure of endurance performance or endurance exercise health-related outcome pre- and post-acute (i.e., immediate or short-term) or chronic (i.e., long-term or training) endurance exercise intervention; and 5) were published in English. Trials were excluded if they contained dietary or weight loss interventions, purposely induced dehydration, involved substance abuse, or only reported *ACE* associations at baseline and not the change of the measure of performance post- versus pre-exercise intervention to minimize sample selection bias (7, 8, 36). Furthermore, any study whose *ACE* allelic distributions were not in Hardy–Weinberg equilibrium was excluded.

Potential reports were screened by LMLC for title, abstract, and full text review to determine if they qualified. In addition, reference lists of 13 qualifying narrative and systematic reviews and meta-analyses (8, 16, 34, 35, 42, 45, 46, 68–72, 76) were manually searched for primary level trials and assessed for possible inclusion. The search yielded 383 reports, of which 29 primary level trials qualified. Details of the trial selection process appear in Figure 17.2. Of these primary level qualifying trials, 20 involved *ACE* and endurance performance (1, 2, 4, 9, 10, 13, 15, 18, 22, 23, 29, 60, 62–66, 73, 74, 77), five involved *ACE* and endurance exercise health-related

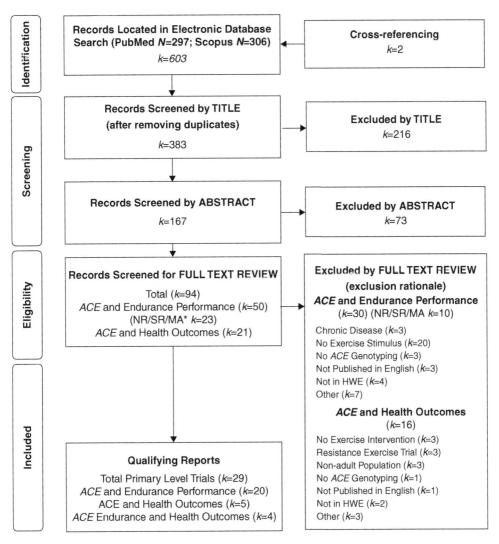

Figure 17.2 Flow chart detailing systematic search of potentially qualifying primary level trials and systematic reviews and meta-analysis that examined *ACE* and endurance and/or endurance performance related outcomes. ACE=angiotensin-converting enzyme; HWE=Hardy–Weinberg equilibrium; *k*=number of trials; MA=meta-analysis; NR=narrative review; SR=systematic review. *k*=13 qualifying NR/SR/MAs were disaggregated and individual trials were assessed for inclusion. The final sample reflects all qualifying primary level trials.

outcomes (6, 20, 26, 43, 54), and four trials reported both endurance performance and health-related outcomes (17, 28, 48, 49, 67); please note references 48 and 49 are from the same trial. Relevant data pertaining to the sample characteristics, endurance performance intervention, and endurance performance or endurance exercise health–related outcomes were extracted by LMLC for each respective trial and appear in Tables 17.1 and 17.2, displayed in their respective sections of this chapter.

Classical and nonclassical renin–angiotensin–aldosterone system in relation to cardiovascular control and endurance exercise performance and health-related outcomes

The classical RAAS, as it pertains to overall cardiovascular control, is stimulated by the release of renin in response to low BP, which catalyzes the conversion of angiotensinogen to angiotensin I. The subsequent conversion of angiotensin I to angiotensin II by ACE then evokes a cascade of actions to raise BP that are largely regulated by the binding of angiotensin II to the angiotensin 1 (AT_1) receptor (24, 53). This pivotal activity by ACE can be increased or decreased according to classical endocrine control (i.e., alterations in circulating levels of renin, angiotensinogen, angiotensin I and II, and ACE), or as more recent evidence suggests, by intracrine, autocrine, and paracrine control in which the components of the RAAS are produced by local tissues and the brain (32, 37, 41, 50, 53, 59). The ensuing downstream pressor actions of angiotensin II include increased sodium and water retention through aldosterone and antidiuretic hormone release; direct vasoconstriction through smooth muscle contraction; stimulation of the sympathetic nervous system to increase norepinephrine release and augment vasoconstriction; and an increase in reactive oxygen species (primarily nicotinamide adenine dinucleotide phosphate (NAD(P)H oxidase)) to reduce nitric oxide (NO) levels and blunt vasodilation. ACE also inhibits the vasodilators bradykinin and kallidin (14, 53), enhancing its role as a pressor enzyme. In addition, RAAS activation is associated with other adverse vascular effects such as cell hypertrophy and proliferation (55).

This classical view of the RAAS has been supplemented by identification of two nonclassical axes. The first nonclassical axis is the involvement of the angiotensin 2 (AT_2) receptor found predominantly in fetal tissue that decreases after birth such that relatively low amounts are typically expressed in adult tissue (50). The AT_2 receptor is associated with antagonistic depressor actions to those regulated by AT_1 binding. These opposing depressor actions to the classical RAAS pressor effects include an increased vasodilatory response through stimulation of endothelial NO synthase to produce NO as well as augmented bradykinin release (14, 53). The second nonclassical axis is the more recent identification of the ACE homolog, ACE2, which binds to a mitochondrial assembly receptor and stimulates a variety of largely antagonistic actions to the classical RAAS pressor actions (14, 31). The actions of ACE2 have not been comprehensively identified and characterized in human models, but appear to be associated with various cardioprotective phenotypes with actions such as vasodilation and antiproliferation (27, 55). An overview of the classical and nonclassical axes of ACE as they relate to cardiorespiratory control is depicted in Figure 17.3.

ACE is a rate-limiting enzyme of the RAAS. Variations in ACE concentrations that are genetically mediated by the *ACE* rs4340 I and D alleles (18, 51, 52) have been hypothesized to play an important role in endurance performance as well as endurance exercise health-related outcomes (8, 16, 39, 40, 45, 57, 69, 73). More recent evidence characterizes the RAAS as a "dual function system" in which the balance between vasoconstrictor and proliferative actions versus vasodilator and antiproliferative actions are influenced by ACE/ACE2 balance (50). For example, individuals with greater ACE concentrations at rest may also shunt more angiotensin II to the ACE homolog, ACE2, for conversion to angiotensin-(1–7), resulting in a lower-than-expected impact on resting BP and sympathetically mediated vasoconstriction (31). Furthermore, the BP response to acute and chronic endurance exercise has been shown to be influenced by the structural variant *ACE* rs4340 and indel *ACE2* rs59272 (6, 20, 21, 26, 30, 48, 54).

The impact of the *ACE* rs4340 genotype on the short- and long-term endurance performance responses is likely mediated by both chronic circulating levels of ACE, as well as

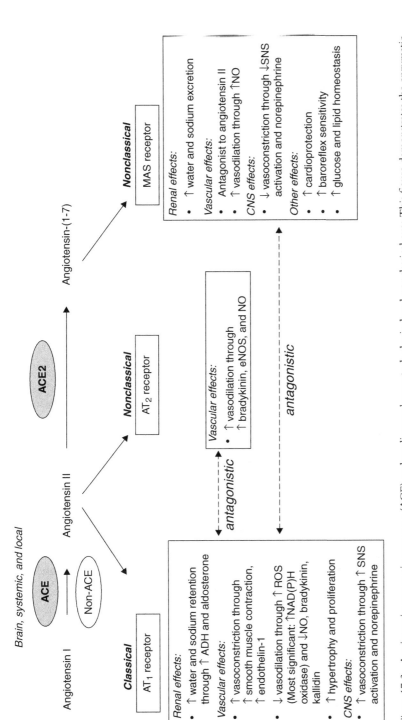

Figure 17.3 Angiotensin-converting enzyme (ACE) and cardiovascular control: classical and nonclassical axes. This figure demonstrates the enzymatic role that ACE, by stimulating the conversion of angiotensin I to angiotensin II, initiates through varied mechanisms that influence cardiovascular control. In the classical axis, the pressor actions result from angiotensin II binding to the AT (angiotensin) 1 receptor (or via the direct inhibitory actions of ACE). In the first nonclassical axis, angiotensin II may bind to AT_2 receptors to evoke antagonistic actions to those stimulated by AT_1 binding. Alternatively, in the second nonclassical axis, ACE2 may convert angiotensin II to angiotensin-(1–7) to bind to the mitochondrial assembly (MAS) receptor, evoking a series of additional antagonistic pathways to those regulated by AT_1 receptor binding and lowering the concentration of angiotensin II available for the classic axis (non-ACE). ACE=angiotensin-converting enzyme; ADH=antidiuretic hormone; AT_1=angiotensin type 1 receptor; AT_2=angiotensin type 2 receptor; eNOS=endothelial nitric oxide synthase; MAS=mitochondrial assembly receptor; NAD(P)H oxidase=nicotinamide adenine dinucleotide phosphate; NO=nitric oxide; ROS=reactive oxygen species; SNS=sympathetic nervous system.

acute exercise-associated increases in ACE and angiotensin II, which are paradoxically higher in individuals with lower resting levels of ACE (65). Under chronic resting conditions, higher concentrations of circulating ACE, as would occur with the presence of the *ACE* rs4340 D allele, are associated with the production of reactive oxygen species, reduced NO-dependent vasodilation, systemic inflammation, sympathetic nervous system activation, and cellular proliferation – responses which are proposed to reduce functional and/or structural cardiorespiratory capacity (5, 37, 53). In contrast, under acute exercise conditions, higher ACE concentrations as associated with the *ACE* rs4340 D allele may serve to enhance sympathetically mediated redirection of muscle blood flow to active muscle, increasing metabolic capacity through improved local vasodilation, capillary perfusion, and muscle metabolism, actions that potentially would improve cardiorespiratory capacity (64, 66). Muscle fiber type composition (i.e., type I vs. type II) also differs by the presence or absence of the *ACE* rs4340 I or D allele (75), raising the possibility of a "cascade" effect, whereby the metabolic outcomes regulated by *ACE* rs4340 are amplified by associated muscle fiber distribution distinctions tied to allelic differences. Surprisingly, there is a paucity of studies linking *ACE* rs4340 and ACE concentrations to measures of acute and chronic endurance performance so that there is an incomplete understanding of how the complexity of the RAAS may regulate endurance performance and health-related outcomes. A final consideration adding to the complexity of the RAAS is that the modulating influence of *ACE* on endurance performance outcomes is likely variable over time, regulated additionally by epigenetic modification through factors such as nutrition, climate, and environment, as well as sex and race (37, 47, 61).

The influence of *ACE* on endurance exercise performance

In total, there were 24 qualifying primary level trials that investigated *ACE* and endurance exercise performance that are detailed in Table 17.1. The subjects in these trials were predominantly young men of various races/ethnicities and levels of cardiorespiratory fitness, ranging from being sedentary to recreational and elite endurance athletes. The types of endurance exercise included submaximal and maximal treadmill walking, running, and cycling, and competitive events in extreme environments such as climbing Mt. Kilimanjaro and the 9-day ascent to Mt. Blanc. The submaximal and maximal measures of endurance performance were varied and included oxygen consumption (VO_2); cardiac output (CO); heart rate (HR); stroke volume (SV); ventilatory threshold; running economy and speed; power output; capillary density, recruitment, and muscle fiber ratio; and mitochondrial volume; among others.

ACE rs4340, plasma ACE concentration/activity, and endurance performance

Rigat et al. found *ACE* rs4340 was strongly associated with circulating plasma ACE levels, with the mean plasma ACE level of DD subjects being about two times that of II subjects, and with ID subjects having intermediate levels between the two homozygous genotypes (51, 52). A long-held supposition has been that varying levels of circulating ACE as mediated by *ACE* rs4340 contribute to differences in physical exercise performance, with carriers of the *ACE* I allele exhibiting lower circulating ACE levels and superior endurance performance compared to those with the D allele (40). Two qualifying trials examined the relationship between plasma ACE concentration/activity and endurance performance by *ACE* rs4340 among different subject populations and endurance exercise performance perturbations (15, 18). Both trials found a strong relationship with *ACE* and circulating ACE activity levels. However, Day et al. (15) found no relationships among *ACE* rs4340, circulating ACE activity levels, and acute submaximal mechanical efficiency and maximal aerobic capacity (VO$_2$max), while Domingo et al. (18) did not report triathlon finishing time by *ACE* genotype nor did they examine the relationships among *ACE* rs4340, plasma ACE concentrations, and measures of endurance performance. Due to limited and disparate findings, no conclusions can be made regarding the role of systemic ACE as genetically modulated by *ACE* rs4340 in endurance performance.

ACE *rs4340, endurance performance, and cardiorespiratory fitness as assessed by maximal or peak oxygen consumption*

A long-held notion has been that the *ACE* I allele is associated with enhanced endurance exercise performance, largely due to greater improvements in VO$_2$max/peak associated with the *ACE* I allele than the D allele. There were 12 qualifying trials that examined associations between the VO$_2$max/peak response to an endurance exercise intervention and *ACE* rs4340 (Table 17.1). Of these, two reported greater increases in VO$_2$max/peak levels with *ACE* II than ID/DD (1, 23), two reported greater increases in VO$_2$max/peak levels with *ACE* DD than ID/II (49, 77), and eight trials found no association between VO$_2$max/peak and *ACE* rs4340 genotype (2, 9, 15, 17, 60, 66, 67, 73). Furthermore, three acute (i.e., short-term or immediate) (1, 23, 77) and one chronic (long-term or training) (49) trial reported associations with *ACE* rs4340 and changes in VO$_2$max/peak, while four acute (9, 15, 60, 67) and four chronic (2, 17, 66, 73) trials did not find associations with *ACE* rs4340 and changes in VO$_2$max/peak (P >0.05). Collectively, due to disparate findings, this literature does not support the working hypothesis of this chapter that *ACE* rs4340, particularly the *ACE* I allele, plays a major role in endurance exercise performance as assessed by VO$_2$max/peak.

ACE *rs4340 and other measures of endurance performance*

In addition to VO$_2$max/peak, other endurance performance phenotypes have been linked to *ACE* and endurance performance (45). Our search resulted in eight qualifying trials that examined associations among these other measures of endurance performance and *ACE* rs4340. Of these, one trial reported greater endurance performance enhancement with moderate intensity (longer duration running among those with *ACE* II than ID and DD (10)), one trial reported greater endurance performance enhancement with higher intensity (shorter duration running among those with *ACE* DD than ID and II) (13), and six trials found no associations with a variety of endurance performances measures that included running efficiency, power output, minute ventilation, and the respiratory exchange ratio, among others (9, 15, 22, 49, 60, 67). Consistent with the literature examining the associations of *ACE* rs4340 with VO$_2$max/peak, the literature on *ACE* and these other measures of endurance performance does not support the working hypothesis of this chapter that *ACE* rs4340, particularly the *ACE* I allele, plays a major role in modifying endurance exercise performance.

ACE *rs4340, endurance performance, and cardiac function*

The RAAS plays a central role in left ventricular remodeling (19, 58). Montgomery and colleagues were the first to note the *ACE* D allele was associated with greater increases in left ventricular mass after endurance exercise training than the I allele (38). There were five trials that examined associations among *ACE* rs4340, endurance performance, and various indices of cardiac function (2, 4, 23, 49, 60). Of these, four trials found no association among *ACE* and measures of cardiac function that included left ventricular mass, CO, SV, and HR, among others

Table 17.1 A summary of the qualifying trials that examined the influence of *ACE* rs4340 on endurance performance*

Author, yr	Sample characteristics		
Valdivieso et al., 2017 (63 BIB-063)	**Untrained** N=24 M (Caucasian) Age=26.3±1.1 yr BMI=24.0±0.7 kg/m^2 %BF=22.2±6.9% BP=124.0±2.3/74.0±2.1 mmHg PPO=293.4±11.4 W VO$_2$peak=48.8±1.7 ml/kg/min	**Trained** N=28 M (Caucasian) Age=28.1±1.2 yr BMI=24.1±0.7 kg/m^2 %BF=14.2±1.3% BP=125.3±2.2/75.3±2.0 mmHg PPO=361.1±11.6 W VO$_2$peak=59.5±1.7 ml/kg/min	
Bueno et al., 2016 (9 BIB-009)	***ACE* II** N=32 M Age=26±3 yr Weight=73.9±8.3 kg Height=175.2±4.8 cm %BF=13±3.6% VO$_2$max=50±5 ml/kg/min RCPspeed=14±1 km/hr RE10=37±6 ml/kg/min RE12=44±3 ml/kg/min	***ACE* ID** N=77 M Age=25±3 yr Weight=78.1±9.7 kg Height=177.2±5.9 cm %BF=14±3.8% VO$_2$max=47±3 ml/kg/min RCPspeed=13±2 kg/hr RE10=36±4 ml/kg/min RE12=42.5±3 ml/kg/min	***ACE* DD** N=41 M Age=24±4 yr Weight=75.8±8.9 kg Height=177.4±5.1 cm %BF=13.1±4.3% VO$_2$max=49±3 ml/kg/min RCPspeed=13.5±2 km/hr RE10=36.5±3 ml/kg/min RE12=43±3 ml/kg/min
Vaughan et al., 2016 (65)	***ACE* II** N=7 Age=23.0±2.9 yr BMI=23.1±0.9 kg/m^2 VO$_2$max=50.13.3 ml/kg/min	***ACE* ID** N=13 Age=31.0±1.4 yr BMI=23.6±0.9 kg/m^2 VO$_2$max=49.0±2.2 ml/kg/min	***ACE* DD** N=11 Age=25.0±1.6 yr BMI=22.1±0.6 kg/m^2 VO$_2$max=55.6±2.2 ml/kg/min

ACE allele distribution^	Intervention characteristics	Results	ACE association
NR	1) Maximal two-legged cycling exercise test 2) Dominant leg, one-legged cycling bout Exercise started with 5-min warm up, pedaling at 80 rpm, followed by 25 min of one-legged cycling at 30% of two-leg PPO. Intensity was increased 10 W every min until fatigue	They measured ACE transcript levels, capillary-to-fiber ratio, fiber cross-sectional area, and decreased muscle glycogen in the *m. vastus lateralis*. ACE II/ID had higher PPO than DD ($P=0.014$). Untrained ACE II/ID carriers had higher capillary CSA (22.6% higher) and fiber ratio than DD ($P=0.040$). Postexercise muscle glycogen was decreased to greater levels among those ACE II/ID than DD ($P=0.010$). There were other favorable adaptations noted among the untrained subjects for proangiogenic factors, ACE transcript levels, and various metabolites with ACE II/ID that were not found for the trained subjects with ACE II/ID. They concluded that regular participation in a training program appeared to override the genetically mediated ACE-dependent angiogenic and metabolic responses to acute endurance exercise they found in the untrained men. Therefore, some of the discrepancies in the ACE rs4340 and endurance performance literature may be related to the training status of the study participants	Yes, ACE II/ID >DD for PPO, capillary CSA and to fiber ratio, and muscle glycogen among untrained but not men
II (21%) ID (52%) DD (27%)	1) Maximal incremental treadmill test with 3 min warm up (8 km/hr), followed by an increase in speed of 1 km/hr every min until failure 2) Two submaximal treadmill tests were conducted at 10 km/hr and 12 km/hr, using 6 min intervals	ACE did not influence VO$_2$max, endurance capacity, or RE at 10 km/hr or 12 km/hr ($P >0.05$)	No, for VO$_2$max, endurance capacity, and RE
II (22.6%) ID (41.9%) DD (35.4)	One-leg cycling bout. Subjects pedaled with the dominant leg at 80 rpm. Warm up was conducted at 15% of the leg max. The exercise portion of the bout was 25 min long at 30% of leg max. The intensity was changed by 10 W until exhaustion followed by a 3 min cool down	They examined associations with ACE rs4340 and capillary volume, mitochondrial density, the capillary fiber ratio, muscle glycogen, and various energy metabolites in the *m. vastus lateralis*. Capillary to fiber ratio, capillary volume, and mitochondrial density were lower in ACE DD than ID/DD (~24%, $P <0.05$), indicating impaired glucose utilization among ACE DD than ID/DD. Subjects with ACE DD showed increased glucose and decreased glycogen levels post exercise compared to ID/D ($P <0.05$). Maximal RER was lower among ACE DD post exercise than ID/II ($P=0.04$). Despite reduced glucose oxidation in the working muscle to an acute bout of one-legged cycling to exhaustion with ACE DD, the authors did not find associations with ACE and measures of endurance exercise performance as assessed by VO$_2$max or marathon completion time	Yes, ACE II >ID/DD capillary to fiber ratio, capillary volume, and mitochondrial density among ACE DD >ID/DD for glucose aerobic metabolic perturbations

(*continued*)

Table 17.1 (Cont.)

Author, yr	Sample characteristics					
Van Ginkel et al., 2015 (64)	N=10 Age=29.6±2.1 yr Weight=76.1±5.6 kg Height=180.9±7.6 cm HR=65.8±9.0 bpm					
	ACE II			***ACE ID/DD***		
	Pre-maximal test			*Pre-maximal test*		
	Capillary recruitment (%)=35.5±5.5%			Capillary recruitment (%)=36.2±6.3%		
	Capillary recruitment=18.3±2.6			Capillary recruitment=15.9±2.7		
	Post-maximal test			*Post-maximal test*		
	Capillary recruitment (%)=43.3±4.6%			Capillary recruitment (%)=23.8±4.1%		
	Capillary recruitment=26.8±2.2			Capillary recruitment=12.9±2.4		
Yau et al., 2014 (74)	***ACE II***		***ACE ID***		***ACE DD***	
	N=12 M		N=21 M		N=12 M	
	Age=28±7 yr		Age=27±8 yr		Age=30±9 yr	
	BMI=23.19±2.38 kg/m²		BMI=25.87±3.94 kg/m²		BMI=24.31±3.54 kg/m²	
	VO₂peak=56.30±8.24 ml/ kg/min		VO₂peak=48.44±8.5 ml/kg/ min		VO₂peak=49.98±12.83 ml/kg/min Urine Osm=459±298 mOsmol/kg	
	Urine Osm=472±311 mOsmol/kg		Urine Osm=502±291 mOsmol/kg			
Verlengia et al., 2014 (67)	**Sedentary**			**Physically active**		
	N=58 W (Caucasian)			N=59 W (Caucasian)		
	Age=23.7±4.5 yr			Age=22.1±4.4 yr		
	BMI=21.9±2.0 kg/m²			BMI=21.5±1.8 kg/m²		
	Supine HR=68.3±8.8 bpm			Supine HR=64.3±9.9 bpm		
	BP=110.6±9.4/71.6±7.9 mmHg			BP=110.4±7.8/74±6.8 mmHg		
	Glucose=72±7.0 mg/dl			Glucose=70±5.0 mg/dl		
	TChol=161±29.0 mg/dl			TChol=175±26.0 mg/dl		
	LDL=109±24.0 mg/dl			LDL=75±23.0 mg/dl		
	HDL=41±8.0 mg/dl			HDL=53±16.0 mg/dl		
	TRIG=92±30.0 mg/dl			TRIG=77±15.0 mg/dl		
	ACE II	***ACE ID***	***ACE DD***	***ACE II***	***ACE ID***	***ACE DD***
	VO₂=29.2± 5.9 ml/ kg/min	VO₂=23.9± 3.1 ml/ kg/min	VO₂=24.6± 2.4 ml/ kg/min	VO₂=33.7± 1.6 ml/ kg/min	VO₂=32.6± 4.0 ml/ kg/min	VO₂=31.0± 3.9 ml/ kg/min
Domingo et al., 2013 (18)	**Fastest triathletes**			**Slowest triathletes**		
	N=72 M (AA)			N=73 M (AA)		
	Age=33.1±6.0 yr			Age=32.9±7.9 yr		
	BMI=23.4±1.6 kg/m²			BMI=24.9±2.4 kg/m²		
	Total Ironman=689±37 min			Total Ironman=860±47 min		
	Swim=64±10 min			Swim=78±13 min		
	Cycle=365±21 min			Cycle=430±28 min		
	Run=253±26 min			Run=332±33 min		
Vaughn et al., 2013 (66)	***ACE II/ID***			***ACE DD***		
	N=21 M			N=14 M		
	Age=33.7±1.9 yr			Age=29.9±2.2 yr		
	BMI=25.5±1.0 kg/m²			BMI=23.0±0.4 kg/m²		
	VO₂max=39.4±1.8 ml/kg/min			VO₂max=47.1±2.3 ml/kg/min		
	Fiber CSA=3586±226 um²			Fiber CSA=3408±242 um²		
	Slow Fiber=51.3±2.4%			Slow Fiber=50.8±4.9%		
	Capillary density=438.9±16.8/mm²			Capillary density=540.4±26.5/mm²		

ACE allele distribution^	Intervention characteristics	Results	ACE association
NR	Three separate exercise sessions on a cycle ergometer: 1) Maximal test, warm up for 3 min at 50 W and increased 25 W each min until failure 2) Cycle at 50 W for 3 min at RCP determined by maximal test 3) Cycle for 12 min at VT determined by maximal test	Angiotensin II increased to greater levels in ACE II than ID/DD. Subjects with ACE II and ACE II had higher capillary recruitment and perfusion than ID/DD ($P < 0.05$)	Yes, ACE II >ID/DD for increased angiotensin II and had higher capillary fiber recruitment and perfusion
II (26.7%) ID (46.7%) DD (26.7)	1) Maximal cycle ergometer exercise test to determine VO_2peak 2) Cycling at 55% VO_2peak, for 60 min	There was no relationship among ACE and body weight, plasma volume, serum osmolality, fluid intake, total sweat loss, or perceptions of thirst ($P > 0.05$)	No, for measures of fluid balance and hydration
Sedentary II (15.5%) ID (48.3%) DD (36.2%) Physically Active II (25.4%) ID (45.8%) DD (28.8%)	Graded exercise test on a cycle ergometer. Subjects had a 4 min warm up at 4 W. Workload was increased by 20–25 W per min until failure or 60 rpm was not sustained	There was no relationship between ACE and VO_2 VCO_2, VE, power output, HR, SBP, and DBP to peak exercise ($P > 0.05$)	No, for VO_2, VCO_2, VE, power output, HR, SBP, and DBP to peak exercise
NR	Compete in South African Ironman Triathlon 2000–2001 that consists of 3.8 km open swim, 180 km cycle, and 42.2 km run	The fastest athletes (top 50%, finishing time=689±37 min) tended to have lower ACE levels (28.8±8.6 mU/ml), whereas the slower athletes (bottom 50%, finishing time=860±47 min) had higher ACE levels (31.6±8.7 mU/ml) ($P=0.055$). ACE II athletes had lower plasma ACE levels than ACE ID or ACE DD genotype athletes ($P < 0.001$). These findings suggest the ACE I allele is associated with lower ACE levels and faster triathlon finishing time compared to the D allele	Yes, ACE II <ID/DD for plasma ACE concentration
NR	1) Cycling, 5 d/wk, 30 min/session, at 90% HRmax for 6 months OR 2) Running, 4 d/wk, 30 min/session at 75% VO_2max for 6 months	They examined associations between ACE and VO_2max, muscle capillary growth, and mitochondrial volume in the m. vastus lateralis. VO_2max not different by ACE. Mitochondrial volume and intramyocellular lipids increased ~3× more among ACE II/ID than DD after training ($P < 0.05$). ACE I allele carriers demonstrated upregulation of 15 transcripts related to glucose and lipid metabolism, among other metabolic processes positively associated aerobic energy utilization. The authors concluded their findings support the hypothesis that	No, VO_2max; Yes, ACE II/ID >DD for mitochondria volume and intramyocellular lipids

(continued)

Table 17.1 (Cont.)

Author, yr	Sample characteristics

Almeidaet al., 2012 (1)	**ACE II**	**ACE ID**	**ACE DD**
	N=17 M (Latino)	N=25 M (Latino)	N=15 M (Latino)
	Age=22.5±3.8 yr	Age=23.7±3.8 yr	Age=22.3±1.3 yr
	Weight=70.5±6.6 kg	Weight=73.2±4.5 kg	Weight=71.3±8.4 kg
	Height=181±4 cm	Height=178±4 cm	Height=177±3 cm
	BMI=21.5±2.2 kg/m²	BMI=23.1 kg/m²	BMI=22.8±2.5 kg/m²
	V1600=258.6±5.4 m/min	V1600=249.1±4.3 m/min	V1600=211.2±8.3 m/min
	VO$_2$max=54.2±0.9 ml/kg/min	VO$_2$max=52.2±0.8 ml/kg/min	VO$_2$max=45.8±1.8 ml/kg/min

Alves et al., 2009 (2)	**ACE II**		**ACE ID/DD**	
	N=18 policemen		N=65 policemen	
	Age=26±1 yr		Age=26±1 yr	
	Pre-training	**Post-training**	**Pre-training**	**Post-training**
	BMI=24±0.5 kg/m²	BMI=23±1 kg/m²	BMI=24± 0.5 kg/m²	BMI=24± 0.5 kg/m²
	VO$_2$peak=51±2 ml/kg/min	VO$_2$peak=55±2 ml/kg/min	VO$_2$peak= 49±1 ml/ kg/min	VO$_2$peak=52±1 ml/kg/min
	MAP=91±1 mmHg	MAP=90±2 mmHg	MAP=91± 1 mmHg	MAP=91±1 mmHg
	HR=74±2 bpm	HR=67±2 bpm	HR=74±2 bpm	HR=70±2 bpm
	LVESD=50.2±0.8 mm	LVESD=31.3±0.8 mm	LVESD=31.5 ±0.8 mm	LVESD=31.2 ±0.5 mm
	LVEDD=31.5±0.8 mm	LVEDD=50.6±0.8 mm	LVEDD=50.2 ±0.8 mm	LVEDD=51.3 ±0.4 mm
	LVM=143±8 g	LVM=149.5±7.5 g	LVM=145±8 g	LVM=159.3±4 g
	LVMI=77.7±4.4 g/m²	LVMI=81.5±4.3 g/m²	LVMI=76±2 g/m²	LVMI=83.5± 2 g/m²

Gomes-Gallego et al., 2009 (22)	**ACE II**	**ACE DD**
	N=13	N=19
	Age=28±1 yr	Age=26±1 yr
	Weight=72.3±1.9 kg	Weight=67.0±1 kg
	Height=183±1.8 cm	Height=176.6±1.2 cm
	VO$_2$max=71.7±1.3 ml/kg/min	VO$_2$max=73.0±0.7 ml/kg/min
	PowerVT=4.3±0.2 W/kg	PowerVT=4.5±0.1 W/kg
	GEVT=23.9±0.0%	GEVT=23.8±0.0%

Kalson et al., 2009 (29)	N=173 (104 M/69 W)
	Age=35.8±11.6 yr
	Weight=69.7±13.5 kg

Cam et al., 2007 (10)	N=55 W (Caucasian)		
	Age=20.7±2 yr		
	ACE II	**ACE ID**	**ACE DD**
	N=12	N=23	N=20
	HRbase=71.8±6.2 bpm	HRbase=75.5±4.1 bpm	HRbase=72.6±7.8 bpm
	HRpost=67.8±4.9 bpm	HRpost=71.9±4 bpm	HRpost=69.7±6.4 bpm
	HRRbase70=161.8±2 bpm	HRRbase70=161.6±2 bpm	HRRbase70=161.5±3 bpm
	HRRpost70=160.6±1.7 bpm	HRRpost70=160.5±2 bpm	HRRpost70=160.6±2.5 bpm
	V30base=9.61±0.78 km/hr	V30base=9.05±0.62 km/hr	V30base=9.4±0.89 km/hr
	V30post=11.57±0.8 km/hr	V30post=10.75±0.84 km/hr	V30post=10.96±1.04 km/hr

ACE allele distribution^	Intervention characteristics	Results	ACE association
		ACE mediated remodeling of aerobic substrate pathways contributes to the superior endurance performance of ACE I allele carriers. However, they did not directly compare the relationships among the various metabolic adaptations to endurance exercise training that they found, ACE, and changes in VO₂max	
NR	1) Maximal incremental treadmill test, incline at 1%, starting speed at 6 km/hr. Increments of 0.75 km/hr per min until failure 2) 1600 m running test on a standard track. Conditions were considered neutral	ACE II had higher VO₂max and 1600 m performance than DD (P <0.05)	Yes, ACE II >DD for VO₂max and 1600 m performance
II (21.6%) ID/DD (78.3%)	Supervised treadmill running was conducted 3 d/wk for 60 min per session for 4 months. Intensity for months 1–2 was moderate, and the last 2 months intensity was above the RCT	There were no associations among ACE and endurance performance echocardiographic cardiac outcomes that included; VO₂peak, LVEDV, LVEDD, AD, LVEF, IVST, LVM, LVMI (P >0.05). Contrary to the long-held hypothesis that individuals with ACE DD would exhibit increased LV mass compared to ACE I allele carriers, there were no significant associations found among changes in cardiac morphology and ACE post vs. pre training	No, for VO₂peak, LVEDV, LVEDD, AD, LVEF, IVST, LVM, LVMI
NR	Maximal cycle ergometer exercise test starting at 25 W starting and increasing by 25 W each minute until failure at 70–90 rpm	For all performance outcomes that included PPO, VT, RCT, and GE, there was no association with ACE (P >0.05).	No, for PPO, VT, RCT, and GE
II (22.0%) ID (52.6%) DD (25.4%)	5 day ascent of Mt. Kilamanjaro. Exercise was gauged as successful/unsuccessful summit ascent	Subjects with ACE DD tended to ascent slower than II/ID (P=0.09). Assessment scores for AMS tended to be higher for those with ACE DD than ACE I allele carriers at an altitude of 2700 m (P=0.07, but not 3700 m (P=0.76) and 4700 m (P=0.14). There was no difference in ACE for those who were successful vs. unsuccessful (P=0.09)	No, for summit ascent success or failure and AMS
II (21.8%) ID (41.8%) DD (36.4%)	1) Maximal treadmill exercise test. Each 2 min stage increased 0.8 km/hr 2) Training was conducted 3 d/wk. Intensity was ~65–80% HRR for a continuous bout of 88 min at the anaerobic threshold, and 36 min of endurance power training at 85–90% HRR. Modality of endurance exercise ranged from treadmill, cross-trainer, and cycle ergometer	30 min and 70% HRR running speed improvements post training were greater among those with ACE II >ID >DD than DD (P=0.05). However, at 90% HRR running speed improvements were greater among those with ACE DD>ID>II (P=0.0001), perhaps due to muscle fiber type	Yes, ACE II >ID >DD for 30 min and 70% HRR running speed; and ACE DD >ID >II for 90% HRR running speed

(continued)

Table 17.1 (Cont.)

Author, yr	Sample characteristics		
Day et al., 2007 (15)	N=62 Age=24±7 yr BMI=23.8±3.2 kg/m^2 VO$_2$max=37.0±6.2 ml/kg/min		
Cerit et al., 2006 (13)	**ACE II** N=31 M (Caucasian) 2400 m Performance Baseline=599.1±33.0 sec Post=541±25.4 sec	**ACE ID** N=86 M (Caucasian) 2400 m Performance Baseline=591.9±33.9 sec Post=532.5±28.0 sec	**ACE DD** N=69 M (Caucasian) 2400 m Performance Baseline=601.0±40.3 sec Post=529.6±28.7 sec
Ashley et al., 2006 (4)	N=85 (62 M/23 W) Age=34±5 yr Weight=74.6±1.2 kg Height=177.7±0.8 cm Body Fat=19.9±0.56% LV=322.53±9.43 g LVMI=168.51±5.59 g/m^2 SV=52.4±1.9 ml CO=5.7±0.21 L/min TPR=1536±109 dyns/sec/cm^5 RR interval=1.08±0.03 ms LF/HF=1.92±0.37		

Jones et al., 2006 (28)	**ACE II**
	N=7
	Age=53±2 yr
	BMI=33±0.8 kg/m^2
	BP (24-hr)=141±2/
	  90±1 mmHg
	VO$_2$max=21±2 ml/kg/min
	CC=89±10 ml/min
	24-Na=123±21 mEq/day
	24-K=52±8 mEq/day
		ACE ID
		N=14
		Age=58±2 yr
		BMI=30±6 kg/m^2
		BP (24-hr)=141±2/
		  83±2 mmHg
		VO$_2$max=22±2 ml/kg/min
		CC=95±10 ml/min
		24-Na=101±8 mEq/day
		24-K=48±7 mEq/day
			ACE DD
			N=10
			Age=52±2 yr
			BMI=33±2 kg/m^2
			BP (24-hr)=135±3/82±3 mmHg
			VO$_2$max=20±2 ml/kg/min
			CC=114±11 ml/min
			24-Na=117±17 mEq/day
			24-K=53±7 mEq/day

Tsianos et al., 2005 (62)	N=1284 (235 M/1049 W) Age=37.0±11.5 yr		

Zhao et al., 2003 (77)	N=67 M (Asian)
	Age=23.2±0.29 yr
	BMI=22.0±0.26 kg/m^2
	ACE II
	N=31
	VO$_2$max=50.48±1.58 ml/
	  kg/min
		ACE ID
		N=27
		VO$_2$max=50.58±1.80 ml/kg/
		  min
			ACE DD
			N=9
			VO$_2$max=57.86±3.5 ml/kg/min

ACE allele distribution^	Intervention characteristics	Results	ACE association
II (23%) ID (40%) DD (37%)	Submaximal test on a cycle ergometer to test for DE and GE40,60, & 80 W mechanical efficiency Maximal exercise treadmill test. Starting speed was 8–10 km/hr at 1% grade. Each stage was 4 min and the speed was increased by 1 km/hr each stage	ACE was associated with plasma ACE activity, with ACE DD (33.8+8.9 nM His-Leu/ml) having greater levels than ID (25.9+5.5 nM His-Leu/ml) followed by II (20.5+4.1 nM His-Leu/ml) (P <0.0005). No associations were found between plasma ACE and VO₂max, DE, and GE40,60, & 80 W	Yes, ACE II <ID <DD for ACE activity; No, for VO₂max, DE, and GE
II (16.7%) ID (46.2%) DD (37.1%)	1) 2400 m middle-distance run at baseline and post-training, measured in sec 2) Exercise training consisted of 2 sessions/d, 6 d/wk for 6 months. The program was military-style flexibility, circuit training and 2400 or 3000 m run on the track	Post-training 2400 m performance time improvements were greatest for ACE DD>ID>II (P=0.001), perhaps due to muscle fiber type	Yes, ACE DD > ID >II for improvements in 2400 m performance time
II (23%) ID (46%) DD (31%)	Adrenalin Rush Adventure Race. The race is run in teams of 4, consists of 300 miles of trekking, mountain biking, kayaking, climbing fixed ropes, and swimming. The race can last for multiple days without rest	ACE predicted LV dysfunction after extreme endurance exercise measured by echocardiography and impedance cardiography. ACE II had a greater decrease in fractional shortening than ID >DD. ACE DD had greater LF:HF ratio than ID>II after the race measured by HR variability. The authors concluded that increased sympathetic system dominance contributed to less LV decline post-race among athletes with ACE DD than I allele carriers (56)	Yes, ACE II >ID >DD for decreases in fractional shortening time; ACE DD> Yes, ACE ID >DD for increases in LF:HF ratio
II (23%) ID (45%) DD (32%)	Supervised treadmill walking at 65% HRR with a 10 min warm up, 30 min walk, 5 min rest, then an additional 20 min walk and 10 min cool down for 7 or 8 consecutive days	Levels of sodium excreted in mEq/day, after exercise was greater for ACE II >ID/DD (II 114±22 vs. 169±39 mEq/day, ID 100±8 vs. 133±17 mEq/day, DD 113±18 vs. 138±11 mEq/day). ACE did not associate with changes in SBP, DBP, or MAP. For ACE II the increase in sodium excretion was inversely correlated with decreases in ambulatory 24 hr DBP (r=−0.88, P=0.02) and MAP (r=−0.95, P=0.004). They postulated that ACE dependent effects in sodium excretion may be due to gene to gene interactions, termed epistasis, with ACE and other renal variants that impact sodium resorption in the kidney	Yes, ACE II >ID/DD for sodium excretion; No, for ambulatory SBP, DBP, and MAP
II (19.7%) ID (50.0%) DD (30.3%)	9 day ascent of Mt. Blanc. Exercise was gauged as successful/unsuccessful summit ascent	Frequency of those who made the summit with the ACE I allele was higher than those who failed to reach the summit (47% vs. 21%, P=0.01). No relationship was noted for ACE and development of AMS	Yes, ACE II/ID > DD for summit completion; No, for AMS
II (46.3%) ID (40.3%) DD (13.4%)	Graded exercise treadmill test. 5 min warm up at 9 km/hr and 1% incline. The speed was increased 1 km/min until failure	VO₂max was higher among those with ACE DD than ID or II (P=0.04).	Yes, ACE DD>ID/II for VO₂max

(continued)

Table 17.1 (Cont.)

Author, yr	Sample characteristics

Author, yr	Sample characteristics		
Dengel et al., 2002 (17)	**ACE II** N=8 3 M/5 W (White) Age=63±2 yr BMI=28.5±1.8 kg/m^2 %BF=37.8±1.5 WHR=0.88±0.03 BP=155±4/89±4 mmHg VO$_2$max=19.1±1.2 ml/kg/min	**ACE ID** N=20 8 M/12 W N=4 AA, N=16 white Age=62±2 yr BMI=28.1±0.9 kg/m^2 %BF=38.4±2.3 WHR=0.87±0.03 BP=149±2/88±2 mmHg VO$_2$max=18.1±0.9 ml/kg/min	**ACE DD** N=7 3 M/4 W N=1 AA, N=4 white Age=62±2 yr BMI=32.4±1.8 kg/m^2 %BF=41.7±3.2 WHR=0.85±0.02 BP=155±5/88±2 mmHg VO$_2$max=16.3±1.0 ml/kg/min
Woods et al., 2002 (73)	N=50 *ACE* II (N=24), *ACE* DD (N=26) Age=18.9±0.4 yr Weight=73.4±1.3 kg Height=178±10 cm		
Hagberg et al., 2002 (23)	**ACE II** N=12 W Age=62±1 yr Body fat=33±2% VO$_2$max=32±1 ml/kg/min HRmax=172±4 bpm submaximal Hemodynamics BP=160±4/82±2 mmHg HR=124±4 bpm CO=9.1±0.4 L/min SV=74±3 ml TPR=1030±60 dyn/sec/cm^2	**ACE ID** N=33 W Age=63±1 yr Body fat=33±1% VO$_2$max=29±1 ml/kg/min HRmax=162±2 bpm Submaximal hemodynamics BP=151±2/78±1 mmHg HR=113±2 bpm CO=87±0.3 L/min SV=77±2 ml TPR=990±40 dyn/sec/cm^5	**ACE DD** N=17 W Age=66±1 yr Body fat=30±2% VO$_2$max=27±1 ml/kg/min HRmax=162±3 bpm Submaximal hemodynamics BP=156±3/76±2 mmHg HR=116±3 bpm CO=8.3±0.4 L/min SV=72±3 ml TPR=1060±50 dyn/sec/cm^5
Sonna et al., 2001 (60)	N=147 (62 M/85 W) Age=21.7±3.6 yr BMI=23.1±3.1 kg/m^2 Body fat=27.9±6.1%		

	ACE II		**ACE ID**		ACE DD		
	Men	**Women**	**Men**	**Women**	**Men**		**Women**
	N=17	N=10	N=26	N=29	N=13		N=22
	PreVO$_2$peak =50.5±1.5 ml/kg/ min PostVO$_2$peak =52.3±1.3 ml/kg/ min	PreVO$_2$peak= 39.4±1.0 ml/ kg/min PostVO$_2$peak =42.1±1.5 ml/ kg/min	PreVO$_2$peak= 51.8±1.5 ml/ kg/min PostVO$_2$peak= 52.5±1.1 ml/ kg/min	PreVO$_2$peak = 39.7±1.0 ml/ kg/min PostVO$_2$peak = 42.2±0.9 ml/ kg/min	PreVO$_2$peak= 49.8±1.4 ml/ kg/min PostVO$_2$peak= 51.8±1.3 ml/ kg/min		PreVO$_2$peak= 40.2±1.3 ml/ kg/min PostVO$_2$peak= 43.8±1.2 ml/ kg/min

ACE allele distribution^	Intervention characterization	Results	ACE association
II (23%) ID (57%) DD (20%)	24 wk of supervised treadmill walking, 3 d/wk, at 75–85% HRR for 40 min per session. Adherence to the intervention was 91%	There were no interactions in the training response in VO_2max, BMI, BF, fat mass, WHR, SBP, and DBP by ACE ($P >0.05$). Individuals with ACE II ($2.5+0.8\ \mu U \times 10^{-4}$/min/ml) exhibited improved insulin sensitivity than ID/DD ($0.7+0.2\ \mu U \times 10^{-4}$/min/ml) as assessed with a GTT ($P=0.011$)	No, for VO_2max, BMI, BF, fat mass, WHR, SBP, and DBP; Yes, for ACE II >ID/DD improved insulin sensitivity
II (23%) ID (54%) DD (23%)	The endurance training program consisted of running, marching, and circuit training in squads for 11 wk. Maximal (40 W increments every 3 min until exhaustion) and submaximal (pedaled for 3 min at 60 rpm in 20 W increments) cycle ergometer exercise test	No significant interaction between ACE and VO_2max, or HR after training. However, the decrease in submaximal VO_2 was greater for ACE II than DD ($P=0.02$)	No, VO_2max or HR; Yes, for ACE II >DD for reduced submaximal VO_2 at 80 W
II (19.4%) ID (53.3%) DD (27.4%)	Graded maximal and submaximal (40%, 60%, and 80% VO_2max) treadmill exercise test	Subjects with ACE II has greater increases in VO_2max and submaximal (9–11 bpm) and maximal HR (10 bpm) than ID/DD, but there were no overall ACE associations with CO, SV, TPR, or the a–VO_2diff	Yes, ACE II > ID/DD for VO_2max and HR; No for CO, SV, TPR, or a–VO_2diff
Men II (30.3%) ID (46.4%) DD (23.3%) Women II (16.4%) ID (47.5%) DD (36.1%)	Before and after basic training, peak treadmill exercise test with a 5 min warm up at 0% grade, speed was 2.68 m/sec (women), and 2.24 m/sec (men) and performance on the APFT. Speed was increased by 0.45 m/sec and 2% grade every 3 min until failure	There was no relationship among ACE and VO_2peak, CO, VE, RER, and %HRmax and any APFT measure	No, for VO_2peak, CO, VE, RER, and %HRmax

(continued)

Table 17.1 (Cont.)

Author, yr	Sample characteristics			
Rankinen et al., 2000 (49)	**Caucasian parents (N=177)** Age=52.9±5.2 yr BMI=27.9±4.6 kg/m² HRmax=174.2± 12.9 bpm Wmax=158±50 watt VO₂max=2.15±0.62 L/min	**Caucasian offspring (294)** Age=25.4± 6.2 yr BMI=24.6±4.7 kg/m² HRmax=192.2± 9.0 bpm Wmax=199± 60 W VO₂max=2.64± 0.74 L/min	**AA parents (N=65)** Age=48.4±7.1 yr BMI=28.6±5.2 kg/m² HRmax=171.9±15.8 bpm Wmax=127±36 watt VO₂max=1.78±0.41 L/min	**AA offspring (182)** Age=28.0±7.4 yr BMI=27.6±6.2 kg/m² HRmax=185.4±12.2 bpm Wmax=156±49 W VO₂max=2.18±0.65 L/min

ACE allele distribution[^]	Intervention characteristics	Results	ACE association
Caucasian (N=476) II/ID (46.8%) DD (53.2%) AA (N=248) II/ID (41.6%) DD (58.4%)	The HEalth, RIsk factors, exercise Training And GEnetics (HERITAGE) family training study consisted of 20 wk of supervised training on a cycle ergometer 3 days per wk at 55% VO_2max (wk 1–2) and gradually increased to 75% VO_2max (wk 14–20) (monitored by HR) for 30 min per session. Pre- and post-training endurance performance outcomes were measured with submaximal and maximal cycle ergometer tests	Measured 54 endurance performance phenotypes in 4 groups of subjects, with only 11 showing significant associations. Caucasian DD offspring > II for increased VO_2max after training (+0.48±0.02 L/min vs. +0.42±0.03 L/min, P=0.042), and submaximal VO_2, VE (ACE II >ID/DD), and VT (ACE II >ID/DD), and a greater decrease in submaximal HR at 50 W. No associations for Caucasian parents or AA parents or offspring. No associations for maximal and submaximal CO, SV, and blood lactate	Yes, for ACE DD>ID/II for VO_2max, and submaximal VO_2, VE, VT, and HR; No, for maximal and submaximal CO, SV, and blood lactate

Note: Data are presented as reported by authors. Data is reported as mean±SD unless otherwise noted. AA=African American. ACE=angiotensin-converting enzyme. AD=auricular diameter. AMS=acute mountain sickness. APFT=Army Physical Fitness Test. a–VO_2diff=arterial venous oxygen difference. Base=baseline. %BF=body fat percentage. BMI=body mass index. BP=blood pressure. bpm=beats per minute. CC=creatinine clearance. CRF=cardiorespiratory fitness. CO=cardiac output. CSA=cross-sectional area. D=deletion. DE=delta efficiency. DBP=diastolic blood pressure. GE40,60 & 80 W=gross mechanical efficiency. GTT=glucose tolerance test. HDL=high density lipoprotein. HR=heart rate. HR0=HR at time 0. HR120=heart rate at 120 minutes after exercise. HRmax=maximum heart rate. HRpeak=peak heart rate. HRR=heart rate reserve. I=insertion. IVST=intraventricular septum thickness. K=potassium. Kg=kilogram. LF:HF=low and high frequency domains of heart rate variability. LDL=low density lipoproteins. LVEDD=left ventricular end diastolic diameter. LVEF=left ventricular ejection fraction. LVESD=left ventricular end systolic diameter. LVEDV=left ventricular end diastolic volume. LVM=left ventricular mass. LVMI=left ventricular mass index. M=meter. MAP=mean arterial pressure. mEq=milliequivalents. min=minute. mOsmol=milliosmols. Na=sodium. NO=nitric oxide. Osm=osmolality. PEH=postexercise hypotension. PowerVT=power at ventilator threshold. PPO=peak power output. PSI=physiological strain index. RCT=respiratory compensation threshold. RE=running economy. RER=respiratory exchange rate. S=heat storage. SBP=systolic blood pressure. SD=standard deviation. SE=standard error. Sec=second. SV=stroke volume. rpm=revolutions per minute. TChol=total cholesterol. TG=triglycerides. TPR=total peripheral resistance. V=velocity. VE=minute ventilation. VCO_2=carbon dioxide output. VO_2max=maximal oxygen consumption. VO_2peak=peak oxygen consumption. VT=ventilatory threshold. WC=waist circumference.

[^]ACE distribution appears when authors report the % of each genotype present in the sample and whether the sample was in Hardy–Weinberg equilibrium. Trials that did not provide both components are listed as NR.

*Data are reported as mean±SD/SE.

(2, 23, 49, 60), and one trial (4) found a greater decrease in fractional shortening among athletes with *ACE* II than ID and DD and an increase in sympathetic system dominance as assessed by HR variability among athletes with *ACE* DD than ID and II after 120 min of continuous extreme exercise. Collectively, these trials do not support the working hypothesis that the *ACE* I allele plays a major role in endurance exercise performance as assessed by measures of cardiac function.

ACE *rs4340, endurance performance, and muscle metabolism*

Angiotensin II elevates BP due to its vasoconstrictor properties, and restricts blood from entering nonactive muscles, thereby allowing blood flow to be redirected from nonactive to metabolically active tissues as occurs with enhanced energy turnover during exercise. Furthermore, angiotensin II promotes angiogenesis, facilitating exercise-induced capillary growth in human skeletal muscle. Those with the *ACE* I allele have lower resting levels of angiotensin II than carriers of the D allele. It has been hypothesized that the *ACE* I allele is associated with superior endurance performance partially due to enhanced oxygen delivery and extraction in the skeletal muscle capillary beds that may result from greater increases in exercise-induced serum angiotensin II levels than with the *ACE* D allele, effects that are overridden at the local level during exercise (54, 64). There were four trials that examined associations among *ACE* rs4340, endurance performance, and muscle metabolism (63–66). Of these, two trials from the same investigative team (65, 66) and two trials from different groups (63, 64) all reported positive associations with the *ACE* I allele and increased capillary density or volume, capillary to fiber ratio, capillary recruitment/perfusion, and/or mitochondrial density or volume compared to *ACE* DD, that varied by training status (63). Furthermore, Vaughan et al. (66) found that *ACE* I allele carriers demonstrated upregulation of 15 mRNA transcripts related to glucose and lipid metabolism, among other metabolic processes positively associated with aerobic energy utilization. Yet, collectively these investigative teams did not comment on how these favorable aerobic metabolic adaptations that appeared to be mediated by the *ACE* I allele related to measures of endurance exercise performance. Therefore, no definitive conclusions can be made from this series of studies regarding whether these favorable genetically mediated skeletal muscle metabolic and vascular adaptations associated with the *ACE* I allele contribute to the purported superior endurance exercise performance of *ACE* I allele carriers than those with the D allele.

ACE *rs4340, endurance exercise performance, and fluid electrolyte balance*

Adequate fluid consumption/replacement during exercise is critical for successful performance (3, 12). Water loss or body mass loss during or after exercise that reaches at least 3% is detrimental to endurance performance. Furthermore, fluid intake is tightly linked to sodium balance, an electrolyte with a prominent role in BP regulation, nerve and muscle function, and various other metabolic processes (e.g., glucose metabolism). The RAAS is a critical regulatory system of fluid and electrolyte balance. There were two trials that examined the association among *ACE* rs4340, endurance performance, and indicators of fluid electrolyte balance (28, 74). These two investigative teams found conflicting findings regarding associations with biomarkers of fluid and electrolyte balance and *ACE* rs4340 so that no conclusions can be made regarding *ACE*, fluid and electrolyte balance, and endurance performance.

ACE *rs4340 and endurance performance at high altitude*

It has been postulated that the *ACE* I allele is associated with lower rates of acute mountain sickness among successful mountaineering athletes (33, 35). Lower levels of circulating ACE among *ACE* I allele carriers are thought ultimately to limit actions of the RAAS that are implicated in the etiology of acute mountain sickness that include vasoconstriction of pulmonary arteries via angiotensin II, dysregulation of fluids and electrolytes, and inhibition of cardiac and pulmonary growth and remodeling. Two trials examined associations between indicators of performance at high altitude that included successful or unsuccessful mountain ascent and assessments of acute mountain sickness by *ACE* (29, 62). The authors reported conflicting findings regarding successful or unsuccessful mountain ascent time, and both found no associations with *ACE* and acute mountain sickness so that no conclusions can be made regarding *ACE* and endurance performance at high altitude.

ACE rs4340 and endurance exercise health-related outcomes

There were nine qualifying primary levels trials that investigated *ACE* rs4340 and endurance exercise health-related outcomes that are detailed in Table 17.2. The subjects in these trials were predominantly middle-aged to older men and women of various races/ethnicities who were sedentary at baseline and then completed either a moderate to vigorous intensity treadmill or cycling exercise training program or acute treadmill, walking, or cycle ergometer exercise bout. The endurance exercise health-related outcomes were varied and included BP, measures of body composition, and various hormone and inflammatory markers.

ACE *rs4340 and the blood pressure response to endurance exercise*

The RAAS is a major BP regulatory pathway due to its vasoactive actions, maintenance of fluid and electrolyte balance, and angiogenic properties (Figure 17.3). ACE is a key enzyme in this pathway, whose circulating levels vary by the *ACE* I and D alleles as discussed previously (15, 18, 51), that converts biologically inactive angiotensin I into angiotensin II, a potent vasopressor, whose actions include vasoconstriction, renal sodium reabsorption, and aldosterone production. For this reason, *ACE* is an ideal candidate gene to explore for associations with the BP response to acute (short-term or immediate, termed *postexercise hypotension* (PEH)) and chronic (long-term or training) endurance exercise. Five trials examined the influence of *ACE* on PEH (6, 20, 43, 54, 67) and four trials investigated the influence of *ACE* on the BP response to endurance exercise training (17, 26, 28, 48).

Of the five trials that examined associations with *ACE* and PEH, four found associations with *ACE* and BP, but with conflicting results (6, 20, 43, 54), and one found no association (67). It should be noted that due to the small sample size, the results of the study by Pescatello et al. (43) should be interpreted with caution. Nonetheless, these investigators utilized deep-exon sequencing of *ACE* and instituted other important methodological strategies to bolster the statistical power to detect PEH–renal genotype associations (7, 8, 36). These other strategies included: 1) a randomized controlled repeated-measure design with 19 hourly time points per subject who served as their own control; 2) a focused inquiry of variants with a prioritized panel of genes that reduced the search space within the genome; 3) high-throughput exon sequencing to focus on functional gene regions; 4) the same standardized protocols from their earlier studies that used the clinical gold standard of BP assessment, ambulatory BP monitoring; 5) a closely monitored, well-controlled exercise exposure; and 6) adjustment for multiple testing based on

Table 17.2 A summary of the qualifying trials that examined the influence of *ACE* rs4340 on endurance exercise health-related outcomes*

Author, yr	Sample characteristics					
Pescatello et al., 2016 (43)	**Caucasian** N=9 M/W Age=45.1±7.8 yr BMI=30.5±1.8 kg/m² Waist Circumference=98.0±7.2 cm VO₂peak=29.7±6.4 ml/kg/min Awake BP=139.3±7.0/85.0±5.1 mmHg Glucose=96.4±12.2 mg/dl Insulin=13.1±10.1 uIU/ml HOMA=3.1±2.2 TChol=207.8±31.1 mg/dl LDL=129.4±20.3 mg/dl HDL=44.1±109 mg/dl Trig=170.8±88.8 mg/dl Nitrate/nitrite=23.3±37.0 umol/L CRP=1.1±1.0 mg/dl Endothelin=0.22±0.21 pmol/L PRA=1.7±1.1 ng/ml/hr		**African American/black** N=14 M/W Age=39.9±10.6 yr BMI=31.1±4.5 kg/m² Waist Circumference=88.3±9.4 cm VO₂peak=25.3±5.7 ml/kg/min Awake BP=140.2±12.3/84.3±6.9 mmHg Glucose=97.2±10.3 mg/dl Insulin=9.4±6.0 uIU/ml HOMA=2.3±1.5 TChol=178.5±27.3 mg/dl LDL=53.9±14.8 mg/dl HDL=53.9±14.8 mg/dl Trig=83.7±35.8 mg/dl Nitrate/nitrite=10.9±13.1 umol/L CRP=2.8±3.5 mg/dl Endothelin=0.38±0.66 pmol/L PRA=0.95±0.84 ng/ml/hr			
Goessler et al., 2015 (20)	***ACE* II/ID** N=24 8 M/16 W Age=62.9±2.1 yr BMI=28.5±1.2 kg/m² BP=133.8±3.0/84.3±1.8 mmHg (70.8% BP medications, 8.3% with diabetes)		***ACE* DD** N=10 Age=58.2±3.1 yr BMI=31±0.9 kg/m² BP=128±5.3/84.5±3.8 mmHg (70% BP medications, 10% with diabetes)			
Verlengia et al., 2014 (67)	**Sedentary** N=58 W (Caucasian) Age=23.7±4.5 yr BMI=21.9±2.0 kg/m² Supine HR=68.3±8.8 bpm BP=110.6±9.4/71.6±7.9 mmHg Glucose=72±7.0 mg/dl TChol=161±29.0 mg/dl LDL=109±24.0 mg/dl HDL=41±8.0 mg/dl TRIG=92±30.0 mg/dl			**Physically Active** N=59 W (Caucasian) Age=22.1±4.4 yr BMI=21.5±1.8 kg/m² Supine HR=64.3±9.9 bpm BP=110.4±7.8/74±6.8 mmHg Glucose=70±5.0 mg/dl TChol=175±26.0 mg/dl LDL=75±23.0 mg/dl HDL=53±16.0 mg/dl TRIG=77±15.0 mg/dl		
	***ACE* II** VO₂=29.2±5.9 ml/kg/min	***ACE* ID** VO₂=23.9±3.1 ml/kg/min	***ACE* DD** VO₂=24.6±2.4 ml/kg/min	***ACE* II** VO₂=33.7±1.6 ml/kg/min	***ACE* ID** VO₂=32.6±4.0 ml/kg/min	***ACE* DD** VO₂=31.0±3.9 ml/kg/min
Izzicupo et al., 2013 (26)	***ACE* II/ID** N=21 W (postmenopausal) Age=56.0±4.6 yr BMI=25.9±4.5 kg/m² %BF=33.2±6.7 WC=82.6±10.5 cm WHR=0.82±0.06 METs_{m/die}=1.54±0.25 ml/kg/min BP=122.1±14/78.1±9.0 mmHg HR=64.7±8.9 bpm TNF-α=34.0±22.1 pg/ml DHEA-S=1.13±0.69 pg/ml Cortisol=123.7±54.2 pg/ml		***ACE* DD** N=15 W (postmenopausal) Age=56.0±3.9 yr BMI=27.9±3.8 kg/m² %BF=36.8±4.8 WC=88.7±9.2 cm WHR=0.84±0.67 METs_{m/die}=1.41±0.23 ml/kg/min BP=133.7±17.7/81.7±7.2 mmHg HR=69.6±6.3 bpm TNF-α=60.0±36.2 pg/ml DHEA-S=0.66±0.35 pg/ml Cortisol=122.5±58.9 pg/ml			

ACE allele distribution^	Intervention characteristics	Results	ACE association
NR	Subjects completed a cardiopulmonary cycle ergometer exercise test to exhaustion (100% VO_2peak), a 20 min session of cycling at 60% VO_2peak with a 5 min warm up and cool down to total 30 min, and a control session of seated rest. Deep-sequenced exons from *ACE*, adducin 1 (*ADD1*), angiotensin II type 1 receptor (*AGTR1*), and the aldosterone synthase (*CYP11B2*) genes	After vigorous intensity over 19 hr among *ACE*, *AGTR1*, *CYP11B2*, and *ADD1* variants passing multiple testing thresholds, as the #MA of increased, SBP and/or DBP decreased 12 (P=4.5E-05) to 30 mmHg (P=6.4E-04) among African Americans only. In contrast, after moderate intensity over 19 hr among *ACE* and *CYP11B2* variants passing multiple testing thresholds, as the #MA increased, SBP *increased* 21 (P=8.0E-04) to 22 mmHg (P=8.2E-04) among African Americans only. Of note, although several *ACE* variants emerged as significantly associated with PEH in this study, *ACE* rs4340 did not, and our significant findings were observed only among African Americans and after vigorous intensity	Yes, *ACE* minor<major alleles for 19 hr ambulatory SBP and DBP
II/ID (70.6%) DD (29.4%)	An acute 45 min walking bout at 60–75% HRR with a 5 min warm up and cool down to total 55 min	Ambulatory DBP was lowered to greater levels following the walking session among individuals with *ACE* II/ID (−6.3+1.9 mmHg) than *ACE* DD (−2.9+1.9 mmHg) for 5 hr (P=0.002), with similar trends for ambulatory SBP (P=0.02), although the SBP data were not provided	Yes, for *ACE* II/ID <DD for SBP and DBP
Sedentary II (15.5%) ID (48.3%) DD (36.2%) Physically Active II (25.4%) ID (45.8%) DD (28.8%)	Graded exercise test on a cycle ergometer. Subjects had a 4 min warm up at 4 W. Workload was increased by 20–25 W per min until failure or 60 rpm was not sustained	There was no relationship among *ACE* and VO_2 VCO_2, VE, power output, HR, SBP, and DBP at peak exercise (P >0.05)	No, for VO_2, VCO_2, VE, power output, HR, SBP, and DBP at peak exercise
NR	13 wk 4 d/wk for 40 min/d (wk 1–4) progressing to 50 min per session (wk 5–13) of walking at a RPE 11 (wk 1–9) and RPE 12/13 (wk 10–13)	After walking, SBP, MAP, and the double product (i.e., HR × SBP) were lower by *ACE* DD <II/ID. There were no differences in the response of TNF-α, DHEA-S, or cortisol by *ACE* (P <0.05)	Yes, *ACE* DD <II/ID for SBP, MAP, and the double product

(continued)

Table 17.2 (Cont.)

Author, yr	Sample characteristics			
Santana et al., 2011 (54)	**ACE II/ID** N=10/10 Age=70.4±6.2 yr BMI=25.9±3.0 kg/m² Glucose=86.9±13.1 mg/dl BP=129.0±17.0/77.0±8.0 mmHg NO=294.4±176.5 uM Wpeak=62.3±21.4 watt VO₂peak=20.5±4.3 ml/kg/min HRpeak=148.0±21.0 bpm 20% on diuretics		**ACE DD** N=10 Age=70.6±5.8 yr BMI=25.4±3.2 kg/m² Glucose=79.6±17.1 mg/dl BP=125.0±14.0/77.0±7.0 mmHg NO=278.2±159.0 uM Wpeak=57.0±19.7 watt VO₂peak=20.1±3.0 ml/kg/min HRpeak=142.7±19.6 bpm 20% on diuretics	

Jones et al., 2006 (28)	**ACE II**
	N=7
	Age=53±2 yr
	BMI=33±0.8 kg/m²
	BP (24-hr)=141±2/
	  90±1 mmHg
	VO₂max=21±2 ml/
	  kg/min
	CC=89±10 ml/min
	24-Na=123±21 mEq/day
	24-K=52±8 mEq/day
		ACE ID
		N=14
		Age=58±2 yr
		BMI=30±6 kg/m²
		BP (24-hr)=141±2/
		  83±2 mmHg
		VO₂max=22±2 ml/kg/min
		CC=95±10 ml.min
		24-Na=101±8 mEq/day
		24-K=48±7 mEq/day
			ACE DD
			N=10
			Age=52±2 yr
			BMI=33±2 kg/m²
			BP (24-hr)=135±3/
			  82±3 mmHg
			VO₂max=20±2 ml/kg/min
			CC=114±11 ml/min
			24-Na=117±17 mEq/day
			24-K=53±7 mEq/day
				II (23%)
				ID (45%)
				DD (32%)

Blanchard et al., 2006 (6)	N=47 M (Caucasian) Age=43.8±1.4 yr BMI=29.4±0.7 kg/m² BP (awake)=145.0±1.5/85.8±1.1 mmHg (hypertension) WC=101.8±2.0 cm VO₂max=31.3±0.9 ml/kg/min			

Dengel et al., 2002 (17)	**ACE II**
	N=8 3 M/5 W (White)
	Age=63±2 yr
	BMI=28.5±1.8
	  kg/m²
	%BF=37.8±1.5
	WHR=0.88±0.03
	BP=155±4/89±4 mmHg
	VO₂max=19.1±1.2 ml/
	  kg/min
		ACE ID
		N=20 8 M/12 W
		N=4 AA, N=16 white
		Age=62±2 yr
		BMI=28.1±0.9 kg/m²
		%BF=38.4±2.3
		WHR=0.87±0.03
		BP=149±2/88±2 mmHg
		VO₂max=18.1±0.9 ml/
		  kg/min
			ACE DD
			N=7 3 M/4 W
			N=1 AA, N=4 white
			Age=62±2 yr
			BMI=32.4±1.8 kg/m²
			%BF=41.7±3.2
			WHR=0.85±0.02
			BP=155±5/88±2 mmHg
			VO₂max=16.3±1.0 ml/kg/min	

ACE allele distribution[^]	Intervention characteristics	Results	ACE association
NR	Acute maximal to exhaustion and a submaximal constant load cycle ergometer exercise test at 90% AT and RPE for 20 min vs. a 20 min control session without exercise	After the maximal ($-7.4+8.4$/ $-4.2+6.0$ mmHg) and submaximal ($2.2+5.9$ mmHg/$-1.1+3.9$) tests, SBP and MAP were reduced, respectively, and NO was increased to greater levels for ACE II/ ID >DD	Yes, ACE II/ ID>DD for SBP, MAP, and NO
	Supervised treadmill walking at 65% HRR with a 10 min warm up, 30 min walk, 5 min rest, then an additional 20 min walk and 10 min cool down for 7 or 8 consecutive days	Levels of sodium excreted in mEq/day, after exercise was greater for ACE II >ID/ DD (II 114±22 vs. 169±39 mEq/day, ID 100±8 vs. 133±17 mEq/day, DD 113±18 vs. 138±11 mEq/day). ACE did not associate with changes in SBP, DBP, or MAP. For ACE II the increase in sodium excretion was inversely correlated with decreases in ambulatory 24 hr DBP ($r=-0.88$, $P=0.02$) and MAP ($r=-0.95$, $P=0.004$)	Yes, ACE II >ID/ DD for sodium excretion; No, for ambulatory SBP, DBP, and MAP
NR	30 min acute bouts of cycle ergometer exercise at 40% VO$_2$max or 60% VO$_2$max with a 5 min warm-up and cool down to total 40 min compared to a control session of rest. Examined the epistatic interactions of ACE, and polymorphisms in angiotensin II type 1 receptor (AGTR1) and the aldosterone synthase (CYP11B2) genes	After the 40% VO$_2$max bout, 14 hr ambulatory SBP was lower in ACE DD than ACE II/ID (132.4 vs. 128.1 mmHg) ($P=0.047$). After the 60% VO$_2$max bout, there were no differences in the BP by ACE. After the 40% VO$_2$max bout, men with 3 RAAS minor alleles lowered SBP and DBP more than men with 0–2 minor alleles	Yes, ACE DD <II/ID for 14 hr ambulatory SBP after 40% VO$_2$max
II (23%) ID (57%) DD (20%)	24 wk of supervised treadmill walking, 3 d/ wk, at 75–85% HRR for 40 min per session. Adherence to the intervention was 91%	There were no interactions among the training response of VO$_2$max, BMI, BF, Fat Mass, WHR, SBP, and DBP by ACE ($P >0.05$). They hypothesized ACE DD is associated with increased ACE activity, which would lead to increased production of angiotensin II, and a decreased half-life of bradykinin, a vasodilator, that would result in decreased glucose delivery to the muscle. They found individuals with ACE II ($2.5+0.8$ μU ×10^{-4}/min/ml) exhibited improved insulin sensitivity than ID/DD ($0.7+0.2$ μU × 10^{-4}/min/ml) as assessed with a GTT ($P=0.011$)	No, for VO$_2$max, BMI, BF, Fat Mass, WHR, SBP, and DBP; Yes, for ACE II >ID/DD improved insulin sensitivity

(continued)

Table 17.2 (Cont.)

Author, yr	Sample characteristics					
Rankinen et al.,2000 (48)	**ACE II**		**ACE ID**		**ACE DD**	
	Men	**Women**	**Men**	**Women**	**Men**	**Women**
	N=54	N=59	N=101	N=117	N=69	N=66
	Age=36.4± 1.0 yr	Age=35.0± 0.9 yr	Age=36.4± 1.0 yr	Age=35.0± 0.9 yr	Age=36.4± 1.0 yr	Age=35.0±0.9 yr
	BMI=26.7± 0.3 kg/m^2	BMI=25.1± 0.3 kg/m^2	BMI=26.7± 0.3 kg/m^2	BMI=25.1± 0.3 kg/m^2	BMI=26.7± 0.3 kg/m^2	BMI=25.1±0.3 kg/m^2
	BP=148.4± 2.1/72.4± 1.3 mmHg	BP=144.9± 2.0/70.3±1.1 mmHg	BP=145.9± 1.5/71.7± 0.9 mmHg	BP=141.0± 1.4/69.3±0.8 mmHg	BP=145.2± 1.9/70.5±1.1 mmHg	BP=144.5±1.9/ 68.4±1.0 mmHg
	BP Response= −5.7±1.3/ −2.8±0.7 mmHg	BValdiviesP Response= −9.7±1.3/− 3.6±0.8 mmHg	BP Response= −5.8±0.9/ −2.4±0.5 mmHg	BP Response= −6.8±0.9/− 3.5±0.6 mmHg	BP Response= −7.1±1.1/ −4.4±0.6 mmHg	BP Response= −7.6±1.2/−4.0±0.8 mmHg

ACE allele distribution[^]	Intervention characteristics	Results	ACE association
Men II (24.1%) ID (45.1%) DD (30.8%) Women II (24.4%) ID (48.3%) DD (27.2%)	20 wk of supervised training on a cycle ergometer 3 days per wk at 55% VO$_2$max (wk 1–2) and gradually increased to 75% VO$_2$max (wk 14–20) (monitored by HR) for 30 min per session. BP was measured pre- and post-training with submaximal and maximal cycle ergometer tests	Men with *ACE* DD marginally lowered DBP to greater levels ~2 mmHg during the submaximal test than II/ID (2.8 (P=0.05)	Yes, for *ACE* DD <II/ID for DBP

Note: Data are presented as reported by authors. Data is reported as mean±*SD* unless otherwise noted. ACE=angiotensin-converting enzyme. %BF=body fat percentage. BMI=body mass index. BP=blood pressure. bpm=beats per minute. CC=creatinine clearance. CRF=cardiorespiratory fitness. CRP=C-reactive protein. D=deletion. DBP=diastolic blood pressure. DHEA-S=dehydroepiandrosterone-sulfate conjugate. HOMA=homeostatic model assessment. HR=heart rate. HRmax=maximum heart rate. HRpeak=peak heart rate. HRR=heart rate reserve. I=insertion. METs$_{m/die}$=daily mean of metabolic equivalent of task. min=minute. NO=nitric oxide. NR=not reported. #MA=number of minor alleles. PEH=postexercise hypotension. PRA=plasma renin activity. SBP=systolic blood pressure. SD=standard deviation. SE=standard error. TChol=total cholesterol. TG=triglycerides. TNF-α=tumor necrosis factor alpha. VE=expiratory minute ventilation. VO$_2$max=maximal oxygen consumption. VO$_2$peak=peak oxygen consumption. WC=waist circumference. wk=week. WHR=waist to hip ratio. Wmax=maximum power. Wpeak=peak power. Yr=year. *ACE* polymorphism distribution denotes the percentage (%) of the sample with the following genotypes: II=homozygous for the insertion. ID=heterozygous. DD=homozygous for the deletion.

★Data are reported as mean±SD/SE.

^ACE distribution appears when authors report the % of each genotype present in the sample and whether the sample was in Hardy–Weinberg equilibrium. Trials that did not provide both components are listed as NR.

+ACE and PEH associations only for rs1055086.

genetic variants exhibiting variability in the number of minor alleles and with unique genotypic values. Of the four trials that examined associations with *ACE* rs4340 and the BP response to endurance exercise training, two found associations with *ACE* and BP (26, 48), and one of these was marginal, and two found no association (17, 28). Collectively, these acute and chronic trials tend to show BP is lowered to greater levels with *ACE* DD than I allele carriers. However, due to the disparate nature of the findings, no definitive conclusions can be made regarding the BP response to either acute or chronic endurance exercise.

ACE rs4340 and the response of other endurance exercise health-related outcomes

Pharmacological ACE inhibitors have been shown to improve insulin resistance, and the D allele has been associated with alterations in exercise-induced glucose metabolism that resemble a prediabetic state (65). Dengal et al., in addition to BP mentioned previously, examined the association with insulin resistance as assessed by an intravenous glucose tolerance test and *ACE* rs4340 (17). They found subjects with *ACE* II showed greater improvements in insulin sensitivity than D allele carriers ($P=0.011$). These findings are consistent with the more recent findings of Vaughan et al. (65), showing the genetically mediated exercise-induced adaptations in the skeletal muscle by *ACE* lead to improved capillarization and glucose and lipid metabolism among I allele carriers. Yet, how these alterations would lead to *ACE* genetically mediated differences in endurance performance are not clear.

Conclusion

For the many reasons discussed in this chapter, *ACE* rs4340 is a biologically plausible candidate gene to explore for its associations with endurance exercise performance and health-related outcomes. To this end, the working hypothesis of this chapter is, adults with the *ACE* I allele exhibit superior endurance exercise performance than adults with the D allele. In contrast to this hypothesis, we conclude there is limited evidence (44) to suggest that *ACE* rs4340 *does not* play a major role in endurance exercise performance regarding exercise-induced changes in cardio-respiratory fitness as assessed by VO₂max/peak and other measures of endurance performance, cardiac morphology and function, fluid and electrolyte balance, and acute mountain sickness. The evidence is moderate (44) indicating that *ACE does* play a role in the acute and chronic exercise-induced adaptations that occur in the skeletal muscle relating to improved capillary perfusion and aerobic energy utilization. Yet, how these more favorable exercise-induced skeletal muscle effects associated with the *ACE* I allele translate into superior endurance performance remains unclear due to the paucity of studies linking *ACE* rs4340 and ACE concentrations to measures of acute and chronic endurance performance. Accordingly, this systematic review *does not* support the working hypothesis of this chapter that adults with the *ACE* I allele exhibit superior endurance exercise performance than adults with the D allele.

These evidence-based conclusions are somewhat surprising due to the extensive volume of literature on this topic that reflects the general level of scientific interest in *ACE* rs4340 and human physical performance (Figure 17.1). Yet, this systematic review, as well as our recent meta-analysis (8) of candidate gene association studies examining the BP response to acute and chronic endurance exercise, highlight the significant limitations of candidate gene association studies. For, they often: 1) have small sample sizes; 2) examine a small number of polymorphisms, and in the case of this systematic review, the focus was on *ACE* rs4340; 3) are subject to sample selection bias; 4) are not sufficiently powered to examine possible confounding sample features; and 5) do not employ statistical corrections for multiple comparisons. Other contributing factors include: 1) endurance exercise performance is a polygenic trait so that it is unlikely that one structural variant such as *ACE* rs4340 would have a major effect; 2) several dbSNP entries exist all tagging *ACE* rs4340 that include: rs4343, rs4341, rs1799752, rs4646994, and rs13447447 suggesting the possibility that *ACE* rs4340 is in linkage disequilibrium with other variants as well as possible epistatic interactions with other genes having stronger effects; 3) the lack of utilization of a systems approach that integrates "omic" high-throughput technology of the genome, transcriptome, proteome, and/or epigenome that would better capture genetically mediated exercise-induced adaptations over time; and 4) the major heterogeneity of this literature in terms of the types of endurance exercise interventions and subject populations.

When Montgomery and colleagues first began to examine the influence of *ACE* rs4340 on human physical performance (39), the RAAS was thought to be a hormonal system occurring exclusively in the circulation. The RAAS is now regarded as a complex "dual functioning system" balancing agonist and antagonist pathways which have intracrine, autocrine, and paracrine actions in virtually every organ in the body (32, 37, 41, 50, 53, 59). Because of the wide-reaching and counterregulatory effects of the RAAS, as well as the other reasons stated above, it is not likely *ACE* rs4340 plays a major role in endurance exercise performance as we have concluded in this chapter. Nonetheless, the *ACE* and endurance exercise performance literature sets the stage for future exercise systems genetic studies that integrate "omic" high-throughput technology that will better inform the genetic basis for what constitutes superior endurance performance.

References

1. **Almeida JA, Boullosa DA, Pardono E, Lima RM, Morais PK, Denadai BS, Souza VC, Nobrega OT, Campbell CS** and **Simoes HG.** The influence of ACE genotype on cardiovascular fitness of moderately active young men. *Arquivos Brasileiros de Cardiologia* 98: 315–320, 2012.

2. **Alves GB, Oliveira EM, Alves CR, Rached HR, Mota GF, Pereira AC, Rondon MU, Hashimoto NY, Azevedo LF, Krieger JE** and **Negrao CE.** Influence of angiotensinogen and angiotensin-converting enzyme polymorphisms on cardiac hypertrophy and improvement on maximal aerobic capacity caused by exercise training. *European Journal of Cardiovascular Prevention and Rehabilitation* 16: 487–492, 2009.

3. **Armstrong LE, Casa DJ, Maresh CM** and **Ganio MS.** Caffeine, fluid-electrolyte balance, temperature regulation, and exercise-heat tolerance. *Exercise and Sport Sciences Reviews* 35: 135–140, 2007.

4. **Ashley EA, Kardos A, Jack ES, Habenbacher W, Wheeler M, Kim YM, Froning J, Myers J, Whyte G, Froelicher V** and **Douglas P.** Angiotensin-converting enzyme genotype predicts cardiac and autonomic responses to prolonged exercise. *Journal of the American College of Cardiology* 48: 523–531, 2006.

5. **Azevedo ER, Mak S, Floras JS** and **Parker JD.** Acute effects of angiotensin-converting enzyme inhibition versus angiotensin II receptor blockade on cardiac sympathetic activity in patients with heart failure. *American Journal of Physiology – Regulatory, Integrative and Comparative Physiology* 313: R410–R417, 2017.

6. **Blanchard BE, Tsongalis GJ, Guidry MA, LaBelle LA, Poulin M, Taylor AL, Maresh CM, Devaney J, Thompson PD** and **Pescatello LS.** RAAS polymorphisms alter the acute blood pressure response to aerobic exercise among men with hypertension. *European Journal of Applied Physiology* 97: 26–33, 2006.

7. **Bouchard C.** Overcoming barriers to progress in exercise genomics. *Exercise and Sport Sciences Reviews* 39: 212–217, 2011.

8. **Bruneau ML, Jr, Johnson BT, Huedo-Medina TB, Larson KA, Ash GI** and **Pescatello LS.** The blood pressure response to acute and chronic aerobic exercise: a meta-analysis of candidate gene association studies. *Journal of Science and Medicine in Sport* 19: 424–431, 2016.

9. **Bueno S, Pasqua LA, de Araujo G, Eduardo Lima-Silva A** and **Bertuzzi R.** The association of ACE genotypes on cardiorespiratory variables related to physical fitness in healthy men. *PLoS One* 11: e0165310, 2016.

10. **Cam S, Colakoglu M, Colakoglu S, Sekuri C** and **Berdeli A.** ACE I/D gene polymorphism and aerobic endurance development in response to training in a non-elite female cohort. *Journal of Sports Medicine and Physical Fitness* 47: 234–238, 2007.

11. **Cambien F, Alhenc-Gelas F, Herbeth B, Andre JL, Rakotovao R, Gonzales MF, Allegrini J** and **Bloch C.** Familial resemblance of plasma angiotensin-converting enzyme level: the Nancy Study. *American Journal of Human Genetics* 43: 774–780, 1988.

12. **Casa DJ, Stearns RL, Lopez RM, Ganio MS, McDermott BP, Walker Yeargin S, Yamamoto LM, Mazerolle SM, Roti MW, Armstrong LE** and **Maresh CM.** Influence of hydration on physiological function and performance during trail running in the heat. *Journal of Athletic Training* 45: 147–156, 2010.

13. **Cerit M, Colakoglu M, Erdogan M, Berdeli A** and **Cam FS.** Relationship between ace genotype and short duration aerobic performance development. *European Journal of Applied Physiology* 98: 461–465, 2006.

14. **Chappell MC.** Nonclassical renin-angiotensin system and renal function. *Comprehensive Physiology* 2: 2733–2752, 2012.

15. **Day SH, Gohlke P, Dhamrait SS** and **Williams AG.** No correlation between circulating ACE activity and VO2max or mechanical efficiency in women. *European Journal of Applied Physiology* 99: 11–18, 2007.

16. **De MC** and **Slocombe R.** The use of angiotensin-I converting enzyme I/D genetic polymorphism as a biomarker of athletic performance in humans. *Biosensors* 2: 396–404, 2012.

17. **Dengel DR, Brown MD, Ferrell RE, Reynolds TH,** 4th and **Supiano MA.** Exercise-induced changes in insulin action are associated with ACE gene polymorphisms in older adults. *Physiological Genomics* 11: 73–80, 2002.

18. **Domingo R, Sturrock ED** and **Collins M.** ACE activity and endurance performance during the South African Ironman triathlons. *International Journal of Sports Medicine* 34: 402–408, 2013.

19. **Ferrario CM.** Cardiac remodelling and RAS inhibition. *Therapeutic Advances in Cardiovascular Disease* 10: 162–171, 2016.

20. **Goessler KF, Cornelissen VA, de Oliveira EM, de F Mota G** and **Polito MD.** ACE polymorphisms and the acute response of blood pressure to a walk in medicated hypertensive patients. *Journal of the Renin-Angiotensin-Aldosterone System* 16: 720–729, 2015.

21. **Goessler KF, Polito MD, Mota GF, de Oliveira EM** and **Cornelissen VA.** Angiotensin converting enzyme 2 polymorphisms and postexercise hypotension in hypertensive medicated individuals. *Clinical Physiology and Functional Imaging* 38: 206–212, 2018.

22. **Gomez-Gallego F, Santiago C, Gonzalez-Freire M, Muniesa CA, Fernandez Del Valle M, Perez M, Foster C** and **Lucia A.** Endurance performance: genes or gene combinations? *International Journal of Sports Medicine* 30: 66–72, 2009.

23. **Hagberg JM, McCole SD, Brown MD, Ferrell RE, Wilund KR, Huberty A, Douglass LW** and **Moore GE.** ACE insertion/deletion polymorphism and submaximal exercise hemodynamics in postmenopausal women. *Journal of Applied Physiology* 92: 1083–1088, 2002.

24. **Herichova I** and **Szantoova K.** Renin-angiotensin system: upgrade of recent knowledge and perspectives. *Endocrine Regulations* 47: 39, 2013.

25. **Hubert C, Houot AM, Corvol P** and **Soubrier F.** Structure of the angiotensin I-converting enzyme gene. Two alternate promoters correspond to evolutionary steps of a duplicated gene. *Journal of Biological Chemistry* 266: 15377–15383, 1991.

26. **Izzicupo P, Ghinassi B, D'Amico MA, Di Blasio A, Gesi M, Napolitano G, Gallina S** and **Di Baldassarre A.** Effects of ACE I/D polymorphism and aerobic training on the immune-endocrine network and cardiovascular parameters of postmenopausal women. *Journal of Clinical Endocrinology & Metabolism* 98: 4187–4194, 2013.

27. **Jiang F, Yang J, Zhang Y, Dong M, Wang S, Zhang Q, Liu FF, Zhang K** and **Zhang C.** Angiotensin-converting enzyme 2 and angiotensin 1–7: novel therapeutic targets. *Nature Reviews Cardiology* 11: 413–426, 2014.

28. **Jones JM, Park JJ, Johnson J, Vizcaino D, Hand B, Ferrell R, Weir M, Dowling T, Obisesan T** and **Brown M.** Renin-angiotensin system genes and exercise training-induced changes in sodium excretion in African American hypertensives. *Ethnicity & Disease* 16: 666–674, 2006.

29. **Kalson NS, Thompson J, Davies AJ, Stokes S, Earl MD, Whitehead A, Tyrrell-Marsh I, Frost H** and **Montgomery H.** The effect of angiotensin-converting enzyme genotype on acute mountain sickness and summit success in trekkers attempting the summit of Mt. Kilimanjaro (5,895 m). *European Journal of Applied Physiology* 105: 373–379, 2009.

30. **Khurana E, Fu Y, Chakravarty D, Demichelis F, Rubin MA** and **Gerstein M.** Role of non-coding sequence variants in cancer. *Nature Reviews Genetics* 17: 93–108, 2016.

31. **Kuczeriszka M, Kompanowska-Jezierska E, Sadowski J, Prieto M** and **Navar LG.** Modulating role of Ang1–7 in control of blood pressure and renal function in AngII-infused hypertensive rats. *American Journal of Hypertension* 31: 504–511, 2018.

32. **Leenen FH.** Actions of circulating angiotensin II and aldosterone in the brain contributing to hypertension. *American Journal of Hypertension* 27: 1024–1032, 2014.

33. **Luo Y, Chen Y, Zhang Y** and **Gao Y.** The association of angiotensin-converting enzyme gene insertion/deletion polymorphisms with acute mountain sickness susceptibility: a meta-analysis. *High Altitude Medicine & Biology* 13: 252–257, 2012.

34. **Ma F, Yang Y, Li X, Zhou F, Gao C, Li M** and **Gao L.** The association of sport performance with ACE and ACTN3 genetic polymorphisms: a systematic review and meta-analysis. *PLoS One* 8: e54685, 2013.

35. **MacInnis MJ, Koehle MS** and **Rupert JL.** Evidence for a genetic basis for altitude illness: 2010 update. *High Altitude Medicine & Biology* 11: 349–368, 2010.

36. **Mattsson CM, Wheeler MT, Waggott D, Caleshu C** and **Ashley EA.** Sports genetics moving forward: lessons learned from medical research. *Physioogical Genomics* 48: 175–182, 2016.

37. **Mirabito Colafella KM** and **Danser AHJ.** Recent advances in angiotensin research. *Hypertension* 69: 994–999, 2017.

38. **Montgomery H** and **Dhamrait S.** ACE genotype and performance. *Journal of Applied Physiology* 92: 1774–5, 2002.

39. **Montgomery HE, Marshall R, Hemingway H, Myerson S, Clarkson P, Dollery C, Hayward M, Holliman DE, Jubb M, World M, Thomas EL, Brynes AE, Saeed N, Barnard M, Bell JD, Prasad K, Rayson M, Talmud PJ** and **Humphries SE.** Human gene for physical performance. *Nature* 393: 221–222, 1998.

40. **Montgomery H** and **Safari L.** Genetic basis of physical fitness. *Annual Review of Anthropology* 36: 391–405, 2007.

41. **Nakagawa P** and **Sigmund CD.** How is the brain renin-angiotensin system regulated? *Hypertension* 70: 10–18, 2017.

42. **Pelliccia A** and **Thompson PD.** The genetics of left ventricular remodeling in competitive athletes. *Journal of Cardiovascular Medicine* 7: 267–270, 2006.

43. **Pescatello LS, Schifano ED, Ash GI, Panza GA, Lamberti L, Chen MH, Deshpande V, Zaleski A, Farinatti P, Taylor BA** and **Thompson PD.** Deep-targeted exon sequencing reveals renal polymorphisms associate with postexercise hypotension among African Americans. *Physiology Reports* 4: e12992, 2016.

44. **Physical Activity Guidelines Advisory Committee.** *2018 Physical Activity Guidelines Advisory Committee Scientific Report.* Washington, DC: US Department of Health and Human Services, 2018.

45. **Puthucheary Z, Skipworth JR, Rawal J, Loosemore M, Van Someren K** and **Montgomery HE.** The ACE gene and human performance: 12 years on. *Sports Medicine* 41: 433–448, 2011.

46. **Qi Y, Sun J, Zhu T, Wang W, Liu J, Zhou W, Qiu C** and **Zhao D.** Association of angiotensin-converting enzyme gene insertion/deletion polymorphism with high-altitude pulmonary oedema: a meta-analysis. *Journal of the Renin-Angiotensin-Aldosterone System* 12: 617–623, 2011.

47. **Raleigh SM.** Epigenetic regulation of the ACE gene might be more relevant to endurance physiology than the I/D polymorphism. *Journal of Applied Physiology* 112: 1082–1083, 2012.

48. **Rankinen T, Gagnon J, Perusse L, Chagnon YC, Rice T, Leon AS, Skinner JS, Wilmore JH, Rao DC** and **Bouchard C.** AGT M235T and ACE ID polymorphisms and exercise blood pressure in the HERITAGE Family Study. *American Journal of Physiology – Heart and Circulatory Physiology* 279: H368–74, 2000.

49. **Rankinen T, Perusse L, Gagnon J, Chagnon YC, Leon AS, Skinner JS, Wilmore JH, Rao DC** and **Bouchard C.** Angiotensin-converting enzyme ID polymorphism and fitness phenotype in the HERITAGE Family Study. *Journal of Applied Physiology* 88: 1029–1035, 2000.

50. **Ribeiro-Oliveira A**, Jr, **Nogueira AI**, **Pereira RM**, **Boas WW**, **Dos Santos RA** and **Simoes e Silva AC.** The renin-angiotensin system and diabetes: an update. *Vascular Health and Risk Management* 4: 787–803, 2008.

51. **Rigat B**, **Hubert C**, **Alhenc-Gelas F**, **Cambien F**, **Corvol P** and **Soubrier F.** An insertion/deletion polymorphism in the angiotensin I-converting enzyme gene accounting for half the variance of serum enzyme levels. *Journal of Clinical Investigation* 86: 1343–1346, 1990.

52. **Rigat B**, **Hubert C**, **Corvol P** and **Soubrier F.** PCR detection of the insertion/deletion polymorphism of the human angiotensin converting enzyme gene (DCP1) (dipeptidyl carboxypeptidase 1). *Nucleic Acids Research* 20: 1433, 1992.

53. **Rush JW** and **Aultman CD.** Vascular biology of angiotensin and the impact of physical activity. *Applied Physiology, Nutrition, and Metabolism* 33: 162–172, 2008.

54. **Santana HA**, **Moreira SR**, **Neto WB**, **Silva CB**, **Sales MM**, **Oliveira VN**, **Asano RY**, **Espindola FS**, **Nobrega OT**, **Campbell CS** and **Simoes HG.** The higher exercise intensity and the presence of allele I of ACE gene elicit a higher post-exercise blood pressure reduction and nitric oxide release in elderly women: an experimental study. *BMC Cardiovascular Disorders* 11: 71, 2011.

55. **Santos RA**, **Ferreira AJ**, **Verano-Braga T** and **Bader M.** Angiotensin-converting enzyme 2, angiotensin-(1–7) and Mas: new players of the renin-angiotensin system. *Journal of Endocrinology* 216: R1–R17, 2013.

56. **Sassi R**, **Cerutti S**, **Lombardi F**, **Malik M**, **Huikuri HV**, **Peng CK**, **Schmidt G** and **Yamamoto Y.** Advances in heart rate variability signal analysis: joint position statement by the e-Cardiology ESC Working Group and the European Heart Rhythm Association co-endorsed by the Asia Pacific Heart Rhythm Society. *Europace* 17: 1341–1353, 2015.

57. **Sećerović A**, **Gurbeta L**, **Omanović-Miklićanin E** and **Badnjević A.** Genotype association with sport activity: the impact of ACE and ACTN3 gene polymorphism on athletic performance. *International Journal of Engineering Research and Technology* 6: 859–863, 2017.

58. **Silva SD**, Jr, **Zampieri TT**, **Ruggeri A**, **Ceroni A**, **Aragao DS**, **Fernandes FB**, **Casarini DE** and **Michelini LC.** Downregulation of the vascular renin-angiotensin system by aerobic training – focus on the balance between vasoconstrictor and vasodilator axes. *Circulation Journal* 79: 1372–1380, 2015.

59. **Siragy HM** and **Carey RM.** Protective role of the angiotensin AT2 receptor in a renal wrap hypertension model. *Hypertension* 33: 1237–1242, 1999.

60. **Sonna LA**, **Sharp MA**, **Knapik JJ**, **Cullivan M**, **Angel KC**, **Patton JF** and **Lilly CM.** Angiotensin-converting enzyme genotype and physical performance during US Army basic training. *Journal of Applied Physiology* 91: 1355–1363, 2001.

61. **Touyz RM** and **Montezano AC.** Angiotensin-(1–7) and vascular function: the clinical context. *Hypertension* 71: 68–69, 2018.

62. **Tsianos G**, **Eleftheriou KI**, **Hawe E**, **Woolrich L**, **Watt M**, **Watt I**, **Peacock A**, **Montgomery H** and **Grant S.** Performance at altitude and angiotensin I-converting enzyme genotype. *European Journal of Applied Physiology* 93: 630–633, 2005.

63. **Valdivieso P**, **Vaughan D**, **Laczko E**, **Brogioli M**, **Waldron S**, **Rittweger J** and **Fluck M.** The metabolic response of skeletal muscle to endurance exercise is modified by the ACE-I/D gene polymorphism and training state. *Frontiers of Physiology* 8: 993, 2017.

64. **van Ginkel S**, **Ruoss S**, **Valdivieso P**, **Degens H**, **Waldron S**, **de Haan A** and **Fluck M.** ACE inhibition modifies exercise-induced pro-angiogenic and mitochondrial gene transcript expression. *Scand J Med Sci Sports* 26: 1180–1187, 2016.

65. **Vaughan D**, **Brogioli M**, **Maier T**, **White A**, **Waldron S**, **Rittweger J**, **Toigo M**, **Wettstein J**, **Laczko E** and **Fluck M.** The angiotensin converting enzyme insertion/deletion polymorphism modifies exercise-induced muscle metabolism. *PLoS One* 11: e0149046, 2016.

66. **Vaughan D**, **Huber-Abel FA**, **Graber F**, **Hoppeler H** and **Fluck M.** The angiotensin converting enzyme insertion/deletion polymorphism alters the response of muscle energy supply lines to exercise. *European Journal of Applied Physiology* 113: 1719–1729, 2013.

67. **Verlengia R**, **Rebelo AC**, **Crisp AH**, **Kunz VC**, **Dos Santos Carneiro Cordeiro MA**, **Hirata MH**, **Crespo Hirata RD** and **Silva E.** Lack of association between ACE indel polymorphism and cardiorespiratory fitness in physically active and sedentary young women. *Asian Journal of Sports Medicine* 5: e22768, 2014.

68. **Wang QQ**, **Yu L**, **Huang GR**, **Zhang L**, **Liu YQ**, **Wang TW**, **Lin H**, **Ren Q**, **Liu P**, **Huang L**, **Qin J**, **Wu GM**, **Li QN**, **Li YF** and **Xiong HY.** Polymorphisms of angiotensin converting enzyme

and nitric oxide synthase 3 genes as risk factors of high-altitude pulmonary edema: a case-control study and meta-analysis. *Tohoku Journal of Experimental Medicine* 229: 255–266, 2013.

69. **Woods D.** Angiotensin-converting enzyme, renin-angiotensin system and human performance. *Medicine and Sport Science* 54: 72–87, 2009.

70. **Woods DR, Brull D** and **Montgomery HE.** Endurance and the ACE I/D polymorphism. *Science Progress* 83: 317–336, 2000.

71. **Woods DR, Humphries SE** and **Montgomery HE.** The ACE I/D polymorphism and human physical performance. *Trends in Endocrinology and Metabolism* 11: 416–420, 2000.

72. **Woods DR** and **Montgomery HE.** Angiotensin-converting enzyme and genetics at high altitude. *High Altitude Medicine & Biology* 2: 201–210, 2001.

73. **Woods DR, Pollard AJ, Collier DJ, Jamshidi Y, Vassiliou V, Hawe E, Humphries SE** and **Montgomery HE.** Insertion/deletion polymorphism of the angiotensin I-converting enzyme gene and arterial oxygen saturation at high altitude. *American Journal of Respiratory and Critical Care Medicine* 166: 362–366, 2002.

74. **Yau AM, Moss AD, James LJ, Gilmore W, Ashworth JJ** and **Evans GH.** The influence of angiotensin converting enzyme and bradykinin receptor B2 gene variants on voluntary fluid intake and fluid balance in healthy men during moderate-intensity exercise in the heat. *Applied Physiology, Nutrition, and Metabolism* 40: 184–190, 2015.

75. **Zhang B, Tanaka H, Shono N, Miura S, Kiyonaga A, Shindo M** and **Saku K.** The I allele of the angiotensin-converting enzyme gene is associated with an increased percentage of slow-twitch type I fibers in human skeletal muscle. *Clinical Genetics* 63: 139–144, 2003.

76. **Zhang T, Zhang CF, Jin F** and **Wang L.** Association between genetic factor and physical performance. *Yi Chuan* 26: 219–226, 2004.

77. **Zhao B, Moochhala SM, Tham S, Lu J, Chia M, Byrne C, Hu Q** and **Lee LK.** Relationship between angiotensin-converting enzyme ID polymorphism and VO(2max) of Chinese males. *Life Sciences* 73: 2625–2630, 2003.

SECTION 4

Systems genetics of muscle mass, strength, and trainability

Section 3 explored the systems genetics underlying endurance and endurance-related traits. Now we shift gears away from endurance and towards muscle-related traits such as muscle size, strength, and power. These traits not only contribute to performance in a myriad of sports, but also heavily influence quality of life and health outside of sport. Again, each author was tasked particularly to review traits at baseline (untrained state) and following acute and chronic exercise training, to highlight gaps in our knowledge and to provide a foundation for future research related to sport and exercise genetics research.

Chapter 18 kicks off Section 4 with a discussion of heritability of muscle strength and size from Dr. Martine Thomis. Readers will quickly realize that "strength" is not a single trait – and the complexity of measuring and interpreting muscle functional data will become clear. Dr. Monica Hubal and colleagues provide a primer for muscle strength in Chapter 19, and start to discuss molecular and genetic drivers of strength variability. It is somewhat impossible to discuss strength without considering muscle size, which is a key component of function. In Chapter 20, Dr. Philip Atherton and colleagues continue the specific discussion of muscle size, again highlighting variation in size at baseline and discussing changes in size following resistance training. It is important to notice similarities and differences between acute bouts of resistance training and chronic exercise training. Both acute and chronic training affect muscle in large part via modulation of neuroendocrine factors such as various growth hormones. Chapter 21 reviews these neuroendocrine modulators and is expertly crafted by Dr. William Kraemer (a pioneer in this field) and colleagues.

As noted in Section 3, a few genetic variations have been studied enough to warrant their own chapters. In Section 4, we explore two such variations: genetic variations related to the potent muscle regulator protein myostatin (*MSTN*; reviewed by Dr. Dustin Hittel in Chapter 22) and a common variation in the fast-twitch muscle gene alpha-actinin-3 (*ACTN3*), reviewed by Dr. Peter Houweling and colleagues in Chapter 23. Each of these mutations is quite interesting to the general public – for example, natural mutations in myostatin have been noted in nature as grossly hypertrophied animal breeds such as the bully whippet or the Belgian Blue cow and myostatin has been under intense study by pharmaceutical companies to try to develop therapies to combat muscle wasting.

Together, the chapters in Section 4 provide a comprehensive review of traits underlying strength and size-related traits both at baseline and following training, highlight gaps in our current knowledge, and provide a solid foundation for future work to inform systems models.

18

HERITABILITY OF MUSCLE SIZE AND STRENGTH TRAITS

Martine Thomis

Muscle mass, strength, and power contribute to athletic performance of extraordinary levels. In the general aging population, high levels of muscular fitness prolong the ability to perform activities of daily living (28) and are related to high levels of physical and psychological well-being (39). Low or weak muscular fitness is associated with higher prevalence of all-cause mortality (29), type 2 diabetes, cardiovascular disease, and osteoarthritis (51). Recent data show grip strength as a stronger predictor of cardiovascular and all-cause mortality than systolic blood pressure (29). Dynapenia (age-associated loss of muscle strength) and sarcopenia (age-associated loss of muscle mass) (36) have an increasing impact on healthcare costs in aging populations (23). On the other hand, gene hunting for "elite power performance" shows high interest in identifying genetic endowments related to strength and or power excellence in sports (43) (see Chapters 19–23).

Skeletal muscle mass, strength, and power are multifactorial traits influenced by a wide range of genetic and environmental factors. This chapter aims to describe studies that have estimated the heritability of skeletal muscle mass and skeletal muscle strength and power, both at baseline and in response to exercise. The following chapters will focus on explaining specific biological pathways that play a role in muscle mass and strength and their responses to progressive resistance training (Chapters 19–21).

Heritability of muscle mass

The increase in muscle mass with age due to fiber hypertrophy is fairly linear from young childhood until puberty, with small but consistent advantages in boys. The sex difference enlarges during and after puberty, driven primarily by the differences in sex steroids (5). Muscle mass remains rather stable during the third and fourth decade of life; nonetheless, after about the age of 50, muscle mass declines at a rate of approximately 1%/year in men and 0.5%/year in women (36). In elite athletes, muscle mass and muscle fiber type composition is related to the specific demands of the sport (63). Skeletal muscle mass is mainly indirectly measured or estimated, by using whole-body lean tissue (dual X-ray absorptiometry (DXA) or magnetic resonance imaging (MRI)) scans to determine whole-body muscle mass (11), or regional measures using computed tomography (CT)/MRI, ultrasonography, or anthropometric measures (skinfold-corrected circumferences) (17). Muscle fiber type distribution (types I, IIa, and IIx) is, among other qualitative factors, related to specific strength, power, and muscular endurance performances and shows large variation in elite performers (63) and in the general population. Muscle biopsies from vastus lateralis muscle are most widely studied, although noninvasive techniques have also emerged (4).

Heritability of regional muscle mass based on circumferences – anthropometric measures

Loos et al. (31) reported heritability estimates in the range of 87–95% for circumferences at the upper- and forearm, and thigh and calf of 10–14-year-old twins in the Leuven Longitudinal Twin Study. Different multivariate models showed age- and sex-dependent genetic covariation in an "arm–leg" or "proximal–distal" pattern. Other twin studies indicate strong evidence for a genetic component of circumference measurements, with heritability estimates ranging between 0.53 and 0.75 (6, 10, 13). In a sample of 748 young, Belgian, male siblings from 335 families, upper-limit heritabilities (including genetic and shared environmental variances) were estimated at 89% and 91% for anthropometrically estimated muscle plus bone cross-sectional area of the arm and thigh, respectively (21).

Heritability of regional and total muscle mass based on imaging techniques

Significant sibling correlations for muscle diameter measures from radiographic analyses in preschool children (r_{males}=0.56 and $r_{females}$=0.63) and monozygotic twin (MZ) intraclass correlations (r_{males}=0.83 and $r_{females}$=0.85) in adolescents indicate an important genetic contribution in calf muscle mass (16, 19). In 41 young adult, male twins, the contribution of additive genetic factors on muscle cross-sectional area of the mid-upper arm determined by CT scans was estimated at 92% (95% confidence interval (CI) 79–97%) (56). In 227 pairs of MZ and 126 pairs of dizygotic (DZ) postmenopausal twins, total body lean mass was measured by a Hologic QDR–2000 DXA scanner (Hologic Inc., Waltham, MA, USA). Heritability was estimated using the Falconer formula and showed that 56% (95% CI 24–88%) of variation in age, height, and weight-corrected whole-body lean mass was attributable to genetic factors (1). Appendicular lean mass (ALM; sum of lean body mass measured at the four limbs) was determined by DXA (QDR 4500W system; Hologic, Inc) in a large sample of adult (51.8 ± 13.7 years) women within the TwinsUK Adult Twin Registry (1196 individuals: 119 DZ and 428 MZ twin pairs and 102 singletons, 56 MZ and 46 DZ twins without sibling measurements). The heritability estimate obtained using variance decomposition analysis was 0.81 ± 0.05 (30). Family members (men, N=580; women, N=766, 327 pedigrees) in the Framingham Osteoporosis Study had leg lean mass (LLM) measured by DXA. Age-adjusted LLM (and estrogen status in women) was highly heritable (upper-limit heritability), with a significant h^2 estimate of 69%. After adjustment for height and body mass index, h^2 decreased to 42% (24). Similar family-based heritability estimates were reported within 244 families ascertained for two adult siblings having type 2 diabetes in the Diabetes Heart Study (20). Estimations of the upper-limit heritability were 0.63 and 0.67 for whole-body lean mass and ALM, respectively, with phenotypes controlled for covariates age, sex, ethnicity, height, diabetes status, smoking, dietary intake, and physical activity.

Heritability of muscle fiber type distribution

Early reports presented high heritability estimates (h^2=0.93) for the proportion of type I fibers in skeletal muscle (26). Komi et al. found that MZ twins (N=15) were almost identical in the percentage of type I fibers in the vastus lateralis muscle, while DZ twins (N=16) were quite variable. Also, high MZ twin intrapair correlations for type I fiber composition (r=0.94) (35) are indicative of a high genetic contribution in young adult males. However, Lortie et al. (32) showed less evidence for high genetic contributions in a study on 32 pairs of brothers and 35 pairs of MZ twins. Significant F-ratios in brothers and MZ twins indicated a significant biological resemblance for type I fiber percentage. The contribution of nongenetic factors was estimated at 30% of the variance in MZ fiber type I distribution, while another 12% of the variance was accounted for by sampling variability and technical error. There was no significant resemblance in brothers for any of the fiber type areas, while MZ twins only exhibited a significant resemblance in type I fiber area. With the inclusion of an additional set of 32 male and 20 female DZ twins to these data, estimates of heritability were based on several estimation formulas and indicated no significant genetic effect for the distribution of fiber type I, IIa, and IIx fibers or fiber areas. In a review on this topic, variation in type I fiber distribution was decomposed in three sources: variance due to sampling variability and technical errors (15%), environmental variance (40%), and genetic variance (40–50%) (49). In 78 sedentary subjects from 19 families of the HERITAGE Family Study, results suggested a weak familial aggregation (F-test for comparison of within and between family variance) for type I fiber areas in the sedentary state (F=2.4, P=0.007). There was some evidence for familial resemblance in the number of capillaries around type I (F=1.9, P=0.039) and type IIa fibers (F=1.9, P=0.044), and in the fiber area per capillary in type I (P=0.011) and type IIa fibers (P=0.042) in the sedentary state (45).

Baguet et al. (3) investigated carnosine as a stable muscle metabolite measured by proton magnetic resonance spectroscopy in a twin cohort (N=25 MZ, N=22 DZ). The content of this metabolite is closely related to the muscle fiber type distribution in human gastrocnemius and soleus muscle (4). In soleus muscle, intratwin similarities were higher for MZ twins compared to DZ twins, suggesting that muscle carnosine levels and fiber type distribution are highly heritable (AE model: h^2=85%). However, these observations could not be observed in gastrocnemius muscle. Although part of the large interindividual variability in proportions of different fiber types in human mixed muscles is genetically determined, its specific contribution and additional role of epigenetic factors (2) still need to be resolved.

Heritability of muscle strength

Muscle strength-related phenotypes are used as an overall term to indicate the different subtypes and evaluation methods to study aspects of contractile outcomes of activated muscle (see Chapter 19 for further details). In general, muscle strength is subdivided into static or isometric strength (force generated at a specific joint angle without lengthening or shortening of the muscle fibers), dynamic concentric contractions (shortening of the muscle fibers at a specific contraction velocity), dynamic eccentric contractions (fibers are lengthened against an external force), muscle power (maximal dynamic strength delivered in the shortest possible time), and muscular endurance (e.g., repeated muscle contractions). Evaluation of each of these characteristics can be based on a wide variety of test protocols.

Recently, two meta-analyses have been performed on heritability estimates of muscle strength-related phenotypes. Schutte et al. (47) reported the weighted mean heritability of (isometric) handgrip strength in 9–25-year-olds (N=4516) at 63% (95% CI 47–73%, five studies) and explosive strength (vertical jump; N=874) at 62% (95% CI 47–77%, four studies) in adolescent twin samples. Zempo et al. (60) included 24 studies (with 58 measurements) on heritability of human muscle strength-related phenotypes in their meta-analysis based on a systematic literature search before August 2016.

Heritability of handgrip strength

Handgrip strength is a widely used measure of isometric strength applied over a large age range. Ten studies based on twin or family data reported (upper-limit) heritability estimates for grip strength (N=320,588 in total, average ages between 9 and 70.5 years) between 0.36 and 0.88, with a weighted mean heritability of 0.56 (95% CI 0.46–0.67) (1, 14, 22, 25, 27, 34, 37, 44, 47, 48, 57). A significant degree of heterogeneity in these studies was further explored and showed a significant negative correlation of grip-strength heritability with age (r=−0.70) and sex (males >females, P <0.05).

Heritability of other isometric strength tests

Other isometric or maximal static strength tests include elbow flexion/extension, knee extension/flexion, or trunk flexion/extension tests using standardized dynamometers, ankle plantar flexion, or arm pull tests. Zempo et al. (60) included 16 measurements from 11 studies for isometric strength measures (21, 27, 33, 38, 42, 48, 56, 57, 59, 62). The weighted h^2 was 0.49 (95% CI 0.47–0.52). Although there was a considerable degree of heterogeneity, there was no significant relationship between age and reported h^2 or sex. Part of the variability in heritability estimates might come from the force–length relationship that determines the optimal strength performance over a range of motion. Thomis et al. (56) found a similar, slightly "mirrored" pattern of h^2 estimates for elbow flexor strength at different elbow angles compared to the observed mean torque values. Different contributions of unique environmental variation might correspond to the degree of variability in muscle activation and performance discomfort at each angle. Also, genetic factors related to the moment arm (tendon insertions and bone structures) might contribute differently at different muscle lengths. However, muscle activation as measured by the maximal value of the filtered differences of the transformed electromyograms during maximal isometric flexion at 140° and 110° elbow flexion was highly determined by genetic factors (h^2=0.78–0.83) (56).

Heritability of isokinetic torque

Isokinetic tests aim to measure the ability of contracting muscle to generate force at a preset speed of contraction – though only over a limited range of motion during shorting (concentric) or lengthening (eccentric) of the muscle. A subset of three studies (12, 21, 46) measuring mainly elbow isokinetic flexion were included in the overview by Zempo et al. (60) and showed a weighted mean h^2 of 0.49 (95% CI 0.37–0.61). Dynamic strength depends on the speed of contraction (lower strengths/torques at higher speeds) and type of contraction (eccentric torques exceeding concentric torques). This force–velocity and contraction type specificity was also partially observed when studying elbow flexor strength at different velocities in both concentric and eccentric contraction types in 41 male twins (56). A trend was observed that heritabilities for eccentric contraction torques were higher than isometric and concentric contractions, and that heritabilities for contraction torques at higher concentric speeds were lower compared to contractions at slower speeds. Also for torques at the elbow, knee, and trunk it was found that dynamic isometric torques showed lower upper-heritability values (63–87%) compared to isometric strength test (82–96%) at a same muscle length in 748 males siblings from 335 families from the Leuven Genes for Muscular Strength project (21).

Heritability of power and jump test performance

Muscle contractions employing as much strength as possible in the shortest possible time, also indicated as "power," are often quantified through jumps or specific dynamometer tests. Six studies (7, 9, 27, 33, 37, 47) including 30–498 young subjects (average ages between 9 and 23.8 years) from (extended) twin designs estimated the contribution of genetic factors to individual variation in jump performance between 0.49 and 0.86 (meta-analysis average h^2=0.55; 95% CI 0.45–0.65). Heritability estimates for leg extension tests and back lifting work were between 0.37 and 0.60 in middle-aged twins (1, 46, 59).

Heritability of muscle functional tests

More functional strength tests that measure components of dynamic strength endurance (e.g., push-ups, sit-ups, bent arm hang, leg lifts, elbow flexion one-repetition maximum (1RM) tests) are mostly studied in younger twins and families. Since contraction type and velocity can be mixed within such tests and different between tests, estimation of an average heritability by means of meta-analysis might be less informative. Zempo et al. (60) included nine measurements from five studies and reported a meta-analysis average h^2 of 0.49 (95% CI 0.32–0.67).

The weighted mean of h^2 for muscle strength-related phenotypes (effects of additive genetic and genetic dominance effects summed) over all selected studies and measurements – different strength phenotypes or different estimates for males and females were included as separate entries in the meta-analysis – was 0.52 (95% CI 0.48–0.56) (60). This analysis showed significant heterogeneity (I^2=91.0%, P <0.001) and was further explored by meta-regression analysis. Only age was a significant contributor to the heterogeneity, with lower heritability estimates in older samples (r=−0.43; specifically for handgrip r=−0.70). The mean h^2 for strength-related phenotypes tended to be higher in men than in women, which only became significant for the sex difference in heritability of handgrip strength. This meta-analysis did not show significant differences between h^2 estimates for the different subphenotypes (grip, isometric, dynamic, isotonic, jump tests), upper or lower body strength, type of SEM model reported, or cohort type (60).

Multivariate heritability studies for muscle mass and strength

Differences in the broad set of strength-related subphenotypes seem not to vary independently from each other within and between individuals. Statistical evidence for a "strength generality" factor is suggested by moderate to high correlations between different strength tests (18). Whether observed phenotypic correlations are based on shared genetic (additive genetic, A; or genetic dominance, D) and/or shared environmental (environmental factors common within families, C; or specific to each individual, E) factors can be explored using multivariate twin models.

Schutte et al. (47) estimated a genetic correlation between handgrip and vertical jump of r_G=0.46 (95% CI 0.27–0.65) in 227 17.2 ± 1.2 year-old twins. Elbow strength measured at a flexion angle of 110° during maximum concentric and eccentric contractions at 120°/s, as well as isometrically, was related to the muscle cross-sectional area (MCSA) at the mid-upper arm in a study of 41 young adult male twins (22.4 ± 3.7 year) (12). A model with a "general" (Ac) genetic factor and a general specific environmental factor (Ec) together with phenotype-specific genetic (AS1–4) and environmental factors (ES1–4) fitted the data best. The shared genetic and environmental component, accounted for 43% and 6% in MCSA (h^2=81%), 47% and 20% in eccentric (h^2=65%), 58% and 4% in isometric (h^2=70%), and 32% and 1% in concentric strength (h^2=32%), respectively. Contraction type-specific and muscle cross-sectional area-specific genetic and environmental effects, accounted for 38% and 14% in MCSA, 18% and 15% in eccentric, 12% and 26% in isometric, and 0% and 67% in concentric strength, respectively. These results support a shared pleiotropic gene action for MCSA, eccentric, isometric, and concentric strength, with a moderate to high genetic contribution to the variability of these characteristics. In the same set of Flemish male twins, covariation in MCSA and static elbow torques in at different muscle lengths (at 140°, 110°, and 80° elbow flexion) could also be explained by a set of shared genetic factors explaining 82% (MSCA), 66% (at 140°), 61% (at 110°), and 50% (at 80°) of the variance (54). An additional torque-specific genetic factor was also included (explaining an additional 6–24% of variance in the elbow flexion torques).

In an older, female twin sample (101 MZ, 116 DZ, 63–76 years) within the Finnish Twin Study on Aging (FITSA), knee extension power and maximal isometric knee extension strength were analyzed in a bivariate reduced ACE Cholesky decomposition model (58). A shared genetic component accounted for 32% of the total variance in leg extensor power and 48% in isometric knee extensor strength. A nonshared environmental effect shared by both phenotypes accounted for 4% of the variance in power and 52% in isometric strength. For leg extensor power, common environmental factors were also significant (28%). Environmental sources of variation might include general levels of physical activity or nutritional choices that act upon the development of muscle mass and all measures of strength (isometric, dynamic, power) and therefore contribute to the shared sets of unique environmental factors. However, specificity of training effects might contribute to the different contributions of environmental factors in different types of muscle contraction. As for genes contributing to multiple forms of muscular strength, candidates can be found in structural elements of muscle and contractile proteins or fiber type distribution. Specific genetic contributions might also relate to the importance of fiber type distribution (e.g., related more strongly to muscle power than muscle strength), and passive elastic components that are contributing to torques in specific muscle contraction types (e.g., eccentric torques).

Back strength was evaluated by an isometric trunk extensor endurance test, isokinetic lifting force, and power and psychophysical lifting test in 122 MZ and 131 DZ male, middle-aged (49.9 ± 7.7 years) twins (46). A general additive genetic factor was included in the model and explained 57–92% of the covariance among the three back tests and 31% of the covariance between isokinetic lifting force and work. Genetic dominance was significantly shared between isokinetic lifting work and force and isokinetic lifting work had a specific dominance factor. Common environmental factors contributed test-specifically to variance in psychophysical lifting force (18%) and isometric trunk extensor endurance (34%). Unique environmental factors were shared between the four phenotypes (explaining between 1% and 49% of the variance) and had test-specific contributions (between 20% and 60%). Covariation explained by unique environmental factors showed much variation between the tests (r_e=0.03–0.43). Broad heritability (sum of A and D sources) was highest for isokinetic lifting force (65%) and work (60%), and lowest for psychophysical lifting force (33%) and the trunk extensor endurance test (5%). A set of models including measured environmental determinants were tested and showed significance for participation in power sports and body weight for isokinetic force and power, but limited contributions of other factors (health compared to others, type of job, doing aerobic sports) in the other back strength measures.

Heritability of muscle mass and strength from longitudinal studies

Sex differences in the intercept and slope of growth in handgrip strength were the focus of variance components analysis using a latent growth curve model analysis in a study of 2513 same-sex twins from 11.8 years (baseline) to 17.8 years of age (second follow-up) (22). High heritabilities were reported for the variability in handgrip strength at 11 years of age (intercept) (males=88%, females=79%). Additive genetic effects accounted for most (80%) of the variance around the slope in males but were of less importance in females (h^2=28%). The absolute genetic variance around the slope (increased by age) was nearly ninefold higher in males. Variation in timing of the adolescent growth spurt is a confounding factor when studying development of muscle mass and strength and its genetic and environmental components during adolescence. Longitudinal models were applied to study the tracking in isometric (arm pull) (41) and explosive (vertical jump) (40) strength in 105 female and male twins of the Leuven Longitudinal Twins Study, between 10 and 18 years of age. All measurements were aligned according to the age at peak height velocity (APHV) for each individual. A model including genetic and environmental innovation and transmission paths could account for the tracking observed in these measurements during adolescence. Arm pull strength 3 years after peak height velocity could be explained by genetic (44.3% in males, 22.5% in females) and environmental factors (31.2% in males, 44.5% in females) transmitted from previous time points (41). In males, new genetic factors seem to increase the overall variance by age, specifically at the time around APHV (innovation A=30.7%). Heritability estimates in vertical jump performance ranged between 60.8% (95% CI 37.7–77.2%) and 87.3% (95% CI 74.2–94.0%) for boys and between 76.5% (95% CI 56.7–89.0%) and 88.6% (95% CI 77.8–94.1%) for girls. Up to 56.4% and 62.8% of the total variation 3 years after APHV was explained by additive genetic factors that already explained a significant amount of variation at previous measurement occasions in boys and girls respectively (40). It thus can be concluded that the observed stability of strength during adolescence is caused by a stable genetic influence, more so in boys than in girls.

Longitudinal genetic modeling in other age periods are limited. One study reported 10-year aging effects on handgrip strength in 77 MZ and 75 DZ twin pairs at mean ages of 63 and 73 years. A bivariate ACE Cholesky decomposition model was used to explore the observed stability in handgrip strength (r=0.62). Shared genetic factors accounted for 35% of the phenotypic correlation, while shared familial environmental effects accounted for 48% of the stability (8). In middle-aged siblings (N=115 subjects from 48 families, age at baseline 44.8 ± 7 years) upper-limit heritability estimates for changes in knee strength over 2.4 years (−2.8 ± 8.6%/ year) were between 54% and 74% (depending on the correction for covariates related to bone and cartilage characteristics related to osteoarthritis) (61).

Role of genetic factors in muscle mass and strength responses to exercise

Few studies have used a family or twin design to investigate the role of genetic factors in the interindividual responses in muscle mass and strength after resistance/strength training. The MZ twin design to explore genotype–training interaction effects was applied in five MZ pairs (17–26 years) in response to 10 weeks of maximal isokinetic knee flexion/extension training (52). No significant genotype–training interaction could be found for the response in peak torque (mean ± SD: 24% ± 12%), although the response in oxoglutarate dehydrogenase activity showed significant intrapair resemblance (r=0.76). Male MZ (N=25) and DZ (N=16) twins (22.4 ± 3.7 years) participated in a 10-week resistance training program for the elbow flexors (55). The evidence for genotype–training interaction, or association of interindividual differences in training effects with the genotype, was tested by a two-way ANOVA in the MZ twins and using a bivariate model-fitting approach on pre- and post-training phenotypes in MZ and DZ twins. Evidence for genotype–training interaction was found for 1RM and isometric strength, with MZ intrapair correlations of 0.46 and 0.30, respectively. Bivariate model-fitting indicated that about 20% of the variation in post-training 1RM, isometric strength, and concentric moment at 120°/s was explained by training-specific genetic factors that were independent from genetic factors that explained variation in the pretraining phenotype (30–77%). A hypertrophic response of arm cross-sectional muscle area (CT) was significant and varied between subjects (2.2 cm^2 ± 2.7); however, no significant genotype–training interaction effect was found. Compared to studies in which anaerobic/intermittent or endurance training were used as exercise regimens (15, 50), strength responses seem to show lower/smaller evidence for genotype–training interaction.

The studies summarized in this chapter indicate that individual differences in muscle mass, muscle strength and power, and responses to resistance training are partially determined by genetic factors. Although heritability estimates vary according to sample characteristics (age, sex), heritability estimation technique, specific strength test, and characteristic (isometric, isotonic, dynamic, functional, eccentric, concentric, strength endurance), it has pushed the field into the search for specific gene variants that underlie the heritability of these traits (53). Environmental factors are mainly identified as unique to the individual and less often "shared" by family members, however, these specific factors (e.g., nutrition, occupation, type of exercise activities, etc.) can be shared between different types of muscle strength. Covariation and uniqueness of multiple types of muscle contraction and strength tests have been explored in multivariate genetic and environmental models. Although shared genetic variation indicated pleiotropic gene actions in most of these analyses, genetic variation specific to each subtrait of strength also indicate specific gene sets for specific strength characteristics. Stability of strength characteristics over time in adolescence and in older age also show a genetic component. In summary, twin and family studies have indicated that genetic factors significantly (>0.50–0.70) contribute to the observed differences in muscle mass and strength characteristics in young and old, males and females and that efforts to investigate DNA sequence variation in candidate gene or genome-wide approaches was merited.

References

1. **Arden NK** and **Spector TD.** Genetic influences on muscle strength, lean body mass, and bone mineral density: a twin study. *J Bone Miner Res* 12: 2076–2081, 1997.
2. **Baar K.** Epigenetic control of skeletal muscle fibre type. *Acta Physiol (Oxf)* 199: 477–487, 2010.
3. **Baguet A, Everaert I, Achten E, Thomis M** and **Derave W.** The influence of sex, age and heritability on human skeletal muscle carnosine content. *Amino Acids* 43: 13–20, 2012.
4. **Baguet A, Everaert I, Hespel P, Petrovic M, Achten E** and **Derave W.** A new method for non-invasive estimation of human muscle fiber type composition. *Plos One* 6: e21956, 2011.
5. **Bouchard C, Malina R** and **Bar-Or O.** *Growth, Maturation, and Physical Activity.* Champaign, IL: Human Kinetics Publishers, 2004.
6. **Byard PJ, Sharma K, Russell JM** and **Rao DC.** A family study of anthropometric traits in a Punjabi community: II. An investigation of familial transmission. *Am J Phys Anthropol* 64: 97–104, 1984.

7. **Calvo M, Rodas G, Vallejo M, Estruch A, Arcas A, Javierre C, Viscor G** and **Ventura JL.** Heritability of explosive power and anaerobic capacity in humans. *Eur J Appl Physiol* 86: 218–225, 2002.
8. **Carmelli D** and **Reed T.** Stability and change in genetic and environmental influences on hand-grip strength in older male twins. *J Appl Physiol (1985)* 89: 1879–1883, 2000.
9. **Chatterjee S** and **Das N.** Physical and motor fitness in twins. *Jpn J Physiol* 45: 519–534, 1995.
10. **Clark PJ.** The heritability of certain anthropometric characters as ascertained from measurements of twins. *Am J Hum Genet* 8: 49–54, 1956.
11. **Culjkovic-Kraljacic B, Baguet A, Volpon L, Amri A** and **Borden KL.** The oncogene eIF4E reprograms the nuclear pore complex to promote mRNA export and oncogenic transformation. *Cell Rep* 2: 207–215, 2012.
12. **De Mars G, Thomis MAI, Windelinckx A, Van Leemputte M, Maes HH, Blimkie CJ, Claessens AL, Vlietinck R** and **Beunen G.** Covariance of isometric and dynamic arm contractions: multivariate genetic analysis. *Twin Res Hum Genet* 10: 180–190, 2007.
13. **Dupae E, Defrise-Gussenhoven E** and **Susanne C.** Genetic and environmental influences on body measurements of Belgian twins. *Acta Genet Med Gemellol (Roma)* 31: 139–144, 1982.
14. **Frederiksen H, Gaist D, Petersen HC, Hjelmborg J, McGue M, Vaupel JW** and **Christensen K.** Hand grip strength: a phenotype suitable for identifying genetic variants affecting mid- and late-life physical functioning. *Genet Epidemiol* 23: 110–122, 2002.
15. **Hamel P, Simoneau JA, Lortie G, Boulay MR** and **Bouchard C.** Heredity and muscle adaptation to endurance training. *Med Sci Sports Exerc* 18: 690–696, 1986.
16. **Hewitt D.** Sib resemblance in bone, muscle and fat measurements of the human calf. *Ann Hum Genet* 22: 213–221, 1958.
17. **Heymsfield SB, Adamek M, Gonzalez MC, Jia G** and **Thomas DM.** Assessing skeletal muscle mass: historical overview and state of the art. *J Cachexia Sarcopenia Muscle* 5: 9–18, 2014.
18. **Hortobagyi T, Katch FI** and **LaChance PF.** Interrelationships among various measures of upper body strength assessed by different contraction modes. Evidence for a general strength component. *Eur J Appl Physiol Occup Physiol* 58: 749–755, 1989.
19. **Hoshi H, Ashizawa K, Kouchi M** and **Koyama C.** On the intra-pair similarity of Japanese monozygotic twins in some somatological traits. *Okajimas Folia Anat Jpn* 58: 675–686, 1982.
20. **Hsu FC, Lenchik L, Nicklas BJ, Lohman K, Register TC, Mychaleckyj J, Langefeld CD, Freedman BI, Bowden DW** and **Carr JJ.** Heritability of body composition measured by DXA in the diabetes heart study. *Obes Res* 13: 312–319, 2005.
21. **Huygens W, Thomis MA, Peeters MW, Vlietinck RE** and **Beunen GP.** Determinants and upper-limit heritabilities of skeletal muscle mass and strength. *Can J Appl Physiol* 29: 186–200, 2004.
22. **Isen J, McGue M** and **Iacono W.** Genetic influences on the development of grip strength in adolescence. *Am J Phys Anthropol* 154: 189–200, 2014.
23. **Janssen I, Shepard DS, Katzmarzyk PT** and **Roubenoff R.** The healthcare costs of sarcopenia in the United States. *J Am Geriatr Soc* 52: 80–85, 2004.
24. **Karasik D, Zhou Y, Cupples LA, Hannan MT, Kiel DP** and **Demissie S.** Bivariate genome-wide linkage analysis of femoral bone traits and leg lean mass: Framingham study. *J Bone Miner Res* 24: 710–718, 2009.
25. **Katzmarzyk PT, Gledhill N, Perusse L** and **Bouchard C.** Familial aggregation of 7-year changes in musculoskeletal fitness. *J Gerontol A Biol Sci Med Sci* 56: B497–502, 2001.
26. **Komi PV, Viitasalo JH, Havu M, Thorstensson A, Sjodin B** and **Karlsson J.** Skeletal muscle fibres and muscle enzyme activities in monozygous and dizygous twins of both sexes. *Acta Physiol Scand* 100: 385–392, 1977.
27. **Kovar R.** Genetic analysis of motor performance. *J Sports Med Phys Fitness* 16: 205–208, 1976.
28. **Landers KA, Hunter GR, Wetzstein CJ, Bamman MM** and **Weinsier RL.** The interrelationship among muscle mass, strength, and the ability to perform physical tasks of daily living in younger and older women. *J Gerontol A Biol Sci Med Sci* 56: B443–448, 2001.
29. **Leong DP, Teo KK, Rangarajan S, Lopez-Jaramillo P, Avezum A, Jr., Orlandini A, Seron P, Ahmed SH, Rosengren A, Kelishadi R, Rahman O, Swaminathan S, Iqbal R, Gupta R, Lear SA, Oguz A, Yusoff K, Zatonska K, Chifamba J, Igumbor E, Mohan V, Anjana RM, Gu H, Li W, Yusuf S** and **Prospective Urban Rural Epidemiology Study investigators**. Prognostic value of grip strength: findings from the Prospective Urban Rural Epidemiology (PURE) study. *Lancet* 386: 266–273, 2015.

30. **Livshits G, Gao F, Malkin I, Needhamsen M, Xia Y, Yuan W, Bell CG, Ward K, Liu Y, Wang J, Bell JT** and **Spector TD.** Contribution of heritability and epigenetic factors to skeletal muscle mass variation in United Kingdom twins. *J Clin Endocrinol Metab* 101: 2450–2459, 2016.

31. **Loos R, Thomis M, Maes HH, Beunen G, Claessens L, Derom C, Legius E, Derom R** and **Vlietinck R.** Gender-specific regional changes in genetic structure of muscularity in early adolescence. *J Appl Physiol (1985)* 82: 1802–1810, 1997.

32. **Lortie G.** Muscle fiber type composition and enzyme activities in brothers and monozygotic twins. In: *Sports and Human Genetics*, edited by Malina R and Bouchard C. Champaign, IL: Human Kinetics, 1986, p. 147–153.

33. **Maes HHM, Beunen GP, Vlietinck RF, Neale MC, Thomis M, VandenEynde B, Lysens R, Simons J, Derom C** and **Derom R.** Inheritance of physical fitness in 10-yr-old twins and their parents. *Med Sci Sports Exerc* 28: 1479–1491, 1996.

34. **Malina RM** and **Mueller WH.** Genetic and environmental influences on the strength and motor performance of Philadelphia school children. *Hum Biol* 53: 163–179, 1981.

35. **Masschelein E, Van Thienen R, Thomis M** and **Hespel P.** High twin resemblance for sensitivity to hypoxia. *Med Sci Sports Exerc* 47: 74–81, 2015.

36. **Mitchell WK, Williams J, Atherton P, Larvin M, Lund J** and **Narici M.** Sarcopenia, dynapenia, and the impact of advancing age on human skeletal muscle size and strength; a quantitative review. *Front Physiol* 3: 260, 2012.

37. **Okuda E, Horii D** and **Kano T.** Genetic and environmental effects on physical fitness and motor performance. *Int J Sport Health Sci* 3: 1–9, 2005.

38. **Pajala S, Era P, Koskenvuo M, Kaprio J, Tolvanen A, Heikkinen E, Tiainen K** and **Rantanen T.** Contribution of genetic and environmental effects to postural balance in older female twins. *J Appl Physiol (1985)* 96: 308–315, 2004.

39. **Payne N, Gledhill N, Katzmarzyk PT, Jamnik V** and **Ferguson S.** Health implications of musculoskeletal fitness. *Can J Appl Physiol* 25: 114–126, 2000.

40. **Peeters MW, Thomis MA, Maes HH, Loos RJ, Claessens AL, Vlietinck R** and **Beunen GP.** Genetic and environmental causes of tracking in explosive strength during adolescence. *Behav Genet* 35: 551–563, 2005.

41. **Peeters MW, Thomis MA, Maes HHM, Beunen GP, Loos RJF, Claessens AL** and **Vlietinck R.** Genetic and environmental determination of tracking in static strength during adolescence. *J Appl Physiol (1985)* 99: 1317–1326, 2005.

42. **Perusse L, Lortie G, Leblanc C, Tremblay A, Theriault G** and **Bouchard C.** Genetic and environmental sources of variation in physical fitness. *Ann Hum Biol* 14: 425–434, 1987.

43. **Pitsiladis Y, Wang G, Wolfarth B, Scott R, Fuku N, Mikami E, He Z, Fiuza-Luces C, Eynon N** and **Lucia A.** Genomics of elite sporting performance: what little we know and necessary advances. *Br J Sports Med* 47: 550–555, 2013.

44. **Reed T, Fabsitz RR, Selby JV** and **Carmelli D.** Genetic influences and grip strength norms in the NHLBI twin study males aged 59–69. *Ann Hum Biol* 18: 425–432, 1991.

45. **Rico-Sanz J, Rankinen T, Joanisse DR, Leon AS, Skinner JS, Wilmore JH, Rao DC, Bouchard C** and **Study HF.** Familial resemblance for muscle phenotypes in the HERITAGE Family Study. *Med Sci Sports Exerc* 35: 1360–1366, 2003.

46. **Ropponen A, Levalahti E, Videman T, Kaprio J** and **Battie MC.** The role of genetics and environment in lifting force and isometric trunk extensor endurance. *Phys Ther* 84: 608–621, 2004.

47. **Schutte NM, Nederend I, Hudziak JJ, de Geus EJ** and **Bartels M.** Differences in adolescent physical fitness: a multivariate approach and meta-analysis. *Behav Genet* 46: 217–227, 2016.

48. **Silventoinen K, Magnusson PK, Tynelius P, Kaprio J** and **Rasmussen F.** Heritability of body size and muscle strength in young adulthood: a study of one million Swedish men. *Genet Epidemiol* 32: 341–349, 2008.

49. **Simoneau JA** and **Bouchard C.** Genetic determinism of fiber type proportion in human skeletal muscle. *FASEB J* 9: 1091–1095, 1995.

50. **Simoneau JA, Lortie G, Boulay MR, Marcotte M, Thibault MC** and **Bouchard C.** Inheritance of human skeletal muscle and anaerobic capacity adaptation to high-intensity intermittent training. *Int J Sports Med* 7: 167–171, 1986.

51. **Strollo SE, Caserotti P, Ward RE, Glynn NW, Goodpaster BH** and **Strotmeyer ES.** A review of the relationship between leg power and selected chronic disease in older adults. *J Nutr Health Aging* 19: 240–248, 2015.

52. **Thibault MC, Simoneau JA, Cote C, Boulay MR, Lagasse P, Marcotte M** and **Bouchard C.** Inheritance of human muscle enzyme adaptation to isokinetic strength training. *Hum Hered* 36: 341–347, 1986.

53. **Thomis M.** Genes and strength and power phenotypes. In: *Genetic and Molecular Aspects of Sport Performance*, edited by Bouchard C and Hoffman EP. Chichester: Wiley-Blackwell, 2011, p. 159–176.

54. **Thomis MA, VanLeemputte M, Maes HH, Blimkie CJR, Claessens AL, Marchal G, Willems E, Vlietinck RF** and **Beunen GP.** Multivariate genetic analysis of maximal isometric muscle force at different elbow angles. *J Appl Physiol (1985)* 82: 959–967, 1997.

55. **Thomis MAI, Beunen GP, Maes HH, Blimkie CJ, Van Leemputte M, Claessens AL, Marchal G, Willems E** and **Vlietinck RF.** Strength training: importance of genetic factors. *Med Sci Sports Exerc* 30: 724–731, 1998.

56. **Thomis MAI, Beunen GP, Van Leemputte M, Maes HH, Blimkie CJ, Claessens AL, Marchal G, WIllems E** and **Vlietinck RF.** Inheritance of static and dynamic arm strength and some of its determinants. *Acta Physiol Scand* 163: 59–71, 1998.

57. **Tiainen K, Sipila S, Alen M, Heikkinen E, Kaprio J, Koskenvuo M, Tolvanen A, Pajala S** and **Rantanen T.** Heritability of maximal isometric muscle strength in older female twins. *J Appl Physiol (1985)* 96: 173–180, 2004.

58. **Tiainen K, Sipila S, Alen M, Heikkinen E, Kaprio J, Koskenvuo M, Tolvanen A, Pajala S** and **Rantanen T.** Shared genetic and environmental effects on strength and power in older female twins. *Med Sci Sports Exerc* 37: 72–78, 2005.

59. **Tiainen KM, Perola M, Kovanen VM, Sipila S, Tuononen KA, Rikalainen K, Kauppinen MA, Widen EI, Kaprio J, Rantanen T** and **Kujala UM.** Genetics of maximal walking speed and skeletal muscle characteristics in older women. *Twin Res Hum Genet* 11: 321–334, 2008.

60. **Zempo H, Miyamoto-Mikami E, Kikuchi N, Fuku N, Miyachi M** and **Murakami H.** Heritability estimates of muscle strength-related phenotypes: A systematic review and meta-analysis. *Scand J Med Sci Sports* 27: 1537–1546, 2017.

61. **Zhai G, Ding C, Stankovich J, Cicuttini F** and **Jones G.** The genetic contribution to longitudinal changes in knee structure and muscle strength: a sibpair study. *Arthritis Rheum* 52: 2830–2834, 2005.

62. **Zhai G, Stankovich J, Ding C, Scott F, Cicuttini F** and **Jones G.** The genetic contribution to muscle strength, knee pain, cartilage volume, bone size, and radiographic osteoarthritis: a sibpair study. *Arthritis Rheum* 50: 805–810, 2004.

63. **Zierath JR** and **Hawley JA.** Skeletal muscle fiber type: influence on contractile and metabolic properties. *PLoS Biol* 2: e348, 2004.

19

GENETIC CONTRIBUTIONS TO MUSCLE STRENGTH

Matthew D. Barberio, Emidio E. Pistilli, and Monica J. Hubal

Muscular strength is defined as the ability to generate force against a resistance and can be thought of in terms of force output by an individual skeletal muscle or a group of skeletal muscles exerting force in a coordinated pattern. Strength is influenced by both intrinsic (i.e., genetic) and extrinsic (i.e., environmental) factors. This book's previous chapter (Chapter 18) explored the heritability of muscle size and strength traits at baseline and changes in these traits following exercise training. This chapter will further explore muscular strength as a multifaceted trait that is affected by underlying components such as muscle mass, neuromuscular activity patterns, and executable skill in performing a variety of tasks. Muscle size and strength are generally positively related to one another (especially at baseline), but this relationship is complex with high intersubject variability, especially during training or detraining. This chapter will serve as a primer to identify important components of muscle strength, highlight biological pathways that modify strength at baseline and strength changes with training, and identify molecular and genetic modifiers of strength. We refer the reader to later chapters for expanded discussions of modifiers of complementary traits such as muscle size (Chapter 20) and neuroendocrine status (Chapter 21).

Muscular strength primer

Skeletal muscle strength is a key determinant of overall functional capacity, and progressive resistance training can stimulate significant gains in muscular strength in both men and women at any stage of life (1–3). In exploring the muscle strength trait, defining a set of commonly used terms is useful. In terms of muscle actions performed during resistance exercise training, three types of action are possible (4, 5). A *concentric contraction* occurs when activated muscle shortens and produces greater force than the external resistance. An *eccentric* or *lengthening action* occurs when activated muscle lengthens rather than shortens because the external resistance is greater than the force that muscle can generate. An *isometric contraction* occurs when activated muscle does not change length as the external force matches the internal force generation. Due to muscle's length–tension relationship, the magnitude of force production during these types of muscle actions are eccentric >isometric >concentric (6). Also, force is inversely related to contraction speed (7). *Absolute strength* is a measure of the total amount of weight that can be lifted by a muscle or group of muscles during a given task. In contrast, *relative strength* is a measure of the amount of weight lifted by a muscle or group of muscles normalized to some measure of body size. One common method to determine absolute strength is to quantify a *repetition maximum* (RM). For example, a one-repetition maximum would be the maximal weight that a person can lift for one repetition when performing a resistance exercise task. Adding a time aspect to strength, *power output* is the rate of doing work, defined as force output applied over a given distance and time (4, 5). Although often used interchangeably, muscular strength and muscular power refer to different types of adaptations that can result from resistance training. *Muscular endurance* is the ability to repeatedly contract a muscle against a resistance while maintaining force output over time. Strength training programs can be designed to target these different aspects of muscle strength. For example, increases in absolute strength could be achieved by lifting maximal weights for very few repetitions (i.e., 1–3 repetitions), while muscular endurance can be trained by lifting submaximal weights for a higher number of repetitions (i.e., 20 repetitions).

Unlike other types of fitness (e.g., cardiovascular, flexibility), strength should not be thought of as a single factor (6). Resistance exercise training can be used to enhance many different expressions of muscular strength, such as maximal muscle force, muscular power, contraction velocity, or muscular endurance, and no single strength training program could enhance all of these factors simultaneously. In other words, muscle performance adaptations in response to strength training are specific to the strength training program utilized. In a similar way, the underlying molecular adaptations within skeletal muscles that occur in response to different resistance training programs are also generally protocol-specific (8, 9). For example, training for muscular endurance would evoke more changes in mitochondrial volume and activity compared to maximal weight/low-repetition training.

Strength training programs can be designed to specifically focus on strength adaptations in individual muscles or on the performance of a coordinated movement task. Resistance training programs that are designed to promote strength and size of individual skeletal muscles are referred to as "*structural*" resistance training programs, while programs aimed at initiating a performance increase are referred to as "*functional*" resistance training programs (6). With this in mind, it is important to note that maximal strength production requires not only contraction of the skeletal muscles involved in the movement, but also the maximal activation of all motor units available in those contracting skeletal muscles by the nervous system. Siff states that a "fundamental principle of strength training is that all strength increases are initiated by neuromuscular stimulation" (6). Therefore, the interaction of the nervous system and the skeletal muscles must be considered in the overall training program if the goal is the development of maximal strength. For readers interested in an extended view of neuroendocrine responses to training, Chapter 21 of this book will discuss this topic at length.

Composition of skeletal muscle

Skeletal muscle is a complex tissue that is composed of multiple layers that each contribute to muscle contraction and force production (reviewed in 10, 11). At the molecular level, individual myosin heads interact with binding sites on actin filaments to form crossbridges, and these crossbridges perform the myosin power stroke using the energy of ATP hydrolysis. The coordinated, and asynchronous, movement of individual crossbridges results in shortening of sarcomeres, which are the basic units of muscle contraction. As sarcomeres shorten, the actin and myosin filaments slide past each other (i.e., sliding filament theory). Sarcomeres are lined up in series within myofibrils, and multiple myofibrils are contained within skeletal muscle fibers.

Skeletal muscle fibers are the cells of skeletal muscle. Numerous muscle fibers are packaged into whole skeletal muscles and, architecturally, can either run from tendon to tendon (i.e., fusiform muscle) or at angles to the line of pull (i.e., pennate muscle). During a concentric contraction, the myosin power stroke and resultant force output of each individual crossbridge is summated within all the sarcomeres in a myofibril, for all myofibrils within each muscle fiber, and for all muscle fibers in a skeletal muscle, which gives rise to muscle contraction and skeletal muscle force output.

Baseline muscle strength in humans and the muscle strength responses to training both display high intersubject variability, due to various factors such as muscle composition, training status, age, and sex. In vastus lateralis muscle biopsies obtained from untrained, sedentary humans, the percentage of type I and type II fiber expression is approximately 50% (reviewed in 12). Although muscle fiber type expression is a dynamic process and is influenced by training stimuli, there is a limit to the extent that fiber type changes can be manipulated by training alone. Genetic predisposition for a specific muscle fiber type distribution is heritable and can influence muscle strength and athletic performance. Genetic predisposition for a greater expression of type II muscle fibers is associated with greater baseline muscle strength and enhanced responses to strength training programs, while a greater expression of type I muscle fibers is associated with enhanced adaptations to endurance training programs (13–16). Heritability and the genetic basis for muscle strength and size traits at baseline and in response to exercise training were explored to a greater extent in Chapter 18 of this book.

Development of muscular strength

In the seminal paper by Moritani and DeVries (17), the time course for development of muscular strength upon initiation of resistance training was established (also reviewed in 18). Early increases in strength in response to resistance exercise training are ascribed to adaptations in the nervous system, as a neuromuscular program is imprinted to the new movement patterns being performed. During this initial period of time, as muscle strength increases in response to the resistance exercise training, minimal muscle hypertrophy is observed. With continuation of resistance training, however, strength continues to increase via muscle hypertrophy. Adaptations in the nervous system are thought to be responsible for the gains in strength that occur within the first 3–5 weeks of starting resistance exercise training (17). After this initial period of time, muscle hypertrophy becomes more evident, which coincides with further strength increases. However, muscle hypertrophy is not infinite, and there are plateaus in both strength and size development, even in those who continue to train for a number of years.

Adaptations in the nervous system that contribute to increases in muscular strength are well established in the literature (reviewed in 19, 20). For example, DeLorme and Watkins (21), first noted that "this initial increase in strength on progressive resistance exercise occurs at a rate far greater than can be accounted for by changes in the muscle." Studies have observed that increases in strength from resistance training within the first few weeks of training are quantifiable despite minimal measurable increases in muscle size (22, 23). In further support of the ability of the nervous system to induce strength gains, unilateral resistance training is associated with gains in strength in the untrained limb (24, 25). This was documented in the Functional Single Nucleotide Polymorphisms Associated with Human Muscle Size and Strength (FAMuSS) study (26, 27), in which 12 weeks of resistance training targeting the upper arm of the nondominant arm was associated with a 54% increase in strength in the trained arm and an 11% increase in strength in the nontrained arm. These post-training increases in strength were associated with a

19% increase in size of the trained arm, compared to a 1.4% increase in size of the nontrained arm (28), supporting a complex relationship between strength and size with training.

Continued increases in muscle strength, following early adaptations in the nervous system, are ascribed to exercise-induced muscle hypertrophy. Muscle hypertrophy can be induced through the activation of numerous signaling pathways (reviewed in 29). Resistance exercise initiates increases in protein accumulation, which is mainly due to greater protein synthesis and slowed protein degradation (30). Greater protein accumulation within skeletal muscle gives rise to larger and more abundant myofibrils within skeletal muscle fibers. In addition, resistance exercise training stimulates the proliferation of satellite cells, which also contribute to increases in muscle size. Following resistance training, the number of myonuclei is increased relative to pretraining numbers (31). Therefore, resistance training stimulates protein synthesis that leads directly to larger myofibrils, a greater number of myofibrils (9), as well as an increase in myonuclear number (31–33). Multiple molecular pathways are upregulated in response to resistance training and help to facilitate increases in muscle size and strength. However, genetic variability in the molecules at play in these pathways can lead to variability in the responses to resistance training (i.e., muscle strength, muscle hypertrophy). More information about factors that underlie muscle mass and its changes with training can be found in Chapter 20.

Genetic variations associated with muscular strength – methodological approaches

Many factors mediate muscle strength (size, neuromuscular efficiency, training history, etc.), making it difficult to isolate individual genetic variations or molecular pathways as being important drivers of muscle strength, yet strength as a phenotype is moderately to highly heritable (34). Approaches to identifying genetic contributions to strength include both global (genome-wide) and targeted (selected gene/variant) association studies. In the early 2000s, with the publication of the human genome, there was a plethora of studies targeting genes related to subcomponents of strength such as muscle size (examples include myostatin, insulin-like growth factor 1 (*IGF1*), alpha-actinin-3 (*ACTN3*), etc.). We briefly review some of the stronger associations later in this chapter, and other literature reviews of single nucleotide polymorphisms and strength traits are available (26, 35, 36). However, many of these studies suffered from lack of statistical power, lack of adequate controls, lack of validation/replication, and other problems related to population genetics studies (for review, see 37). In addition, there are few studies that adopt a systems biology approach to strength genetics – following up association studies with detailed molecular studies to demonstrate functional consequences of genetic variation (though there are some exceptions to this, such as *ACTN3*, further discussed in this book in Chapter 23). Attempting these types of studies in trained populations adds in additional problems, given that training introduces a large new amount of variability to the strength phenotype. One of the largest training studies to date was the FAMuSS study, which tested strength and size gains following 12 weeks of unilateral resistance training in approximately 750 subjects. We refer the reader to reviews of findings from FAMuSS related to size and strength (26, 27).

Because many of the associations reported in these early studies either have small effect sizes or have not been consistently replicated (especially in trained athletes), single-gene variant association studies have fallen out of favor in the literature, replaced by more complex multigene variant models or genome-wide association studies (GWAS). The multigene variant model approach has yet to be applied well to the phenotype of muscle strength, so it will not be addressed further here. Future work from large consortia such as the Molecular Transducers of Physical Activity (MoTrPAC) will likely shed light on genetic contributions to strength using multivariant modeling. Likewise, future studies using the GWAS approach should be informative. Unfortunately, the GWAS approach requires extremely large population sizes, as well as large validation and replication sets, to identify loci associated with a particular trait. GWAS have not lived up to the expectation that once scientists could look across the entire genome at once, that disease- or trait-associated loci would be easily identified. In the largest (N=195,180) GWAS study to date to specifically examine strength (38), 16 loci were deemed significantly associated with grip strength, all in genes that were largely untargeted by previous studies but that represent new areas of exploration, including neuronal maintenance and signaling and psychomotor skills.

As we await more results from large, well-controlled studies of genetic associations with strength, we will conclude this chapter with a summary of cellular and molecular pathways that play direct or indirect roles in muscle strength and how genetic variation in pathway subcomponents contribute to strength variability. By necessity, these results overlap somewhat with pathways that control muscle growth, due to the overall relationship between strength and size.

Cellular pathways related to muscle strength

The functional relationship between strength and muscle size at the molecular level is best explained by the relationship between protein synthesis and protein degradation. Depending on the health status of the population, a single bout of resistance exercise can result in significantly increased rates of protein synthesis as early as 1 hour after exercise which persist for up to 48 hours. Protein degradation is also upregulated in response to resistance exercise, though proportionally less so than protein synthesis resulting in a net protein accretion. The molecular drivers and contributors to regulating protein synthesis and protein degradation pathways are complex and not fully understood. Here we will explore major growth, inflammatory, and neuromuscular pathways that are responsive to tension/load stimuli and their role in the development of muscular strength.

Regulation of muscle size and strength by growth factors

While there are numerous pathways associated with regulation of protein synthesis, the central, and most well understood, pathway is the phosphatidylinsositol-3-kinase (PI3K)/protein kinase B (Akt)/mammalian target of rapamycin (mTOR) axis. It should be noted that these pathways, independent of other signaling molecules, are activated by mechanotransduction, but are further augmented by naturally occurring proteins called growth factors. Figure 19.1 shows an integrated, but not comprehensive, schematic of the major growth factor signaling cascades in regulating protein synthesis and degradation. We discuss a few key elements of the PI3K/Akt/mTOR pathway in the following subsections.

Insulin-like growth factor 1

Both skeletal muscle and liver cells produce IGF1, though paracrine/autocrine actions of skeletal muscle-derived IGF1 appear more critical for skeletal muscle growth than circulating levels (39). IGF1, upon stimulation of the IGF1 receptor, stimulates the activation of PI3K/Akt that promotes skeletal muscle growth through both the activation of protein synthesis and inhibition of protein degradation pathways (40). IGF1-stimulated activation of Akt indirectly promotes protein synthesis through activation of mTOR, resulting in further activation

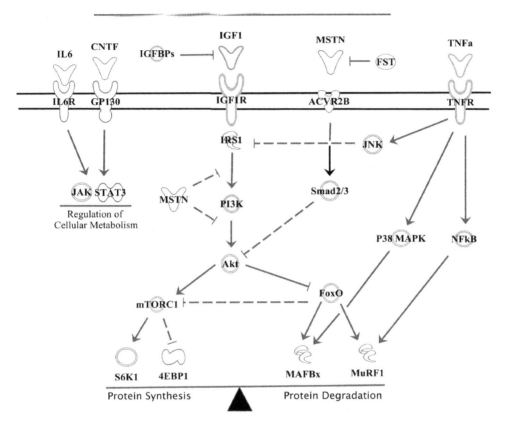

Figure 19.1 Molecular pathways involved in the regulation and balance of protein synthesis and protein degradation. Skeletal muscle contraction (tension/load) during resistance exercises stimulates both protein synthesis and protein degradation. These processes are primarily modulated through the PI3K/Akt/mTOR signaling axis. Growth factors, such as IGF1, increase Akt/mTOR signaling in response to contractile activity, which enhances protein production through regulation of translational regulators such as eukaryotic translation initiation factor 4E-binding protein (4E-BP1). Protein degradation pathways are controlled by forkhead box proteins (FoxO). Other growth factors, such as circulating or skeletal muscle-produced MSTN, inhibit this pathway, resulting in protein degradation. Inflammatory mediators, also increased as a result of contractile activity, such a TNFα, may indirectly regulate PI3K/Akt/mTOR signaling through c-Jun N-terminal kinases (JNK) and also stimulate protein degradation pathways through p38 MAPK and NFkB signaling.

of the translational protein S6 kinase (S6K1) and by inactivating inhibitory eIF4E-binding proteins (4EBPs), allowing for activation of eukaryotic translation initiation factor 4E (eIF4E) (40). Simultaneously, activation of Akt also results in inhibition of protein degradation pathways through phosphorylation and repression of forkhead box O (FoxO) transcriptional factors (40).

The effect of resistance exercise on IGF1 expression is less clear. A number of studies have resulted in conflicting results for *IGF1* mRNA expression in skeletal muscle. Resistance exercise studies have shown upregulation (41–43), downregulation (44), and no changes (45) in *IGF1* mRNA expression. However, transgenic animal models have provided direct evidence of its role in promoting increased muscle mass and preservation of motoneurons during age-related loss, both of which would likely result in increased strength (46, 47). Furthermore, human studies using recombinant human IGF1 administration demonstrated improved strength in older females (48). Thus, IGF1 is certainly involved in the regulation of skeletal muscle mass and strength, though the role of resistance exercise in increasing IGF1 expression and its subsequent role in resistance exercise-induced strength improvements is less clear.

One reason there may be conflicting responses between resistance exercise studies and IGF1 is the role of other interacting proteins and signaling pathways in its mechanism of action. First, a binding protein, IGF-binding protein 3 (IGFBP3) is responsible for extending the half-life of circulating IGF1 and IGF2. Increasing the half-life would serve to augment their interactions with surface receptors on skeletal muscle and cardiomyocytes (49, 50). However, other IGFBPs are responsible for inhibiting its interactions with the surface receptor. Furthermore, IGF1-induced hypertrophy in both skeletal and cardiac tissue is largely influenced by signaling pathways independent of the PI3K/Akt/mTOR axis previously described. Specifically, the protein phosphatase calcineurin is involved in the Ca^{2+}-dependent calcineurin signaling pathway, which influences IGF1-induced growth (51). Lastly, the timing and developmental phase of the tissue may be critical as well. During fetal growth, IGF2 acts as the primary skeletal muscle tissue growth factor and is later involved in regulation of skeletal muscle satellite cells (52).

As previously mentioned, expression levels of IGF1 following resistance exercise have provided conflicting results, making interpretation of its role in resistance exercise-induced strength changes complicated. However, the nature of the *IGF1* gene itself may be partially responsible for these conflicting results. Splice variants of the *IGF1* gene give rise to multiple mature protein products, one of which is IGF-1Ec, also known as mechanogrowth factor (MGF). MGF has been shown to increase the proliferative capacity of skeletal muscle progenitor cells (53) as well as myotubes *in vitro* (54), thus, providing a clear role in the development of muscle mass. However, animal and human models of skeletal muscle overload using synergistic ablation (55) and resistance exercise (56) have shown an age-dependent upregulation of *MGF* mRNA.

Myostatin

Myostatin (MSTN), previously known as growth differentiation factor-8 (GDF-8), is a highly conserved negative regulator of muscle development (57). This negative regulation has been shown to occur through multiple signaling pathways: circulating MSTN activates activin type IIa and IIb receptors (ACVR2A and ACVR2B) (58, 59) while skeletal muscle-produced MSTN has been shown to inhibit IGF1-induced PI3K/Akt/mTOR signaling (57). Naturally occurring loss of MSTN in humans (60), as well as in multiple animal models, results in significantly more muscle mass in comparison to genetic wild types (61–64). A number of studies have explored circulating and tissues levels of MSTN in response to single or repeated bouts of resistance training. Kim et al. (65) demonstrated reductions of *MSTN* mRNA in the vastus lateralis following a single bout of resistance training in both old and young males and females. The resistance exercise-induced reduction was blunted in older females however. A study by Dalbo et al. (66) showed reduced *MSTN* mRNA expression in old, but not young, men following three bouts of resistance exercise. Furthermore, older participants also showed upregulation of follistatin (FST), which is known to inhibit circulating MSTN activity by preventing binding with the ACVR2A and ACVR2B receptors. Roth et al. (67) showed 9 weeks of heavy exercise reduced vastus lateralis *MSTN* mRNA expression by 37% in men and women. Expression levels in this study were not correlated to any measure of skeletal muscle mass or strength at any time point. An extended review of MSTN's role in muscle size is presented in Chapter 22 of this handbook.

Regulation of muscle strength and size by inflammatory factors

The inflammatory response to various exercise modalities plays a role in systemic and cellular adaptation. The cellular and systemic mediators of this response are a class of proteins called cytokines. While numerous, a key subset of cytokines has been of particular interest to those trying to understand their role in protein accretion and degradation. Tumor necrosis factor-alpha (TNFα), interleukin (IL)-6, and IL-15 are some of the most well studied to date. Independently these cytokines result in distinct cellular signaling cascades, but also work synergistically and in opposition to each other as well as growth factors.

Tumor necrosis factor-alpha

Originally identified as "cachectin" (due to elevated systemic levels in muscle wasting during cancer cachexia) (68), TNFα is a proinflammatory mediator of skeletal muscle protein degradation (69). TNFα exerts its proteolytic actions through activation of multiple signaling pathways. TNFα activates the classical proinflammatory protein complex nuclear factor kappa-light-chain-enhancer of activated B cells (NF-κB) (70). Activation of TNFα membrane-bound receptors, TNFR1 and TNFR2, results in phosphorylation and degradation of the enzyme complex IκB kinase (IKK). Degradation of this complex results in activation and nuclear translocation of NF-κB which signals for further production of proinflammatory cytokines, including TNFα, and the proteolytic E3 ubiquitin-ligase MuRF1 (71). Studies have also demonstrated a non-NF-κB dependent proteolytic pathway activated by TNFα. P38 mitogen-activated protein kinase (p38) is activated through TNFα receptor signaling which results in activation of the proteolytic E3 ubiquitin ligase muscle atrophy F box (MAFbx/Atrogin-1) protein (72). Lastly, TNFα has been demonstrated to inhibit both the expression and protein activity of growth factors such as IGF1 (73, 74).

The proteolytic actions of TNFα can be demonstrated or correlated at the cellular and whole-organ level. Blockade of TNFα signaling mitigates loss of muscle mass in models of muscle wasting such as cancer or sepsis (75, 76). Li and Reid (77) also demonstrated the role of NF-κB-mediated TNFα-induced protein loss in C_2C_{12} myoblasts. Although there is a high degree of variability in the TNFα response to resistance training, circulating levels of TNFα have been shown to decrease following strength training and have an inverse relationship to strength gains (78). However, skeletal muscle expression of TNFα following resistance exercise has been demonstrated to increase for up to 12 hours (79, 80). Louis et al. (80) also demonstrated that elevations in TNFα resulted in upregulation of MuRF1 and MAFbx expression for up to 4 hours after resistance exercise. These studies, as well as observational studies (78, 81), clearly demonstrate a relationship between TNFα and muscle mass and muscle strength in disease states and during strength training-induced adaptations. The early upregulation in expression of TNFα and downstream effectors following a resistance exercise load indicates it is likely involved in the exercise-induced increase in protein degradation, which is outpaced by the protein synthesis resulting in a net protein accretion.

Interleukin-6 and ciliary neurotrophic factor

Similar to TNFα, an inverse relationship between circulating levels of IL-6 and measures of muscle mass and muscle strength in older men and women has been demonstrated (78, 81, 82). However, the role of IL-6 in regulating the balance between protein synthesis and degradation is less clear. Due to skeletal muscle being a primary site of synthesis and release in response to exercise, IL-6 has been termed a myokine (83). Traditionally a regulator of the acute phase response to various cellular and systemic stressors, IL-6 synthesis and release from skeletal muscle is regulated by the contractile process (84). Once into circulation, IL-6 can interact with either the interleukin 6 receptor (IL-6R) or the glycoprotein 130 (GP130) cytokine receptor, which results in the activation of JAK/STAT3 signaling and transcription. Multiple studies of resistance exercise demonstrate an acute upregulation of IL-6 expression, with one showing a biphasic response over 24 hours (79, 80). Circulating levels of IL-6 are highly variable between individuals and are highly influenced by age and health status. Furthermore, circulating levels following exercise are highly dependent on exercise modality, intensity, and duration (83). While there is evidence that IL-6 may interfere with the anabolic actions of IGF1 (85), it is possible that the IL-6 relationship to protein balance is indirect, likely through a negative regulation of TNFα.

Ciliary neurotrophic factor (CNTF) shares a similar molecular structure with IL-6 and is able to bind to the GP130 membrane receptor, resulting in activation of the STAT3 and AMPK signaling pathways (86). Interest in CNTF as a regulator of muscle mass and strength is based on its ability to promote increased cellular growth and survival of neurons (87). Multiple resistance training studies (88, 89) have identified a positive correlation between *CNTF* expression in skeletal muscle and resistance training outcomes. Furthermore, these studies also identified an age effect on *CNTF* expression, with older individuals expressing less. However, use of recombinant human CNTF for treatment of amyotrophic lateral sclerosis (ALS), a neurodegenerative disease, did not attenuate loss of isometric grip strength (90).

Interleukin-15

IL-15 was originally identified as a growth factor after it was demonstrated to increase myoblast proliferation and muscle-specific myosin heavy chain composition (91). Further *in vitro* (92) and overexpression (93) studies supported the role of IL-15 in promoting increased protein accretion as well as preventing protein degradation. More recent studies in mice have altered this view of IL-15, instead focusing on its role in mitochondrial biogenesis and fiber type composition. Overexpression of *IL-15* results in a more oxidative skeletal muscle phenotype (94), while loss of the IL-15 receptor α subunit of the IL-15 plasma membrane receptor increased endurance capacity and resistance to fatigue (95).

Limitations, practical applications, and future directions

In this chapter, we have provided a primer for understanding the muscular strength trait at baseline and following training and have explored molecular pathways that can contribute to variations in strength within a population. We noted that while the heritability of strength is moderate to high, genetic contributions can be quite varied due to the complex nature of the strength trait. We discussed current limitations to identifying genetic associations with strength, including limited sample sizes and the introduction of variability during training. With a few exceptions (such as *ACTN3* and *MSTN*, discussed further in their own chapters), both targeted and global association studies have yet to identify strong single gene–strength interactions, and it is likely that multivariant modeling will be needed to explain currently missing strength heritability. This will be enabled by efforts such as MoTrPAC and other large consortia projects, though results from these studies are likely years away. In the meantime, there is strong evidence that pathway modification of underlying strength components such as muscle size accounts for significant variability in baseline strength and in functional gains with training. Understanding these to a greater extent should help develop training programs that optimize gains among a variety of different people.

References

1. **Campos, G.E.**, et al., Muscular adaptations in response to three different resistance-training regimens: specificity of repetition maximum training zones. *Eur J Appl Physiol*, 2002. 88(1–2): p. 50–60.
2. **Chilibeck, P.D.**, et al., Twenty weeks of weight training increases lean tissue mass but not bone mineral mass or density in healthy, active young women. *Can J Physiol Pharmacol*, 1996. 74(10): p. 1180–5.
3. **Peterson, M.D., A. Sen**, and **P.M. Gordon**, Influence of resistance exercise on lean body mass in aging adults: a meta-analysis. *Med Sci Sports Exerc*, 2011. 43(2): p. 249–58.
4. **Harman, E.**, Biomechanics of resistance training, in *Essentials of Strength Training and Conditioning*, T.R. Baechle and R.W. Earle, Editors. 2008, Human Kinetics.
5. **Knuttgen, H.G.** and **P.V. Komi**, Basic definitions for exercise, in *Strength and Power in Sport*, P.V. Komi, Editor. 1992, Blackwell Science.
6. **Siff, M.C.**, *Supertraining*. 5th ed. 2000, Supertraining Institute.
7. **Wilkie, D.R.**, The relation between force and velocity in human muscle. *J Physiol*, 1949. 110(3–4): p. 249–80.
8. **Goldspink, G.**, Cellular and molecular aspects of adaptation in skeletal muscle, in *Strength and Power in Sport*, P.V. Komi, Editor. 1992, Blackwell Science.
9. **Bickel, C.S.**, et al., Time course of molecular responses of human skeletal muscle to acute bouts of resistance exercise. *J Appl Physiol (1985)*, 2005. 98(2): p. 482–8.
10. **Caiozzo, V.J.**, The muscular system: structural and functional plasticity, in *ACSM's Advanced Exercise Physiology*, P.A. Farrell, M.J. Joyner, and V.J. Caiozzo, Editors. 2012, Lippincott Williams & Wilkens.
11. **Billeter, R.** and **H. Hoppeler**, Muscular basis of strength, in *Strength and Power in Sport*, P.V. Komi, Editor. 1992, Blackwell Science.
12. **Saltin, B.** and **P.D. Gollnick**, Skeletal muscle adaptability: significance for metabolism and performance, in *Handbook of Physiology: Skeletal Muscle*, L.D. Peachey, R.H. Adrian, and R.S. Geiger, Editors. 1983, Williams & Wilkins.
13. **Simoneau, J.A.** and **C. Bouchard**, Genetic determinism of fiber type proportion in human skeletal muscle. *FASEB J*, 1995. 9(11): p. 1091–5.
14. **Simoneau, J.A.** and **C. Bouchard**, Human variation in skeletal muscle fiber-type proportion and enzyme activities. *Am J Physiol*, 1989. 257(4 Pt 1): p. E567–72.
15. **Simoneau, J.A.**, et al., Inheritance of human skeletal muscle and anaerobic capacity adaptation to high-intensity intermittent training. *Int J Sports Med*, 1986. 7(3): p. 167–71.
16. **Prud'homme, D.**, et al., Sensitivity of maximal aerobic power to training is genotype-dependent. *Med Sci Sports Exerc*, 1984. 16(5): p. 489–93.
17. **Moritani, T.** and **H.A. deVries**, Neural factors versus hypertrophy in the time course of muscle strength gain. *Am J Phys Med*, 1979. 58(3): p. 115–30.
18. **Moritani, T.**, Time course of adaptations during strength and power training, in Strength and Power in Sport, P.V. Komi, Editor. 1992, Blackwell Science.
19. **Sale, D.G.**, Neural adaptations to strength training, in Strength and Power in Sport, P.V. Komi, Editor. 1992, Blackwell Science.
20. **Aagaard, P.**, Training-induced changes in neural function. *Exerc Sport Sci Rev*, 2003. 31(2): p. 61–7.
21. **DeLorme, T.L.** and **A.L. Watkins**, *Progressive Resistance Exercise*. 1951, Appleton Century Inc.
22. **DeVries, H.A.**, "Efficiency of electrical activity" as a physiological measure of the functional state of muscle tissue. *Am J Phys Med*, 1968. 47(1): p. 10–22.
23. **Bowers, L.**, Effects of autosuggested muscle contraction on muscular strength and size. *Res Q*, 1966. 37(3): p. 302–12.
24. **Hellebrandt, F.A., A.M. Parrish**, and **S.J. Houtz**, The influence of unilateral exercise on the contralateral limb. *Arch Phys Med Rehabil*, 1947. 28(2): p. 76–85.
25. **Coleman, E.A.**, Effect of unilateral isometric and isotonic contractions on the strength of the contralateral limb. *Res Q*, 1969. 40: p. 490–495.
26. **Pescatello, L.S.**, et al., Highlights from the functional single nucleotide polymorphisms associated with human muscle size and strength or FAMuSS study. *Biomed Res Int*, 2013. 2013: p. 643575.

27. **Thompson, P.D.**, et al., Functional polymorphisms associated with human muscle size and strength. *Med Sci Sports Exerc*, 2004. 36(7): p. 1132–9.
28. **Hubal, M.J.**, et al., Variability in muscle size and strength gain after unilateral resistance training. *Med Sci Sports Exerc*, 2005. 37(6): p. 964–72.
29. **Tsika, R.**, The muscular system: the control of muscle mass, in *ACSM's Advanced Exercise Physiology*, P.A. Farrell, M.J. Joyner, and V.J. Caiozzo, Editors. 2012, Lippincot Williams and Wilkens.
30. **Biolo, G.**, et al., Increased rates of muscle protein turnover and amino acid transport after resistance exercise in humans. *Am J Physiol*, 1995. 268(3 Pt 1): p. E514–20.
31. **Allen, D.L., R.R. Roy**, and **V.R. Edgerton**, Myonuclear domains in muscle adaptation and disease. *Muscle Nerve*, 1999. 22(10): p. 1350–60.
32. **Petrella, J.K.**, et al., Potent myofiber hypertrophy during resistance training in humans is associated with satellite cell-mediated myonuclear addition: a cluster analysis. *J Appl Physiol (1985)*, 2008. 104(6): p. 1736–42.
33. **Verdijk, L.B.**, et al., Skeletal muscle hypertrophy following resistance training is accompanied by a fiber type-specific increase in satellite cell content in elderly men. *J Gerontol A Biol Sci Med Sci*, 2009. 64(3): p. 332–9.
34. **Zempo, H.**, et al., Heritability estimates of muscle strength-related phenotypes: A systematic review and meta-analysis. *Scand J Med Sci Sports*, 2017. 27(12): p. 1537–1546.
35. **Rankinen, T.**, et al., Advances in exercise, fitness, and performance genomics. *Med Sci Sports Exerc*, 2010. 42(5): p. 835–46.
36. **Venezia, A.C.** and **S.M. Roth**, Recent research in the genetics of exercise training adaptation. *Med Sport Sci*, 2016. 61: p. 29–40.
37. **Bouchard, C.**, Exercise genomics – a paradigm shift is needed: a commentary. *Br J Sports Med*, 2015. 49(23): p. 1492–6.
38. **Willems, S.M.**, et al., Large-scale GWAS identifies multiple loci for hand grip strength providing biological insights into muscular fitness. *Nat Commun*, 2017. 8: p. 16015.
39. **Adams, G.R., F. Haddad**, and **K.M. Baldwin**, Time course of changes in markers of myogenesis in overloaded rat skeletal muscles. *J Appl Physiol (1985)*, 1999. 87(5): p. 1705–12.
40. **Schiaffino, S.** and **C. Mammucari**, Regulation of skeletal muscle growth by the IGF1-Akt/PKB pathway: insights from genetic models. *Skelet Muscle*, 2011. 1(1): p. 4.
41. **Bamman, M.M.**, et al., Cluster analysis tests the importance of myogenic gene expression during myofiber hypertrophy in humans. *J Appl Physiol (1985)*, 2007. 102(6): p. 2232–9.
42. **Deldicque, L.**, et al., Increased IGF mRNA in human skeletal muscle after creatine supplementation. *Med Sci Sports Exerc*, 2005. 37(5): p. 731–6.
43. **Greig, C.A.**, et al., Skeletal muscle IGF-I isoform expression in healthy women after isometric exercise. *Growth Horm IGF Res*, 2006. 16(5–6): p. 373–6.
44. **Psilander, N., R. Damsgaard**, and **H. Pilegaard**, Resistance exercise alters MRF and IGF-I mRNA content in human skeletal muscle. *J Appl Physiol (1985)*, 2003. 95(3): p. 1038–44.
45. **Coffey, V.G.** and **J.A. Hawley**, The molecular bases of training adaptation. *Sports Med*, 2007. 37(9): p. 737–63.
46. **Messi, M.L.** and **O. Delbono**, Target-derived trophic effect on skeletal muscle innervation in senescent mice. *J Neurosci*, 2003. 23(4): p. 1351–9.
47. **Gonzalez, E.**, et al., Insulin-like growth factor-1 prevents age-related decrease in specific force and intracellular Ca2+ in single intact muscle fibres from transgenic mice. *J Physiol*, 2003. 552(Pt 3): p. 833–44.
48. **Boonen, S.**, et al., Musculoskeletal effects of the recombinant human IGF-I/IGF binding protein-3 complex in osteoporotic patients with proximal femoral fracture: a double-blind, placebo-controlled pilot study. *J Clin Endocrinol Metab*, 2002. 87(4): p. 1593–9.
49. **Ferry, R.J.**, Jr., et al., Cellular actions of insulin-like growth factor binding proteins. *Horm Metab Res*, 1999. 31(2–3): p. 192–202.
50. **Jones, J.I.** and **D.R. Clemmons**, Insulin-like growth factors and their binding proteins: biological actions. *Endocr Rev*, 1995. 16(1): p. 3–34.
51. **Musaro, A.**, et al., IGF-1 induces skeletal myocyte hypertrophy through calcineurin in association with GATA-2 and NF-ATc1. *Nature*, 1999. 400(6744): p. 581–5.
52. **Goldberg, A.L.**, et al., Mechanism of work-induced hypertrophy of skeletal muscle. *Med Sci Sports*, 1975. 7(3): p. 185–98.

53. **Kandalla, P.K.**, et al., Mechano growth factor E peptide (MGF-E), derived from an isoform of IGF-1, activates human muscle progenitor cells and induces an increase in their fusion potential at different ages. *Mech Ageing Dev*, 2011. 132(4): p. 154–62.

54. **Philippou, A.**, et al., Expression of IGF-1 isoforms after exercise-induced muscle damage in humans: characterization of the MGF E peptide actions in vitro. *In Vivo*, 2009. 23(4): p. 567–75.

55. **Owino, V., S.Y. Yang**, and **G. Goldspink**, Age-related loss of skeletal muscle function and the inability to express the autocrine form of insulin-like growth factor-1 (MGF) in response to mechanical overload. *FEBS Lett*, 2001. 505(2): p. 259–63.

56. **Hameed, M.**, et al., Expression of IGF-I splice variants in young and old human skeletal muscle after high resistance exercise. *J Physiol*, 2003. 547(Pt 1): p. 247–54.

57. **Morissette, M.R.**, et al., Myostatin inhibits IGF-I-induced myotube hypertrophy through Akt. *Am J Physiol Cell Physiol*, 2009. 297(5): p. C1124–32.

58. **Lee, S.J.**, et al., Regulation of muscle growth by multiple ligands signaling through activin type II receptors. *Proc Natl Acad Sci U S A*, 2005. 102(50): p. 18117–22.

59. **Lee, S.J.** and **A.C. McPherron**, Regulation of myostatin activity and muscle growth. *Proc Natl Acad Sci U S A*, 2001. 98(16): p. 9306–11.

60. **Schuelke, M.**, et al., Myostatin mutation associated with gross muscle hypertrophy in a child. *N Engl J Med*, 2004. 350(26): p. 2682–8.

61. **Clop, A.**, et al., A mutation creating a potential illegitimate microRNA target site in the myostatin gene affects muscularity in sheep. *Nat Genet*, 2006. 38(7): p. 813–8.

62. **McPherron, A.C.** and **S.J. Lee**, Double muscling in cattle due to mutations in the myostatin gene. *Proc Natl Acad Sci U S A*, 1997. 94(23): p. 12457–61.

63. **Mosher, D.S.**, et al., A mutation in the myostatin gene increases muscle mass and enhances racing performance in heterozygote dogs. *PLoS Genet*, 2007. 3(5): p. e79.

64. **Szabo, G.**, et al., A deletion in the myostatin gene causes the compact (Cmpt) hypermuscular mutation in mice. *Mamm Genome*, 1998. 9(8): p. 671–2.

65. **Kim, J.S., J.M. Cross**, and **M.M. Bamman**, Impact of resistance loading on myostatin expression and cell cycle regulation in young and older men and women. *Am J Physiol Endocrinol Metab*, 2005. 288(6): p. E1110–9.

66. **Dalbo, V.J.**, et al., Acute loading and aging effects on myostatin pathway biomarkers in human skeletal muscle after three sequential bouts of resistance exercise. *J Gerontol A Biol Sci Med Sci*, 2011. 66(8): p. 855–65.

67. **Roth, S.M.**, et al., Myostatin gene expression is reduced in humans with heavy-resistance strength training: a brief communication. *Exp Biol Med (Maywood)*, 2003. 228(6): p. 706–9.

68. **Beutler, B.**, et al., Purification of cachectin, a lipoprotein lipase-suppressing hormone secreted by endotoxin-induced RAW 264.7 cells. *J Exp Med*, 1985. 161(5): p. 984–95.

69. **Argiles, J.M.** and **F.J. Lopez-Soriano**, The role of cytokines in cancer cachexia. *Med Res Rev*, 1999. 19(3): p. 223–48.

70. **von Haehling, S.**, et al., Cachexia: a therapeutic approach beyond cytokine antagonism. *Int J Cardiol*, 2002. 85(1): p. 173–83.

71. **Bodine, S.C.**, et al., Identification of ubiquitin ligases required for skeletal muscle atrophy. *Science*, 2001. 294(5547): p. 1704–8.

72. **Li, Y.P.**, et al., TNF-alpha acts via p38 MAPK to stimulate expression of the ubiquitin ligase atrogin1/MAFbx in skeletal muscle. *FASEB J*, 2005. 19(3): p. 362–70.

73. **Fernandez-Celemin, L.**, et al., Inhibition of muscle insulin-like growth factor I expression by tumor necrosis factor-alpha. *Am J Physiol Endocrinol Metab*, 2002. 283(6): p. E1279–90.

74. **Langen, R.C.**, et al., Inflammatory cytokines inhibit myogenic differentiation through activation of nuclear factor-kappaB. *FASEB J*, 2001. 15(7): p. 1169–80.

75. **Breuille, D.**, et al., Pentoxifylline decreases body weight loss and muscle protein wasting characteristics of sepsis. *Am J Physiol*, 1993. 265(4 Pt 1): p. E660–6.

76. **Costelli, P.**, et al., Tumor necrosis factor-alpha mediates changes in tissue protein turnover in a rat cancer cachexia model. *J Clin Invest*, 1993. 92(6): p. 2783–9.

77. **Li, Y.P.** and **M.B. Reid**, NF-kappaB mediates the protein loss induced by TNF-alpha in differentiated skeletal muscle myotubes. *Am J Physiol Regul Integr Comp Physiol*, 2000. 279(4): p. R1165–70.

78. **Schaap, L.A.**, et al., Higher inflammatory marker levels in older persons: associations with 5-year change in muscle mass and muscle strength. *J Gerontol A Biol Sci Med Sci*, 2009. 64(11): p. 1183–9.

79. **Buford, T.W., M.B. Cooke**, and **D.S. Willoughby**, Resistance exercise-induced changes of inflammatory gene expression within human skeletal muscle. *Eur J Appl Physiol*, 2009. 107(4): p. 463–71.

80. **Louis, E.**, et al., Time course of proteolytic, cytokine, and myostatin gene expression after acute exercise in human skeletal muscle. *J Appl Physiol (1985)*, 2007. 103(5): p. 1744–51.

81. **Visser, M.**, et al., Relationship of interleukin-6 and tumor necrosis factor-alpha with muscle mass and muscle strength in elderly men and women: the Health ABC Study. *J Gerontol A Biol Sci Med Sci*, 2002. 57(5): p. M326–32.

82. **Schaap, L.A.**, et al., Inflammatory markers and loss of muscle mass (sarcopenia) and strength. *Am J Med*, 2006. 119(6): p. 526 e9–17.

83. **Pedersen, B.K.**, et al., Role of myokines in exercise and metabolism. *J Appl Physiol (1985)*, 2007. 103(3): p. 1093–8.

84. **Pedersen, B.K.** and **M.A. Febbraio**, Muscle as an endocrine organ: focus on muscle-derived interleukin-6. *Physiol Rev*, 2008. 88(4): p. 1379–406.

85. **Lazarus, D.D., L.L. Moldawer**, and **S.F. Lowry**, Insulin-like growth factor-1 activity is inhibited by interleukin-1 alpha, tumor necrosis factor-alpha, and interleukin-6. *Lymphokine Cytokine Res*, 1993. 12(4): p. 219–23.

86. **Watt, M.J.**, et al., CNTF reverses obesity-induced insulin resistance by activating skeletal muscle AMPK. *Nat Med*, 2006. 12(5): p. 541–8.

87. **Ip, N.Y.** and **G.D. Yancopoulos**, Ciliary neurotrophic factor and its receptor complex. *Prog Growth Factor Res*, 1992. 4(2): p. 139–55.

88. **Dennis, R.A.**, et al., Aging alters gene expression of growth and remodeling factors in human skeletal muscle both at rest and in response to acute resistance exercise. *Physiol Genomics*, 2008. 32(3): p. 393–400.

89. **Dennis, R.A.**, et al., Muscle expression of genes associated with inflammation, growth, and remodeling is strongly correlated in older adults with resistance training outcomes. *Physiol Genomics*, 2009. 38(2): p. 169–75.

90. **Group, A.C.T.S.**, A double-blind placebo-controlled clinical trial of subcutaneous recombinant human ciliary neurotrophic factor (rHCNTF) in amyotrophic lateral sclerosis. *Neurology*, 1996. 46(5): p. 1244–9.

91. **Quinn, L.S., K.L. Haugk**, and **K.H. Grabstein**, Interleukin-15: a novel anabolic cytokine for skeletal muscle. *Endocrinology*, 1995. 136(8): p. 3669–72.

92. **Furmanczyk, P.S.** and **L.S. Quinn**, Interleukin-15 increases myosin accretion in human skeletal myogenic cultures. *Cell Biol Int*, 2003. 27(10): p. 845–51.

93. **Quinn, L.S.**, et al., Overexpression of interleukin-15 induces skeletal muscle hypertrophy in vitro: implications for treatment of muscle wasting disorders. *Exp Cell Res*, 2002. 280(1): p. 55–63.

94. **Quinn, L.S.**, et al., IL-15 overexpression promotes endurance, oxidative energy metabolism, and muscle PPARdelta, SIRT1, PGC-1alpha, and PGC-1beta expression in male mice. *Endocrinology*, 2013. 154(1): p. 232–45.

95. **Pistilli, E.E.**, et al., Loss of IL-15 receptor alpha alters the endurance, fatigability, and metabolic characteristics of mouse fast skeletal muscles. *J Clin Invest*, 2011. 121(8): p. 3120–32.

20

GENETIC CONTRIBUTIONS TO SKELETAL MUSCLE SIZE

Philip J. Atherton, Jessica Cegielski, and Daniel J. Wilkinson

Resistance exercise training and muscle hypertrophy

The main physiological adaptive feature of resistance exercise training (RET) is increased muscle mass, which manifests as an increase in the dimensions of whole muscle groups as a result of growth of individual muscles. These gross physiological changes in skeletal muscle mass are most commonly determined using imaging techniques such as dual-energy X-ray absorptiometry (DXA), computed tomography (CT), magnetic resistance imaging (MRI), or ultrasonography (43). Muscle hypertrophy can also be measured on a single-fiber level by estimation of individual myofiber cross-sectional area in biopsy samples using histological techniques coupled to imaging software analysis to determine hypertrophy on a cell-by-cell level (20). It is believed that postnatal growth of skeletal muscle occurs via the process of hypertrophy, which represents an increase in cross-sectional area of *existing* post-mitotic muscle cells, rather than through fiber splitting or hyperplasia (61).

RET-induced hypertrophy is reliant on a number of different components and is regulated through complex and integrated gene–environment interactions. Moreover, using standard muscle loading regimens, approximately 20% of adults do not demonstrate measurable increases in muscle mass (6, 23, 74) even after months of resistance training; this intersubject variability is important to keep in mind when considering the various potential mediators of skeletal muscle cell hypertrophy (ensuing sections). Muscle mass in adults is maintained through the diurnal pattern of building muscle proteins via muscle protein synthesis (MPS) following periods of feeding, with dietary amino acids (AAs) replenishing muscle proteins that are broken down via muscle protein breakdown (MPB) during periods of fasting. Under normal healthy circumstances, diurnal MPS matches MPB and muscle mass is maintained. In contrast, in chronic periods of growth (e.g., adolescence) or RET-induced hypertrophy, MPS >MPB, while in situations of skeletal muscle wasting (e.g., catabolic disease or ageing), MPS <MPB (15).

Resistance exercise training-induced effects on muscle protein synthesis and muscle protein breakdown

In the immediate period following a single bout of resistance exercise (RE), MPS is markedly increased approximately two- to fourfold above baseline rates (at rest, human muscle proteins turnover at approximately 0.05%/hour or 1.2%/day) (55). The magnitude of increase in MPS in response to RE displays a dose-dependent increase in MPS, reaching near maximal rates at approximately 60% of one-repetition maximum (1RM) (55), beyond which no additional stimulation is observed. Despite this observation, this does not mean exercising at lower intensities is of no benefit (when it comes to muscle size and hypertrophy that is), since increases in acute MPS at 30% 1RM are equivalent to those at 90% 1RM, but only when RE is performed to failure (17). This is likely due to increased type II muscle fiber recruitment through fatiguing contractions (Hennemen's size principle) (42), resulting in maximal fiber recruitment and hence maximal recruitment and thereby anabolic stimulation of that muscle.

It is the accumulation of postexercise increases in MPS that, over a period of RET, ultimately creates a greater sustained positive net protein balance (i.e., MPS >MPB) culminating in muscle growth or hypertrophy (13, 14). Few studies have addressed the temporal nature of MPS response throughout a RET program due to traditional measurement approaches requiring constant infusions of AA tracers, limiting studies to hours rather than days or weeks. However, recent advances using the D_2O stable isotope tracer have allowed further understanding of the cumulative, temporal nature of MPS responses over progressive RET programs. What can be observed from these studies is that the major hypertrophic responses to (unaccustomed) RET occurs during the early phase of RET, with significant increases in D_2O-derived MPS only observed over 0–3 weeks of a 6-week resistance exercise program. No significant increase was observed between 3 and 6 weeks (13). These conclusions are supported by a number of RET studies showing pronounced increases in muscle mass using CT, DXA, and ultrasonography, during the early phases of RET, which curtail within the later weeks (9, 25, 85). Despite the idea of "early hypertrophy" still being considered a somewhat controversial idea by some, based on findings from acute MPS tracer studies, conceptually it makes perfect sense. Indeed, early acute stable isotope tracer studies highlighted that following a single bout of RET, MPS responses were more pronounced in individuals unaccustomed to RET as compared with those accustomed to regular RET (77). Moreover, following unilateral RET, MPS responses are reduced within the trained versus untrained leg (75), with this training-induced attenuation of MPS beginning following only a few RET bouts (22, 89, 94). These findings support the idea of rapid remodeling and growth in the early phases due to heightened MPS responses to RE, followed by a period of sustained maintenance and neuromuscular adaptations.

Nutrient interactions with resistance exercise training for regulation of muscle size

The impact of nutrients on muscle protein turnover is now very well established (see 5, 15, 24, 65, 71). In terms of muscle protein turnover, it is the essential amino acid (EAA) components of a mixed meal that are the primary driver behind increases in MPS in the postprandial phase, reverting the muscle to a net positive balance and replenishing the protein lost during the previous fasted/postabsorptive period (5, 67, 86, 87). In particular, the branched-chain AA leucine has been found to have potent anabolic properties, acting as both a substrate and a signal for muscle protein synthesis (12, 40, 95, 96). In terms of MPB, the release of insulin – either through the carbohydrate content of a mixed meal, or via AA-mediated insulin release (36) – helps to suppress MPB, augmenting the shift to positive protein balance further. However, the acute response to nutrition is finite; MPS peaks at about 1.5 hours following feeding and then rapidly returns to baseline values, once the fasted loss of protein has been replenished in the fed state, a term known as "muscle full" (4, 66). Once this is complete, these energetically demanding metabolic processes can be shut down until required again. While muscle size is dependent on adequate nutrition, nutrition alone does not regulate muscle size, growth, or hypertrophy – at least in adult muscle. It is the important interaction between nutrition and exercise that is key to regulating growth.

It should also be noted, that RE *in the absence of nutrition* is actually a significant catabolic stressor. Following an acute bout of RE, MPB increases by as much as 50%, which, despite concomitant increases in MPS in the postabsorptive state (i.e., absence of nutrition), leads to an overall negative net balance (54, 55, 76). Crucially, nutrition plays a significant facilitating role in RE-induced anabolism, helping to suppress the exercise-induced increase in MPB (via insulin-mediated mechanism discussed above) while also potentiating the RE-induced increase in MPS (8). Thus, in terms of protein turnover, while postexercise increases in MPS are the major determinants of adaptive hypertrophy, the potentiation of this MPS response through interactions with dietary protein intake rich in EAAs, alongside the associated attenuation of MPB, is necessary to maximize positive net protein balance and muscle gains. Following RE, MPS can remain elevated for up to, and potentially beyond, 24 hours, essentially "sensitizing" the muscle to future anabolic stimuli, such as food intake (16, 64, 76). This interaction between nutrient intake and RE has led to the investigation of whether there may be an optimal dosage or timing of nutrient intake allied to RE-induced anabolism (71). It appears that, as with protein intake alone, there is a "muscle-full" effect, whereby MPS response is near maximal following the provision of between 0.25 and 0.4 g/kg (~20–30g of protein for the average size male) (69), with higher doses providing no additional benefit and only leading to increased AA oxidation (69, 98). Nonetheless, due to the extended anabolic window provided following RE, many have investigated whether the timing of protein ingestion is an important consideration; however, little evidence suggests that anything other than providing protein in the post-RE period close to the cessation of exercise is of any additional benefit (68).

Intramuscular sensing and signaling regulating resistance exercise training-induced muscle hypertrophy

Of all the signaling pathways associated with RET response, the mechanistic target of rapamycin, complex 1 (mTORC1: composed of the genes *mTOR, raptor, PRAS40, Deptor,* and *LST8*) is considered a "master" determinant of the regulation of RET-induced hypertrophy (33). For instance, experiments where rapamycin, an inhibitor of mTORC1, was administered to humans revealed a complete blockade of RE-mediated increases in MPS (28). The notion that activation of mTORC1 might represent a central node communicating RE to MPS can be reconciled by the number of substrates associated with mRNA translation. Indeed, activation of mTORC1 is associated with the phosphorylation of multiple translational initiation factors substrates including 4E-binding protein (4EBP1), ribosomal protein S6 kinase (p70S6K1), and eukaryotic initiation factors 4 G/A/B (eIF4G/A/B), that facilitate formation of an eIF3F scaffold and assembly of a "competent" 48S pre-initiation complex. In a parallel pathway, activation of the guanine exchange factor, eukaryotic initiation factor 2B (eIF2B), shuttles the initiator tRNA (Met-tRNAi) to the ribosome during formation of the 48S pre-initiation complex, thereby promoting "global" MPS (mRNA translation) and thus coordinately enhancing translational efficiency (see 45 for control of translation). Practically all of these factors have been shown to be stimulated in response to RE, and many are used as a proxy for mTORC1 signaling (e.g., p70S6K1) since kinase activity of mTORC1 is a complex combination of cellular localization, affinity to its multiple binding partners, and phosphorylation events.

Upstream signaling to mTORC1 in response to resistance exercise

While the mTORC1 signaling pathway is thought to be an affirmed central regulator of MPS and hypertrophy, the proximal mechanisms involved in the activation of mTORC1 by RE remain incompletely defined. In the most basic sense, "upstream" signals triggered by RE cause the activation of intracellular signaling pathways that are responsible for modulating post-translational control of MPS and also that of muscle mRNA expression. Like any form of physical activity, RE triggers complex physiochemical events (i.e., mechanotransduction (33), endocrine (41), and auto/paracrine (7) responses) which combine to determine the net adaptive responses. The genetic bases of neurohormonal responses to RET are further discussed in Chapter 21. Much of the early preclinical (10) and cell culture work (78) implicated insulin-like growth factor (IGF) canonical signaling in RE-mediated alterations in MPS and hypertrophy. Increases in the expression of IGF-1 and its splice variants (mechanogrowth factor, liver IGF-1 isoforms) bind the insulin-like growth factor 1 receptor (IGF-1R), which in turn yields activation of a classical insulin-mediated PI3K-protein kinase B (AKT)–mTORC1 signaling pathway. However, it is now thought that canonical IGF-1R–AKT–mTOR signaling is an oversimplification of the complex regulation of RE-induced muscle hypertrophy. An example of this can be found in one elegant study, where adult human volunteers performed RE either in arm muscles alone or concurrently in arm and leg muscles; the rationale being to create either a high (i.e., arm and leg exercise) or a low (i.e., arm exercise alone) systemic hormone milieu based on differences in recruitment of absolute muscle mass. Despite markedly different systemic concentrations of growth hormone, testosterone and IGF-1 between groups, there was no difference in mTORC1-signaling or in MPS – or critically – chronic adaptations to training in terms of muscle mass/strength gains (92, 93). These data indicate that modulating the systemic concentrations of IGF-1 or testosterone and growth hormone (GH, the latter of which acts via inducing IGF-1 expression rather than having any direct effect on MPS in adult humans) (27) within the physiological range might not play a role in adaptive hypertrophy and challenges the classic view of canonical insulin-signaling pathway. This does not however preclude that IGF-1 regulates AKT-mTOR signaling via "local" autoparacrine signaling mechanisms undetectable by measuring serum abundance of IGF-1. That being said, IGF-1R knockout did not attenuate functional loading-induced muscle hypertrophy in animal models (88) (synergist ablation model), once again suggesting that neither IGF-1 canonical signaling, nor perhaps, systemic hormone milieu can explain RE-induced hypertrophy (i.e., there must be other mechanisms at play).

The absence of accord over the role of canonical signaling from exogenous (to the muscle) IGF-1 (or other circulating hormones) has led to new hypotheses surrounding the mechanistic basis of RET-induced hypertrophy with greater focus on it being a process both arising from and being regulated within the muscle. The intrinsic mechanisms by which this is thought to occur is via mechanotransduction; the process of converting mechanical signals sensed in response to cellular movement into molecular signals. One mechanoresponsive target was recently highlighted, where activation of phospholipase D (PLD) enzymes increases production of the lipid second messenger phosphatidic acid (PA) in a mechanosensitive manner. Mechanistically, it has been demonstrated that PA signaling is upstream of contraction-induced activation of mTOR, since pharmacological inhibition of PLD effectively ablated activation of mTOR in response to contractions (73). While pharmacological inhibitors are rarely entirely selective, this perhaps represents at least one line of evidence for a mechanism by which muscle can adapt independently of systemic hormones and/or a canonical IGF-1 pathway.

Another possible mechanosensitive pathway is that of the muscle attachment, or focal adhesion complexes: macromolecular structures situated in the sarcolemma of muscle fibers, that link the extracellular matrix to the cytoplasmic cytoskeleton, consisting of a variety of extracellular matrix receptors/integrins and intracellular cytoskeletal and signaling molecules (52). Indeed, interactions of extracellular matrix proteins with integrin receptors stimulate intracellular signaling pathways important in cell growth and migration in adult skeletal muscle (84). Moreover, activation of integrin receptors appears to be a common feature of muscle remodeling in response to a variety of conditions including endurance training and muscular dystrophy (90). Focal adhesion kinase (FAK) is a nonreceptor tyrosine kinase that localizes to focal adhesion complexes and is thought to represents a key component of integrin-mediated signaling (19). Engagement of integrin receptors induces phosphorylation of FAK at Tyr397, which correlates with its activation (18) and a growing body of evidence has associated FAK activation with the hypertrophic response to mechanical stress in skeletal muscle (29). Indeed, expression patterns of FAK have been reported to be load-dependent, i.e., phosphorylation of FAK was lowered following hindlimb suspension in rodents (34), immobilization in humans (11), and increased in models of overload (31, 35) and following RE training in humans (97). Finally, local overexpression of FAK (FAK pLKO.1 plasmid electroporation) *in vivo* in rodents was shown to stimulate muscle hypertrophy (52), suggesting FAK is a genuine mechanosensitive component of muscle hypertrophy. This notion is further supported by recent work demonstrating that FAK is associated with skeletal muscle remodeling in response to RET in humans, with its activation being associated with areas of most significant RET-induced hypertrophy (32).

PGC1 and myostatin as regulators of RET-induced muscle hypertrophy

The identification of splice variants of peroxisome proliferator-activated receptor gamma coactivator 1-alpha (PGC1α: α1, α2, α3, and α4,) in muscle has led to the suggestion that PGC1α4 is critical for the regulation of muscle hypertrophy through upregulation of IGF-1 signaling and inhibition of myostatin (80) in mice. However, translation of these findings were questioned in a study which reported no differential upregulation of PGC1α splice variants in response to acute exercise of contrasting type and effects on muscle hypertrophy (resistance vs. endurance) (99). Moreover, exercise-induced expression of PGC1α variants following 5 weeks of unilateral RET showed no correlation with increases in muscle size and strength (57), casting doubt upon a role of such splice variants regulating human muscle growth in responses to RET. In terms of other key purported regulators, myostatin remains the most potent (negative) regulator of muscle mass since its discovery about 20 years ago (63). Yet, despite the compelling studies in animals revealing the gross musculature of animals in which myostatin itself or its endogenous serum binding partners (follistatin, G protein-coupled receptor- associated sorting protein (GASP-1), myostatin propeptide) were genetically manipulated, the role of myostatin in human muscle hypertrophy remains poorly understood with studies in humans aimed at defining the role of myostatin in hypertrophy yielding contentious data. Indeed, while downregulation of myostatin would be expected in relation to hypertrophy-inducing exercise, some studies have shown this (3, 44, 51, 83), while others have noted no differences, or a poor association with resulting muscle hypertrophy (50, 56). Much of the problem associated with studying the role of myostatin may be due to its complex post-translational processing (62), which makes accurate protein identification problematic. In addition to its purported effects on anabolic signaling, inhibition of myostatin has also been suggested as a mediator of satellite cell activity (satellite cells represent a pool of muscle "stem cells" able to contribute to muscle repair or growth). However, while the use of a soluble activin receptor 2B antagonist was associated with muscle growth, this was associated with minimal labelling of satellite cell-derived nuclei, suggesting that myostatin acts on myofibers, rather than satellite cell to influence muscle hypertrophy (91). Therefore, while myostatin remains a therapeutic target for muscle growth, its physiological role in human muscle hypertrophy remains unclear. It could be postulated that while myostatin is important in development, its homeostatic role in the regulation and maintenance of adult skeletal muscle is limited, thereby limiting scope for any downregulation to have effects. Myostatin is described in greater detail in Chapter 22.

Genetic contributors to muscle mass/strength

As alluded to earlier, there is marked intersubject variation in an individual's response to RET in terms of mass and strength gains. It is therefore intuitive that this variation may be associated with genetic variability in individuals, and the presence of common inherited mutations (or polymorphisms). There have been a number of studies investigating this, and a number of potential candidate genes and gene variants have been proposed; for example, angiotensin-converting enzyme (*ACE*; more detail in Chapter 17) insertion/deletion polymorphism, *ACTN3* (detailed in Chapter 23), ciliary neurotrophic factor (*CNTF*) and receptor, myostatin-related genes (*MSTN*; detailed in Chapter 22), and the vitamin D receptor (*VDR*), as highlighted by Kostek et al. (53) and Roth et al. (79). Nevertheless, findings have been somewhat inconclusive and lacking in reproducibility, such that definitive conclusions are difficult to draw as to whether these gene variants are important for heritability in mass and strength or not. As such, there remains a great deal of work to be done to investigate relationships between heritability and muscle mass/strength. There has been some progress however, with one of the first large-scale genome-wide association meta-analyses studies being performed and identifying five single nucleotide polymorphisms in/near hydroxysteroid 17-beta dehydrogenase 11 (*HSD17B11*), veriscan (*VCAN*), a disintegrin-like and metalloprotease domain with thrombospondin type-1 motifs-like-3 (*ADAMTSL3*), insulin receptor substrate-1 (*IRS1*), and fat-mass and obesity associated gene (*FTO*), which were associated with lean body mass, and with successful replication across multiple different cohorts (100). This perhaps provides an important breakthrough in our attempts to understand the genetic variation in skeletal muscle size and strength. Due to the complexity of analysis in "omics" and the study sizes needed to explore this complexity, it still remains to be seen as to whether these gene variants can explain the heterogeneous responses to RET in humans.

Relationships between muscle mass and strength gains in response to resistance exercise training

As described in Chapter 19, the positive relationship between muscle strength and muscle size (cross-sectional area (CSA) and muscle volume), is well established (2, 46, 47). However, numerous studies utilizing RET have shown early increases in strength where muscle hypertrophy is not yet evident (21, 81), suggesting that other variables contribute to strength gain, such as changes to neural drive or a change in fiber composition. Moreover, classical studies comparing strength and muscle CSA in sprinters and endurance runners (59) have shown that sprinters produced higher maximal knee extensor voluntary isometric force compared to endurance runners, despite there being no significant difference in muscle CSA between the two. In addition, numerous studies have compared the effects of RET in relation to training status (i.e., between trained and untrained individuals) (1, 60). The results of such studies suggest that despite comparable muscle CSA, greater gains in strength (from baseline) are found in untrained individuals (38). This is likely due to trained subjects already possessing forms of favorable neuromuscular or morphological adaptations (e.g., altered fiber type composition and/or muscle architecture), in comparison with the untrained such that the untrained individuals have a greater potential for adaptation and thus a more pronounced gain in strength (58). This demonstrates that strength is not solely dependent on muscle mass; instead, there are many adaptations contributing to strength outcomes (i.e., neuromuscular/architectural/fiber type).

As discussed above, neuromuscular adaptations are an important contributor to strength changes. These adaptations can occur at the neuromuscular junction or central nervous system (30, 49). Electromyography (EMG) allows for the investigation of neural adaptations in response to exercise (26, 70, 72). Using surface electrodes, motor unit (MU) activation can be recorded as an integral of the electrical activity measured (iEMG), before, during and after contraction (39, 82). (For a more detailed review on EMG methods, see 82.) As previously described, studies have identified that initial increases in strength correlate with increases in iEMG (i.e., MU activation) during early periods of training where muscle hypertrophy was not evident. Therefore, these increases in strength are due to increased neural adaptations, such as increased MU recruitment. In addition to changes in muscle strength following RET in a trained limb, a phenomenon termed "cross-education" or "cross-training effect" was identified whereby increases in strength were also detected in the contralateral untrained limb (47). Consequently, it was hypothesized that neural adaptations had to be occurring more centrally to elicit such effects on the contralateral untrained limb. It is since known that with long-term RET, neural adaptations occur in the primary motor cortex, M1 (49). Similarly, neuromuscular plasticity can also be observed during detraining. Narici et al. (72) observed similar rates of change in CSA, iEMG, and maximum voluntary contraction during the training and detraining period. Conversely, Ishida et al. (48) observed a significant increase in maximum voluntary contraction during training but an insignificant decrease during the detraining period. This suggested that there were potential strength training adaptations that remained. It was proposed that this was due to enzyme activity in the muscle, as described by Guy and Snow (37), or that it was as a result of changes in the size of sarcoplasmic reticulum or release of calcium ions. The latter is a crucial component of the excitation–contraction coupling cascade.

Conclusion

Muscle hypertrophy is the most recognized feature of adaptation to RET, governed by both genetic and environmental factors. The general time-course of RET-induced hypertrophy is one of rapid onset in the first weeks, before gradual slowing, despite pursuing progressive regimens (adjusting loads for strength gains). The upstream mechanisms triggering sustained increases in MPS (the driver of protein accretion) has been related to induction of systemic hormones and contraction-induced mechanotransduction within muscle; with the latter perhaps being more critical. Either way, the activation of proximal signaling to mTORC1 is a critical step since its substrates are linked to global mRNA translation and enhanced MPS. Nonetheless, responses are highly variable among individuals, albeit for poorly defined reasons. This variation may relate to impaired activation of MPS, or satellite cell recruitment, and be driven by genetic predisposition to trainability; nonetheless, any gene variants regulating hypertrophic responses to RET and its variation remain to be robustly identified. Strength gains accompany muscle hypertrophy and are related to the degree of muscle hypertrophy, but also neuromuscular adaptations, perhaps at the level of the brain and spinal cord – but also – at the level of individual motor units and the excitation–contraction coupling apparatus.

References

1. **Ahtiainen JP, Pakarinen A, Alen M, Kraemer WJ, Häkkinen K**. Muscle hypertrophy, hormonal adaptations and strength development during strength training in strength-trained and untrained men. *Eur J Appl Physiol* 89: 555–563, 2003.

2. **Akagi R, Takai Y, Ohta M, Kanehisa H, Kawakami Y, Fukunaga T**. Muscle volume compared to cross-sectional area is more appropriate for evaluating muscle strength in young and elderly individuals. *Age Ageing* 38: 564–569, 2009.

3. **Aoki MS, Soares AG, Miyabara EH, Baptista IL, Moriscot AS**. Expression of genes related to myostatin signaling during rat skeletal muscle longitudinal growth. *Muscle Nerve* 40: 992–999, 2009.

4. **Atherton PJ, Etheridge T, Watt PW, Wilkinson D, Selby A, Rankin D, Smith K, Rennie MJ**. Muscle full effect after oral protein: time-dependent concordance and discordance between human muscle protein synthesis and mTORC1 signaling. *Am J Clin Nutr* 92: 1080–1088, 2010.

5. **Atherton PJ, Wilkinson DJ, Smith K**. Feeding modulation of amino acid utilization: role of insulin and amino acids in skeletal muscle. In: *The Molecular Nutrition of Amino Acids and Proteins*, edited by Dardevet D. London: Academic Press, 2016, p. 109–124.

6. **Bamman MM, Petrella JK, Kim JS, Mayhew DL, Cross JM**. Cluster analysis tests the importance of myogenic gene expression during myofiber hypertrophy in humans. *J Appl Physiol* 102: 2232–2239, 2007.

7. **Bamman MM, Shipp JR, Jiang J, Gower BA, Hunter GR, Goodman A, McLafferty CL, Urban RJ**. Mechanical load increases muscle IGF-I and androgen receptor mRNA concentrations in humans. *Am J Physiol Endocrinol Metab* 280: E383–E390, 2001.

8. **Biolo G, Tipton KD, Klein S, Wolfe RR**. An abundant supply of amino acids enhances the metabolic effect of exercise on muscle protein. *Am J Physiol* 273: E122–E129, 1997.

9. **Blazevich AJ, Cannavan D, Coleman DR, Horne S**. Influence of concentric and eccentric resistance training on architectural adaptation in human quadriceps muscles. *J Appl Physiol* 103: 1565–1575, 2007.

10. **Bodine SC, Stitt TN, Gonzalez M, Kline WO, Stover GL, Bauerlein R, Zlotchenko E, Scrimgeour A, Lawrence JC, Glass DJ, Yancopoulos GD**. Akt/mTOR pathway is a crucial regulator of skeletal muscle hypertrophy and can prevent muscle atrophy in vivo. *Nat Cell Biol* 3: 1014–1019, 2001.

11. **de Boer MD, Selby A, Atherton P, Smith K, Seynnes OR, Maganaris CN, Maffulli N, Movin T, Narici M V, Rennie MJ**. The temporal responses of protein synthesis, gene expression and cell signalling in human quadriceps muscle and patellar tendon to disuse. *J Physiol* 585: 241–251, 2007.

12. **Bonfils G, Jaquenoud M, Bontron S, Ostrowicz C, Ungermann C, De Virgilio C**. Leucyl-tRNA synthetase controls TORC1 via the EGO complex. *Mol Cell* 46: 105–110, 2012.

13. **Brook M, Wilkinson D, Mitchell W, Lund J, Szewczyk NJ, Greenhaff P, Smith K, Atherton P**. Skeletal muscle hypertrophy is most active during early resistance exercise training responses, matching long term deuterium oxide (D2O)-derived measures of muscle protein synthesis and mTORc1-signaling. *FASEB J* 29: 4485–4496, 2015.

14. **Brook MS, Wilkinson DJ, Mitchell WK, Lund JN, Phillips BE, Szewczyk NJ, Greenhaff PL, Smith K, Atherton PJ**. Synchronous deficits in cumulative muscle protein synthesis and ribosomal biogenesis underlie age-related anabolic resistance to exercise in humans. *J Physiol* 594: 7399–7417, 2016.

15. **Brook MS, Wilkinson DJ, Phillips BE, Perez-Schindler J, Philp A, Smith K, Atherton PJ**. Skeletal muscle homeostasis and plasticity in youth and ageing: impact of nutrition and exercise. *Acta Physiol* 216: 15–41, 2016.

16. **Burd NA, West DWD, Moore DR, Atherton PJ, Staples AW, Prior T, Tang JE, Rennie MJ, Baker SK, Phillips SM**. Enhanced amino acid sensitivity of myofibrillar protein synthesis persists for up to 24 h after resistance exercise in young men. *J Nutr* 141: 568–573, 2011.

17. **Burd NA, West DWD, Staples AW, Atherton PJ, Baker JM, Moore DR, Holwerda AM, Parise G, Rennie MJ, Baker SK, Phillips SM**. Low-load high volume resistance exercise stimulates muscle protein synthesis more than high-load low volume resistance exercise in young men. *PLoS One* 5: e12033, 2010.

18. **Calalb MB, Polte TR, Hanks SK, Calalb MB Polte TR HSK**. Tyrosine phosphorylation of focal adhesion kinase at sites in the catalytic domain regulates kinase activity: a role for Src family kinases. *Mol Cell Biol* 15: 954–963, 1995.

19. **Cary LA, Guan JL**. Focal adhesion kinase in integrin-mediated signaling. *Front Biosci* 4: D102–D113, 1999.

20. **Ceglia L, Niramitmahapanya S, Price TJ, Harris SS, Fielding RA, Dawson-Hughes B**. An evaluation of the reliability of muscle fiber cross-sectional area and fiber number measurements in rat skeletal muscle. *Biol Proced Online* 15: 6, 2013.

21. **Chilibeck PD, Caldera W, Sale DG, Webber CE**. A comparison of strength and muscle mass increases during resistance training in young women. *Eur J Appl Physiol Occup Physiol* 77: 170–175, 1998.

22. **Damas F, Phillips S, Vechin FC, Ugrinowitsch C**. A review of resistance training-induced changes in skeletal muscle protein synthesis and their contribution to hypertrophy. *Sports Med* 45: 801–807, 2015.

23. **Davidsen PK, Gallagher IJ, Hartman JW, Tarnopolsky MA, Dela F, Helge JW, Timmons JA, Phillips SM**. High responders to resistance exercise training demonstrate differential regulation of skeletal muscle microRNA expression. *J Appl Physiol* 110: 309–317, 2011.

24. **Deane CS, Wilkinson DJ, Phillips BE, Smith K, Etheridge T, Atherton PJ**. "Nutraceuticals" in relation to human skeletal muscle and exercise. *Am J Physiol – Endocrinol Metab* 312, E282–E299, 2017.

25. **DeFreitas JM, Beck TW, Stock MS, Dillon MA, Kasishke PR**. An examination of the time course of training-induced skeletal muscle hypertrophy. *Eur J Appl Physiol* 111: 2785–2790, 2011.

26. **DeVries HA**. "Efficiency of electrical activity" as a physiological measure of the functional state of muscle tissue. *Am J Phys Med* 47: 10–22, 1968.

27. **Doessing S, Heinemeier KM, Holm L, Mackey AL, Schjerling P, Rennie M, Smith K, Reitelseder S, Kappelgaard A-M, Rasmussen MH, Flyvbjerg A, Kjaer M**. Growth hormone stimulates the collagen synthesis in human tendon and skeletal muscle without affecting myofibrillar protein synthesis. *J Physiol* 588: 341–351, 2010.

28. **Drummond MJ, Fry CS, Glynn EL, Dreyer HC, Dhanani S, Timmerman KL, Volpi E, Rasmussen BB**. Rapamycin administration in humans blocks the contraction-induced increase in skeletal muscle protein synthesis. *J Physiol* 587: 1535–1546, 2009.

29. **Durieux AC, Desplanches D, Freyssenet D, Fluck M**. Mechanotransduction in striated muscle via focal adhesion kinase. *Biochem Soc Trans*. 35: 1312–1313, 2007.

30. **Fang Y, Siemionow V, Sahgal V, Xiong F, Yue GH**. Greater movement-related cortical potential during human eccentric versus concentric muscle contractions. *J Neurophysiol* 86: 1764–1772, 2001.

31. **Flück M, Carson JA, Gordon SE, Ziemiecki A, Booth FW**. Focal adhesion proteins FAK and paxillin increase in hypertrophied skeletal muscle. *Am J Physiol* 277: C152–C162, 1999.

32. **Franchi MV, Ruoss S, Valdivieso P, Mitchell KW, Smith K, Atherton PJ, Narici MV, Flück M**. Regional regulation of focal adhesion kinase after concentric and eccentric loading is related to remodelling of human skeletal muscle. *Acta Physiol* 223: e13056, 2018.

33. **Goodman CA, Frey JW, Mabrey DM, Jacobs BL, Lincoln HC, You J-S, Hornberger TA**. The role of skeletal muscle mTOR in the regulation of mechanical load-induced growth. *J Physiol* 589: 5485–5501, 2011.

34. **Goodman CA, Mabrey DM, Frey JW, Miu MH, Schmidt EK, Pierre P, Hornberger TA**. Novel insights into the regulation of skeletal muscle protein synthesis as revealed by a new nonradioactive in vivo technique. *FASEB J* 25: 1028–1039, 2011.

35. **Gordon SE, Flück M, Booth FW**. Selected Contribution: skeletal muscle focal adhesion kinase, paxillin, and serum response factor are loading dependent. *J Appl Physiol* 90: 1174–1183, 2001.

36. **Greenhaff PL, Karagounis LG, Peirce N, Simpson EJ, Hazell M, Layfield R, Wackerhage H, Smith K, Atherton P, Selby a, Rennie MJ**. Disassociation between the effects of amino acids and insulin on signaling, ubiquitin ligases, and protein turnover in human muscle. *Am J Physiol Endocrinol Metab* 295: E595–E604, 2008.

37. **Guy PS, Snow DH**. The effect of training and detraining on muscle composition in the horse. *J Physiol* 269: 33–51, 1977.

38. **Häkkinen K, Komi P., Tesch P**. Effect of combined concentric and eccentric strength training and detraining on force-time, muscle fiber and metabolic characteristics of leg extensor muscles. *Scand J Med Sci Sport* 3: 50–58, 1981.

39. **Häkkinen K, Kraemer WJ, Newton RU, Alen M**. Changes in electromyographic activity, muscle fibre and force production characteristics during heavy resistance/power strength training in middle-aged and older men and women. *Acta Physiol Scan* 171: 51–62, 2001.

40. **Han JM, Joong SJ, Park MC, Kim G, Kwon NH, Kim HK, Ha SH, Ryu SH, Kim S**. Leucyl-tRNA synthetase is an intracellular leucine sensor for the mTORC1-signaling pathway. *Cell* 149: 410–424, 2012.

41. **Hansen S, Kvorning T, Kjaer M, Sjøgaard G**. The effect of short-term strength training on human skeletal muscle: the importance of physiologically elevated hormone levels. *Scand J Med Sci Sports* 11: 347–354, 2001.

42. **Henneman E**. Relation between size of neurons and their susceptibility to discharge. *Science* 126: 1345–1347, 1957.

43. **Heymsfield SB, Gallagher D, Visser M, Nuñez C, Wang ZM**. Measurement of skeletal muscle: laboratory and epidemiological methods. *J Gerontol A Biol Sci Med Sci* 50: 23–29, 1995.

44. **Hulmi JJ, Tannerstedt J, Selänne H, Kainulainen H, Kovanen V, Mero AA**. Resistance exercise with whey protein ingestion affects mTOR signaling pathway and myostatin in men. *J Appl Physiol* 106: 1720–1729, 2009.

45. **Iadevaia V, Huo Y, Zhang Z, Foster LJ, Proud CG**. Roles of the mammalian target of rapamycin, mTOR, in controlling ribosome biogenesis and protein synthesis. *Biochem Soc Trans* 40: 168–172, 2012.

46. **Ikai M, Fukunaga T**. Calculation of muscle strength per unit cross-sectional area of human muscle by means of ultrasonic measurement. *Int Zeitschrift für Angew Physiol Einschließlich Arbeitsphysiologie* 26: 26–32, 1968.

47. **Ikai M, Fukunaga T**. A study on training effect on strength per unit cross-sectional area of muscle by means of ultrasonic measurement. *Int Zeitschrift für Angew Physiol Einschließlich Arbeitsphysiologie* 28: 173–180, 1970.

48. **Ishida K, Moritani T, Itoh K**. Changes in voluntary and electrically induced contractions during strength training and detraining. *Eur J Appl Physiol Occup Physiol* 60: 244–248, 1990.

49. **Kami A, Meyer G, Jezzard P, Adams MM, Turner R, Ungerleider LG**. Functional MRI evidence for adult motor cortex plasticity during motor skill learning. *Nature* 377: 155, 1995.

50. **Kim J-S, Petrella JK, Cross JM, Bamman MM**. Load-mediated downregulation of myostatin mRNA is not sufficient to promote myofiber hypertrophy in humans: a cluster analysis. *J Appl Physiol* 103: 1488–1495, 2007.

51. **Kim J, Cross JM, Bamman MM**. Impact of resistance loading on myostatin expression and cell cycle regulation in young and older men and women. *Am J Physiol Endocrinol Metab* 288: E1110–E1119, 2005.

52. **Klossner S, Durieux A-C, Freyssenet D, Flueck M**. Mechano-transduction to muscle protein synthesis is modulated by FAK. *Eur J Appl Physiol* 106: 389–398, 2009.

53. **Kostek M, Hubal MJ, Pescatello LS**. The role of genetic variation in muscle strength. *Am J Lifestyle Med* 5: 156–170, 2011.

54. **Kumar V, Atherton P, Smith K, Rennie MJ**. Human muscle protein synthesis and breakdown during and after exercise. *J Appl Physiol* 106: 2026–2039, 2009.

55. **Kumar V, Selby A, Rankin D, Patel R, Atherton P, Hildebrandt W, Williams J, Smith K, Seynnes O, Hiscock N, Rennie MJ**. Age-related differences in the dose-response relationship of muscle protein synthesis to resistance exercise in young and old men. *J Physiol* 587: 211–217, 2009.

56. **Kvorning T, Andersen M, Brixen K, Schjerling P, Suetta C, Madsen K**. Suppression of testosterone does not blunt mRNA expression of myoD, myogenin, IGF, myostatin or androgen receptor post strength training in humans. *J Physiol* 578: 579–593, 2007.

57. **Lundberg TR, Fernandez-Gonzalo R, Norrbom J, Fischer H, Tesch PA, Gustafsson T**. Truncated splice variant PGC-1α4 is not associated with exercise-induced human muscle hypertrophy. *Acta Physiol (Oxf)* 1: e00140, 2014.

58. **Mangine GT, Gonzalez AM, Townsend JR, Adam J, Beyer KS, Miramonti AA, Ratamess NA**. Influence of baseline muscle strength and size measures on training adaptations in resistance-trained men. *Int J Exerc Sci* 11: 198–213, 2018.

59. **Maughan RJ, Watson JS, Weir J**. Relationships between muscle strength and muscle cross-sectional area in male sprinters and endurance runners. *Eur J Appl Physiol Occup Physiol* 50: 309–318, 1983.

60. **Maughan RJ, Watson JS, Weir J**. Muscle strength and cross-sectional area in man: a comparison of strength-trained and untrained subjects. *Br J Sports Med* 18: 149–157, 1984.

61. **McCall GE, Byrnes WC, Dickinson A, Pattany PM, Fleck SJ**. Muscle fiber hypertrophy, hyperplasia, and capillary density in college men after resistance training. *J Appl Physiol* 81: 2004–2012, 1996.

62. **McFarlane C, Langley B, Thomas M, Hennebry A, Plummer E, Nicholas G, McMahon C, Sharma M, Kambadur R**. Proteolytic processing of myostatin is auto-regulated during myogenesis. *Dev Biol* 283: 58–69, 2005.

63. **McPherron AC, Lawler AM, Lee SJ**. Regulation of skeletal muscle mass in mice by a new TGF-beta superfamily member. *Nature* 387: 83–90, 1997.

64. **Miller BF, Olesen JL, Hansen M, Døssing S, Crameri RM, Welling RJ, Langberg H, Flyvbjerg A, Kjaer M, Babraj JA, Smith K, Rennie MJ**. Coordinated collagen and muscle protein synthesis in human patella tendon and quadriceps muscle after exercise. *J Physiol* 567: 1021–1033, 2005.

65. **Mitchell W, Wilkinson D, Phillips B, Lund J, Smith K, Atherton P**. Human skeletal muscle protein metabolism responses to amino acid nutrition. *Adv Nutr* 7: 828S–838S, 2016.

66. **Mitchell WK, Phillips BE, Williams JP, Rankin D, Lund JN, Smith K, Atherton PJ**. A dose-rather than delivery profile-dependent mechanism regulates the "muscle-full" effect in response to oral essential amino acid intake in young men. *J Nutr* 145: 207–214, 2015.

67. **Mitchell WK, Wilkinson DJ, Phillips BE, Lund JN, Smith K, Atherton PJ**. Human skeletal muscle protein metabolism responses to amino acid nutrition. *Adv Nutr* 7: 828S–838S, 2016.

68. **Moore DR, Churchward-Venne TA, Witard O, Breen L, Burd NA, Tipton KD, Phillips SM**. Protein ingestion to stimulate myofibrillar protein synthesis requires greater relative protein intakes in healthy older versus younger men. *J Gerontol Ser A Biol Sci Med Sci* 70: 57–62, 2015.

69. **Moore DR, Robinson MJ, Fry JL, Tang JE, Glover EI, Wilkinson SB, Prior T, Tarnopolsky MA, Phillips SM**. Ingested protein dose response of muscle and albumin protein synthesis after resistance exercise in young men. *Am J Clin Nutr* 89: 161–168, 2009.

70. **Moritani T, de Vries HA**. Neural factors versus hypertrophy in the time course of muscle strength gain. *Am J Phys Med* 58: 115–130, 1979.

71. **Morton RW, McGlory C, Phillips SM**. Nutritional interventions to augment resistance training-induced skeletal muscle hypertrophy. *Front Physiol* 6: 245, 2015.

72. **Narici M V., Roi GS, Landoni L, Minetti AE, Cerretelli P**. Changes in force, cross-sectional area and neural activation during strength training and detraining of the human quadriceps. *Eur J Appl Physiol Occup Physiol* 59: 310–319, 1989.

73. **O'Neil TK, Duffy LR, Frey JW, Hornberger TA**. The role of phosphoinositide 3-kinase and phosphatidic acid in the regulation of mammalian target of rapamycin following eccentric contractions. *J Physiol* 587: 3691–3701, 2009.

74. **Phillips BE, Williams JP, Gustafsson T, Bouchard C, Rankinen T, Knudsen S, Smith K, Timmons JA, Atherton PJ**. Molecular networks of human muscle adaptation to exercise and age. *PLoS Genet* 9: e1003389, 2013.

75. **Phillips SM, Parise G, Roy BD, Tipton KD, Wolfe RR, Tamopolsky MA**. Resistance-training-induced adaptations in skeletal muscle protein turnover in the fed state. *Can J Physiol Pharmacol* 80: 1045–1053, 2002.

76. **Phillips SM, Tipton KD, Aarsland a, Wolf SE, Wolfe RR**. Mixed muscle protein synthesis and breakdown after resistance exercise in humans. *Am J Physiol* 273: E99–E107, 1997.

77. **Phillips SM, Tipton KD, Ferrando AA, Wolfe RR**. Resistance training reduces the acute exercise-induced increase in muscle protein turnover. *Am J Physiol* 276: E118–E124, 1999.

78. **Rommel C, Bodine SC, Clarke BA, Rossman R, Nunez L, Stitt TN, Yancopoulos GD, Glass DJ**. Mediation of IGF-1-induced skeletal myotube hypertrophy by PI(3)K/Akt/mTOR and PI(3)K/Akt/GSK3 pathways. *Nat Cell Biol* 3: 1009–13, 2001.

79. **Roth SM, Rankinen T, Hagberg JM, Loos RJF, Pérusse L, Sarzynski MA, Wolfarth B, Bouchard C**. Advances in exercise, fitness, and performance genomics in 2011. *Med Sci Sports Exerc* 44: 809–817, 2012.

80. **Ruas JL, White JP, Rao RR, Kleiner S, Brannan KT, Harrison BC, Greene NP, Wu J, Estall JL, Irving BA, Lanza IR, Rasbach KA, Okutsu M, Nair KS, Yan Z, Leinwand LA, Spiegelman BM**. A PGC-1α isoform induced by resistance training regulates skeletal muscle hypertrophy. *Cell* 151: 1319–1331, 2012.

81. **Rutherford OM, Jones DA**. The role of learning and coordination in strength training. *Eur J Appl Physiol Occup Physiol* 55: 100–105, 1986.

82. **Sale DG**. Neural adaptation to resistance training. *Med Sci Sport Exerc* 20: 135–145, 1988.

83. **Saremi A, Gharakhanloo R, Sharghi S, Gharaati MR, Larijani B, Omidfar K**. Effects of oral creatine and resistance training on serum myostatin and GASP-1. *Mol Cell Endocrinol* 317: 25–30, 2010.

84. **Schlaepfer DD, Hauck CR, Sieg DJ**. Signaling through focal adhesion kinase. *Prog Biophys Mol Biol* 71: 435–478, 1999.

85. **Seynnes OR, de Boer M, Narici M V**. Early skeletal muscle hypertrophy and architectural changes in response to high-intensity resistance training. *J Appl Physiol* 102: 368–373, 2007.

86. **Smith K, Barua JM, Watt PW, Scrimgeour CM, Rennie MJ**. Flooding with L-[1-13C]leucine stimulates human muscle protein incorporation of continuously infused L-[1–13C]valine. *Am J Physiol* 262: E372–E376, 1992.

87. **Smith K, Reynolds N, Downie S, Patel a, Rennie MJ**. Effects of flooding amino acids on incorporation of labeled amino acids into human muscle protein. *Am J Physiol* 275: E73–E78, 1998.

88. **Spangenburg EE, Le Roith D, Ward CW, Bodine SC**. A functional insulin-like growth factor receptor is not necessary for load-induced skeletal muscle hypertrophy. *J Physiol* 586: 283–291, 2008.

89. **Tang JE, Perco JG, Moore DR, Wilkinson SB, Phillips SM**. Resistance training alters the response of fed state mixed muscle protein synthesis in young men. *Am J Physiol Regul Integr Comp Physiol* 294: R172–R178, 2008.

90. **Timmons JA, Larsson O, Jansson E, Fischer H, Gustafsson T, Greenhaff PL, Ridden J, Rachman J, Peyrard-Janvid M, Wahlestedt C, Sundberg CJ**. Human muscle gene expression responses to endurance training provide a novel perspective on Duchenne muscular dystrophy. *FASEB J* 19: 750–760, 2005.

91. **Wang Q, McPherron AC**. Myostatin inhibition induces muscle fibre hypertrophy prior to satellite cell activation. *J Physiol* 590: 2151–2165, 2012.

92. **West DWD, Burd NA, Tang JE, Moore DR, Staples AW, Holwerda AM, Baker SK, Phillips SM**. Elevations in ostensibly anabolic hormones with resistance exercise enhance neither training-induced muscle hypertrophy nor strength of the elbow flexors. *J Appl Physiol* 108: 60–67, 2010.

93. **West DWD, Kujbida GW, Moore DR, Atherton P, Burd NA, Padzik JP, De Lisio M, Tang JE, Parise G, Rennie MJ, Baker SK, Phillips SM**. Resistance exercise-induced increases in putative anabolic hormones do not enhance muscle protein synthesis or intracellular signalling in young men. *J Physiol* 587: 5239–5247, 2009.

94. **Wilkinson DJ, Franchi M V, Brook MS, Narici M V, Williams JP, Mitchell WK, Szewczyk NJ, Greenhaff PL, Atherton PJ, Smith K**. A validation of the application of D2O stable isotope tracer techniques for monitoring day-to-day changes in muscle protein subfraction synthesis in humans. *Am J Physiol Endocrinol Metab* 306: E571–E579, 2014.

95. **Wilkinson DJ, Hossain T, Hill DS, Phillips BE, Crossland H, Williams J, Loughna P, Churchward-Venne TA, Breen L, Phillips SM, Etheridge T, Rathmacher J a, Smith K, Szewczyk NJ, Atherton PJ**. Effects of leucine and its metabolite β-hydroxy-β-methylbutyrate on human skeletal muscle protein metabolism. *J Physiol* 591: 2911–2923, 2013.

96. **Wilkinson DJ, Hossain T, Limb MC, Phillips BE, Lund J, Williams JP, Brook MS, Cegielski J, Philp A, Ashcroft S, Rathmacher JA, Szewczyk NJ, Smith K, Atherton PJ**. Impact of the calcium form of β-hydroxy-β-methylbutyrate upon human skeletal muscle protein metabolism. *Clin Nutr* 37: 2068–2075, 2017.

97. **Wilkinson SB, Phillips SM, Atherton PJ, Patel R, Yarasheski KE, Tarnopolsky MA, Rennie MJ**. Differential effects of resistance and endurance exercise in the fed state on signalling molecule phosphorylation and protein synthesis in human muscle. *J Physiol* 15: 3701–3717, 2008.

98. **Witard OC, Jackman SR, Breen L, Smith K, Selby A, Tipton KD**. Myofibrillar muscle protein synthesis rates subsequent to a meal in response to increasing doses of whey protein at rest and after resistance exercise. *Am J Clin Nutr* 99: 86–95, 2014.

99. **Ydfors M, Fischer H, Mascher H, Blomstrand E, Norrbom J, Gustafsson T**. The truncated splice variants, NT-PGC-1α and PGC-1α4, increase with both endurance and resistance exercise in human skeletal muscle. *Physiol Rep* 1: e00140, 2013.

100. **Zillikens MC, Demissie S, Hsu Y-H, Yerges-Armstrong LM, Chou W-C, Stolk L, Livshits G, Broer L, Johnson T, Koller DL, Kutalik Z, Luan J, Malkin I, Ried JS, Smith A V., Thorleifsson G, Vandenput L, Hua Zhao J, Zhang W, Aghdassi A, Åkesson K, Amin N, Baier LJ, Barroso I, Bennett DA, Bertram L, Biffar R, Bochud M, Boehnke M, Borecki IB, Buchman AS, Byberg L, Campbell H, Campos Obanda N, Cauley JA, Cawthon PM, Cederberg H, Chen Z, Cho NH, Jin Choi H, Claussnitzer M, Collins F, Cummings SR, De Jager PL, Demuth I, Dhonukshe-Rutten RAM, Diatchenko L, Eiriksdottir G, Enneman AW, Erdos M, Eriksson JG, Eriksson J, Estrada K, Evans DS, Feitosa MF, Fu M, Garcia M, Gieger C, Girke T, Glazer NL, Grallert H, Grewal J, Han B-G, Hanson RL, Hayward C, Hofman A, Hoffman EP, Homuth G, Hsueh W-C, Hubal MJ, Hubbard A, Huffman KM, Husted LB, Illig T, Ingelsson E, Ittermann T, Jansson J-O, Jordan JM, Jula A, Karlsson M, Khaw K-T, Kilpeläinen TO, Klopp N, Kloth JSL, Koistinen HA, Kraus WE, Kritchevsky S, Kuulasmaa T, Kuusisto J, Laakso M, Lahti J, Lang T, Langdahl BL, Launer LJ, Lee J-Y, Lerch MM, Lewis JR, Lind**

L, Lindgren C, Liu Y, Liu T, Liu Y, Ljunggren Ö, Lorentzon M, Luben RN, Maixner W, McGuigan FE, Medina-Gomez C, Meitinger T, Melhus H, Mellström D, Melov S, Michaëlsson K, Mitchell BD, Morris AP Mosekilde L, Newman A, Nielson CM, O'Connell JR, Oostra BA, Orwoll ES, Palotie A, Parker SCJ, Peacock M, Perola M, Peters A, Polasek O, Prince RL, Räikkönen K, Ralston SH, Ripatti S, Robbins JA, Rotter JI, Rudan I, Salomaa V, Satterfield S, Schadt EE, Schipf S, Scott L, Sehmi J, Shen J, Soo Shin C, Sigurdsson G, Smith S, Soranzo N, Stančáková A, Steinhagen-Thiessen E, Streeten EA, Styrkarsdottir U, Swart KMA, Tan S-T, Tarnopolsky MA, Thompson P, Thomson CA, Thorsteinsdottir U, Tikkanen E, Tranah GJ, Tuomilehto J, van Schoor NM, Verma A, Vollenweider P, Völzke H, Wactawski-Wende J, Walker M, Weedon MN, Welch R, Wichmann H-E, Widen E, Williams FMK, Wilson JF, Wright NC, Xie W, Yu L, Zhou Y, Chambers JC, Döring A, van Duijn CM, Econs MJ, Gudnason V, Kooner JS, Psaty BM, Spector TD, Stefansson K, Rivadeneira F, Uitterlinden AG, Wareham NJ, Ossowski V, Waterworth D, Loos RJF, Karasik D, Harris TB, Ohlsson C, Kiel DP. Large meta-analysis of genome-wide association studies identifies five loci for lean body mass. *Nat Commun* 8: 80, 2017.

21

GENETIC CONTRIBUTIONS TO NEUROENDOCRINE RESPONSES TO RESISTANCE TRAINING

William J. Kraemer, Nicholas A. Ratamess, and Jakob L. Vingren

Introduction

The endocrine system plays a substantial role in mediating the acute responses to resistance exercise (RE) as well as influencing subsequent baseline resistance training (RT) adaptations. Hormonal signals play a variety of roles in anabolism (tissue growth, substrate restoration, recovery) and catabolism (tissue breakdown, metabolic regulation). The interactions of hormonal signals with the cells' genetic machinery are complex and the understanding of this area is still in its infancy. Recent discoveries show that multiple pathways relay hormonal signals to affect nuclear targets (48) and thus induce acute and chronic anabolic or catabolic effects on target cells (3, 71). Our evolving understanding of RE-induced hormonal influences must be put into context of an individual's training state, RE protocols used, and inherent genetic potential for adaptive changes in specific phenotypic characteristics (17, 40, 45, 46) (Figure 21.1). However, hormones do not function within an isolated setting. Rather, a specific hormonal response must be viewed within the context of the entire endocrine system and its relationship with other physiological systems (some of which are depicted in Figure 21.1).

It is clear that genetics substantially contribute to an individual's baseline adaptability in muscle strength, power, endurance, and hypertrophy from RT. Several candidate genes (i.e., *ACTN3*, *PPARA*, *CNTF*, *ACE*, and *VDR*) have been identified that contribute to a strength phenotype where either a specific polymorphism(s) has been associated with baseline muscle strength and mass or with the magnitude of muscle strength increases and hypertrophy from training (8). Heritability studies have shown that genetics account for 31–83% of variability in muscle strength and lean tissue mass (11, 60) (see Chapter 18 for further details). From a neuroendocrine perspective, genetics contribute to the amount of each hormone produced through regulation of enzymes in biosynthetic pathways, the quantity/activity/affinity of transport proteins, coregulatory proteins, hormone receptors, and molecular pathway intermediates, all of which affect the magnitude of adaptations. Epigenetics and transcriptional modifications increase the complexity of genetic control over neuroendocrine function. A genetic polymorphism of a receptor can strengthen or weaken its affinity for hormone binding and thus be associated with responder or nonresponder status for a given trait. RT influences genetic expression of many

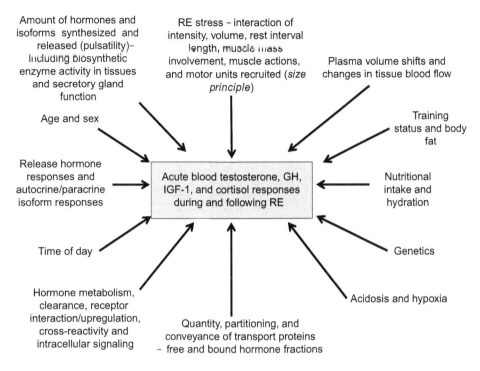

Figure 21.1 Factors influencing the acute hormonal responses to resistance exercise. RE=resistance exercise.

genes thereby affecting mRNA and increasing synthesis of several critical proteins involved in adaptation. In addition, gene doping has the potential to target anabolic hormone DNA (i.e., insulin-like growth factor-1 (IGF-1)) to elicit further gains in muscle strength and hypertrophy. Specific pathways that play roles in muscle strength (Chapter 19) and hypertrophy (Chapter 20) are covered previously in this book. Here, we explore genetic contributions of key anabolic hormones (androgens, growth hormone (GH) superfamily, IGF-1), glucocorticoids (cortisol), and their receptors to acute RE responses and adaptations to RT.

Androgens

Testosterone (T) is the primary anabolic androgen that interacts with androgen receptors (ARs) within skeletal muscle; whereas, the more potent dihydrotestosterone (DHT) primarily acts within sex-linked tissues with a secondary role in skeletal muscle. T is released from the Leydig cells of the testes (in men) under the control of gonadotropin releasing hormone (GnRH)-stimulated release of luteinizing hormone (LH) via neural stimulation and kisspeptin. Kisspeptins, produced from the *KISS1* gene, regulate GnRH. Kisspeptin neurons are found in the arcuate nucleus and anteroventral periventricular nucleus of the brain (26). Mutations and polymorphisms of the *KISS1* gene and kisspeptin receptor (*KISS1R*) genes alter sexual maturation and can lead to early onset puberty (72). How these gene polymorphisms affect muscular performance has yet to be elucidated. Other sources of T synthesis include the adrenal cortex, ovaries, and skeletal muscle (77). Skeletal muscle T may act in an intracrine rather

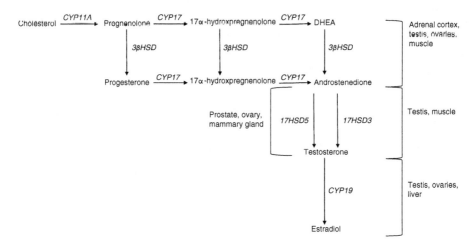

Figure 21.2 Testosterone biosynthesis. Key enzymes catalyzing androgen biosynthesis from cholesterol include cytochrome P450 cholesterol side chain cleavage enzyme (CYP11A); cytochrome P450 17α-hydroxylase/17,20 lyase (CYP17), 3ß-hydroxysteroid dehydrogenase (3ßHSD, types 1 and 2), 17ß-hydroxysteroid dehydrogenases (17ßHSD, types 3 and 5 (AKR1C3)). Aromatase cytochrome P450 (CYP19) catalyzes the conversion of T to estradiol; whereas, 5α-reductase catalyzes the conversion of T to the more potent DHT (not shown).

than endocrine manner. Testosterone is synthesized from cholesterol in a series of steps that involve the intermediate formation of weaker steroids including DHEA, androstenedione, and androstenediol (Figure 21.2). T is released into circulation upon synthesis where it is transported bound to binding proteins, primarily sex hormone-binding globulin (SHBG). Free (unbound, ~2% of total T in circulation) testosterone (FT) is taken up at the tissue level for potential binding to ARs. A change in SHBG concentrations may influence the magnitude of FT available for diffusion across the cell membrane.

Acute testosterone responses and chronic adaptations to resistance training

RE can elicit elevations in T and FT concentrations for up to 30 minutes after exercise in men with either small or no increases in women (41, 79). Acute elevations in androstenedione, DHEA sulfate, and SHBG, as well as delayed increases in LH have also been reported. The magnitude of the acute androgen response is affected by the exercise selection and muscle mass involvement, the interaction of intensity, volume, and rest interval lengths, nutritional intake, metabolic demand, age, and training experience (41, 45, 46). A few studies have shown augmented acute T responses following a period of RT. The ramifications of acute elevations in androgens with RE are unclear as some studies show relationships between T elevations and AR upregulation and strength and hypertrophy enhancement whereas others do not (45). Thus, acute T responses must be viewed within the context of multiple skeletal muscle signaling pathway adaptations as well as how it coincides with other androgen, GH, IGF-1, insulin, and cortisol responses.

Findings for effects of RT on resting T are inconsistent and may be confounded by other variables (i.e., diurnal variations, nutritional interventions, and the time blood sample was obtained relative to last workout), thereby making interpretation difficult. Most studies have shown no changes in resting T or FT concentrations following RT while some have found elevations or reductions (41, 45). Other resting androgen (DHT, DHEA or DHEA sulfate, androstenedione) or SHBG concentrations may decrease or not change (41, 45). Because diurnal T concentrations are tightly regulated, it is unlikely for a permanent change to occur as regulatory mechanisms are quickly re-engaged after acute RE (41). Rather, an elevation/reduction may reflect a transient change that will return to a normal circadian pattern soon thereafter.

Androgen biosynthesis and skeletal muscle steroidogenesis

Androgen biosynthesis (Figure 21.2) is affected by other hormones including insulin and IGF-1 (31). Several genes encode for these biosynthetic enzymes, resulting in varied concentrations of androgens and other steroids in multiple tissues. For example, mutations in the *HSD17B3* gene encoding the enzyme 17β-HSD3 cause male pseudo-hermaphroditism during fetal development due to low T and DHT (51). Polymorphisms of genes encoding for 17β-HSD3 and 17β-HSD5 have been related to increased risk for diseases such as polycystic ovary syndrome and cancer. Although some polymorphisms are associated with increased androgen levels, their potential effects on muscle performance are poorly understood.

Of recent interest is the investigation of steroidogenic enzymes in skeletal muscle capable of synthesizing T from DHEA, androstenedione, and androstenediol. Steroidogenic enzyme content and T concentrations in skeletal muscle appear to be similar between men and women (77). RE has been shown to increase skeletal muscle DHEA, FT, DHT, 3β-HSD, 17β-HSD, and 5α-reductase type I content in older men (65) but not in resistance-trained young men and women within 70 minutes of exercise (77). Statistical trends for increased muscle concentrations of T and DHT have been observed 3 and 24 hours after RE. Sato et al. (65) showed significant correlations between muscle DHEA, FT, and 5α-reductase concentrations and isokinetic strength and muscle cross-sectional area (CSA) in older men. These findings indicate that skeletal muscle is a source of T, albeit the effects of RE remain unclear but could be a mechanism to help counteract circulating T reductions in older men.

Androgen signaling

Androgens affect acute performance and increase CSA of type I and II muscle fibers, strength, power, and endurance via several molecular pathways (Figure 21.3). Androgens increase protein synthesis, alter fiber types, increase lactate transport via upregulation of monocarboxylate transporter 1 (MCT1) and 4 (MCT4) proteins, increase satellite cell activation, proliferation, differentiation, and incorporation into skeletal muscle as myonuclei, differentiation of mesenchymal pluripotent cells, follistatin expression, myotube formation, increase polyamine synthesis, GH, muscle mechanogrowth factor (MGF), and IGF-1Ea mRNA, downregulate and upregulate myostatin gene expression, downregulate Acvr2b receptor mRNA and Ankrd1, inhibit forkhead box O (FoxO) family of transcription factors, and downregulate glucocorticoid receptor expression (46). Nongenomic actions are rapid and result in a rise in intracellular calcium and may lead to PI3K/Akt/mTORC1/S6K1 pathway-induced muscle hypertrophy.

Androgen receptor genetic variations

The androgen receptor gene (*AR*) is located on the q arm of chromosome X at position 11–12 (Figure 21.4) and is widely expressed in most tissues. The first exon contains several regions of repetitive DNA sequences, one of which is the CAG triplet repeat that begins at codon 58, with the length varying between 8 and 35 repeats. Polymorphisms yielding a variety of repeats are associated with a variety of conditions including male infertility, prostate and testicular cancer, bone disease, and cardiovascular disease. Long CAG repeats may interfere with androgen

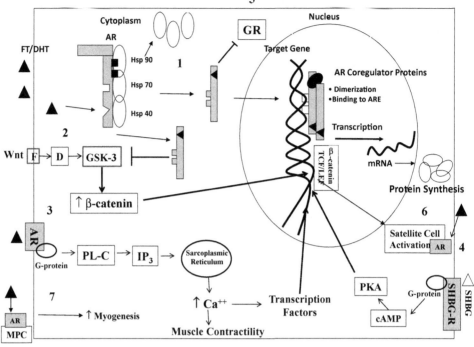

Figure 21.3 A simplified model of intracellular androgen signaling in skeletal muscle. A truncated model of anabolic and anticatabolic actions of androgens is shown. Pathway 1 depicts classical genomic activation. FT or DHT diffuses through the cell membrane and binds to an AR in the cytoplasm – binding dissociates heat shock proteins (HSP) stabilizing the AR; the FT-AR complex translocates to the nucleus and binds to specific DNA elements (androgen response elements or AREs). Coactivators, general transcription factors, and RNA polymerase II are recruited, transcription is increased, and protein synthesis increases. Pathway 2 depicts a secondary genomic pathway, canonical Wnt-β-catenin signaling. Wnt binds to frizzled (F) receptors and activates Dishevelled (D) and inhibits glycogen synthase kinase-3 (GSK-3) reducing β-catenin degradation. The FT-AR complex inhibits GSK-3 and increases β-catenin where it translocates to the nucleus, binds to DNA response elements (T-cell factor/lymphoid enhancer factor 1 (TCF/LEF)), increases transcription, and activation of muscle satellite cells. Pathway 3 depicts a nongenomic pathway where FT binds to a membrane-bound AR that is coupled with a pertussis toxin (PTX)-sensitive G protein that activates phospholipase C (PL-C) and increases IP_3. IP_3 binds to specific receptors on the sarcoplasmic reticulum (SR) and increases intracellular calcium. Calcium may mediate/augment muscle contraction or activate several pathways including Src/Ras/ERK/MAPK/ mTOR to increase transcription. Pathway 4 depicts the SHBG receptor (SHBG-R) activation upon binding of SHBG-T activating a G-protein to form cyclic AMP (cAMP), activation of protein kinase A (PKA), and increased transcriptional activation of nuclear AR. Pathway 5 depicts T/DHT ability to decrease glucocorticoid receptor (GR) expression and increase competitive binding between androgen-AR complex and common response elements between AR and GR shared cistromes on target genes. Pathway 6 depicts androgen-AR binding on satellite cells increases proliferation, mobilization, differentiation, and incorporation into skeletal muscle. T/AR binding to myogenic intermediates may also occur, favoring increased differentiation. Pathway 7 depicts androgen-AR binding on mesenchymal pluripotent cells (MPC) increases propensity towards myogenesis in skeletal muscle. Crosstalk between pathways, muscle steroidogenesis, and other noncortisol hormone-receptor interactions are not shown thereby showing the vast nature of androgen signaling.

actions (reduce interaction between the N and C termini), whereas short repeats are associated with increased AR protein expression and enhance androgen action through stronger binding yielding greater transcriptional activity.

The potential relationship between CAG repeat number and muscle strength and lean body mass (LBM) might be critical. *AR* gene polymorphisms affecting CAG repeat length could help explain the concept of responders and nonresponders to RT in addition to the physiological responses to exogenous T administration. However, contradictory results have been reported where CAG repeat number was positively related, inversely related, or not related to LBM, T or FT concentrations, and muscle strength in young and older men (12, 69, 81). In a study examining a large number of young men aged 20–29 years, Nielsen reported significant inverse relationships between CAG repeat number and thigh and trunk muscle size (52). Reductions in repeats of ten equaled increases of muscle size of 6–11 cm². Thus, performance phenotypes based on *AR* candidate gene polymorphisms remain unclear but is an area of great RT.

Androgen receptor structure

The nuclear AR is a 110 kD receptor consisting of 919 amino acids, 12 α-helices, and 2 ß-sheets that belongs to a large family of nuclear transcription factors (Figure 21.4). A truncated

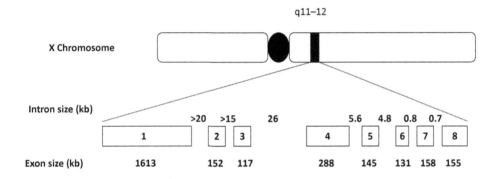

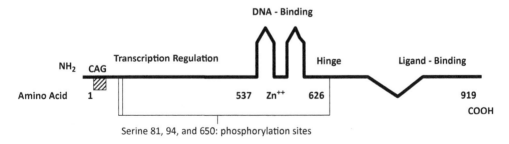

Figure 21.4 The androgen receptor gene and protein. The *AR* gene (upper panel) is oriented with the 5′ end toward the centromere and spans approximately 90 kb of DNA containing eight exons that code for approximately 2757-base pair open reading frames within a 10.6 kb mRNA (14). The first exon codes for the N-terminus domain; exons 2–3 code for the central DNA binding domain; exons 4–8 code for the C terminus ligand-binding domain (14). The AR (lower panel) forms ligand-induced homodimers that bind to inverted repeat DNA response elements and consist of four functional domains: a C-terminal ligand-binding domain (LBD; comprises amino acids 662–919), a DNA-binding domain that is built with two zinc finger motifs (amino acids 538–611), a hinge region (amino acids 612–661), and a N-terminus transcription activation domain (amino acids 1–537) (10).

AR protein (87 kD) with similar function has been identified. Androgen binding (or binding by selective androgen receptor modulators (SARMs)) to AR is part of a complex signaling system (Figure 21.3). Androgen binding stabilizes the AR in a dose-dependent manner and this stabilization is critical to modifying AR content. The half-life of AR without androgen binding is 1 hour whereas the formation of the AR–androgen complex extends the half-life to 6 hours (32). T dissociates from the AR three times faster than DHT or synthetic androgens and is less effective for stabilizing the AR (86), which helps explains the greater potency of these compounds. The AR is capable of undergoing multiple bouts of recycling (at least four times) between the nucleus and cytoplasm after ligand binding and dissociation (62).

Androgen receptor adaptations to training

Androgens and RE each upregulate AR protein content. *AR* gene expression in skeletal muscle has correlated with FT concentrations and a few studies have shown relationships between exercise-induced T and FT elevations and AR content from 1 to 48 hours post RE (45,46). AR quantity is related to muscle strength and CSA (61). The importance of androgens in mediating training-induced hypertrophy was shown in multiple studies (41). In male *AR* gene knockout mice (but not female), significant reductions in muscle mass (up to 25%) and strength were reported (49). Ninety-three genes were up- (*N*=47) or downregulated (*N*=46; including several regulating muscle cytoskeletal proteins) in male AR knockout mice (49) showing the complexity of androgen signaling across several pathways.

Single and sequential bouts of RE may increase AR protein or mRNA expression with the magnitude and time course mediated by the volume of RE, muscle mass involvement, nutritional consumption, and the quantity of circulating T in the blood (45). Initially, downregulation or no change may occur in men and women but upregulation appear to follow within 3 hours post RE and may persist for up to 48 hours post RE (45,61). Baseline AR protein content or mRNA may not change over long-term RT, suggesting that the acute cyclical upregulation in response to sequential RE bouts may play a critical role in mediating androgen-induced muscular adaptations. AR up- and downregulation may be cross-regulated via hormonal or growth factor (e.g., IGF-1, cortisol, and the GH superfamily) interactions with other receptors. Such cross-regulation demonstrates the importance of several molecular pathways in AR regulation and provides a combinatorial mechanism for hormone-specific positive and/or negative modulation of different genes.

Growth hormone(s)

Our understanding of GH has evolved significantly over the years (33, 43, 50). The single 191-amino acid 22 kD monomer is not the only form found in anterior pituitary somatotrophs or in circulation (4, 5, 55); hence, the concept of the GH "superfamily" of isoforms with different molecular heterogeneity. Considering the diversity of GH isoforms, a host of questions remain regarding the effects of RE on GH-family molecules. Different immunoassays were used to assay GH during RE in the 1990s as research focused on GH responses to a variety of exercise protocols, the concept of pulsatility, and sexual dimorphism. Bioassays of GH revealed concentration differences from radioimmunoassays. This created the concept that there is a difference between the "bioactive" versus "immunoreactive" assay signals. Concerns about GH drug use dramatically increased and stimulated various controversies regarding drug testing and if GH was, in fact, an effective anabolic hormone in skeletal muscle (25).

Basic growth hormone cybernetics

Multiple pathways are involved with regulating the release of GH. The control of GH release starts with neural stimulation of a pulsatile release of the hypothalamic GH releasing hormone (GHRH) contained in arcuate neurons of the neurosecretory nerve terminals into hypothalamo-hypophyseal portal circulation to the anterior pituitary where it interacts with GHRH-receptors, a class II G protein-coupled receptor, and via an extensive signaling system mediate the release of GH (13). The 22 kD monomer assayed by immunoassay (IGH) is released in a pulsatile manner similar to its trophic hormone (76). The larger bioactive GH aggregates (BGH) assay signals have not shown pulsatility. Somatostatin opposes the stimulation of GHRH and is released from periventricular somatostatin neurons, carried by the same portal circulation to the anterior pituitary where it inhibits GH secretion. This dynamic is thought to contribute to the pulsatile release of IGH. The hypothalamus acts as the primary pulse generator of various hormones. Interestingly, with high-volume RE, IGH reduces pulsatility in the first half of sleep followed by higher pulsatility in the second half of sleep, indicating pulse generation and the types of GH released may vary from the 22 kD monomer (54). Such an effect may be due to an increased somatostatin influence or more provocatively a greater synthesis of aggregated forms of BGH, limiting the production and release of IGH from band I somatotrophs.

A series of steps initiate the synthesis of the 22 kD monomer in the somatotrophs of the anterior pituitary. GHRH binds to its receptor and creates a conformational change in the alpha Gs subunit of the G-protein complex in the intracellular side (80). From here, a series of cAMP pathways are stimulated ending with the transcription of *GH* by the interactions of cAMP response elements with the promoter region of the *GH* gene. This produces the 191-amino acid, 22 kD monomer secreted from the somatotrophs. Increased transcription of the *GHRHR* gene creates the well-known positive feedback loop.

Somatotroph types and growth hormone isoforms

Two distinctly different somatotrophs of GH have been identified (20): band I contains lower-molecular-weight forms of GH (predominantly 22 kD) whereas band II contains higher-molecular-weight isoforms of GH (i.e., aggregates or BGH) (Figure 21.5). Aggregates may be formed via zinc, disulfide, and hydrostatic bindings as partial degradation of the aggregates' disulfide bonds increases the 22 kD monomer concentration reflecting one of these aggregate binding mechanisms (30, 63). Additionally, tibial peptide, found in the granules and somatotrophs, has biological functions with the tibial growth plate and possibly other unknown cellular interfaces (29).

Growth hormone in circulation

GH has the potential for post-translational processing within the periventricular space (e.g., GH to prolactin). Hosts of molecular GH isoforms, splice variants, and fragments have been assayed in plasma (4, 5). There is a unique circulatory pathway directly into the brain potentially allowing for the GH superfamily to influence neuroplasticity and function (7). Both high- and low-affinity binding proteins have been identified with the high-affinity GH binding protein (GHBP), considered to be the principal binding protein in circulation. GHBP arises from proteolytic cleavage of the extracellular domain of the GH receptor (85). This process occurs mostly in the liver, which is the most GH receptor-rich tissue, but could occur wherever GH receptors exists. It has been suggested that GHBP may play a role in GH supply and receptor

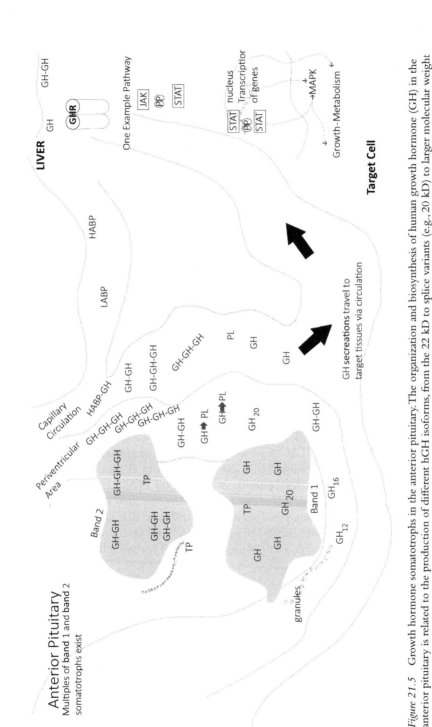

Figure 21.5 Growth hormone somatotrophs in the anterior pituitary. The organization and biosynthesis of human growth hormone (GH) in the anterior pituitary is related to the production of different hGH isoforms, from the 22 kD to splice variants (e.g., 20 kD) to larger molecular weight aggregates (e.g., dimers GH–GH; trimers GH–GH–GH etc.). Band 1 and 2 somatotrophs have been identified (20) and GH isoforms are organized and stored for release into the circulation through a microtubular transport system. Release into the periventricular area also allows for last minute, post-translational processing of GH prior to being released into circulation (e.g., GH to prolactin (PL)). High– and low-affinity binding proteins derived from the liver also may bind with GH, yet their functions remain unclear. GH can have direct effects on the target tissues and need not be mediated via IGF-1. Multiple pathways exist and there is a great deal of signal complexity (33). One common pathway is shown. GHR=growth hormone receptor; JAK–STAT=Janus kinase signal transducer and activator of transcription proteins; MAPK=mitogen–activated protein kinase; P=phosphate.

function (67). Interestingly, with heavy RE, significant increases in GHBP were observed in both sedentary and trained men indicating training does not augment the GHBP response to RE. The BGH response indicates that some molecular weight fractions are more responsive than others to RE. Nevertheless, signal strength varies with the type of assay used, e.g., IGH or BGH (28). GH receptors are present in many different tissues including skeletal muscle and are coded by the GH receptor gene. Ultimately, GH binds to the GH receptor resulting in receptor dimerization, activating intra- and intercellular transduction signal pathways influencing metabolism and growth (33).

Resistance exercise responses

RE alters plasma IGH concentrations more consistently than BGH (see Table 21.1). Our understanding of RE effects has become complicated given the varieties of different assays used to measure GH (28, 43). The RE protocol influences the IGH response with higher volume of work, 10RM resistances, and short rest resulting in the greatest increases in men and women (37, 38) likely because reduced pH mediates such responses (18). McCall et al. (50) first observed that BGH was responsive to RE and had an inherent neurological afferent feedback mechanism with unloading. Later, whole-body RE protocols in women were found to elicit increases in IGH, whereas BGH was unchanged (30). Only with long-term (6 months) RT in women did BGH concentrations significantly increase (42) but still with little or no response to acute exercise. Interestingly, stronger women have been found to have higher concentrations of BGH (38) and older women to have lower BGH than younger women post RE (19).

Health issues may also be reflected in the BGH signal. Obesity results in a lower BGH assay signal in younger men at rest and during RE, implicating reduced function of the band II somatotrophs (73). Recent findings of a lack of BGH signal in resting blood samples of older men and women (60–95 years) with no age relationships suggest that somatotrophs' functionality is not guaranteed (44).

Insulin-like growth factors

IGFs are structurally related to insulin. IGFs are small polypeptide hormones (70 and 67 amino acids for IGF-1 and IGF-2, respectively) synthesized from a larger precursor peptide that is post-translationally processed into its active form. Of the two, IGF-1 has been most extensively studied and is secreted by the liver in response to GH stimulation. Only 2% of IGF-1 circulates in its free form; most circulates as a binary (20–25%) or ternary complex (~75%) (53–56). In its binary form, IGF-1 circulates with one of seven binding proteins whereas in its ternary form, IGF-1 circulates with IGFBP-3 and its acid labile subunit (ALS). IGF-1 is a systemic anabolic and metabolic hormone and also produced locally (i.e., autocrine and paracrine mechanisms) in tissues and cells. IGF-1 acts as both a cell cycle initiation and progression factor and facilitates satellite cell activation, proliferation, survival, and differentiation; increases myotube size and number of nuclei per myotube; stimulates amino acid uptake and protein synthesis and muscle hypertrophy, neuronal myelinization, axonal sprouting, and damage repair; reduces chronic inflammatory response; increases free fatty acid utilization; and enhances insulin sensitivity upon receptor binding and subsequent intracellular signaling and glucose metabolism (22, 46). Much of the hypertrophy-induced effects of IGF-1 occur via effects on satellite cells. Because of these critical anabolic functions, IGF genes have been considered a potential target for gene therapies and for gene doping in athletes (23). While liver-derived IGF-1 is under direct regulation of GH, local mechanical-stretch mechanisms can activate IGF-1 synthesis in

Table 21.1 Comparison of assay signal concentrations from immunoassays and bioassays during resistance exercise. Postexercise (PE) concentrations were determined between 0 and 15 minutes in young men (M) and women (W)

Study (reference)	Sex	Program	Immunoassay (IGH) µg/L		Bioassay total (BGH) µg/L	
			Pre-exercise	PE	Pre-exercise	PE
McCall et al. (50)	M	Isometric plantar flexion 5 min at 30% MVC	12.0	14.0	1300.0	3300.0*
McCall et al. (50)	M	Isometric plantar flexion 1 min at 80% MVC (B)	12.0	13.0	1100.0	2300.0*
Kraemer et al. (37)	M	8 EX, 10RM 1 min RI	2.2	23.9*	–	–
Kraemer et al. (37)	M	8 EX, 5 RM 3 min RI	2.1	5.2*	–	–
Kraemer et al. (38)	W	8 EX, 10RM 1 min RI	7.6	16.5*	–	–
Kraemer et al. (38)	W	8 EX, 5 RM 3 min RI	7.1	5.6	–	–
Hymer et al. (30)	W	Squat 6 × 10 80% 1RM, 2 min RI	7.7	26.3*	3927.0	3787.0
Kraemer et al. (42)	W	Squat 6 × 10 80% 1RM, 2 min RI	2.6	11.2*	2450	3300
Thomas et al. (73)	M	3 × 10 reps: 85–95% of 10 RM for squat, bench press, leg curls, dumbbell rows, dumbbell shoulder press, and dumbbell step-up	1.2	9.9*	6000.0	11,000.0

*=P ≤0.05 from corresponding pre-exercise value; EX=exercises; MVC=maximal voluntary contraction; RM=repetition maximum; RI=rest interval.

tissues. The potency of circulating IGF-1 remains unclear and needs to be viewed in context with its binding proteins that regulate bioavailability as several studies have shown systemic elevations in IGF-1 produced no elevations in protein synthesis or hypertrophy during RT whereas upregulation in the muscle isoform was linked to significant muscle hypertrophy (22).

IGF and IGFBP genes

The IGF-1 gene is shown in Figure 21.6. Some IGF-1 gene variants (i.e., cytosine adenine dinucleotide repeats in the promoter region) have been reported and associated with greater

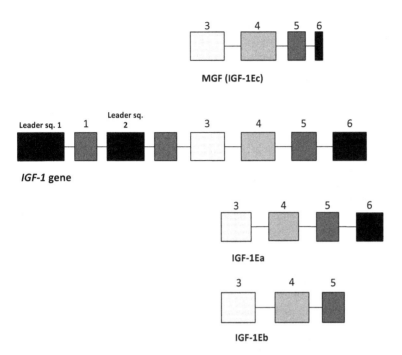

Figure 21.6 IGF-1 isoforms. The *IGF-1* gene is mapped to the long arm of chromosome 12 (12q22–q24.1) and the short arm of chromosome 11 (11p15). The gene contains two promoters and six exons which could be spliced to produce at least six mRNAs. Exons 1 and 2 determine the protein class, exons 3 and 4 encode the mature peptide and ligand-binding site, and exons 5 and 6 determine the E domain peptide and polyadenylating signals. The gene produces IGF-1Ea, IGF-1Eb, and IGF-1Ec (mechanogrowth factor (MGF)) (23).

strength changes during RT (34). This same polymorphism has been associated with baseline muscle power, i.e., lower power outputs for those homozygous for the 192-allele compared to other genotypes, but not with power increases accompanying RT (70). The C−1245T (rs35767) is a single nucleotide polymorphism (SNP) found in the promoter region and has been associated (the minor T allele) with systemic IGF-1 concentrations, muscle strength, response to eccentric exercise, bone mineral density, LBM, and left ventricular hypertrophy, in addition to being found in a small percent (5%) of endurance and power athletes compared to other genotypes (6,35). Carriers of the GA genotype with the rs6220 SNP have shown greater strength than AA homozygotes and CC homozygotes of the SNP rs7136446 showed greater strength (by 9%) compared to TT and TC genotypes (27). No such relationships have been found for the rs2854744 SNP of the *IGFBP-3* gene (27). Polymorphisms of the *IGF-2* gene (e.g., ApaI) have been associated with muscle strength. In men, the *IGF-2* SNPs G13790C, C16646T, and ApaI were significantly associated with strength loss, creatine kinase activity, and soreness following eccentric exercise (9).

Acute responses and chronic adaptations of IGFs to resistance training

The systemic liver-induced IGF-1 response to RE is unclear as elevations (during and up to 30 minutes after exercise), decreases, and no changes have been found (41). A lack of change may be attributed to, at least in part, the delay in secretion of IGF-1 (i.e., 3–9 hours) following GH stimulation (41). Despite the anabolic actions of IGF-1, a direct link between RE-induced elevations and muscle strength and hypertrophy has been difficult to determine. Some evidence indicates that the role of systemic IGF-1 may lie more as a "regulator or amplifier" of muscle remodeling (46). Of importance is the response of IGFBPs, which have generated more consistent responses with RE acutely elevating IGFBP-3 (41). Nindl et al. (54) monitored overnight IGF-1 following heavy RE and showed IGF-1 concentrations remained unchanged but IGFBP-2 increased and ALS decreased, suggesting that binding protein partitioning, rather than changes in systemic IGF-1, was critical. Other studies have shown IGFBP-1 was sensitive to exercise duration, but not exercise mode. Using microdialysis to measure IGF-1 in interstitial fluid, Nindl et al. (56) showed total and free IGF-1 and IGFBP-3 were elevated; whereas, IGF-1 in interstitial fluid was unaltered following high-power exercise. Furthermore, IGF-1 receptor phosphorylation was not increased, and IGF mRNA content and Akt phosphorylation were increased (56), reinforcing the concept that skeletal muscle adaptation is not dependent on systemic IGF-1, but rather the interplay across biocompartments. Chronic RT studies examining resting circulating IGF-1 concentrations have shown reductions, no change, and elevations with no change or reductions in IGFBP-1 and IGFBP-3 (41). No significant changes in IGF-1, IGFBP-1, or IGFBP-3 were found in subjects who were considered extreme responders to 16 weeks of RT versus nonresponders, although a trend was shown where IGFBP-3 in extreme responders tended to be lower than nonresponders (58). Resistance-trained men were shown to have higher resting IGF-1 concentrations than untrained men (64). Thus, the contributions and ramifications of single-data point circulating IGF-1 chronic measures remain unclear.

Of greater significance may be the training responses of locally produced IGF-1 isoforms. RE of sufficient intensity and volume increases IGF-1 and MGF mRNA for up to 48 hours post RE (41,59). IGF-1 and MGF mRNA have increased 2 hours post exercise (but not 6 hours) after a single bout of moderate- (65% of 1RM; 18–20 repetitions) and moderately high-intensity (85% of 1RM; 8–10 repetitions) RE (82). Other studies show MGF acts independently, is expressed earlier than other IGF-1 isoforms in response to RE, and may have greater anabolic potency (15). Overloaded muscle and mechanical damage from RT are potent stimuli for local production of IGF-1.

IGF-1 receptor and intracellular signaling

The endocrine, autocrine, and paracrine effects of IGF-1 are mediated through binding to the IGF-1 receptor (IGF-1R), a ligand-activated receptor tyrosine kinase. The *IGF-1R* gene is mapped to chromosome 15q25–26. Two receptor types have been identified (type 1 and 2). IGF-1 binds with greater affinity to type 1 than to type 2 or the insulin receptor whereas IGF-2 binds with greater to affinity to the type 2 receptor (see Figure 21.7). IGF-1R phosphorylation may be sensitive to RE favoring high-volume over high-intensity protocols 1 hour after exercise (16) and moderate- and moderately high-intensity RE has been shown to increase *IGF-1R* mRNA 2 hours after RE (82).

Glucocorticoids

Glucocorticoids (GCs) are steroids synthesized primarily in the adrenal cortex (with minimal amounts produced in other tissues such as the brain, thymus, skin, and gastrointestinal tract). The primary glucocorticoid is cortisol (~95% of GC activity), synthesized from pregnenolone via P450c17 17α-hydroxylation and a few other intermediate steps. Cortisol secretion is under neuroendocrine control via hypothalamic secretion of corticotropin-releasing hormone (CRH), the activation of gene transcription of pro-opiomelanocortin (POMC) in the anterior

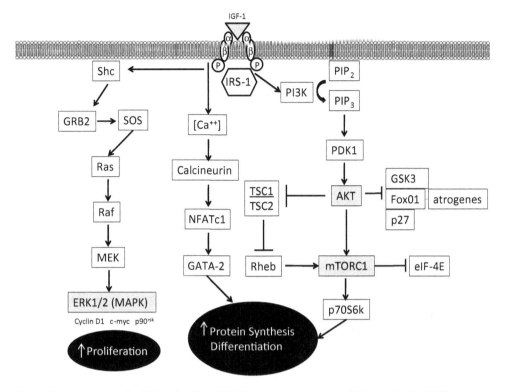

Figure 21.7 Intramuscular IGF-1 signaling. IGF-1R contains two extracellular α subunits (IGF-1 binding sites) and two transmembrane β subunits that upon binding to IGF-1 autophosphorylate the tyrosine residues which stimulates intermediates such as the IRS family (IRS-1 in skeletal muscle) and Shc proteins. The two main intracellular signaling pathways involve the phosphatidyl-inositol 3-kinase (PI3)/ Akt kinase pathway and the mitogen-activated protein kinase (MAPK)/ERK pathway (55). A calcium-dependent calcineurin pathway has been identified resulting in the activation of the transcription factor GATA-2 whose upregulation is associated with muscle hypertrophy (59). IGF-1 has also been shown to increase DHP receptor concentrations in skeletal muscle suggesting that IGF-1 may influence excitation–contraction coupling and subsequent recovery of muscle following damage (59). In addition, IGF-1 may increase cyclin D1 mRNA thereby enhancing proliferation and the myogenic response and inhibit "atrogenes" (59). Lastly, IGF-1 interaction with IGF-1R is influenced by other hormone–receptor interactions and negatively affected by proinflammatory cytokines such as TNFα, IL-1, and IL-6 (1).

pituitary, and subsequent release of its fragment adrenocorticotropic hormone (ACTH) which, in turn, induces cortisol release in the adrenal cortex. Cortisol is released in response to several stimuli including the stress of RE. Cortisol binds mostly to corticosteroid-binding globulin (CRG; ~75%), albumin (~15%), while 10% of circulating cortisol is free. Similar to androgens, GCs diffuse through the cell membrane, and bind to their nuclear receptors, but elicit catabolic effects on skeletal muscle especially in type II muscle fibers. As for androgens, rapid nongenomic effects of GC have also been reported (24).

Acute responses and chronic adaptations of glucocorticoids to resistance training

Several studies have shown significant elevations in cortisol and ACTH from an acute bout of RE with the response similar between men and women (41). The acute cortisol response correlates to blood lactate and protocols high in volume, moderate-to-high intensity with short rest periods tend to elicit the most substantial cortisol increase (11). Resting cortisol concentrations reflect a long-term training stress and RT has been shown to produce no change, reductions, and elevations (41). It appears that the acute cortisol response may reflect metabolic stress, whereas chronic changes (or lack of change) may be involved with tissue homeostasis involving protein metabolism.

Glucocorticoid signaling

Glucocorticord/Glucocorticord Receptor (GR) interaction increases protein degradation, decreases protein synthesis, decreases transport of amino acids, and causes atrophy, mainly of type muscle II fibers. Of interest is the potential competitive signaling between GC/GR and androgens/AR. In fact, the homologies of the DNA-binding and ligand-binding domains between the AR and GR are 79% and 50%, respectively, and both AR and GR can bind to the same *cis*-element on a shared androgen and GC DNA response element, i.e., 5′-AGAACAnnnTGTTCT-3′ (21). Thus, competitive binding in this region could help mediate, in part, anabolic versus catabolic signaling within muscle.

Signaling pathways are vast and catabolism may occur in a variety of ways. Glucocorticoids inhibit the anabolic actions of androgens, insulin, IGF-1, and amino acids (leucine) (66). Glucocorticoids stimulate major proteolytic pathways such as the ubiquitin proteasome, lysosomal (autophagy), and calpain systems. Glucocorticoids have also been shown to inhibit the PI3/Akt pathway (that mediates insulin and IGF-1 signaling) via reduced IRS-1 and increased p85α and miR1 expression, increase *FOXO-1* and *FOXO-3a* gene expression, activate "atrogenes" such as *Atrogin-1*, *MuRF-1*, and *Cathepsin-L*, inhibit mTORC1 via increased transcription of REDD1 and KLF-15, increase C/EBPβ and p300, stimulate glycogen synthase kinase 3β (GSK3β) (and decrease β-catenin), inhibit production of muscle IGF-1 isoforms, increase *Pdk4* gene expression (and inhibit pyruvate dehydrogenase), reduce circulating T concentrations, and increase myostatin (*MSTN*) gene expression and mRNA with a concomitant decrease in MHC II protein expression (47, 66).

Glucocorticoid receptor

The GR gene (*NR3C1*) is located on chromosome 5q31–32. It encodes the GR, which belongs to the nuclear receptor superfamily of ligand-dependent transcription factors. *NR3C1* contains NH_2-terminal transactivation, DNA-binding, and ligand-binding domains as well as a hinge region. Coactivators, chromatin remodeling enzymes, and RNA polymerase II assist with hormone interaction and transcription processes. The GR DNA-binding domain binds to specific DNA sequences in the promoter region of target genes. Multiple isoforms of the GR are expressed in various tissues (24). GC binding to the GR dissociates heat shock proteins and the cortisol/GR complex is chaperoned to the nucleus via a protein complex along the microtubules. Chromatin remodeling occurs via pioneering transcription factors enabling the hormone/GR complex binding to the genomic target sequence. The ligand-bound GR can then regulate gene expression.

Several polymorphisms of the *GR* gene have been identified and shown to relate to various health indices. Van Rossum and colleagues (74) examined the ER22/23EK polymorphism and reported associations with LBM and muscle strength in young men but not women. This polymorphism has been associated with GC resistance, lower cholesterol, and increased insulin sensitivity (75). A follow-up study showed that the ER22/23EK and N363S polymorphisms modified the inverse relationships seen between serum cortisol and muscle mass and strength in older adults (57). The Bcll polymorphism in intron 2 of the *GR* gene showed higher incidences of obesity and insulin resistance (74,75). The N363S polymorphism has been associated with lower bone mineral density and increased insulin resistance and body mass index (74,75). Ash and colleagues (2) studied *GR* polymorphisms prior to and following 12 weeks of RT and reported that men with the 2722 G>A and 1887 GG genotypes gained 16% less strength than AA homozygotes and 6% greater strength gains than A alleles, respectively (accounting for 3.2% and 2.4% of the variance of strength changes respectively), with no effects on muscle size. In women, only those carrying the 1017 T>C allele gained more muscle size than CC homozygotes (accounting for 1.7% of the variance of relative size). No genotypes were associated with baseline strength or muscle size. Thus, some polymorphisms of *GR* mediate the sensitivity of the GC response and can partially affect strength and hypertrophy adaptions to RT.

Acute changes in *GR* mRNA or protein content and potential long-term up- or downregulation play a role in tissue remodeling and muscle damage repair following RE and could mediate part of the anabolic/catabolic processes seen during RT. Willoughby et al. (83) reported significant upregulation of GR protein content 6 and 24 hours following an eccentric RE protocol in untrained men with an attenuated response from the same protocol 3 weeks later. However, in RT men and women no change was found in GR content 10 and 70 minutes following a RE protocol (78). Interestingly, women had higher GR content than men at all time points. These studies suggest that training status plays a critical role in GR training response. Willoughby (84) also reported higher GR content following 6 and 12 weeks of RT; however, samples were taken in close proximity to training so the chronic adaptation is difficult to surmise. In contrast, 6 weeks of intense run training in military cadets (leading to increased muscle mass) induced a significant 6.3% reduction in *GR* mRNA (68). Thus, reduced GC sensitivity may be seen over time during training but the acute response may be determined by training status and the extent of muscle damage incurred.

Summary

Testosterone, GH superfamily, IGF-1, and cortisol play a substantial role in mediating the acute responses to RE and subsequent RT adaptations. Genetics substantially contributes to these responses and adaptations via the amount of each hormone produced through regulation of enzymes in biosynthetic pathways, the quantity/activity/affinity of transport proteins, coregulatory proteins, hormone receptors, and molecular pathway intermediates. Several candidate genes have been identified that contribute to a strength and power performance phenotype. Further study is needed to investigate more specific performance phenotypes based on genetic variability.

References

1. **Adams GR**. Insulin-like growth factor 1 signaling in skeletal muscle and the potential for cytokine interactions. *Medicine and Science in Sports and Exercise* 42: 50–57, 2010.
2. **Ash GI**, **Kostek MA**, **Lee H,** et al. Glucocorticoid receptor (NR3C1) variants associate with the muscle strength and size response to resistance training. *PLoS One* 11: e0148112, 2016.
3. **Bajer B**, **Vlcek M**, **Galusova A**, **Imrich R**, **Penesova A**. Exercise associated hormonal signals as powerful determinants of an effective fat mass loss. *Endocrine Regulation*. 49: 151–163, 2015.

4. **Baumann G**. Growth hormone heterogeneity: genes, isohormones, variants, and binding proteins. *Endocrine Reviews* 12: 424–449, 1991.

5. **Baumann G**. Growth hormone isoforms. *Growth Hormone & IGF Research* 19: 333–340, 2009.

6. **Ben-Zaken S, Meckel Y, Nemet D, Eliakim A**. Can IGF-1 polymorphism affect power and endurance athletic performance? *Growth Hormone & IGF Research* 23: 175–178, 2013.

7. **Bergland R, Blume H, Hamilton A, Monica P, Paterson R**. Adrenocorticotropic hormone may be transported directly from the pituitary to the brain. *Science* 31: 541–543, 1980.

8. **Bray MS, Hagberg JM, Perusse L, Rankinen T, Roth SM, Wolfarth B, Bouchard C**. The human gene map for performance and health-related fitness phenotypes: the 2006–2007 update. *Medicine and Science in Sports and Exercise* 41: 34–72, 2009.

9. **Devaney JM, Hoffman EP, Gordish-Dressman H, Kearns A, Zambraski E, Clarkson PM**. IGF-II gene region polymorphisms related to exertional muscle damage. *Journal of Applied Physiology* 102: 1815–1823, 2007.

10. **Eder IE, Culig Z, Putz T, Menardi CN, Bartsch G, Klocker H**. Molecular biology of the androgen receptor: from molecular understanding to the clinic. *European Urology* 40: 241–251, 2001.

11. **Eynon N, Hanson ED, Lucia A, Houwelling PJ, Garton F, North KN, Bishop DJ**. Genes for elite power and sprint performance: *ACTN3* leads the way. *Sports Medicine* 43: 803–817, 2013.

12. **Folland JP, McCauley TM, Phypers C, Hanson B, Mastana SS**. The relationship of testosterone and AR CAG repeat genotype with knee extensor muscle function of young and older men. *Experimental Gerontology* 47: 437–443, 2012.

13. **Gaylin BD**. Growth hormone releasing hormone receptor. *Receptors Channels* 8: 155–162, 2002.

14. **Gelman EP**. Molecular biology of the androgen receptor. *Journal of Clinical Oncology* 20: 3001–3015, 2002.

15. **Goldspink G, Wessner B, Tschan H, Bachl N**. Growth factors, muscle function, and doping. *Endocrinology Metabolism Clinics of North America* 39: 169–181, 2010.

16. **Gonzalez AM, Hoffman JR, Townsend JR**, et al. Intramuscular anabolic signaling and endocrine response following high volume and high intensity resistance exercise protocols in trained men. *Physiological Reports* 3: e12466, 2015.

17. **Gonzalez AM, Hoffman JR, Stout JR, Fukuda DH, Willoughby DS**. Intramuscular anabolic signaling and endocrine response following resistance exercise: implications for muscle hypertrophy. *Sports Medicine* 46: 671–685, 2016.

18. **Gordon SE, Kraemer WJ, Vos NH, Lynch JM, Knuttgen HG**. Effect of acid-base balance on the growth hormone response to acute high-intensity cycle exercise. *Journal of Applied Physiology* 76: 821–829, 1994.

19. **Gordon SE, Kraemer WJ, Looney DP, Flanagan SD, Comstock BA, Hymer WC**. The influence of age and exercise modality on growth hormone bioactivity in women. *Growth Hormone and IGF Research* 24: 95–103, 2014.

20. **Grindeland RE, Kraemer WJ, Hymer WC**. Two types of rat pituitary somatotrophs secrete growth hormone with different biological and immunological profiles. *Growth Hormone and IGF Research* 36: 52–56, 2017.

21. **Harada N, Inui H**, and **Yamaji R**. Competitive and compensatory effects of androgen signaling and glucocorticoid signaling. *Receptors and Clinical Investigation* 2: e785, 2015.

22. **Harridge SDR**. Plasticity of human skeletal muscle: gene expression to in vivo function. *Experimental Physiology* 92: 783–797, 2007.

23. **Harridge SDR, Velloso CP**. IGF-1 and GH: potential use in gene doping. *Growth Hormone and IGF Research* 19: 378–382, 2009.

24. **Hartmann K, Koenen M, Schauer S, Wittig-Blaich S, Ahmad M, Baschant U, Tuckerman JP**. Molecular actions of glucocorticoids in cartilage and bone during health, disease, and steroid therapy. *Physiological Reviews* 96: 409–447, 2016.

25. **Hoffman JR, Kraemer WJ, Bhasin S, Storer T, Ratamess NA, Haff GG, Willoughby DS, Rogol AD**. Position stand on androgen and human growth hormone use. *Journal of Strength and Conditioning Research* 23: S1–S59, 2009.

26. **Hooper DR, Kraemer WJ, Focht BC, Volek JS, DuPont WH, Caldwell LK, Maresh CM**. Endocrinological roles for testosterone in resistance exercise responses and adaptations. *Sports Medicine* 47: 1709–1720, 2017.

27. **Huuskonen A, Lappalainen J, Oksala N, Santtila M, Häkkinen K, Kyrolainen H, Atalay M.** Common genetic variation in the *IGF1* associates with maximal force output. *Medicine and Science in Sports and Exercise* 43: 2368–2374, 2011.

28. **Hymer WC, Grindeland RE, Nindl BC, Kraemer WJ.** Growth hormone variants and human exercise In: *The Endocrine System in Sports and Exercise*, edited by Kraemer WJ, Rogol, AD. Malden, MA: Blackwell Publishers, p. 77–93, 2005.

29. **Hymer W, Kirshnan K, Kraemer W, Welsch J, Lanham W.** Mammalian pituitary growth hormone: applications of free flow electrophoresis. *Electrophoresis* 21: 311–317, 2000.

30. **Hymer WC, Kraemer WJ, Nindl BC,** et al. Characteristics of circulating growth hormone in women after acute heavy resistance exercise. *American Journal of Physiology, Endocrinology Metabolism* 281: E878–E887, 2001.

31. **Kempna P, Marti N, Udhane S, Fluck CE.** Regulation of androgen biosynthesis – a short review and preliminary results from the hyperandrogenic starvation NCI-H295R cell model. *Molecular and Cellular Endocrinology* 408: 124–132, 2015.

32. **Kemppainen JA, Lane MV, Sar M, Wilson EM.** Androgen receptor phosphorylation, turnover, nuclear transport, and transcriptional activation. Specificity for steroids and antihormones. *Journal of Biological Chemistry* 267: 968–974, 1992.

33. **Kopchick JJ.** Lessons learned from studies with the growth hormone receptor. *Growth Hormone and IGF Research* 28: 21–25, 2016.

34. **Kostek MC, Delmonico MJ, Reichel JB, Roth SM, Douglass L, Ferrell RE, Hurley BF.** Muscle strength response to strength training is influenced by insulin-like growth factor 1 genotype in older adults. *Journal of Applied Physiology* 98: 2147–2154, 2005.

35. **Kostek MC, Devaney JM, Gordish-Dressman H,** et al. A polymorphism near IGF1 is associated with body composition and muscle function in women from the Health, Aging, and Body Composition Study. *European Journal of Applied Physiology* 110: 315–324, 2010.

36. **Kraemer WJ, Noble BJ, Culver BW, Clark MJ.** Physiologic responses to heavy-resistance exercise with very short rest periods. *International Journal of Sports Medicine* 8: 247–252, 1987.

37. **Kraemer WJ, Marchitelli L, Gordon SE,** et al. Hormonal and growth factor responses to heavy resistance exercise protocols. *Journal of Applied Physiology* 69: 1442–1450, 1990.

38. **Kraemer WJ, Fleck SJ, Dziados JE,** et al. Changes in hormonal concentrations after different heavy-resistance exercise protocols in women. *Journal of Applied Physiology* 75: 594–604, 1993.

39. **Kraemer WJ, Rubin MR, Häkkinen K,** et al. Influence of muscle strength and total work on exercise-induced plasma growth hormone isoforms in women. *Journal of Science and Medicine in Sport* 6: 295–306, 2003.

40. **Kraemer WJ, Ratamess NA.** Fundamentals of resistance training: progression and exercise prescription. *Medicine and Science in Sports and Exercise* 36: 674–688, 2004.

41. **Kraemer WJ and Ratamess NA.** Hormonal responses and adaptations to resistance exercise and training. *Sports Medicine* 35: 339–361, 2005.

42. **Kraemer WJ, Nindl BC, Marx JO,** et al. Chronic resistance training in women potentiates growth hormone in vivo bioactivity: characterization of molecular mass variants. *American Journal of Physiology, Endocrinology, Metabolism* 291: E1177–E1187, 2006.

43. **Kraemer WJ, Dunn-Lewis C, Comstock BA, Thomas GA, Clark JE, Nindl BC.** Growth hormone, exercise, and athletic performance: a continued evolution of complexity. *Current Sports Medicine Reports* 9: 242–252, 2010.

44. **Kraemer WJ, Kennett MJ, Mastro AM,** et al. Bioactive growth hormone in older men and women: its relationship to immune markers and healthspan. *Growth Hormone and IGF Research* 34: 45–54, 2017.

45. **Kraemer WJ, Ratamess NA, Flanagan SD, Shurley JP, Todd JS, Todd TC.** Understanding the science of resistance training: an evolutionary perspective. *Sports Medicine* 47: 2415–2435, 2017.

46. **Kraemer WJ, Ratamess NA, Nindl BC.** Recovery responses of testosterone, growth hormone, and IGF-1 after resistance exercise. *Journal of Applied Physiology* 122: 549–558, 2017.

47. **Kuo T, Harris CA, Wang JC.** Metabolic functions of glucocorticoid receptor in skeletal muscle. *Molecular and Cellular Endocrinology* 380: 79–88, 2013.

48. **Kupr B, Schnyder S, Handschin C.** Role of nuclear receptors in exercise-induced muscle adaptations. *Cold Spring Harbor Perspectives in Medicine* 7: a029835, 2017.

49. **MacLean HE, Chiu WSM, Notini AJ,** et al. Impaired skeletal muscle development and function in male, but not female, genomic *androgen receptor* knockout mice. *FASEB Journal* 22: 2676–2689, 2008.

50. **McCall GE, Goulet C, Grindeland RE, Hodgson JA, Bigbee AJ, Edgerton VR**. Bed rest suppresses bioassayable growth hormone release in response to muscle activity. *Journal of Applied Physiology* 83: 2086–2090, 1997.

51. **Mizrachi D, Auchus RJ**. Androgens, estrogens, and hydroxysteroid dehydrogenases. *Molecular and Cellular Endocrinology* 301: 37–42, 2009.

52. **Nielsen TL, Hagen C, Wraae K, Bathum L, Larsen R**, and **Brixen K**. The impact of the CAG repeat polymorphism of the androgen receptor gene and adipose tissues in 20–29-year-old Danish men: Odense Androgen Study. *European Journal of Endocrinology* 162: 795–804, 2010.

53. **Nindl BC, Hymer WC, Deaver DR, Kraemer WJ**. Growth hormone pulsatility profile characteristics following acute heavy resistance exercise. *Journal of Applied Physiology* 91: 163–172, 2001.

54. **Nindl BC, Kraemer WJ, Marx JO, Arciero PJ, Dohi K, Kellogg MD, Loomis GA**. Overnight responses of the circulating IGF-I system after acute, heavy-resistance exercise. *Journal of Applied Physiology* 90: 1319–1326, 2001.

55. **Nindl BC**. Exercise modulation of growth hormone isoforms: current knowledge and future directions for the exercise endocrinologist. *British Journal of Sports Medicine* 41: 346–348, 2007.

56. **Nindl BC, Urso ML, Pierce JR**, et al. IGF-I measurement across blood, interstitial fluid, and muscle biocompartments following explosive, high-power exercise. *American Journal of Physiology – Regulatory Integrated Comparative Physiology* 303: R1080–R1089, 2012.

57. **Peeters GMEE, van Schoor NM, van Rossum EFC, Visser M, Lips P**. The relationship between cortisol, muscle mass and muscle strength in older persons and the role of genetic variations in the glucocorticoid receptor. *Clinical Endocrinology (Oxford)* 69: 673–682, 2008.

58. **Petrella JK, Kim J, Mayhew DL, Cross JM, Bamman MM**. Potent myofiber hypertrophy during resistance training in humans is associated with satellite cell-mediated myonuclear addition: a cluster analysis. *Journal of Applied Physiology* 104: 1736–1742, 2008.

59. **Philippou A, Halapas A, Maridaki M, Koutsilieris M**. Type I insulin-like growth factor receptor signaling in skeletal muscle regeneration and hypertrophy. *Journal of Musculoskeletal Neuronal Interaction* 7: 208–218, 2007.

60. **Puthucheary Z, Skipworth JRA, Rawal J, Loosemore M, Van Someren K, Montgomery HE**. Genetic influences in sport and physical performance. *Sports Medicine* 41: 845–859, 2011.

61. **Ratamess NA, Kraemer WJ, Volek JS**, et al. Androgen receptor content following heavy resistance exercise in men. *Journal of Steroid Biochemistry Molecular Biology* 93: 35–42, 2005.

62. **Roy AK, Tyagi RK, Song CS, Lavrovsky Y, Ahn SC, Oh TS, Chatterjee B**. Androgen receptor: structural domains and functional dynamics after ligand-receptor interaction. *Annals of the NY Academy of Science* 949: 44–57, 2001.

63. **Rubin MR, Kraemer WJ, Kraemer RR**, et al. Responses of growth hormone aggregates to different intermittent exercise intensities. *European Journal of Applied Physiology* 89: 166–170, 2003.

64. **Rubin MR, Kraemer WJ, Maresh CM**, et al. Response of high-affinity growth hormone binding protein to acute heavy resistance exercise in resistance-trained and untrained men. *Medicine and Science in Sports and Exercise* 37: 395–403, 2005.

65. **Sato K, Iemitsu M, Matsutani K, Kurihara T, Hamaoka T, Fujita S**. Resistance training restores muscle sex steroid hormone steroidogenesis in older men. *FASEB Journal* 28: 1891–1897, 2014.

66. **Schakman O, Kalista S, Barbe C, Loumaye A, Thissen JP**. Glucocorticoid-induced skeletal muscle atrophy. *The International Journal of Biochemistry and Cell Biology* 45: 2163–2172, 2013.

67. **Schilbach K, Bidlingmaier M**. Growth hormone binding protein – physiological and analytical aspects. *Best Practice & Research Clinical Endocrinology & Metabolism* 29: 671–683, 2015.

68. **Silva TS, Longui CA, Rocha MN**, et al. Prolonged physical training decreases mRNA levels of glucocorticoid receptor and inflammatory genes. *Hormone Research in Paediatrics* 74: 6–14, 2010.

69. **Simmons ZL, Roney JR**. Variation in CAG repeat length of the androgen receptor gene predicts variables associated with intrasexual competitiveness in human males. *Hormones and Behavior* 60: 306–312, 2011.

70. **Sood S, Hanson ED, Delmonico MJ**, et al. Does insulin-like growth factor 1 genotype influence muscle power response to strength training in older men and women? *European Journal of Applied Physiology* 112: 743–753, 2012.

71. **Spiering BA, Kraemer WJ, Anderson JM**, et al. Resistance exercise biology: manipulation of resistance exercise programme variables determines the responses of cellular and molecular signaling pathways. *Sports Medicine* 38: 527–540, 2008.

72. **Teles MG, Silveira LF, Tusset C, Latronico AC**. New genetic factors implicated in human GnRH-dependent precocious puberty: the role of kisspeptin system. *Molecular and Cellular Endocrinology* 346: 84–90, 2011.

73. **Thomas GA, Kraemer WJ, Kennett MJ**, et al. Immunoreactive and bioactive growth hormone responses to resistance exercise in men who are lean or obese. *Journal of Applied Physiology* 111: 465–472, 2011.

74. **Van Rossum EF, Voorhoeve PG, te Velde SJ**, et al. The ER 22/23EK polymorphism in the glucocorticoid receptor gene is associated with a beneficial body composition and muscle strength in young adults. *Journal of Clinical Endocrinology and Metabolism* 89: 4004–4009, 2004.

75. **Van Rossum EF, Lamberts SW**. Polymorphisms in the glucocorticoid receptor gene and their associations with metabolic parameters and body composition. *Recent Progress in Hormone Research* 59: 333–357, 2004.

76. **Veldhuis JD, Anderson SM, Shah N**, et al. A neurophysiological regulation and target-tissue impact of the pulsatile mode of growth hormone secretion in the human. *Growth Hormone and IGF Research* 11 Suppl A: S25–S37, 2001.

77. **Vingren JL, Kraemer WJ, Hatfield DL**, et al. Effect of resistance exercise on muscle steroidogenesis. *Journal of Applied Physiology* 105: 1754–1760, 2008.

78. **Vingren JL, Kraemer WJ, Hatfield DL**, et al. Effect of resistance exercise on muscle steroid receptor protein content in strength-trained men and women. *Steroids* 74: 1033–1039, 2009.

79. **Vingren JL, Kraemer WJ, Ratamess NA, Anderson JM, Volek JS, Maresh CM**. Testosterone physiology in resistance exercise and training: the up-stream regulatory elements. *Sports Medicine* 40: 1037–1053, 2010.

80. **Vo N, Goodman RH**. CREB-binding protein and p300 in transcriptional regulation. *Journal of Biological Chemistry* 276: 13505–13508, 2001.

81. **Walsh S, Zmuda JM, Cauley JA**, et al. Androgen receptor CAG repeat polymorphism is associated with fat-free mass in men. *Journal of Applied Physiology* 98: 132–137, 2005.

82. **Wilborn CD, Taylor LW, Greenwood M, Kreider RB, Willoughby DS**. Effects of different intensities of resistance exercise on regulators of myogenesis. *Journal of Strength and Conditioning Research* 23: 2179–2187, 2009.

83. **Willoughby DS, Taylor M, Taylor L**. Glucocorticoid receptor and ubiquitin expression after repeated eccentric exercise. *Medicine and Science in Sports and Exercise* 35 : 2023–2031, 2003.

84. **Willoughby DS**. Effects of heavy resistance training on myostatin mRNA and protein expression. *Medicine and Science in Sports and Exercise* 36: 574–582, 2004.

85. **Zhang Y, Jiang J, Black RA, Baumann G, Frank SJ**. Tumor necrosis factor-α converting enzyme (TACE) is a growth hormone-binding protein (GHBP) sheddase: the metalloprotease TACE/ADAM-17 is critical for (PMA-induced) GH receptor proteolysis and GHBP generation. *Endocrinology* 141: 4342–4348, 2000.

86. **Zhou ZX, Lane MV, Kemppainen JA, French FS, Wilson EM**. Specificity of ligand-dependent androgen receptor stabilization: receptor domain interactions influence ligand dissociation and receptor stability. *Molecular Endocrinology* 9: 208–218, 1995.

22

MYOSTATIN'S ROLE IN GENETIC CONTROL OF MUSCLE SIZE AND STRENGTH

Dustin S. Hittel

Introduction

Previous chapters have described the genetic, molecular, and neuroendocrine underpinnings of skeletal muscle size and strength and their response to exercise training. In this chapter, we discuss the specific role of myostatin, a protein that encompasses these three levels of control over muscle morphology and yet underscores the challenges and opportunities facing the nascent field of sport and exercise systems genetics. The transforming growth factor-beta (TGF-β) superfamily includes a diverse group of growth and differentiation factors that regulate embryonic development and subsequently, tissue homeostasis in adult animals (59). In 1997, Alexandra McPherron and Se-Jin Lee identified growth/differentiation factor-8 (GDF-8), a novel muscle-specific TGF-β family member that is expressed during embryogenesis and continues to be expressed by cells fated to the muscle lineage throughout development and into adulthood (13, 33). McPherron and Lee went on to characterize the developmental role of GDF-8 by disrupting the gene in mice, using targeted inactivation resulting in extremely hypermuscular animals with very low body fat. These findings determined that prenatal loss of GDF-8 liberates skeletal muscle growth through a combination of hypertrophy (an increase in the diameter of individual skeletal muscle fibers) and hyperplasia (an increase in the number of skeletal muscle fibers) (4, 6, 19, 32, 33, 37). Anecdotally, this gene was renamed myostatin (*MSTN*) in homage to a drug first appearing in "The Incredible Hulk" television series, but most likely owes this shared etymology with the Greek description of its role in skeletal muscle homeostasis (*myo-* (of muscle) *stasis-* (inactivity/inhibition)).

The discovery of myostatin subsequently revealed the genetic basis for naturally occurring "double-muscling" phenotypes of significant agricultural interest such as the Piedmontese, Asturiana, Marchigiana, and Belgian Blue cattle breeds (34), with additional natural mutations associated with excess muscle mass in racing dogs (40) and domestic sheep (10). Similarly, humans harboring natural mutations in the myostatin gene exhibit hypermuscularity and low body fat without any obvious deleterious effects (34, 50), which indicates that the role of myostatin in regulating muscle growth development is conserved across species. Hypermuscularity was also evident in adult mice treated with a variety of myostatin-depleting biological drugs (9), whereas postnatal myostatin overexpression is associated with skeletal muscle wasting so dramatic it resembles cachexia (44, 64). Taken together, these studies identify the primary role for myostatin as a powerful negative regulator of skeletal muscle growth and development (3).

Since its discovery, myostatin has generated significant popular interest. One needs only to conduct a cursory Internet search to find hundreds of "myostatin-blocking" supplements targeting athletes seeking to exceed the natural limits of human physiology (13, 57). While the efficacy of these supplements does not survive minimal scientific scrutiny, the development of myostatin-blocking therapies may still hold great promise for patients suffering from muscle wasting disease and cachexia. Apart from regulating skeletal muscle size alone in healthy mice and humans, myostatin has also been implicated in the metabolic deterioration and muscle wasting associated with sarcopenic obesity, heart failure, both type 1 and 2 diabetes, and cancer (13). As such, this chapter will focus on myostatin's impact on muscle size and strength characteristics with particular attention paid to its role in exercise adaptation and muscle wasting. For a broader historical perspective on the discovery and characterization of this fascinating growth factor, the reader is referred to several excellent reviews (3, 13, 29, 52, 56).

Gene expression, secretion, and signaling

The myostatin gene (*MSTN*), located on chromosome 2 in humans, is organized into three exons separated by two introns (Human Genome Assembly GRCh38.p12, chromosome 2: 190,055,697–190,062,729). Among the other members of the TGF-β superfamily, GDF-11 exhibits the highest sequence homology with myostatin, with 90% identity of the carboxy terminal region. Interestingly, parabiosis experiments, the surgical union of two mice allowing sharing of the blood circulation, identified GDF-11 as a potential therapeutic for age-related cardiac and skeletal muscle decrements (21). However, recent experiments showing that supraphysiological levels of GDF-11 cause wasting of both skeletal and cardiac muscle indicate a deleterious role in muscle wasting diseases (21).

Because of the potentially devastating effects of unchecked or aberrant expression (64), the spatiotemporal regulation of myostatin signaling is highly coordinated (11). As with most TGF-β family members, myostatin is initially synthesized as an inactive pro-protein (375 amino acids in humans) with an amino-terminal signal peptide (23 amino acids), pro-domain (242 amino acids), and a carboxy-terminal (108-amino acid) growth factor domain (11). The primary sequence of myostatin is remarkably consistent among vertebrates (~96% identity), supporting a conserved physiological role. After synthesis, the pro-protein forms a disulfide dimer that is subsequently cleaved by furin-like pro-protein convertase (furin) into an amino-terminal inhibitory pro-domain and a dimeric carboxy-terminal active domain (22). Secreted myostatin then circulates as a latent multiprotein complex consisting of the carboxy dimer noncovalently bound to the pro-domain and/or other circulating inhibitory proteins such as follistatin, follistatin-like-3 (FSTL3), and G protein-coupled receptor associated sorting proteins 1 and 2 (GASP-1/2) (22). In addition, decorin, a matrix-associated proteoglycan, also binds myostatin which likewise prevents the interaction of the peptide with its receptor, whereas TCAP/telethonin/limb-girdle muscular dystrophy 2G, a prominent sarcomeric protein, traps myostatin in the Golgi apparatus, possibly preventing its secretion in response to mechanical disruption of muscle sarcomeres (13). Similarly, a pool of unprocessed extracellular pro-myostatin is bound to a large latent complex leading to extracellular sequestration and prevention of furin cleavage (58). Further evidence for proteolytic regulation of myostatin occurs during myoblast differentiation, where the expression of furin mRNA is negatively regulated by myostatin resulting in slower processing of pro-myostatin into its biologically active form (31). This negative-feedback

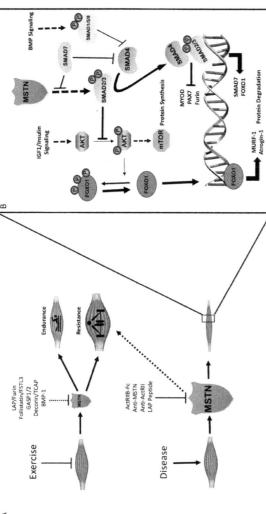

Figure 22.1 The activation (→) and inhibition (−⊣) of myostatin signaling by exercise, disease, and its rescue by pharmacological targeting. (A) A schematic representing how exercise and disease reciprocally affect the expression of myostatin resulting in adaptive or maladaptive changes in skeletal muscle size and strength. Also shown are natural and synthetic (pharmacological) protein modulators of myostatin signaling that dictate the remodeling of healthy muscle in response to exercise and potentially reverse muscle atrophy associated with disease. The blow-up panel (B) describes the primary molecular processes in myostatin–involved muscle atrophy where dashed lines (----) indicate the presence of intermediate steps not included in the figure. Myostatin signaling begins with binding to ActRIIB, which in turn recruits activin type 1 receptors and induces the phosphorylation of SMAD2/3, leading to its binding with SMAD4 and translocation of the complex to the nucleus where it blocks the transcription of genes responsible for the myogenesis (*MYOD, PAX7*) and increases the expression of *FOXO1* and *SMAD7*. SMAD7 attenuates myostatin signaling by blocking the interaction of SMAD2/3 with activin type 1 receptors as well as preventing the formation of the SMAD 2/3 and SMAD4 complex. The phosphorylation of SMAD1/5/8 via the BMP signaling pathway also blocks this complex by competing for SMAD4. AKT phosphorylation occurs in the response to insulin and IGF-1 stimulation. The active/phosphorylated form of AKT in turn activates mTOR leading to increased protein synthesis and the inhibition of FOXO1 by phosphorylation. Under conditions of high myostatin signaling, AKT phosphorylation is inhibited, leading to decreased mTOR activity and to decreased protein synthesis. In addition, activated FOXO1 translocates to the nucleus and induces the transcription of E3 ubiquitin ligases MURF-1 and atrogin-1, increasing protein degradation.

mechanism is thought to regulate myostatin levels during prenatal development to allow for coordinated muscle development (52). Finally, myostatin-binding proteins, regardless of the type or route of delivery, produce a hypermuscular phenotype in adult mice that indicates a common mechanism *in vivo* (Figure 22.1A) (11).

Recent structural characterization of the latent myostatin complex suggests that it circulates in serum in a "spring-loaded" state that can be quickly triggered into activation in the appropriate physiological context (55). Biologically active myostatin is liberated from its inhibitory protein complex by the BMP1/Tolloid (TLD) metalloprotease located in the extracellular matrix of muscle, heart (in humans), and possibly other tissues (55, 61). Free from inhibitory proteins, the approximately 25 kDa mature myostatin dimer binds to the cell surface activin receptor type IIa or IIb (ActIIRA or ActIIRB) and two of either activin type 1 (ALK4) or TGF-β type 1 (ALK5) receptors to form a heterotetrametic complex, which in turn induces the phosphorylation of the Sma- and Mad-related (SMAD) family of transcription factors via the canonical TGF-β signaling pathway (11, 58). SMAD proteins are transcription factors that regulate the expression of hundreds of genes, including those involved in muscle growth (development and exercise) and wasting (atrophy and disease) (29). In addition to the regulation of gene transcription, the phosphorylation of SMAD2/3 also inhibits AKT/protein kinase B phosphorylation leading to low mechanistic/mammalian target of rapamycin (mTOR) activity and hence lower rates of protein synthesis (29). Conversely, the phospho-AKT-mediated activation of mTOR with myostatin inhibition accounts for only half of the resulting increase in muscle mass, revealing the equal importance of the regulation of atrophy-promoting genes (Figure 22.1B) (29).

During myogenesis, the myostatin-induced phosphorylation of SMAD2/3 facilitates binding to SMAD4 and subsequently translocation to the nucleus, where it regulates the transcription of myogenic factors that enable myogenic precursor cells to exit the cell cycle and differentiate into myofibers (15). There is also mounting evidence that mitogenic signaling through the bone morphogenetic protein (BMP) receptor modulates SMAD2/3 signaling by competing for SMAD4 via SMAD1/5/8 phosphorylation (20). For instance, when myostatin signaling is high, SMAD4 binds to SMAD2/3 and then translocates to the nucleus where it can decrease the expression of genes needed for muscle growth and/or increase the expression of genes that drive muscle wasting (Figure 22.1B). However, when BMP signaling is high, SMAD4 preferentially binds SMAD1/5/8 resulting in the increased expression of muscle growth genes and/or the attenuation of myostatin-induced gene expression (15). Furthermore, animals in which SMAD1/5/8 are constitutively activated are resistant to myostatin-induced muscle atrophy suggesting that BMP signaling is dominant over myostatin signaling. Together, these studies demonstrate that the ability of myostatin to regulate muscle growth is dependent on competition for SMAD4 binding.

Another level of control over myostatin signaling is mediated by SMAD7, which is able to block the phosphorylation of SMAD2/3 by competing with the receptor, blocking access to the SMAD proteins (63). Reciprocal autoregulation is also evident as *SMAD7* mRNA expression is induced by myostatin, whereas myostatin mRNA is decreased by SMAD7 in skeletal muscle (Figure 22.1B) (63). Taken together, these findings describe the highly redundant, complex, and elegant regulation of myostatin signaling in the growth and development of healthy skeletal muscle and provide clues about its dysregulation in muscle wasting disease states.

Resistance exercise, size, and strength

Myostatin inhibition was initially considered to be a potential resistance exercise mimetic because of the hypermuscular phenotype it generates across multiple species (3). However, it soon became apparent that muscle from engineered myostatin knockout animals was of poor quality, exhibiting compromised force production, fewer mitochondria, and weaker tendons (5, 36). Notwithstanding these observations in mice, early human studies found that both acute and chronic resistance exercise elicited significant decreases in skeletal muscle myostatin mRNA levels (Figure 22.1A) (46). For example, myostatin mRNA decreased by 2.2-fold in muscle biopsies taken 4 hours after an acute bout of knee extension resistance training and remained 44% below baseline levels in biopsies taken at 24 hours (43). Contradicting these findings, muscle myostatin mRNA, as well as muscle and serum protein levels, were all increased acutely (~15 minutes) after the last bout of a resistance training program. The reason for the discrepancy may reflect variations in/lack of standardization of the training regimens for gene and protein expression studies, as well as differences in biopsy sampling time. Further muddying the waters, a positive correlation between skeletal muscle mass and both local and circulating myostatin levels, the so-called myostatin paradox, is counterintuitive for a negative muscle regulator and likely reflects the larger pool of protein-bound inactive and active myostatin needed to maintain a larger muscle mass (17). Given the extensive post-translational regulation of myostatin, others have attempted to determine whether muscle and circulating protein levels are changed by resistance training. For instance, Walker et al. showed that plasma myostatin protein levels were decreased by approximately 20% following 10 weeks of elbow flexor exercise (54) and Saremi and coworkers identified a modest but significant 10% decrease in serum myostatin levels following 12 weeks of arm- and leg-press resistance training (48). However, Kim et al. reported no change in serum myostatin levels following 16 weeks of knee extensor resistance training and reported high variability in serum myostatin levels even between untrained subjects (25).

Notably, the generation of specific antibodies against GDF8/myostatin has been hampered due to cross-reactivity with other TGF-β family members such as the highly homologous GDF-11. This may account for the high degree of variability in the immunodetection of mature and latent forms of myostatin in serum, plasma and tissue homogenates. This may also account for the withdrawal of the ActRIIB receptor-Fc ligand-trap from phase II trials given that most attempts to block myostatin have been hampered by the cross-reactivity with structurally related TGF-β superfamily growth factors (11). The differences between these studies may also reflect the confounding effects of myostatin efflux and/or clearance from the systemic circulation between subjects or between resistance exercise paradigms (3). Thus, it does not appear that circulating myostatin levels alone can be used as a reliable biomarker for training status nor does it accurately reflect the mass of exercised muscle. Moreover, the exact role of changes in myostatin expression in response to resistance exercise is not clear. But in a cluster analysis on resistance-trained humans, while myostatin mRNA levels significantly decreased in muscle biopsies 24 hours after a single knee extensor resistance exercise bout and 24 hours after completing the final bout of a 16-week training regimen, the decrease was the same for non-, modest, and extreme responders with respect to changes in muscle fiber size, suggesting that the magnitude of decrease in myostatin expression was not associated with greater hypertrophic growth in response to resistance training (25). Thus, it is not clear to what extent decreases in myostatin expression may be a prerequisite for the muscle fiber hypertrophy accompanying resistance training in humans. While myostatin signaling clearly plays an important role in muscle growth and development, its role in load-induced muscle growth remains unclear. As described above, myostatin mRNA levels do not predict load-induced skeletal muscle hypertrophy. Highlighting yet another level of control over myostatin signaling, the laboratory of Barr and colleagues show the transcriptional inhibitor Notch is activated following resistance exercise and translocates to the nucleus where it prevents the transcriptional repression of SMAD2/3. In this way, SMAD activity can be regulated locally within the exercised muscle, resulting in a muscle-specific signal for load-induced skeletal muscle hypertrophy (29).

Recently, Sharples and colleagues investigated genome-wide DNA methylation and gene expression after muscle hypertrophy followed by detraining and later reloading (51). They discovered increased frequency of hypomethylation across the genome after reloading versus earlier loading that corresponded to increased gene expression, suggesting that muscle maintains an epigenetic "memory" of hypertrophy. Although myostatin was not among these genes, nor has it been shown to directly influence their expression, Fan et al. determined that sulforaphane, a compound that is abundant in cruciferous vegetables, is a histone deacetylase and a DNA methyltransferase inhibitor, and significantly represses myostatin expression. This epigenetic repression of myostatin was attributed in part to hypoacetylation of the MyoD binding sites in the myostatin promoter (14). Another epigenetic regulator of myostatin is SIRT6, a member of the sirtuin family of protein deacetylases that regulate gene expression in response to the energy status of the cell. Interestingly, SIRT6 knockout mice display a myostatin-dependent loss of muscle, fat, and bone density, typical characteristics of cachexia and starvation. It was subsequently shown that SIRT6 depletion in cardiac and skeletal muscle cells promotes myostatin expression. Taken together, these findings suggest that SIRT6 may mediate the link between global nutritional status and skeletal muscle mass through the epigenetic regulation of myostatin (47).

The relationship between myostatin and muscle strength remains equivocal. The ratio of amino acid-changing versus nonchanging variants in the human myostatin gene are greater than expected, suggesting that they have been subject to recent positive selection. This, in turn, suggests that human variations in the myostatin gene are associated with functional differences (49). This is somewhat borne out in the observation that myostatin variants are associated with baseline muscle strength among African Americans (27). However, other variants in the myostatin gene are associated with extreme longevity, lower muscle strength, and obesity, suggesting that the selective pressure may be thrifty rather than strength and size promoting (49). Indeed, the high energetic cost to maintain a large muscle mass may explain, in part, the infrequency of inactivating myostatin mutations in the human population. For instance, one of the only humans with a confirmed natural myostatin-null genotype exhibited a muscle mass twice that of sex- and age-matched controls (50). Although this individual was otherwise healthy, heterozygotes in his pedigree also exhibited increased muscle size and strength, but to a lesser degree.

Finally, genetic studies of the canine myostatin gene by Mosher et al. have shown it to be responsible for the double-muscling phenotype seen in "bully" whippets (39). Furthermore, the loss of one functional myostatin allele confers a competitive advantage to racing whippets (over ~300 metres), providing evidence that loss of myostatin function can enhance athletic performance. The degree to which loss of function mutations in myostatin contributes to elite athletic performance phenotypes in humans will become apparent in the current era of population-scale genome sequencing.

Endurance exercise

Studies of the relationship between myostatin and endurance exercise adaptation have generally demonstrated a decrease in gene and protein expression following exercise (Figure 22.1A) (3).

For example, 12 weeks of cycling endurance exercise training decreased myostatin mRNA by 50% in human muscle biopsies (26). In addition, muscle and plasma myostatin protein levels decreased after 6 months of low-intensity aerobic training in prediabetic subjects (23). Myostatin mRNA levels also decrease in response to a single bout of endurance exercise training. For instance, myostatin mRNA levels were decreased approximately three- to fourfold in gastrocnemius biopsies after a single bout of running for 30 minutes at 75% VO_2max (28). High-intensity interval training (HIIT) can elicit similar adaptations to endurance exercise and may offer a time-saving alternative to traditional endurance exercise (16). Early evidence seems to indicate that HIIT exercises result in lower myostatin mRNA to levels similar to those seen after longer endurance training; however, more studies are needed to support these findings (16, 42). Taken together, these results suggest that a decrease in myostatin expression in humans is a hallmark of both acute and chronic endurance exercise.

Although muscle from myostatin-null animals is grossly hypertrophied, it exhibits compromised force production and fewer mitochondria (5, 36). It was therefore not surprising that myostatin null mice show reduced involuntary treadmill time to exhaustion compared to wild-type mice (30). One possible reason for decreased endurance performance in myostatin null mice is a greater percentage of fatigable fast-twitch glycolytic fibers compared to wild-type animals (18). Despite this, muscle from myostatin null mice were able to increase mitochondrial enzymes in response to run and swim training (30) showing that myostatin inactivation does not adversely affect the metabolic adaptations accompanying endurance exercise training (3).

In summary, a decrease in myostatin mRNA and protein levels in muscle is a characteristic of endurance exercise training in humans and rodents regardless of the exercise modality, intensity, or dose. However, germline inactivation of myostatin limits aerobic exercise performance in mice, possibly due to a larger proportion of glycolytic fibers, while myostatin inactivation combined with exercise training in older adult mice appears to increase endurance exercise performance. Together, these findings indicate that myostatin plays a central role in integrating anabolic and catabolic responses to exercise (Figure 22.1B).

Obesity, insulin resistance, and diabetes

There is mounting evidence that myostatin has effects on metabolism that are associated with obesity and insulin resistance (3). For instance, muscle and circulating myostatin protein levels are increased in obese human subjects, as is myostatin secretion from myotubes derived from myoblasts isolated from muscle biopsies of obese compared to nonobese women (24). Conversely, myostatin mRNA levels decreased in muscle biopsies from obese human patients following weight loss due to either biliopancreatic diversion or gastric bypass surgery (3). In addition, the manipulation of myostatin signaling can dramatically impact the development of obesity in mice. For instance, muscle-specific overexpression of myostatin caused a decrease in muscle mass and an increase in epididymal fat pad mass similar to sarcopenic obesity (44). This may be explained, in part, by the role of myostatin in the regulation of fat mass. Following the pioneering work of Allen et al. (2), others have identified the expression of myostatin and *ActIIRB* mRNA in adipose tissue, although it has not been established if adipose-derived myostatin is secreted into the circulating endocrine pool of latent and active myostatin. That being said, possessing an intact activin signaling pathway predisposes adipose cells and tissue to regulation by myostatin. For instance, myostatin stimulates 3T3-L1 adipocyte proliferation by increasing the expression of cell-proliferation-related genes and yet inhibits their differentiation resulting in deceased lipid accumulation and promoting the expression of lipolytic enzymes (62). Further, myostatin has recently been shown to inhibit the differentiation of brown preadipocytes and that the amount of subcutaneous fat and leaf fat of myostatin null pigs were significantly decreased mainly due to the browning of subcutaneous adipose (8). Therefore, excess myostatin signaling promotes both the loss of muscle mass and accumulation of poor quality adipose tissue resulting in a diabetogenic metabolic profile.

Conversely, many studies have shown that inactivation of myostatin can prevent the development of obesity in mice. For instance, crossing myostatin null mice with genetically obese ob/ob mice attenuated the increased adipose mass, hyperglycemia, hyperlipidemia, and hyperinsulinemia typically observed in these animals (35). Whereas, postnatal injection of mice with the ActRIIB-Fc ligand trap increased muscle mass and decreased fat mass in mice fed a high-fat diet (1). Taken together, these studies clearly demonstrate that the inhibition of myostatin can greatly arrest or reverse the development of obesity and its adverse health consequences in mice.

Recent evidence suggests that myostatin may play a role in the development of diabetes in addition to, and perhaps independent of, its effect on obesity. For instance, transcriptomic analysis revealed that myostatin mRNA levels were elevated in skeletal muscle biopsies from type 2 diabetics, as well as from nonobese hyperinsulinemic relatives of type 2 diabetics (41). In addition, both muscle and plasma myostatin protein levels in insulin-resistant middle-aged men were decreased by aerobic exercise training and were strongly correlated with insulin sensitivity (23). These subjects experienced decreases in circulating myostatin, insulin, and glucose levels that were not accompanied by any change in fat mass or body mass index following exercise training, strongly suggesting that these changes were not secondary to a change in adipose mass. Furthermore, Bernardo et al. (7) showed improvements in fed and fasted blood glucose levels without any change in adipose mass in ob/ob mice injected for 6 weeks with a neutralizing antibody to myostatin. Lastly, injection of recombinant myostatin decreased insulin sensitivity in healthy male mice and in mice harbouring a loss-of-function mutation to myostatin on a high-fat diet without a corresponding change in body mass in either study (23, 60). Together these studies indicate that increased myostatin expression is inversely related to insulin sensitivity independent of obesity status.

Atrophy and cachexia

Loss of muscle mass is observed after trauma, with neuromuscular disorders and catabolic diseases such as cancer, diabetes, renal failure, cardiorespiratory insufficiency, and sepsis (53). Furthermore, muscle atrophy also occurs with starvation, immobilization, microgravity, and sarcopenia, the age-related loss of skeletal muscle that is associated with frailty (Figure 22.1B) (38). Regardless of the pathophysiological or environmental causes, myostatin-associated wasting of skeletal muscle results from both decreased protein synthesis and increased ubiquitin-mediated protein degradation of contractile proteins (52). Myostatin also inhibits paired box 7 (PAX7) expression resulting in the inhibition of myogenic precursor cell proliferation and satellite cell renewal and thereby blunting the cellular basis for muscle regeneration. Myostatin also induces the AKT-mediated activation of the transcription factor forkhead box O1 (FOXO1) which in turn, increases the expression of the ubiquitin E3 ligases atrogin-1 and MuRF1. This results in the ubiquination and degradation of sarcomeric proteins when combined with myostatin/mTORC1-associated suppression of muscle structural protein expression results in the rapid loss of skeletal muscle mass (Figure 22.1B).

Cachexia is a multifactorial syndrome associated with chronic disease that is characterized by skeletal muscle wasting with associated asthenia (loss of muscle strength), loss of body fat, and a dramatic catabolic shift in lipid, carbohydrate, and protein metabolism (52, 53). Cancer-cachexia is exhibited by about 80% of all patients who possess advanced tumors of pancreatic, lung, and gastric origin. Not surprisingly, elevated levels of circulating myostatin correlate with the progression of cancer-associated cachexia in part because several tumor cell lines produce and secrete myostatin (53). Given the highly visible and personally devastating effects of cancer cachexia, it is a high priority target for myostatin-neutralizing therapies in humans (Figure 22.1A).

Myostatin upregulation is observed in muscle of hypoxemic patients with severe chronic obstructive pulmonary disease (COPD). Myostatin is similarly increased with hypoxia-induced atrophy in rats and in human myotubes treated with hypoxia-mimicking agents (45). It is therefore not surprising that approximately 40% of people with COPD eventually develop significant muscle wasting with a dramatic decline in oxidative muscle phenotype of the remaining muscle, resulting in reduced energy output loss of function (52). In addition, muscle myostatin-mediated expression of the ubiquitin proteasome E3 ligases atrogin-1 and MuRF-1 have been show to be the primary drivers of muscle wasting in COPD patients (Figure 22.1B) compared with healthy controls suggesting a mechanistic link that could be targeted with antimyostatin therapeutics.

Chronic inflammation of the liver caused by alcohol, diet, or disease eventually results in cirrhosis and loss of skeletal muscle mass secondary to hyperammonemia (12). As with cancer and COPD, mounting evidence implicates myostatin is a key factor involved in muscle wasting seen in patients with liver disease. Indeed, higher levels of circulating myostatin were noted in patients with end-stage liver disease and in skeletal muscle of patients with cirrhosis (39).

As with cancer, COPD, and liver disease, one of the comorbidities associated with chronic kidney disease is the rapid onset of muscle wasting (52). Increased protein breakdown, insulin resistance, excessive glucocorticoid production, and a significant increase in the expression of muscle myostatin track with the loss of muscle mass in these patients. Subsequent pharmacological inhibition of myostatin reversed the loss of body weight and muscle mass in mice, making chronic kidney disease an ideal target for myostatin-neutralizing therapies in humans.

Myostatin inhibitors

Although the targeted inhibition of myostatin has been successfully used to increase muscle growth in food animals and in the burgeoning "clean meat" market, its therapeutic use in humans faces considerable technical and ethical challenges. For instance, several myostatin-neutralizing biological agents have been withdrawn due to safety concerns and failure to meet primary clinical endpoints (9). This is due in part to the cross-reactivity of myostatin antagonists with structurally related growth factors. While this underscores the challenges faced when developing new drugs, a number of recent studies may provide new insights for the design of the next generation of myostatin inhibitors. First, to investigate the molecular mechanisms by which pro-myostatin remains latent, Cotton et al. have resolved the structure of unprocessed pro-myostatin and analyzed the properties of the protein in its latent and active forms (11). A high-resolution structure of myostatin may guide the development of inhibitors with lower cross-reactivity and higher specificity. Second, blockade of individual ActRII receptors using anti-ActRIIA or anti-ActRIIB antibodies has been shown to produce only a small (~15%) increase in muscle mass in animals (38). However, Morvan et al. demonstrate that maximal anabolic/hypertrophic response is achieved with simultaneous blockade of both receptors (38).

Third, an alternative spliced 129-amino acid isoform of avian myostatin inhibits proteolytic processing of pro-myostatin, and thereby reduces the release of mature myostatin in cell culture and *in vivo* (9). Myostatin inhibition using such peptides is an emerging area of interest in both agricultural animals to increase meat production as well as human medicine (Figure 22.1A).

Although myostatin inhibitors are a promising new class of therapeutics for the treatment of muscle wasting, they are also very tempting as performance-enhancing drugs and cosmetic agents. While no myostatin inhibitors have obtained clinical approval, the proactive development of detection methods for emerging doping agents represent a key aspect of prevention. For instance, Bimagrumab (Novartis) is a human anti-ActRII antibody which was found to increase muscle mass and function by blocking ActRII signaling. As it has considerable potential for being misused as a doping agent in sports, a rapid mass spectrometric detection assay has been developed in concert with the drug manufacturer to discourage use and abuse by athletes (57).

Summary

Since the discovery of myostatin over 20 years ago, considerable progress has been made in understanding its impact on the growth and maintenance of skeletal muscle mass. In keeping with its negative role in myogenesis, myostatin expression is highly regulated at several levels including epigenetic, transcriptional, post-transcriptional, and post-translational. Mutations in and around the myostatin gene have taught us much about the role of lean body mass in combating obesity as well as the neuroendocrine response to exercise training and disease. Recent insights about the structure and regulation of myostatin have revealed novel exploits for the development of the next generation of myostatin antagonists to combat muscle wasting disease and cachexia. Finally, besides its impact on muscle, myostatin plays an important role in metabolism and as a facilitator of muscle–organ crosstalk in both in health and disease. Future studies of myostatin will tease out the molecular mechanisms by which myostatin balances anabolic and catabolic responses of skeletal muscle in both health and disease.

References

1. **Akpan I, Goncalves MD, Dhir R** et al. The effects of a soluble activin type IIB receptor on obesity and insulin sensitivity. *Int J Obes (Lond)*. 2009;33(11):1265–73.
2. **Allen DL, Cleary AS, Speaker KJ** et al. Myostatin, activin receptor IIb, and follistatin-like-3 gene expression are altered in adipose tissue and skeletal muscle of obese mice. *Am J Physiol Endocrinol Metab*. 2008;294(5):E918–27.
3. **Allen DL, Hittel DS, McPherron AC**. Expression and function of myostatin in obesity, diabetes, and exercise adaptation. *Med Sci Sports Exerc*. 2011;43(10):1828–35.
4. **Amthor H, Macharia R, Navarrete R** et al. Lack of myostatin results in excessive muscle growth but impaired force generation. *Proc Natl Acad Sci U S A*. 2007;104(6):1835–40.
5. **Amthor H, Macharia R, Navarrete R** et al. Lack of myostatin results in excessive muscle growth but impaired force generation. *Proc Natl Acad Sci U S A*. 2007;104(6):1835–40.
6. **Bellinge RH, Liberles DA, Iaschi SP, O'Brien PA, Tay GK**. Myostatin and its implications on animal breeding: a review. *Anim Genet*. 2005;36(1):1–6.
7. **Bernardo BL, Wachtmann TS, Cosgrove PG** et al. Postnatal PPARdelta activation and myostatin inhibition exert distinct yet complimentary effects on the metabolic profile of obese insulin-resistant mice. *PloS One*. 2010;5(6):e11307.
8. **Cai C, Qian L, Jiang S** et al. Loss-of-function myostatin mutation increases insulin sensitivity and browning of white fat in Meishan pigs. *Oncotarget*. 2017;8(21):34911–22.
9. **Chen PR, Lee K**. Invited review. Inhibitors of myostatin as methods of enhancing muscle growth and development. *J Anim Sci*. 2016;94(8):3125–34.

10. **Clop A, Marcq F, Takeda H** et al. A mutation creating a potential illegitimate microRNA target site in the myostatin gene affects muscularity in sheep. *Nat Genet.* 2006;38(7):813–8.

11. **Cotton TR, Fischer G, Wang X** et al. Structure of the human myostatin precursor and determinants of growth factor latency. *EMBO J.* 37: 367–383, 2018.

12. **Dasarathy S**. Myostatin and beyond in cirrhosis: all roads lead to sarcopenia. *J Cachexia Sarcopenia Muscle.* 2017;8(6):864–9.

13. **Dschietzig TB**. Myostatin – from the mighty mouse to cardiovascular disease and cachexia. *Clin Chim Acta.* 2014;433:216–24.

14. **Fan H, Zhang R, Tesfaye D** et al. Sulforaphane causes a major epigenetic repression of myostatin in porcine satellite cells. *Epigenetics.* 2012;7(12):1379–90.

15. **Gaarenstroom T, Hill CS**. TGF-beta signaling to chromatin: how Smads regulate transcription during self-renewal and differentiation. *Semin Cell Dev Biol.* 2014;32:107–18.

16. **Gillen JB, Gibala MJ**. Is high-intensity interval training a time-efficient exercise strategy to improve health and fitness? *Appl Physiol Nutr Metab.* 2014;39(3):409–12.

17. **Gilson H, Schakman O, Combaret L** et al. Myostatin gene deletion prevents glucocorticoid-induced muscle atrophy. *Endocrinology.* 2007;148(1):452–60.

18. **Girgenrath S, Song K, Whittemore LA**. Loss of myostatin expression alters fiber-type distribution and expression of myosin heavy chain isoforms in slow- and fast-type skeletal muscle. *Muscle Nerve.* 2005;31(1):34–40.

19. **Girgenrath S, Song K, Whittemore LA**. Loss of myostatin expression alters fiber-type distribution and expression of myosin heavy chain isoforms in slow- and fast-type skeletal muscle. *Muscle Nerve.* 2005;31(1):34–40.

20. **Goodman CA, Hornberger TA**. New roles for Smad signaling and phosphatidic acid in the regulation of skeletal muscle mass. *F1000Prime Rep.* 2014;6:20.

21. **Hammers DW, Merscham-Banda M, Hsiao JY, Engst S, Hartman JJ, Sweeney HL**. Supraphysiological levels of GDF11 induce striated muscle atrophy. *EMBO Mol Med.* 2017;9(4):531–44.

22. **Hill JJ, Davies MV, Pearson AA** et al. The myostatin propeptide and the follistatin-related gene are inhibitory binding proteins of myostatin in normal serum. *J Biol Chem.* 2002;277(43):40735–41.

23. **Hittel DS, Axelson M, Sarna N, Shearer J, Huffman KM, Kraus WE**. Myostatin decreases with aerobic exercise and associates with insulin resistance. *Med Sci Sports Exerc.* 2010;42(11):2023–9.

24. **Hittel DS, Berggren JR, Shearer J, Boyle K, Houmard JA**. Increased secretion and expression of myostatin in skeletal muscle from extremely obese women. *Diabetes.* 2009;58(1):30–8.

25. **Kim JS, Petrella JK, Cross JM, Bamman MM**. Load-mediated downregulation of myostatin mRNA is not sufficient to promote myofiber hypertrophy in humans: a cluster analysis. *J Appl Physiol (1985).* 2007;103(5):1488–95.

26. **Konopka AR, Douglass MD, Kaminsky LA** et al. Molecular adaptations to aerobic exercise training in skeletal muscle of older women. *J Gerontol A Biol Sci Med Sci.* 2010;65(11):1201–7.

27. **Kostek MA, Angelopoulos TJ, Clarkson PM** et al. Myostatin and follistatin polymorphisms interact with muscle phenotypes and ethnicity. *Med Sci Sports Exerc.* 2009;41(5):1063–71.

28. **Louis E, Raue U, Yang Y, Jemiolo B, Trappe S**. Time course of proteolytic, cytokine, and myostatin gene expression after acute exercise in human skeletal muscle. *J Appl Physiol (1985).* 2007;103(5):1744–51.

29. **Marcotte GR, West DW, Baar K**. The molecular basis for load-induced skeletal muscle hypertrophy. *Calcif Tissue Int.* 2015;96(3):196–210.

30. **Matsakas A, Mouisel E, Amthor H, Patel K**. Myostatin knockout mice increase oxidative muscle phenotype as an adaptive response to exercise. *J Muscle Res Cell Motil.* 2010;31(2):111–25.

31. **McFarlane C, Langley B, Thomas M** et al. Proteolytic processing of myostatin is auto-regulated during myogenesis. *Dev Biol.* 2005;283(1):58–69.

32. **McPherron AC, Huynh TV, Lee SJ**. Redundancy of myostatin and growth/differentiation factor 11 function. *BMC Dev Biol.* 2009;9:24.

33. **McPherron AC, Lawler AM, Lee SJ**. Regulation of skeletal muscle mass in mice by a new TGF-beta superfamily member. *Nature.* 1997;387(6628):83–90.

34. **McPherron AC, Lee SJ**. Double muscling in cattle due to mutations in the myostatin gene. *Proc Natl Acad Sci U S A.* 1997;94(23):12457–61.

35. **McPherron AC, Lee SJ**. Suppression of body fat accumulation in myostatin-deficient mice. *J Clin Invest.* 2002;109(5):595–601.

36. **Mendias CL, Bakhurin KI, Faulkner JA.** Tendons of myostatin-deficient mice are small, brittle, and hypocellular. *Proc Natl Acad Sci U S A.* 2008;105(1):388–93.

37. **Mendias CL, Marcin JE, Calerdon DR, Faulkner JA.** Contractile properties of EDL and soleus muscles of myostatin-deficient mice. *J Appl Physiol.* 2006;101(3):898–905.

38. **Morvan F, Rondeau JM, Zou C** et al. Blockade of activin type II receptors with a dual anti-ActRIIA/IIB antibody is critical to promote maximal skeletal muscle hypertrophy. *Proc Natl Acad Sci U S A.* 2017;114(47):12448–53.

39. **Mosher DS, Quignon P, Bustamante CD** et al. A mutation in the myostatin gene increases muscle mass and enhances racing performance in heterozygote dogs. *PLoS Genet.* 2007;3(5):e79.

40. **Mosher DS, Quignon P, Bustamante CD** et al. A mutation in the myostatin gene increases muscle mass and enhances racing performance in heterozygote dogs. *PLoS Genet.* 2007;3(5):e79.

41. **Palsgaard J, Brons C, Friedrichsen M** et al. Gene expression in skeletal muscle biopsies from people with type 2 diabetes and relatives: differential regulation of insulin signaling pathways. *PloS One.* 2009;4(8):e6575.

42. **Pugh JK, Faulkner SH, Jackson AP, King JA, Nimmo MA.** Acute molecular responses to concurrent resistance and high-intensity interval exercise in untrained skeletal muscle. *Physiol Rep.* 2015;3(4).

43. **Raue U, Slivka D, Jemiolo B, Hollon C, Trappe S.** Myogenic gene expression at rest and after a bout of resistance exercise in young (18–30 yr) and old (80–89 yr) women. *J Appl Physiol (1985).* 2006;101(1):53–9.

44. **Reisz-Porszasz S, Bhasin S, Artaza JN** et al. Lower skeletal muscle mass in male transgenic mice with muscle-specific overexpression of myostatin. *Am J Physiol Endocrinol Metab.* 2003;285(4):E876–88.

45. **Rodriguez J, Vernus B, Chelh I** et al. Myostatin and the skeletal muscle atrophy and hypertrophy signaling pathways. *Cell Mol Life Sci.* 2014;71(22):4361–71.

46. **Roth SM, Martel GF, Ferrell RE, Metter EJ, Hurley BF, Rogers MA.** Myostatin gene expression is reduced in humans with heavy-resistance strength training: a brief communication. *Exp Biol Med (Maywood).* 2003;228(6):706–9.

47. **Samant SA, Kanwal A, Pillai VB, Bao R, Gupta MP.** The histone deacetylase SIRT6 blocks myostatin expression and development of muscle atrophy. *Sci Rep.* 2017;7(1):11877.

48. **Saremi A, Gharakhanloo R, Sharghi S, Gharaati MR, Larijani B, Omidfar K.** Effects of oral creatine and resistance training on serum myostatin and GASP-1. *Mol Cell Endocrinol.* 2010;317(1–2):25–30.

49. **Saunders MA, Good JM, Lawrence EC, Ferrell RE, Li WH, Nachman MW.** Human adaptive evolution at Myostatin (GDF8), a regulator of muscle growth. *Am J Hum Genet.* 2006;79(6):1089–97.

50. **Schuelke M, Wagner KR, Stolz LE** et al. Myostatin mutation associated with gross muscle hypertrophy in a child. *N Engl J Med.* 2004;350(26):2682–8.

51. **Seaborne RA, Strauss J, Cocks M** et al. Human skeletal muscle possesses an epigenetic memory of hypertrophy. *Sci Rep.* 2018;8(1):1898.

52. **Sharma M, McFarlane C, Kambadur R, Kukreti H, Bonala S, Srinivasan S.** Myostatin: expanding horizons. *IUBMB Life.* 2015;67(8):589–600.

53. **Smith RC, Lin BK.** Myostatin inhibitors as therapies for muscle wasting associated with cancer and other disorders. *Curr Opin Support Palliat Care.* 2013;7(4):352–60.

54. **Walker KS, Kambadur R, Sharma M, Smith HK.** Resistance training alters plasma myostatin but not IGF-1 in healthy men. *Med Sci Sports Exerc.* 2004;36(5):787–93.

55. **Walker RG, McCoy JC, Czepnik M** et al. Molecular characterization of latent GDF8 reveals mechanisms of activation. *Proc Natl Acad Sci U S A.* 2018.

56. **Walker RG, Poggioli T, Katsimpardi L** et al. Biochemistry and biology of GDF11 and myostatin: similarities, differences, and questions for future investigation. *Circ Res.* 2016;118(7):1125–41.

57. **Walpurgis K, Thomas A, Schanzer W, Thevis M.** Myostatin inhibitors in sports drug testing: detection of myostatin-neutralizing antibodies in plasma/serum by affinity purification and Western blotting. *Proteomics Clin Appl.* 2016;10(2):195–205.

58. **Walton KL, Johnson KE, Harrison CA.** Targeting TGF-beta mediated SMAD signaling for the prevention of fibrosis. *Front Pharmacol.* 2017;8:461.

59. **Wharton K, Derynck R.** TGFbeta family signaling: novel insights in development and disease. *Development.* 2009;136(22):3691–7.

60. **Wilkes JJ, Lloyd DJ, Gekakis N**. Loss-of-function mutation in myostatin reduces tumor necrosis factor alpha production and protects liver against obesity-induced insulin resistance. *Diabetes.* 2009;58(5):1133–43.

61. **Wolfman NM, McPherron AC, Pappano WN** et al. Activation of latent myostatin by the BMP-1/tolloid family of metalloproteinases. *Proc Natl Acad Sci U S A.* 2003;100(26):15842–6.

62. **Zhu HJ, Pan H, Zhang XZ** et al. The effect of myostatin on proliferation and lipid accumulation in 3T3-L1 preadipocytes. *J Mol Endocrinol.* 2015;54(3):217–26.

63. **Zhu X, Topouzis S, Liang LF, Stotish RL**. Myostatin signaling through Smad2, Smad3 and Smad4 is regulated by the inhibitory Smad7 by a negative feedback mechanism. *Cytokine.* 2004;26(6):262–72.

64. **Zimmers TA, Davies MV, Koniaris LG** et al. Induction of cachexia in mice by systemically administered myostatin. *Science.* 2002;296(5572):1486–8.

23

ALPHA-ACTININ-3'S ROLE IN THE GENETIC CONTROL OF MUSCLE STRENGTH AND PERFORMANCE

Jane T. Seto, Fleur C. Garton, Kathryn N. North, and
Peter J. Houweling

Introduction

The α-actinin-3 gene (*ACTN3*) R577X polymorphism is one of the most highly studied genetic variations associated with human skeletal muscle function and performance. More than 1 billion people worldwide are completely deficient in α-actinin-3 due to homozygosity for the null polymorphism (*ACTN3* 577XX). Deficiency of α-actinin-3 is associated with reduced muscle force and power, and frequency of the *ACTN3* 577XX genotype is underrepresented in elite sprint and power athletes compared to population controls. The *ACTN3* 577X allele has undergone strong, recent positive selection during modern human migration out of Africa, suggesting that inheritance of this allele provides a survival advantage for endurance in colder climes. The combination of human studies and research in the *Actn3* knockout (KO) mouse model to date has solidified the association between *ACTN3* R577X and human muscle performance and begun to unravel how *ACTN3* modifies fast-twitch fiber characteristics and muscle function. In this chapter, we summarize the current research in *ACTN3* R577X and discuss the molecular mechanisms that underlie the consequences of α-actinin-3 deficiency, with new insights into implications for the general population beyond athletic performance – in healthy ageing, muscle disuse, and disease.

The α-actinins and skeletal muscle

The α-actinins are a family of four actin-binding proteins (α-actinin 1–4) that have evolved from repeated gene duplication events to perform similar roles in different cell types (35). The skeletal muscle-specific isoforms α-actinin-2 and -3 (encoded by *ACTN2* and *ACTN3*) are highly conserved (81% identical and 91% similar) and are major components of the Z-disk within the skeletal muscle contractile apparatus (sarcomeres). Both sarcomeric α-actinins have a N-terminal actin-binding domain, a rod domain with four spectrin repeats, and a C-terminal region containing calcium-binding EF hand motifs (Figure 23.1) (39). α-Actinin-2 is expressed in all human skeletal muscle fibers, whereas α-actinin-3 has evolved a specialized expression pattern and is only present in type 2 (fast, glycolytic) muscle fibers (50). The sarcomeric α-actinins interact with a vast network of structural, signaling, and metabolic proteins associated

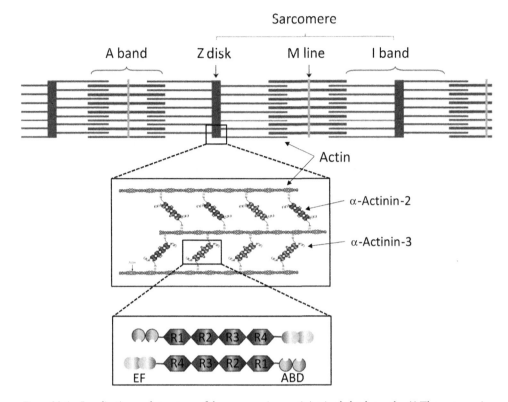

Figure 23.1 Localization and structure of the sarcomeric α-actinins in skeletal muscle. A) The sarcomeric α-actinins are found at the Z-disc (black), where they anchor actin-containing thin filaments (grey) from adjacent sarcomeres. The sarcomeric α-actinins form head to tail dimers to cross-link actin at the Z-disc. Their structure consists of an actin-binding domain (ABD), a rod domain with four spectrin repeats (R1-R4) and an EF-hand domain (EF). Image adapted from (24) and (35).

with the Z-disk (reviewed in 33) and are known to cross-link and stabilize actin thin filaments at the Z-disk during muscle contractions.

The *ACTN3* R577X polymorphism is common in humans

The role of sarcomeric α-actinins in the maintenance of ordered myofibrillar arrays in skeletal muscle make them prime candidate genes for human muscle disease. In 1999, we identified a common null polymorphism in *ACTN3* (a C>T transition in exon 16), which converts an arginine (R) to a premature stop (X) codon at residue 577 (R577X; rs1815739). Homozygosity for the X-allele results in the complete loss of α-actinin-3 but is not associated with overt muscle disease (50, 51).

To determine the frequency of the *ACTN3* 577X allele in the general population, we initially genotyped 485 DNA samples covering four main diversity groups of Asia/Americas, Australasia, Africa, and Europe. The X-allele frequency differs throughout the world, ranging from 10% in African populations to 45% in European and 54% in Asian populations (41). We estimate that approximately 18% of the world's population are completely deficient in α-actinin-3. With a population size of about 7.6 billion people (in 2017), this equates to about 1.4 billion individuals worldwide being completely deficient in α-actinin-3. The high incidence of

ACTN3 577XX globally suggests that α-actinin-3 is potentially redundant – i.e., many of its functions in muscle can be compensated for by the closely related protein α-actinin-2. However, the limited expression of α-actinin-3 in fast, glycolytic muscle fibers and sequence differences from α-actinin-2 suggest that α-actinin-3 may have evolved to play a specialized role in fast fibers that cannot be completely compensated for by α-actinin-2.

ACTN3 577X has undergone strong, recent positive selection

The varied allele frequencies observed between the different ethnic groups and specialized protein expression in fast glycolytic muscle fibers suggest that selective forces may be acting on the *ACTN3* 577X allele during modern human evolution. To explore this, we analyzed *ACTN3* DNA sequence and long-range linkage disequilibrium data around the R577X allele in individuals of European, East Asian, and African ancestry (41). Our analyses found low rates of DNA substitutions and high long-range linkage disequilibrium for recombination among X-allele-containing haplotypes compared with the R-allele in Europeans and Asians, consistent with strong, recent positive selection of the 577X allele in these populations. This suggests that the 577X allele provides an advantage to modern humans adapting to the Eurasian environment, which we estimate to have occurred around 15,000 years ago in Europe and around 30,000 years ago in East Asia. The increase in *ACTN3* 577XX genotype also correlated with a higher global latitude gradient and reduced species richness (18), suggesting that environmental variables related to temperature (cold tolerance), and diet (feast/famine) may influence the observed R577X genotype frequencies worldwide.

The absence of α-actinin-3 is detrimental to elite sprint/power performance

Since α-actinin-3 shows specialized expression in the fast, glycolytic muscle fibers and deficiency does not cause a known muscle disease, we hypothesized that deficiency of α-actinin-3 impacts muscle function at the extremes of muscle performance. In collaboration with the Australian Institute of Sports, we examined the frequency distribution of *ACTN3* R577X in elite sprint and endurance athletes compared to population controls. Elite athletes were defined as those who had qualified to represent Australia internationally either at the Commonwealth/Olympic Games or world championships. A total of 458 elite Australian Caucasian athletes from 14 different sports and 436 healthy Caucasian controls were genotyped for *ACTN3* R577X (74). Analysis of the *ACTN3* R577X genotype in a subset of 107 specialist sprint/power athletes compared to 194 specialist endurance athletes revealed differences in *ACTN3* genotype frequency. Remarkably, sprint/power athletes had an extremely low frequency of 577XX (5% compared to 18% in controls) and a high frequency of RR (50% compared to 30% in controls) (χ^2=19.70, P <0.0001) (Figure 23.2), suggesting that α-actinin-3 deficiency is detrimental to elite sprint/power performance. In contrast, female elite endurance athletes had higher frequencies of 577XX genotype compared to controls (χ^2=6.15, P <0.05), although this effect was not significant when the whole population was examined. Importantly, genotype profiles in sprint/power and endurance athletes deviated in opposite directions and differed from each other (χ^2=19.45, P <0.001) (74).

Our finding that α-actinin-3 deficiency is detrimental in elite sprint/power performance in Caucasians has been independently replicated in 16 elite athlete populations from around the world (Table 23.1). These studies show that male and female sprint/power athletes (across different sport and backgrounds) have a lower frequency of the *ACTN3* 577XX genotype compared to population controls. There are some exceptions, with several studies finding no association between *ACTN3* R577X and strength/power athletic status or performance (23,

Table 23.1 Sprint/power elite athlete association studies

Origin	Sports/events	ACTN3 XX genotype % Athlete vs. controls	Reference
Caucasian			
Australian	Judo, speed skating, swimming, track and field, track cycling	M: XX: 8% vs. XX: 16% F: XX 0% vs. 16%	74
Finnish	Track and field	M & F: XX 0% vs. 9%	48
Greek	Jumping decathlon, throwing, track and field	M & F: XX 16% vs. 18%	52
	Sprinters (100–400 m)	M & F: XX 9% vs. 18%	
Israeli	Sprinters (track 100–200 m)	M & F: XX 14% vs. 18%	15
	Sprinters (track 100–200 m)	M & F: XX 16.7% vs. 18.4%	2
Italian	Artistic gymnasts	M & F: XX 3% vs. 19%	43
Polish	Track sprinters, swimming, weight lifting	M & F: XX 8% vs. 15%	9
Spanish	Track and field	M & F: XX 12% vs. 15%	61
Russian	Alpine skiing and jumping, gymnastics, body building, figure skating, ice hockey, power lifting, soccer, speed skating, swimming, trowing, track and field, volleyball, weight lifting, and wrestling	M: XX 6% vs. 16% F: 6.5% vs. 13%	13
Asian			
Japanese	Wrestling	M: XX 11% vs. 28%	30
	International sprinters ≤400 m	M & F: XX 10% vs. 26%	44
	Track and field	M & F: RR vs. XX; OR 1.59, 95% CI 1.16–2.18; P=0.003	31
Korean	Gymnasts, sprinters, throwers short distance speed skaters, weightlifters and martial arts (Taekwondo)	M: XX 21% vs. 18% F: XX 11% vs. 18%	28
	Weightlifters, sprinters (≤400 m), speed skaters (≤1500 m) and swimmers (≤100 m)	M & F: XX 11.6% vs. 19.1%	32
Taiwanese	Swimmers ≤400 m	M: XX 14% vs. 20% F: XX 11% vs. 20%	7

Table 23.1 (Cont.)

Origin	Sports/events	ACTN3 XX genotype % Athlete vs. controls	Reference
Chinese	Sprinter (100–200 m), cyclists (500 m), throwers, jumpers, shot put, weightlifting	M & F: 5% vs. 34%	76
African			
Jamaican	Track and field	M & F: XX 3% vs. 2%	64
Nigerian	Sprinters (track 100–400 m) and jumpers	M & F: 0% vs. 3%	75
African American	Track and field	M & F: 2% vs. 4%	64
	Bodybuilding and power lifting	M & F: 7% vs. 16%	59

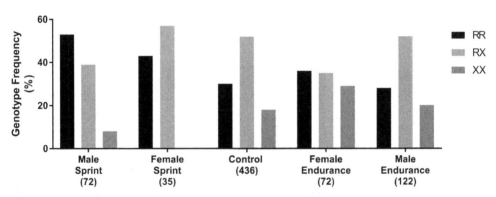

Figure 23.2 Frequency of the *ACTN3* genotype in controls and elite sprint and endurance athletes. Sample size of each group is shown in parentheses. Female and male athletes who had competed at an Olympic level are shown as separate groups for both sprint/power and endurance events. Image adapted from (74).

64, 65). In addition, the *ACTN3* R577X association does not appear to influence sprint/power performance in African athletes. Three African population cohorts (Jamaican and US), two of which included World Champion/Olympic medalists, showed low frequencies of the 577XX genotype in both athletes (2–7%) and controls (2–4%) (59, 64, 75). This precludes the identification of significantly altered frequencies compared to controls but can be interpreted as the African population being more suited to sprint performance (74).

To date, four meta-analyses (1, 20, 38, 73) have explored the association between *ACTN3* R577X with sprint, power, and endurance phenotypes in athletes, and are unanimous that the absence of α-actinin-3 is detrimental to sprint/power performance in Caucasian/Asian athletes – demonstrating that the *ACTN3* R577X association with sprint/power performance is one of the most highly replicable genetic modifiers of muscle strength and power. In our most recent meta-analysis which encompassed raw data from 12 independent studies with similar caliber athletes who competed in similar sprint/power events, we found strong evidence fot a consistent homozygote effect (RR vs. XX; overall per-allele odds ratio (OR)=1.4, 95% confidence interval (CI) 1.3–1.6; between-study standard deviation (s.d.) τ=0.12, 95% CI 0.01–0.31) but there was substantial heterogeneity in the dominance effect (overall OR=0.98, 95% CI 0.73–1.3; between-study s.d. τ=0.40, 95% CI 0.18–0.72), indicative of the effect of heterozygotes being highly variable (20). Therefore, while the absence of α-actinin-3 (*ACTN3* XX) is strongly correlated with reduced elite sprint/power performance, our study indicates that a nonsingle genetic model can explain the association between *ACTN3* R577X and elite sprint/power performance due to the variable effect of the heterozygotes.

The *Actn3* knockout mouse model

α-*Actinin-3 deficiency "slows" fast-twitch muscle fiber characteristics*

Our group established an α-actinin-3 (*Actn3*) KO mouse model in order to understand the mechanisms underlying the positive selection of the 577X allele and the effects of α-actinin-3 deficiency on muscle performance. *Actn3* KO mice recapitulated human α-actinin-3 deficiency and demonstrated reduced grip strength (7.4% lower), hindlimb muscle force generation (10.9% lower), and enhanced endurance running performance as compared to wild-type (WT) controls (6, 40, 41). Electron microscopy shows normal Z-disk ultrastructure and sarcomeric organization in *Actn3* KO mouse muscles (Figure 23.3). Unlike humans, α-actinin-2 is not expressed in all muscle fibers in WT mice (45), but α-actinin-2 is upregulated and expressed in all fiber types in *Actn3* KO muscles, similar to the expression pattern seen in human *ACTN3* XX (Figure 23.4).

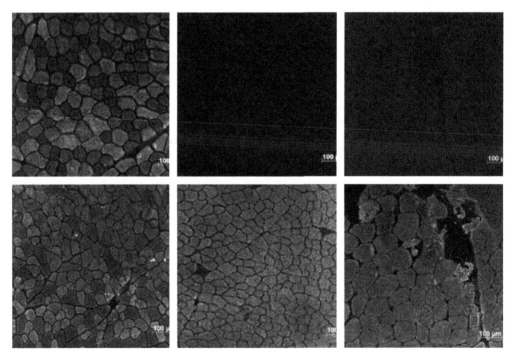

Figure 23.3 α–Actinin-3 deficiency in skeletal muscle. Skeletal muscle cross sections from mouse (WT, *Actn3* KO) and human immuno-stained for α-actinin-3 (top row) and α-actinin-2 (bottom row). α-Actinin-3 deficiency results in up-regulation of α-actinin-2 so that it is expressed in all muscle fibres. Image adapted from (41).

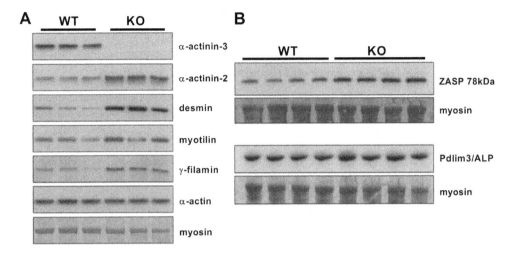

Figure 23.4 Z-disk proteins are upregulated in *Actn3* knockout mice. A) α-Actinin-2, desmin, myotilin, γ-filamin are up-regulated in *Actn3* KO muscle compared to WT muscle; α-actin and myosin as shown as loading controls. B) The expression of the 78kDa isoform of Z-band alternatively spliced PDZ-motif protein (ZASP) is also up-regulated in Actn3 KO muscles, however expression of the ZASP related, actin-associated LIM protein (Pdlim3/ALP) is not altered in KO muscles relative to WT control. Myosin is shown as loading control. Image adapted from (66).

Consistent with reduced muscle force generation, analyses of lean mass by dual-energy X-ray absorptiometry and isolated muscles from WT and *Actn3* KO mice showed that KO muscles are reduced in mass and have smaller fast-twitch fibers. There was no change in fiber type proportions, but analysis of the overall muscle cross-sectional area (CSA) dominated by each fiber type (considering both fiber size and number) showed reduction in 2B CSA and increased 2X CSA in KO muscles relative to WT (21, 40, 67). A number of studies in human cohorts found similar genotype effects. The *ACTN3* 577XX genotype was associated with reductions in lean mass, fat mass, and BMI (72), as well as thigh muscle CSA (77). α-Actinin-3 deficiency was also found to be associated with reduced proportions of fast fibers (71), while other studies assessing active individuals found no association between *ACTN3* genotype and fiber type distribution or fiber size (19, 49).

Enzymatic activities in the anaerobic and aerobic pathways involved in glucose breakdown are also different in *Actn3* KO muscles relative to WT (40, 41). The activity of anaerobic enzyme lactate dehydrogenase (LDH) was reduced by approximately 16% in *Actn3* KO muscle, while mitochondrial enzymes citrate synthase, succinate dehydrogenase, and cytochrome *c* oxidase, were increased by 22–39%. Activities of fatty acid oxidation enzymes, β-hydroxyacyl-CoA dehydrogenase and medium chain acyl-CoA dehydrogenase were also 30–42% higher in *Actn3* KO muscles. These results indicate that deficiency of α-actinin-3 causes fast-twitch muscle fibers to switch to greater reliance on oxidative rather than glycolytic metabolism, consistent with characteristics of a slower-twitch muscle.

The absence of α-actinin-3 also altered the twitch characteristics of fast-twitch muscles. Assessment of the fast fiber-rich, extensor digitorum longus muscles from *Actn3* KO and WT mice showed that *Actn3* KO muscles have longer twitch half-relaxation times and enhanced force recovery following contraction-induced muscle fatigue (6). Single muscle fiber analyses further showed that contractile changes were caused by slower calcium uptake (calcium loading into sarcoplasmic reticulum) in *Actn3* KO fast-twitch fibers compared to WT fibers (5). Together with reduced fast-twitch fiber size and shifts towards oxidative metabolism, these qualities make α-actinin 3-deficient fast-twitch muscles less favorable for rapid, repetitive muscle contractions necessary for sprint/power generation, but beneficial for endurance performance.

ACTN3 genotype and the response to exercise training

Skeletal muscle is capable of adapting to environmental stresses and physiological demands. The baseline phenotypes of the *Actn3* KO mouse confirm that α-actinin-3 plays a key role in the determination of fast-twitch fiber size, fiber type CSA, muscle mass, and metabolism, so it follows that the *Actn3* genotype could also influence how muscle adapts to exercise training. Indeed, elite athletes represent the most well-trained cohorts with decade/s of persistent and specific training – it is conceivable therefore that the effect of the *ACTN3* genotype on elite athletic performance may be enhanced by training.

Consistent with our hypothesis, the shift in fast-twitch fiber properties towards slow-twitch not only predisposed *Actn3* KO mice for endurance performance, but also primed their responsiveness to endurance training. In response to a progressive treadmill running program over 4 weeks, where trained WT mice could run two times further than their untrained counterparts in a maximal incremental run to fatigue (similar to a maximal oxygen consumption (VO_2max) test), trained *Actn3* KO mice were able to run 3.3 times further compared to untrained KO mice (67). Analyses of untrained and trained muscles showed that trained *Actn3* KO muscles had greater 2B to 2X CSA type shifts and higher oxidative enzyme activity compared to trained WT, consistent with enhanced response to endurance training.

The effect of the *ACTN3* genotype on endurance training responsiveness in athletes has so far not been replicated but improved endurance capacity in the general population has been observed in a number of studies (Table 23.2). Similarly, the effect of the *ACTN3* genotype on the response to various resistance training programs has been examined. While some found increased strength gains with 577XX, others observed no clear association with the *ACTN3* genotype (Table 23.2). Overall, there appears to be a positive association between the *ACTN3* 577R allele with higher response to resistance training. This could be reflective of the fast fiber-specific expression of α-actinin-3 and its role in maintaining muscle strength. The response to resistance training has yet to be examined in the *Actn3* mouse model but future investigation could shed light on the mechanism for this training effect in humans. An extensive review of this topic was performed by Garton et al. (19).

α-Actinin-3 influences on muscle strength and performance

To properly understand the phenotypic effects of the *Actn3* KO mouse model, and indeed, α-actinin-3 deficiency in humans, the presence and function of α-actinin-2 in skeletal muscle must also be considered. Total sarcomeric α-actinin content in skeletal muscle is closely regulated; induced overexpression of one sarcomeric α-actinin leads to downregulation of the other (20, 66). The effects of the *Actn3* KO mouse and *ACTN3* 577XX humans must therefore be interpreted as a consequence of the loss of α-actinin-3 and simultaneous upregulation of α-actinin-2 in fast-twitch muscle fibers.

The diverse phenotypes of the *Actn3* KO mouse emphasize the involvement of sarcomeric α-actinins in various systems that govern muscle biology, strength, and performance. As discussed, the sarcomeric α-actinins are components of a sensor machinery through direct protein interactions at both the membrane and the Z-disk (reviewed in 35). Although α-actinin-2 and α-actinin-3 share 80% identity in amino acid sequence (45), functional divergence and fiber type specificity between these closely related proteins are likely mediated by differences in

Table 23.2 ACTN3 genotype and training association studies (endurance and resistance training)

Origin	Sex Age (years)	N	Tested	Significant associations	Reference
Endurance training					
Brazil	M	150	Maximal incremental running test, ventilatory threshold (VT) and respiratory compensation point (RCP)	ACTN3 XX genotype is over-represented in groups with higher VT($P <0.0001$) and respiratory compensation ($P <0.0001$)	53
Estonia	M & F 15–19	58 41 males 17 females	5-year endurance cross-country skiing performance	No significant difference	42
Brazil	M 25 ± 4	206	18 weeks of endurance running training	XX show higher VO_2 at anaerobic threshold, RCP, and exercise peak compared to RR ($P <0.003$). Following training the differences between XX and RR were no longer observed	69
Resistance training					
Spain	F 65.5 ± 8.2	139	2 weeks of high-speed power training on maximal strength (1RM) of the arm and leg muscles, muscle power performance (counter-movement jump), and functional capacity (sit-to-stand test)	Significant genotype-training interaction ($P<0.05$) for all muscular performance indices	56
UK	M 20.3 ± 3.1	51	9-week knee extension resistance training (RT)	ACTN3 R-allele carriers had greater quadriceps femoris muscle volume (Vm), maximum isoinertial strength (1RM), and maximum power (W max) than XX homozygotes at baseline (all $P <0.05$), but responses to RT were independent of ACTN3 genotype (all $P >0.05$)	14

(continued)

Table 23.2 (Cont.)

Origin	Sex Age (years)	N	Tested	Significant associations	Reference
Brazil	F 67	246	Quadriceps isokinetic strength pre and post 24 wks of resistance training	No significant difference	36
Brazil	M 23–31	141	1RM bench press, knee extensors peak torque (60°/s), and knee extensors before and after 11 wks of training	No significant difference	22
		40	Ultrasound muscle thickness before and after 11 wks of training	RR/RX increased muscle thickness after training	
Taiwan	M 11–13	50	12 wks swim training, 25 m and 100 m swim time pre and post, body mass index, % body fat, in young males=serum thyroid, testosterone and growth hormones	In young males; RR had fastest mean before and after training (no *P* value). RX and XX greater improvement in 25 m swim performance vs. RR genotype	7
	M 21–30	38		No significant difference	
US	M 56–74	71	Knee extensor concentric peak power before and after 10 wks of unilateral knee training	Post-training, trend for relative peak power change in RR was higher than XX ($P=0.07$)	11
	F 64	86		Higher peak power and 1RM in XX women at baseline vs. RX/RR. Post-training, relative peak power change in RR was higher than the XX ($P<0.05$)	

binding affinity or selectivity among interaction partners for a specific α-actinin isoform, which could culminate in altered protein complex stability. Based on the known functions of the α-actinin interacting partners, the roles of α-actinin-3 (and α-actinin-2) can be broadly classified into the following categories: structural, signaling, metabolic, and calcium handling.

α-Actinin-3 enhances Z-disk stability

Assessment of *Actn3* WT and KO muscle response to lengthening contractions showed that α-actinin-3 plays a major structural role in the Z-disk. In response to muscle damage induced using repeated eccentric contractions at 30% stretch (equivalent to downhill skiing), *Actn3* KO muscles showed approximately 2.5 times greater force deficits compared to WT (66), indicating that the absence of α-actinin-3 from fast-twitch fibers results in increased susceptibility to eccentric muscle damage. The mechanism underlying the altered Z-disk stability in *Actn3* KO muscles points to an alteration in Z-disk protein composition and interaction. Compensatory upregulation of α-actinin-2 in *Actn3* KO mouse muscles is accompanied by increases in myofibrillar Z-disk proteins γ-filamin, myotilin, and Z-band alternatively spliced PDZ-motif protein (ZASP), as well as the intermediate filament protein desmin (66) (Figure 23.4). These proteins are expressed in both skeletal and cardiac muscle and are known to contribute to Z-disk stability and elasticity. In addition, ZASP, calsarcin-2, titin, and vinculin were shown to preferentially bind to α-actinin-2, while myotilin showed equivalent affinity for α-actinin-2 and α-actinin-3 (66, 67). The interaction between ZASP, titin, and α-actinin-2 is critical for the maintenance of Z-disk integrity during muscle contractions, and titin and vinculin are both involved in the modulation of Z-disk width (33). Together, these findings indicate that α-actinin-3 plays an integral role in stabilizing the Z-disk during lengthening muscle contractions – a role that cannot be fully compensated by increased expression of α-actinin-2 and other Z-disk proteins and tighter protein interactions. As Z-disk rigidity also influences muscle force transmission, changes in protein composition and interactions may also contribute to the reduction in force generation in α-actinin-3-deficient muscles.

Sarcomeric α-actinins regulate calcineurin signaling

Calsarcin-2 (also called myozenin 1 or FATZ) is exclusively expressed in fast-twitch fibers of skeletal muscle and inhibits calcineurin – a calcium/calmodulin-dependent serine, threonine phosphatase that mediates transcription of the slow, oxidative myogenic program in muscle (17). The calsarcin-2 KO mouse demonstrates enhanced calcineurin/NFAT activity, resulting in increases in oxidative metabolism, reduced fast-twitch muscle mass, and increased endurance running capacity – phenotypes similar to the *Actn3* KO mouse model (16). To date, the calsarcin-2 KO and the *Actn3* KO are the only two examples where loss of function resulted in enhanced oxidative phenotype.

This led to our hypothesis that enhanced calcineurin signaling may also occur downstream of α-actinin-3 deficiency (67). Assessment of muscles from the *Actn3* KO mouse model showed significant upregulation of calcineurin activity and expression of the downstream regulator of calcineurin (RCAN1–4) with α-actinin-3 deficiency; these results were also confirmed in human muscle samples. There were no changes in calsarcin-2 expression in WT and *Actn3* KO muscles, but as discussed, calsarcin-2 preferentially binds to α-actinin-2. The calsarcins have overlapping regions that facilitate interaction with α-actinin, γ-filamin, telethonin, and calcineurin that could result in competition for binding with calsarcin (34).

Further investigation of these protein dynamics by co-expressing calsarcin-2, α-actinin-2, and calcineurin in COS cells and co-immunoprecipitation showed that calcineurin is outcompeted for binding with calsarcin-2 in the presence of increasing α-actinin-2 concentrations – resulting in greater release of calcineurin from the inhibitory effects of calsarcin-2 (67). In the context of α-actinin-3 deficiency where α-actinin-2 is overexpressed, the dynamics of these protein interactions thus explain the enhanced calcineurin activity and resultant shifts towards oxidative metabolism in fast-twitch fibers of *Actn3* KO and *ACTN3* 577XX muscles. Increased calcineurin activity at baseline also contributed to the *Actn3* KO muscle adaptive response to endurance training (67).

α-Actinin-3 regulates muscle metabolism through modulation of glycogen phosphorylase activity

The sarcomeric α-actinins also form complexes with a number of metabolic enzymes at the Z-disk, such as glycogen phosphorylase (GPh) (8, 56), fructose 1,6-bisphosphatase, and aldolase (57), suggesting that the sarcomeric α-actinins are likely involved in metabolic sensing with respect to glyconeogenesis and glycogenolysis (34). In the absence of α-actinin-3, GPh activity is significantly reduced by 50%, resulting in almost twice the glycogen content of WT muscles at baseline – suggesting that glycogen breakdown is dysregulated/slower in KO muscles (56). The increase in glycogen content and reduction in GPh activity occurs concomitantly with the changes in glycolytic and mitochondrial enzyme activity and are apparent in *Actn3* KO mouse muscles from at least 4 weeks of age. Together, these results suggest that reduced GPh activity due to α-actinin-3 deficiency necessitates fast-twitch muscle fibers to switch to greater reliance on oxidative metabolism in order to generate ATP at a rate that is sufficient to sustain requirements for rapid force generation. The mechanism by which α-actinin-3 influences GPh activity is yet to be fully uncovered, but proteomic analyses suggest that α-actinin-3 plays a role in the post-translational modification of GPh (56).

Muscle metabolism may indeed be the trait that is most sensitive to changes in α-actinin-3 expression. In our most recent study, we explored the effect of postnatal α-actinin-3 replacement by "gene doping" *Actn3* KO muscles to restore α-actinin-3 expression to WT levels. Contrary to expectations, there were no effects on muscle force generation, muscle mass, fiber size or fiber type, and no changes to Z-disk protein composition or calcineurin signaling (20), but muscle metabolism and response to contraction-induced fatigue were successfully restored to WT levels in rescued *Actn3* KO mice (Figure 23.5). These results suggest that the effect of α-actinin-3 on oxidative metabolism occurs independent of these other traits, or that changes in those traits require expression of α-actinin-3 during muscle development. In contrast, postnatal overexpression of α-actinin-3 in WT muscles caused widespread muscle damage and was detrimental to muscle function and performance.

α-Actinin-3 modifies calcium handling

Intracellular calcium concentration ($[Ca^{2+}]_i$) varies during muscle contraction and relaxation through calcium release and reuptake at the sarcoplasmic reticulum (SR). In addition to modulating glycogenolysis, GPh-a (the serine-14 phosphorylated active form of GPh) is also a negative regulator of SR calcium release – thus providing the functional crosstalk between SR calcium release and ATP generation (25). Consistent with reduced GPh activity, both *Actn3* KO muscle fibers and myotubes in culture show an approximately fourfold higher calcium leak

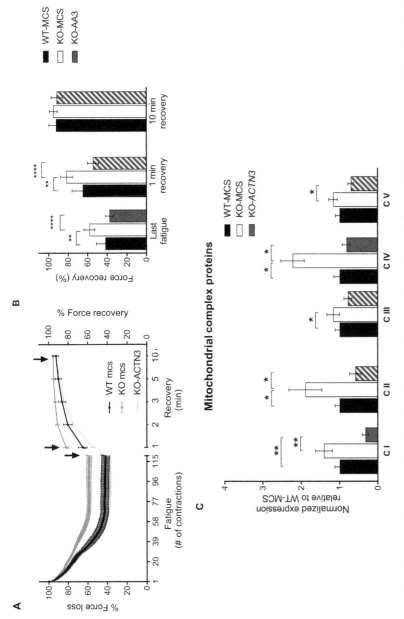

Figure 23.5 Postnatal replacement of α-actinin–3 in *Actn3* knockout muscles restored muscle metabolism and fatigue response to wild-type levels. *Actn3* KO mice received intramuscular injections of recombinant adeno-associated viral vectors (rAAV) carrying human *ACTN3* (KO-*ACTN3*) in the tibialis anterior muscle (TA) of one hindlimb, or empty vector (KO-MCS) in the TA of the contralateral limb. Results were compared to WT muscles injected with empty vector (WT-MCS) at the equivalent dose. A) *In situ* physiology assessments of KO-MCS (red), KO-*ACTN3* (black) and WT-MCS (blue) TA muscles. Muscles were repeatedly and maximally stimulated at 150 Hz (1s on, 1s off) for 2 min and force loss (% maximal force) due to fatigue was recorded. Force recovery was assessed over 1, 2, 3, 5 and 10 mins. Arrows indicate time-points shown in panel B. B) KO-*ACTN3* muscles showed significantly greater force loss and slower force recovery compared to KO-MCS with a force/time profile that is more similar to WT-MCS. C) Protein expression of muscle mitochondrial complexes I–V (CI-V) showed significant upregulation of CII and CIV in KO-MCS compared to WT-MCS, which corresponds to succinate dehydrogenase and cytochrome c oxidase subunit I. Replacement of α-actinin–3 in KO TA muscles (KO-*ACTN3*) resulted in significant decreases in all complexes (I, II, III, IV and V) relative to KO-MCS, to be equal or below WT-MCS levels. Image adapted from (20).

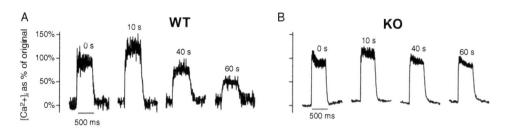

Figure 23.6 WT and *Actn3* knockout [Ca^{2+}]$_i$ transients at 0, 10, 40, and 60 seconds during contraction-induced muscle fatigue. WT muscle fibres show the characteristic pattern of [Ca^{2+}]$_i$ during repeated tetanic stimulation – initially rising, then gradually falling. In contrast, KO fibres maintained [Ca^{2+}]$_i$ longer into the fatigue run. Image adapted from (24).

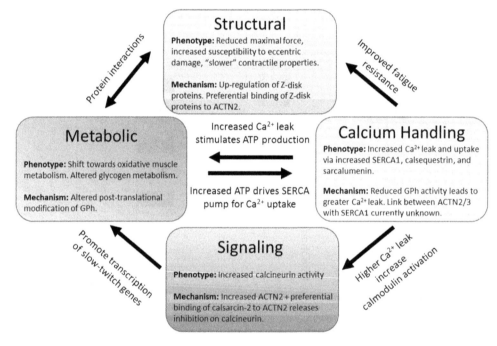

Figure 23.7 Mechanistic insights from *Actn3* knockout mouse model highlighting the structural, metabolic, signaling, and calcium handling pathways. Alterations in all four pathways have been described as a result of α-actinin-3 deficiency. The arrows indicate the cascades between each pathway as well as the phenotype and mechanism thought to be responsible for alterations in each pathway. Image adapted from (33).

compared to WT (24, 56). Calcium reuptake is also approximately threefold higher in KO fibers during twitch relaxation, such that on balance [Ca^{2+}]$_i$ declines more quickly in KO than in WT (24). *Actn3* KO muscles also show slower rate of decay for tetanic [Ca^{2+}]$_i$ compared to WT, in line with increased resistance to fatigue (6, 24, 40) (Figure 23.6). Major proteins associated with the rise of calcium transients (dihydropyridine receptor voltage sensor (DHPR); and ryanodine-receptor Ca^{2+}-release channel (RyR1)), and decay of calcium transients (which includes the calcium buffer parvalbumin, the SR calcium pump SERCA1, and the intraluminal calcium buffers calsequestrin and sarcalumenin) were examined in WT and *Actn3* muscles. Consistent with increased calcium reuptake, *Actn3* KO muscles showed significant increases in SERCA1, calsequestrin, and sarcalumenin. Collectively, these results indicate that α-actinin-3 regulates muscle contractile properties through modulating calcium dynamics.

Mechanistic insights from the Actn3 KO mouse

Our work in the *Actn3* KO mouse is unravelling the complex interplay of the structural, metabolic, signaling, and calcium handling functions of α-actinin-3 and the underlying consequence of α-actinin-3 deficiency that led to the changes in muscle function and performance (Figure 23.7). The primary absence of α-actinin-3 from fast-twitch muscle fibers leads to changes in the recruitment of structural and metabolic proteins at the Z-disk, affecting Z-disk rigidity and force transmission through altered protein composition and binding. This, in turn, enhances calcineurin signaling, as increased α-actinin-2 sequesters calsarcin-2 from its calcineurin inhibitory function. Increased calcineurin activity promotes transcription of slow-twitch genes, which together with reduced GPh activity, drives the metabolic shift toward oxidative metabolism. As part of a continuous cycle, increased mitochondrial respiration supplies the necessary ATP to support increased SERCA1 calcium uptake; the increased demand for ATP signals for greater calcium leak, which in turn stimulates the activities of the tricarboxylic acid cycle enzymes and increases ATP production. Increased calcium leak also induces greater calcium/calmodulin-dependent calcineurin activity, further promoting the maintenance of the slow myogenic program and improving muscle fatigue resistance.

Increased heat generated by ATP hydrolysis as a result of increased SR calcium leakage and pumping in α-actinin-3-deficient muscles would be advantageous in cold environments. Together with improved fatigue resistance and increased mitochondrial activity, *Actn3* KO muscles thus exhibit all the hallmarks of muscles exposed to cold (4), suggesting that *Actn3* KO mice are pre-acclimatized to cold. In addition, the shift towards oxidative muscle metabolism promotes energy efficiency that is beneficial for survival under conditions of famine and enhances endurance capacity. Our findings from the mouse model therefore lend biological support to the positive selection of the *ACTN3* 577X allele during modern human migration out of Africa into colder climates.

Beyond athletics – the role of α-actinin-3 in muscle ageing, disuse, and disease

While the absence of α-actinin-3 does not in itself cause disease, there is accumulating evidence to show that the *ACTN3* genotype is associated with increased morbidity in people who are frail. Several studies have examined the impact of *ACTN3* R577X on skeletal muscle traits and function in the aging population (55). With some exceptions, the general consensus from human and mouse studies is that the effect of the *ACTN3* genotype on some muscle traits and physical performance measures is lifelong, with α-actinin-3 deficiency generally associated with lower muscle mass and strength and higher sarcopenia risk. On this basis, the effect of the *ACTN3* genotype on resistance training response in the elderly is being scrutinized as a way to identify at-risk groups and personalize strategies for sarcopenia prevention and treatment.

The absence of α-actinin-3 also influences how skeletal muscle adapts to disuse. Using the *Actn3* KO mouse model to assess the effects of denervation and immobilization, we found that *Actn3* KO mice exhibit significantly lower levels of muscle and fast 2B fiber atrophy, suggesting that α-actinin-3 deficiency affords a level of protection against muscle wasting (21). Additionally, KO muscles show reduced threshold for fast-to-slow fiber CSA shifts (with immobilization)

Table 23.3 ACTN3 genotype and inherited muscle diseases

Population description (number)	N	Ages (years) Sex	Study results	Reference
Merosin congenital muscular dystrophy (11) Severe childhood autosomal recessive MD (11) Mild limb girdle (13)	54	5–25 M & F	No correlation was found with degree of muscle degeneration or clinical course	70
Neuromuscular disease patients and controls	217	M & F	No difference in the frequency of XX genotypes among individuals with dystrophic, myopathic, neurogenic, or normal muscle histology	51
Human muscle glycogen phosphorylase deficiency (MPL/McArdle's disease)	99	8–81 M & F	No significant relationships identified between clinical severity (daily activity measures) and *ACTN3* genotype	60
	40	34–41 M & F	XX and RX had a higher $V\dot{O}_2$ peak than RR females. No differences in male patients.	37
Inflammatory myopathies Dermatomyositis (DM) (*N*=27) polymyositis (PM) (*N*=10)	37	24–54 M & F	Enhanced proportion XX genotypes in affected group ($P <0.001$). *ACTN3* genotype not related to severity of phenotype or enzyme levels (CPK, LDH, AST, and ALT)	62
Glycogen storage disease type II (GSDII) or Pompe disease	126	58–68 M & F	XX genotype is significantly associated with an early onset of the disease (P=0.024)	10
Duchenne muscular dystrophy (DMD)	61	M	DMD patients with the X-allele show reduced muscle strength and a longer 10 min walk test time	26

and increased threshold for slow-to-fast CSA shifts (with denervation) compared to WT, as well as changes in muscle metabolism and calcineurin signaling with respect to both stimuli that is consistent with maintenance of a "slower" muscle phenotype.

We and others have also examined the role of *ACTN3* R577X in the progression and development of various muscle disorders (Table 23.3). Carriage of the *ACTN3* X-allele was associated with increased exercise tolerance in female patients with McArdle's disease (a disorder of glycogen accumulation) (37), while α-actinin-3 deficiency was associated with increased likelihood of developing inflammatory myopathies (63) and earlier onset of Pompe disease (10). Recently, the *ACTN3* genotype was also correlated with survival in patients with congestive heart failure, with patients carrying the X-allele having 1.72 times higher mortality than patients with the *ACTN3* 577RR genotype (P=0.01) (3).

ACTN3 R577X is a modifier of Duchenne muscular dystrophy.

Duchenne muscular dystrophy (DMD) is an X-linked inherited muscle disease caused by mutations in the dystrophin gene that is characterized by a severe progressive muscle degeneration and weakness. Patients are diagnosed from an early age, typically become wheelchair

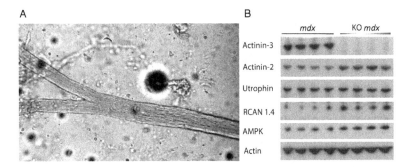

Figure 23.8   Actn3 knockout/*mdx* muscles show slower disease progression compared to *mdx*. A) Fibre branching is a hallmark of damage and regeneration. *Actn3* KO/mdx muscles had markedly fewer complex branched fibres compared to *mdx* muscles. B) Protein expression of a-actinin-2, RCAN1-4 and AMPK is increased in *Actn3* KO/*mdx* (DKO) muscles, consistent with activation of the slow myogenic program. Image adapted from (26).

bound by age 12, and despite careful clinical management, succumb to the disease in their late 20s. The current gold standard therapy for DMD is chronic corticosteroid (prednisone or deflazacort) treatment (47) to slow progression of the disease. There is considerable interpatient variability in DMD onset and progression (12), and much of this variation is thought to arise from the presence of modifier genes that alter disease progression independently from the causative mutations in the *DMD* gene.

Because *ACTN3* R577X is so common and strongly influences muscle function in the general population – both healthy and frail — we hypothesized that the *ACTN3* genotype may also be a disease modifier for DMD. In collaboration with the Cooperative International Neuromuscular Research Group (CINRG) consortium, we examined the association of *ACTN3* R577X with a number of clinical muscle strength and performance measures in 61 young, ambulant patients with DMD (27). Consistent with our hypothesis, patients carrying the *ACTN3* 577X allele showed reduced muscle strength and a longer 10-minute walk test time (Table 23.3). To study the functional implications of the *ACTN3* genotype in DMD, we crossed the *Actn3* KO mouse with the *mdx* mouse (a model for DMD) to generate a double knockout model (*Actn3* KO/*mdx*). Similar to *ACTN3* 577XX patients, *Actn3* KO/*mdx* mice showed reduced muscle strength, but older *Actn3* KO/*mdx* mice showed reduced stretch-induced muscle damage, suggesting that α-actinin-3 deficiency protects dystrophic muscle from contraction induced damage and thereby slows disease progression. Moreover, compared to 12-month-old *mdx* mice, muscle fibers from *Actn3* KO/*mdx* muscles exhibited lower incidence and severity of fiber branching – a hallmark of muscle damage and regeneration (Figure 23.8). Comparison of *Actn3* KO/*mdx* muscles to *mdx* showed no difference in the expression of utrophin, a dystrophin homolog that is highly expressed in developing muscle (68). However, *Actn3* KO/*mdx* muscles showed increased oxidative muscle metabolism compared to *mdx*, which was mediated by significantly higher activation of calcineurin and AMPK signaling. Since slow fibers are less susceptible to damage in the *mdx* mouse (46), the predisposition of "slower" fast-twitch muscles with α-actinin-3 deficiency fibers likely protected *Actn3* KO/*mdx* mice from progressive contraction-induced damage. In addition, enhanced calcineurin signaling is associated with increased regeneration (16). Our combined studies in mice and humans lend support to our hypothesis that the *ACTN3* R577X genotype is a modifier of clinical outcomes in DMD patients.

Therapeutic implications of Actn3 knockout mouse findings for ACTN3 577XX patients

The findings from our muscular dystrophy studies have important implications for clinical management of DMD patients moving forward. Current treatment strategies that aim to replace dystrophin and induce muscle hypertrophy are successful in ameliorating disease (58), but our results from α-actinin-3-deficient muscle suggest that co-delivery of pharmacological interventions that promote slow muscle programming (29) may provide better long-term protective benefits for patients with DMD. Similar strategies could be employed for patients with muscle disuse, since increased shifts towards slow, oxidative metabolism mediated by enhanced calcineurin activity were common in our studies of muscle disuse and muscular dystrophy using the *Actn3* KO mouse model. Continued research in these areas are required and considering the *ACTN3* genotype of patients is likely to inform on their prognosis and develop a more complete clinical picture.

Conclusion

Deficiency of α-actinin-3 is common and its detrimental effect on elite sprint and power performance has been repeatedly demonstrated. The effect of α-actinin-3 deficiency on more vulnerable populations, such as those who are elderly or suffer from muscle disuse or disease, will benefit greatly from further research, especially for conditions that could be treated or ameliorated using exercise training interventions, and for identifying patients who are at greater risk for steeper decline. Phenotypic analysis of the *Actn3* KO mouse model has revealed valuable insights regarding the specialized role of α-actinin-3 and its cooperative functions with α-actinin-2 in regulating muscle structure, cell signaling, metabolism, and calcium handling. Further research into the mechanisms behind α-actinin-3 deficiency could aid identification of therapeutic targets for personalized, precision medicine and provide better understanding towards the positive selection of the *ACTN3* 577X allele and its implications for health in modern society.

References

1. **Alfred T**, et al. ACTN3 genotype, athletic status, and life course physical capability: meta-analysis of the published literature and findings from nine studies. *Hum Mutat* 32: 1008–1018, 2011.
2. **Ben-Zaken S**, et al. ACTN3 polymorphism: comparison between elite swimmers and runners. *Sports Med Open* 1: 13, 2015.
3. **Bernardez-Pereira S**, et al. ACTN3 R577X polymorphism and long-term survival in patients with chronic heart failure. *BMC Cardiovasc Disord* 14: 90, 2014.
4. **Bruton JD**, et al. Increased fatigue resistance linked to Ca2+-stimulated mitochondrial biogenesis in muscle fibres of cold-acclimated mice. *J Physiol* 588: 4275–4288, 2010.
5. **Chan S**, et al. Properties of extensor digitorum longus muscle and skinned fibers from adult and aged male and female Actn3 knockout mice. *Muscle Nerve* 43: 37–48, 2011.
6. **Chan S**, et al. A gene for speed: contractile properties of isolated whole EDL muscle from an alpha-actinin-3 knockout mouse. *Am J Physiol* 295: C897–C904, 2008.
7. **Chiu LL**, et al. ACTN3 genotype and swimming performance in Taiwan. *Int J Sports Med* 32: 476–480, 2011.
8. **Chowrashi P**, et al. Amorphin is phosphorylase; phosphorylase is an alpha-actinin-binding protein. *Cell Motil Cytoskeleton* 53: 125–135, 2002.
9. **Cieszczyk P**, et al. Association of the ACTN3 R577X polymorphism in Polish power-orientated athletes. *J Hum Kinet* 28: 55–61, 2011.

10. **De Filippi P**, et al. Genotype-phenotype correlation in Pompe disease, a step forward. *Orphanet J Rare Dis* 9: 102, 2014.
11. **Delmonico MJ**, et al. Alpha-actinin-3 (ACTN3) R577X polymorphism influences knee extensor peak power response to strength training in older men and women. *J Gerontol A Biol Sci Med Sci* 62: 206–212, 2007.
12. **Desguerre I**, et al. Clinical heterogeneity of Duchenne muscular dystrophy (DMD): definition of sub-phenotypes and predictive criteria by long-term follow-up. *PLoS One* 4: e4347, 2009.
13. **Druzhevskaya AM**, et al. Association of the ACTN3 R577X polymorphism with power athlete status in Russians. *Eur J Appl Physiol* 103: 631–634, 2008.
14. **Erskine RM**, et al. The individual and combined influence of ACE and ACTN3 genotypes on muscle phenotypes before and after strength training. *Scand J Med Sci Sports* 24: 642–648, 2014.
15. **Eynon N**, et al. ACTN3 R577X polymorphism and Israeli top-level athletes. *Int J Sports Med* 30: 695–698, 2009.
16. **Frey N**, et al. Calsarcin-2 deficiency increases exercise capacity in mice through calcineurin/NFAT activation. *J Clin Invest* 118: 3598–3608, 2008.
17. **Frey N**, et al. Calsarcins, a novel family of sarcomeric calcineurin-binding proteins. *Proc Natl Acad Sci U S A* 97: 14632–14637, 2000.
18. **Friedlander SM**, et al. ACTN3 Allele frequency in humans covaries with global latitudinal gradient. *PLoS One* 8: e52282, 2013.
19. **Garton FC** and **North KN**. The effect of heterozygosity for the ACTN3 null allele on human muscle performance. *Med Sci Sports Exerc* 2015.
20. **Garton FC**, et al. The effect of ACTN3 gene doping on skeletal muscle performance. *Am J Hum Genet* 102: 845–857, 2018.
21. **Garton FC**, et al. alpha-Actinin-3 deficiency alters muscle adaptation in response to denervation and immobilization. *Hum Mol Genet* 23: 1879–1893, 2014.
22. **Gentil P**, et al. ACTN3 R577X polymorphism and neuromuscular response to resistance training. *J Sports Sci Med* 10: 393–399, 2011.
23. **Gineviciene V**, et al. Association analysis of ACE, ACTN3 and PPARGC1A gene polymorphisms in two cohorts of European strength and power athletes. *Biol Sport* 33: 199–206, 2016.
24. **Head SI**, et al. Altered Ca2+ kinetics associated with alpha-actinin-3 deficiency may explain positive selection for ACTN3 null allele in human evolution. *PLoS Genet* 11: e1004862, 2015.
25. **Hirata Y**, et al. Mastoparan binds to glycogen phosphorylase to regulate sarcoplasmic reticular Ca2+ release in skeletal muscle. *Biochem J* 371: 81–88, 2003.
26. **Hogarth MW**, et al. Analysis of the ACTN3 heterozygous genotype suggests that alpha-actinin-3 controls sarcomeric composition and muscle function in a dose-dependent fashion. *Hum Mol Genet* 25: 866–877, 2016.
27. **Hogarth MW**, et al. Evidence for ACTN3 as a genetic modifier of Duchenne muscular dystrophy. *Nat Comm* 8: 14143, 2017.
28. **Hong SSJ** and **Jin HJ**. Assessment of association of ACTN3 genetic polymorphism with Korean elite athletic performance. *Genes Genomics* 35: 617, 2013.
29. **Jahnke VE**, et al. Metabolic remodeling agents show beneficial effects in the dystrophin-deficient mdx mouse model. *Skelet Muscle* 2: 16, 2012.
30. **Kikuchi N**, et al. Higher frequency of the ACTN3 R allele + ACE DD genotype in Japanese elite wrestlers. *J Strength Cond Res* 26: 3275–3280, 2012.
31. **Kikuchi N**, et al. ACTN3 R577X genotype and athletic performance in a large cohort of Japanese athletes. *Eur J Sport Sci* 16: 694–701, 2016.
32. **Kim H**, et al. The ACTN3 R577X variant in sprint and strength performance. *J Exerc Nutrition Biochem* 18: 347–353, 2014.
33. **Lee FX**, et al. How does alpha-actinin-3 deficiency alter muscle function? Mechanistic insights into ACTN3, the "gene for speed". *Biochim Biophys Acta* 1863: 686–693, 2016.
34. **Lek M** and **North KN**. Are biological sensors modulated by their structural scaffolds? The role of the structural muscle proteins alpha-actinin-2 and alpha-actinin-3 as modulators of biological sensors. *FEBS Lett* 584: 2974–2980, 2010.
35. **Lek M**, et al. The evolution of skeletal muscle performance: gene duplication and divergence of human sarcomeric α-actinins. *Bioessays* 32: 17–25, 2010.

36. **Lima RM**, et al. ACE and ACTN3 genotypes in older women: muscular phenotypes. *Int J Sports Med* 32: 66–72, 2011.
37. **Lucia A**, et al. The 577X allele of the ACTN3 gene is associated with improved exercise capacity in women with McArdle's disease. *Neuromuscul Disord* 17: 603–610, 2007.
38. **Ma F**, et al. The association of sport performance with ACE and ACTN3 genetic polymorphisms: a systematic review and meta-analysis. *PLoS One* 8: e54685, 2013.
39. **MacArthur DG** and **North KN**. A gene for speed? The evolution and function of alpha-actinin-3. *Bioessays* 26: 786–795, 2004.
40. **MacArthur DG**, et al. An Actn3 knockout mouse provides mechanistic insights into the association between alpha-actinin-3 deficiency and human athletic performance. *Hum Mol Genet* 17: 1076–1086, 2008.
41. **MacArthur DG**, et al. Loss of ACTN3 gene function alters mouse muscle metabolism and shows evidence of positive selection in humans. *Nat Genet* 39: 1261–1265, 2007.
42. **Magi A**, et al. The association analysis between ACE and ACTN3 genes polymorphisms and endurance capacity in young cross-country skiers: longitudinal study. *J Sports Sci Med* 15: 287–294, 2016.
43. **Massidda M**, et al. Association between the ACTN3 R577X polymorphism and artistic gymnastic performance in Italy. *Genet Test Mol Biomarkers* 13: 377–380, 2009.
44. **Mikami E**, et al. ACTN3 R577X genotype is associated with sprinting in elite Japanese athletes. *Int J Sports Med* 35: 172–177, 2014.
45. **Mills M**, et al. Differential expression of the actin-binding proteins, alpha-actinin-2 and -3, in different species: implications for the evolution of functional redundancy. *Hum Mol Genet* 10: 1335–1346, 2001.
46. **Moens P**, et al. Increased susceptibility of EDL muscles from mdx mice to damage induced by contractions with stretch. *J Muscle Res Cell Motil* 14: 446–451, 1993.
47. **Moxley RT**, 3rd, et al. Practice parameter: corticosteroid treatment of Duchenne dystrophy: report of the Quality Standards Subcommittee of the American Academy of Neurology and the Practice Committee of the Child Neurology Society. *Neurology* 64: 13–20, 2005.
48. **Niemi AK**, and **Majamaa K**. Mitochondrial DNA and ACTN3 genotypes in Finnish elite endurance and sprint athletes. *Eur J Hum Genet* 13: 965–969, 2005.
49. **Norman B**, et al. Strength, power, fiber types, and mRNA expression in trained men and women with different ACTN3 R577X genotypes. *J Appl Physiol (1985)* 106: 959–965, 2009.
50. **North KN** and **Beggs AH**. Deficiency of a skeletal muscle isoform of alpha-actinin (alpha-actinin-3) in merosin-positive congenital muscular dystrophy. *Neuromuscul Disord* 6: 229–235, 1996.
51. **North KN**, et al. A common nonsense mutation results in alpha-actinin-3 deficiency in the general population. *Nat Genet* 21: 353–354, 1999.
52. **Papadimitriou ID**, et al. The ACTN3 gene in elite Greek track and field athletes. *Int J Sports Med* 29: 352–355, 2008.
53. **Pasqua LA**, et al. Influence of ACTN3 R577X polymorphism on ventilatory thresholds related to endurance performance. *J Sports Sci* 34: 163–170, 2016.
54. **Pereira A**, et al. ACE I/D and ACTN3 R/X polymorphisms as potential factors in modulating exercise-related phenotypes in older women in response to a muscle power training stimuli. *Age* 35: 1949–1959, 2013.
55. **Pickering C** and **Kiely J**. ACTN3, morbidity, and healthy aging. *Front Genet* 9: 15, 2018.
56. **Quinlan KGR**, et al. Alpha-actinin-3 deficiency results in reduced glycogen phosphorylase activity and altered calcium handling in skeletal muscle. *Hum Mol Genet* 19: 1335–1346, 2010.
57. **Rakus D**, et al. Interaction between muscle aldolase and muscle fructose 1,6-bisphosphatase results in the substrate channeling. *Biochemistry* 43: 14948–14957, 2004.
58. **Rodino-Klapac LR**, et al. Micro-dystrophin and follistatin co-delivery restores muscle function in aged DMD model. *Hum Mol Genet* 22: 4929–4937, 2013.
59. **Roth SM**, et al. The ACTN3 R577X nonsense allele is under-represented in elite-level strength athletes. *Eur J Hum Genet* 16: 391–394, 2008.
60. **Rubio JC**, et al. Genotype modulators of clinical severity in McArdle disease. *Neurosci Lett* 422: 217–222, 2007.
61. **Ruiz JR**, et al. Can we identify a power-oriented polygenic profile? *J Appl Physiol (1985)* 108: 561–566, 2010.
62. **Sandoval-García F**, et al. The ACTN3 R577X polymorphism is associated with inflammatory myopathies in a Mexican population. *Scand J Rheumatol* 41: 396–400, 2012.

63. **Sandoval-Garcia F**, et al. The ACTN3 R577X polymorphism is associated with inflammatory myopathies in a Mexican population. *Scand J Rheumatol* 41: 396–400, 2012.
64. **Scott RA**, et al. ACTN3 and ACE genotypes in elite Jamaican and US sprinters. *Med Sci Sports Exerc* 42: 107–112, 2010.
65. **Sessa F**, et al. Gene polymorphisms and sport attitude in Italian athletes. *Genet Test Mol Biomarkers* 15: 285–290, 2011.
66. **Seto JT**, et al. Deficiency of α-actinin-3 is associated with increased susceptibility to contraction-induced damage and skeletal muscle remodeling. *Hum Mol Genet* 20: 2914–2927, 2011.
67. **Seto JT**, et al. ACTN3 genotype influences muscle performance through the regulation of calcineurin signaling. *J Clin Invest* 123: 4255–4263, 2013.
68. **Seto JT**, et al. Gene replacement therapies for duchenne muscular dystrophy using adeno-associated viral vectors. *Curr Gene Ther* 12: 139–151, 2012.
69. **Silva MS**, et al. Elimination of influences of the ACTN3 R577X variant on oxygen uptake by endurance training in healthy individuals. *Int J Sports Physiol Perform* 10: 636–641, 2015.
70. **Vainzof M**, et al. Deficiency of alpha-actinin-3 (ACTN3) occurs in different forms of muscular dystrophy. *Neuropediatrics* 28: 223–228, 1997.
71. **Vincent B**, et al. The ACTN3 (R577X) genotype is associated with fiber type distribution. *Physiol Genomics* 32: 58–63, 2007.
72. **Walsh S**, et al. ACTN3 genotype is associated with muscle phenotypes in women across the adult age span. *J Appl Physiol* 105: 1486–1491, 2008.
73. **Weyerstrass J**, et al. Nine genetic polymorphisms associated with power athlete status – a meta-analysis. *J Sci Med Sport* 21: 213–220, 2018.
74. **Yang N**, et al. ACTN3 genotype is associated with human elite athletic performance. *Am J Hum Genet* 73: 627–631, 2003.
75. **Yang N**, et al. The ACTN3 R577X polymorphism in East and West African athletes. *Med Sci Sports Exerc* 39: 1985–1988, 2007.
76. **Yang R**, et al. ACTN3 R577X gene variant is associated with muscle-related phenotypes in elite Chinese sprint/power athletes. *J Strength Cond Res* 31: 1107–1115, 2017.
77. **Zempo H**, et al. ACTN3 polymorphism affects thigh muscle area. *Int J Sports Med* 31: 138–142, 2010.

SECTION 5

Systems genetics of sports performance

As we transition into the later sections of the book, we build on the foundational information of the previous chapters and now add substantial complexity. Whereas the previous chapters have looked at the systems genetics underlying particular phenotypes (e.g., physical activity, cardiorespiratory fitness, and muscle size), Section 5 now moves to similar questions related to sport and exercise performance. Performance is remarkably challenging to measure, and by definition elite-level performance is rare. The complexity of performance is in part due to the fact that it is not a trait per se, but an outcome of many traits working in combination. Moreover, performance is generally tied to competition, which additionally imparts elements of environmental conditions and chance that laboratory-based trait measurements are meant to minimize.

The authors contributing to Section 5 are experts in a variety of related fields and provide unique insights into the role of systems genetics on different aspects of sport and exercise performance. In Chapter 24, Dr. Nir Eynon and his team from Victoria University in Australia provide a review of the genetic aspects of sport performance and lay the foundation for the section. Chapter 25, contributed by Drs. Colin Moran, Alun Williams, and Guan Wang from the UK, delves into the use of elite athletes as models for genetic analysis. These unique performers who rise to the very top of their sport can provide unique insights into what makes them so good, yet their small numbers challenge our statistical models. In Chapter 26, Drs. José Maia and Peter Katzmarzyk look at how our familial relations, specifically in the form of twin and family-based genetic studies, can further inform our understanding of genetic contributions to performance and related traits. Chapters 27 and 28 examine a frequent side effect of engagement in sport: injury. While certain sports lend themselves to greater rates of injury, genetic susceptibility has emerged as a contributing factor for certain individuals. Chapter 27, by Drs. Ryan Tierney and Jane McDevitt from Temple University in the US, considers the systems genetics of brain injury, in particular concussion, which has gained public attention across the world in recent years. Chapter 28 focuses below the neck, with Dr. Malcolm Collins and his team from South Africa specifically examining the role of genetic susceptibility to soft tissue injuries, such as tendon and ligament tears. As genetic testing costs shrink and our understanding of genetic susceptibility improves, the push for genetic testing in these areas will increase with the hopes of reducing injury rates in athletes (as we explore more broadly in Section 6).

We end Section 5 with a chapter focused on the broader theme of sex and performance. While we know that performance in men's and women's sport differs in many areas, justifying sex separation in the vast majority of sports leagues, what is less certain is the basis for these underlying differences. In Chapter 29, Dr. Mindy Millard-Stafford and Matthew Wittbrodt from the US review the evidence for sex differences in sport performance and outline the latest hypotheses for why these differences exist.

In total, Section 5 not only provides a bookend for the prior sections of the book, by pulling in the trait-specific analyses of preceding chapters and viewing them through the complex lens of performance, but also opens a door to Section 6, which will examine the ethical questions inherent in advancing sport performance with our growing understanding of systems genetics. We have many gaps in our knowledge, as outlined in these insightful chapters, but as those gaps are narrowed, athletes, coaches, and others will use this information to their advantage to try to pursue performance improvements.

24

SUMMARY FINDINGS ON GENETICS AND SPORT PERFORMANCE

Macsue Jacques, Shanie Landen, Sarah Voisin, and Nir Eynon

Introduction

In the past decades, the genetic basis for athletic performance and response to exercise training (trainability) has become a topic of great interest. Twin and familial studies have shown that part of the interindividual variability reported in sports science studies can be explained by the genetic makeup of individuals (16). Although humans' DNA sequences are similar at 99.9%, genetic mutations are found across the genome at a rate of approximately 1 change per 1000 base pairs. Some of these mutations consist of the replacement of a single nucleotide by another and are referred to as single nucleotide polymorphisms (SNPs). Those SNPs can be rare (occur at a frequency <1%) or common (occur at a frequency >1%) within a given population. Each human carries 3–4 million common variants and 200,000–500,000 rare variants, and some of these variants are involved in athletic performance and trainability. To discover those variants, initially candidate gene approaches and then later genome-wide association studies (GWAS) were conducted (Figure 24.1). To date, more than 200 genetic variants have been associated with athletic performance or trainability in at least one study (1, 10, 14, 22, 52, 53, 65). These findings suggest that athletic performance and trainability are not determined by a single gene but by a plethora of genes and are therefore considered complex traits. In this chapter, we will summarize the findings on genetics and sport performance and we will discuss some of the current research efforts that are undergoing to further characterize "exercise genes."

Exercise performance and heritability

It is common for more than one family member to be an athlete. There is a long list of successful sibling athletes (i.e., the Williams sisters in tennis), and parent and child athletes (i.e., John Kelly and John Kelly Jr. in rowing). Examples like these highlight not only the significance of family support in producing a successful athlete, but also the potential role of genetic predisposition to exceptional athletic performance. In science, the genetic predisposition for a given trait is measured by a quantity called "heritability." Heritability is defined as the proportion of variance in a trait that is explained by heritable factors, for a given population at a given moment in time (7). Heritability in exercise performance was first introduced by twin and family studies in the 1970s–1990s. A pioneering study on 25 pairs of twins found that about 93% of the variation

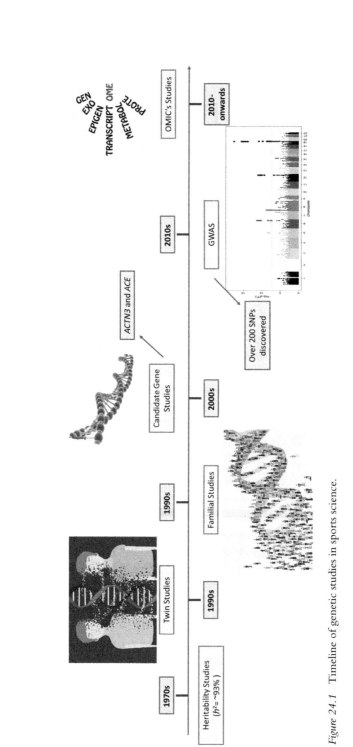

Figure 24.1 Timeline of genetic studies in sports science.

in VO_2max is explained by genetic factors (26). However, this study assumed similar environmental interaction between twin pairs and the absence of gene–environment correlation, which is not necessarily true and may overestimate heritability (19). High heritability estimates were also found for skeletal muscle fiber composition (h^2=96.5%) (26), maximal power (h^2=97%), and maximal isometric force (h^2=83%) (23). Subsequent to these pioneering studies, other twin and family studies also reported high heritability estimates for VO_{2max} (77% (17), 69–87% (31), and 71% (38)). A meta-analysis of eight twin studies found a weighted VO_2max heritability estimate of 72% (50). In addition to those, several other studies in different areas have attempted to estimate heritability in different cohorts and phenotypic traits (28, 29, 34, 35, 57, 58). Although heritability studies did not require genetic testing to create estimations, they played an important role in the full comprehension of the heritability concept, often misunderstood (19). For example, when said that VO_2max h^2=93%, is almost always misinterpreted to mean that 93% of this phenotype is genetically determined and only 7% would be affected to environment stimuli. Heritability only has a meaning at the population level and is irrelevant at an individual level. In addition, heritability varies depending on the studied population (e.g., young, old, healthy, and diseased) and time as the environment can change with time. As previously written:

> [Heritability] describes the extent to which heredity affects the variation of a given attribute in a given population exposed to common environmental influences at a given time. A high heritable attribute does not mean that a phenotype is predetermined and the environment has no effect. It only indicates that the observed individual differences in the given attribute are due to genetic differences and are highly predictable. (19)

Following heritability estimates for aerobic and muscular fitness at a single timepoint, the heritability of *responses* to exercise training (trainability) was also calculated in the large-scale HEalth, RIsk factors, exercise Training And GEnetics (HERITAGE) Family Study in the 1990s. After adjusting for confounders such as age, sex, baseline VO_2max, body mass, and composition, the HERITAGE Family Study reported that approximately 47–50% of the variance in VO_2max improvements following exercise training was due to genetic factors (3). The variance in individual training response between families was 2.5 times higher than within families. As a result of family and twin studies reporting consistently high heritability estimates, a hunt for the genes responsible for both athletic performance and trainability began.

Linkage analyses and the candidate gene approach

The pivotal HERITAGE Family Study (4) and two other twin and family studies (36, 56) performed linkage analysis to detect the chromosomal location of genes associated with athletic status, physical activity level, and trainability. They identified markers on several chromosomes, which were associated with their traits of interest, but few of them were in common. The completion of the Human Genome Project in 2001 (59) allowed for the development of genetic studies based on genes with a specific function. This method, called the "candidate gene approach," was a hypothesis-driven approach whereby the frequency of mutations in genes with a potentially relevant function for exercise was compared between athletes and controls, or associated with aerobic and muscular fitness measures (20). A recent review reported that about 200 SNPs have been associated with performance traits in at least one study, and around 25 SNPs with athletic status (16, 61, 65). These SNPs were found to have an extremely small effect size, which means that their individual contribution to the variability in performance traits and athletic status was tiny, and therefore hard to detect. In addition, only two SNPs showed consistent replication across different studies and populations.

One of them is located in the *ACTN3* gene. The alpha-actinin-3 protein, encoded by the *ACTN3* gene, is almost exclusively expressed in the sarcomeres of fast glycolytic type II fibers that generate powerful, explosive contractions (67). The unique expression pattern and sequence conservation of alpha-actinin-3 over 300 million years in humans, suggest that it has an important function in fast, glycolytic (type IIX) muscle fibers (33). A common SNP in this gene causes the substitution of an R (arginine) for a stop codon (X) at amino acid position 577, resulting in complete deficiency of the alpha-actinin-3 protein (*ACTN3* XX variant) (67). The *ACTN3* R577X variant has been extensively studied in sports performance. The earliest findings reported that fewer Australian sprint elite athletes than healthy controls carried the XX genotype (66). Many replication studies in different cohorts of varying ethnicities found a systematically lower frequency of the XX genotype in strength and power athletes compared with controls and endurance athletes (13, 15, 21, 40, 42, 49, 67). Overall, nearly all studies on *ACTN3* and sports performance reported the same findings: the RR genotype is associated with strength and muscle power, while the XX genotype tends to be associated with endurance performance, but this association is less pronounced (12, 15, 18, 24, 25, 30, 41, 43, 54, 55).

Another gene that has showed consistent replication in exercise science is the angiotensin-converting enzyme (*ACE*) gene. ACE converts the angiotensin I hormone to another form named angiotensin II (46). Angiotensin II helps regulate blood pressure and may also influence skeletal muscle function, although this role is not completely understood (9). A polymorphism in the *ACE* gene that consists of an insertion (I) or a deletion (D) of a segment of DNA (with a length of 287 bp of nucleotides), alters the levels of the ACE enzyme in blood. Individuals can have either zero (DD genotype), one (ID genotype), or two (II genotype) insertions at the *ACE* I/D polymorphism. Of the three genotypes, DD, is associated with the highest levels of ACE in blood (64). DD carriers have a higher proportion of fast-twitch muscle fibers and greater speed (44, 52). However, findings on *ACE* are more conflicting, and less convincing than those on *ACTN3*. The initial findings that II carriers are better at endurance while DD carriers are better at power/strength (37, 46) was not replicated in some studies (8, 51), perhaps due to different cohorts or small sample sizes.

In addition to *ACTN3* and *ACE*, many other genes with diverse functions have been associated with exercise-related traits without showing consistent replication. Some are involved in skeletal muscle function, while others play roles in the production of cellular energy or communication between nerve cells. From the candidate gene approach, the large-scale screening of millions of SNPs and their association with exercise-related traits in genome-wide association studies (GWAS) has greatly advanced the field.

Genome-wide association studies

With advances in microarray-based high-throughput technologies, screening hundreds of thousands, and even millions of SNPs simultaneously has been made possible. The GWAS approach is an unbiased, hypothesis-free design that has led to substantial progress in the field of disease genetics (32) and more recently in the field of sport performance. In fact, this method has identified a plethora of genes, whose variants can be related to physical performance, achievement, and sports results. Unfortunately, this method also revealed that genes influencing exercise performance and their relationships are more complex than previously thought. The HERITAGE Family Study was the first GWAS to identify several SNPs related to VO_2max trainability in an unbiased, hypothesis-free manner (5). However, replications of those SNPs were unsuccessful (19). This lack of replication may be explained by a lack of statistical power in replication studies, as SNPs that influence exercise-related traits have typically very small effect sizes. In other words, those SNPs have such a small effect on the phenotype of interest that it is challenging to detect their effect, thus leading to negative results. A recent GWAS was conducted on a total of 1520 elite athletes and 2760 controls spanning eight different cohorts of athletes from Australia, Ethiopia, Japan, Kenya, Poland, Russia, and Spain (47). Forty-five promising SNPs were found during the discovery phase but failed to pass the replication phase. The study was likely underpowered to identify alleles with small effect sizes, perhaps due to the fact that the technology used was an earlier-generation microarray covering only 195,000 gene markers (48). Another GWAS of 492 strength/power and 227 endurance athletes found that the rare T allele of rs939787 in the dystrophin gene (*DMD*) was overrepresented among strength/power athletes compared with endurance athletes (25% vs. 8.8%) (39). Even more recently, 16 novel genetic loci were associated with handgrip strength (a simple measure of functional strength) in a large-scale GWAS of 195,180 individuals; however, those interesting findings await replication (63). Although candidate gene and GWAS studies have increased our understanding of the genetic contribution to athletic performance, especially with regard to effect sizes, those initial findings need to be replicated. In addition, the molecular mechanisms by which those SNPs act need to be uncovered to have a clear picture of how the genetic makeup shapes the athletic potential and exercise adaptation.

Conclusion and recommendations for future research

To date, neither candidate genes nor genome-wide associations have convincingly validated any of the target genes discovered by the pioneering HERITAGE Family Study (5), and the largest GWAS combining more than 1500 athletes found no evidence of a common DNA variant profile specific to world-class endurance athletes (47). The limited progress in genetics and sports performance achieved today is due to small and mostly heterogeneous cohorts, resulting in doubtful and conflicting findings (19, 62). There is a necessity for larger collective work, with well-defined phenotypes of interest, tightly controlled interventions, and subsequent replication studies to produce robust results. Sports scientists have answered this call by creating the "Athlome Project Consortium" (www.athlomeconsortium.org). This multicentered, international collaborative action intends to create a large databank, with enough expertise and state-of-the-art "omics" technologies from around the world. This project aims to expand knowledge on genetic variants involved in sports performance, trainability, and injury predisposition (more about this project can be found in a recent review, see 62).

Bouchard also argued that there is a need for a paradigm shift in the field (2). Research should be conducted using an unbiased approach, using the full power of genomics, epigenomics, and transcriptomics together with large-scale cohorts and validation studies. Fortunately, the Athlome Consortium meets those suggested criteria, and the project published a GWAS on eight different cohorts of athletes (48) and announced the sequencing of 1000 of the world's greatest athletes as part of the 1000 Athlome Project (45). The field has progressed from heritability models to comprehensive sequencing and genetic screening, but to fully comprehend the mechanism of action of exercise-related variants, it is essential to consider interactions between those genetic variants and the environment. Perhaps the epigenetic response to exercise training will help scientists understand changes in gene function that cannot be explained by changes in DNA sequences (60). Epigenetics is an attractive mechanism to explain the paradoxical findings of identical twins who differ in heritable traits (6, 27). The field of sports and epigenetics is still in its infancy, and the mechanisms that modulate gene expression are not well understood (11).

Great challenges lay ahead in the field of sports and genomics/epigenomics, but it is an exciting future to dissect the role of epigenetic and genetic modifications on sports performance and trainability.

References

1. **Ben-Zaken S, Meckel Y, Nemet D, Eliakim A**. IGF-I receptor 275124A>C (rs1464430) polymorphism and athletic performance. *J Sci Med Sport* 18: 323–327, 2015.
2. **Bouchard C**. Exercise genomics—a paradigm shift is needed: a commentary. *Br J Sports Med* 49: 1492–1496, 2015.
3. **Bouchard C, An P, Rice T, Skinner JS, Wilmore JH, Gagnon J, Perusse L, Leon AS, Rao DC**. Familial aggregation of VO2 max response to exercise training: results from the HERITAGE Family Study. *J Appl Physiol* 87: 1003–1008, 1999.
4. **Bouchard C, Rankinen T, Chagnon YC, Rice T, Pérusse L, Gagnon J, Borecki I, An P, Leon AS, Skinner JS, Wilmore JH, Province M, Rao DC**. Genomic scan for maximal oxygen uptake and its response to training in the HERITAGE Family Study. *J Appl Physiol* 88: 551–559, 2000.
5. **Bouchard C, Sarzynski M a, Rice TK, Kraus WE, Church TS, Sung YJ, Rao DC, Rankinen T**. Genomic predictors of the maximal O_2 uptake response to standardized exercise training programs. *J Appl Physiol* 110: 1160–1170, 2011.
6. **Bouchard T, Lykken D, McGue M, Segal N, Tellegen A**. Sources of human psychological differences: the Minnesota Study of Twins Reared Apart. *Science* 250: 223–228, 1990.
7. **Cesarini D, Visscher PM**. Genetics and educational attainment. *NPJ Sci Learn* 2: 4, 2017.
8. **Day SH, Gohlke P, Dhamrait SS, Williams AG**. No correlation between circulating ACE activity and VO2max or mechanical efficiency in women. *Eur J Appl Physiol* 99: 11–18, 2007.
9. **Djarova T, Bardarev D, Boyanov D, Kaneva R, Atanasov P**. Performance enhancing genetic variants, oxygen uptake, heart rate, blood pressure and body mass index of elite high altitude mountaineers. *Acta Physiol Hung* 100: 289–301, 2013.
10. **Egorova ES, Borisova A V, Mustafina LJ, Arkhipova AA, Gabbasov RT, Druzhevskaya AM, Astratenkova I V, Ahmetov II**. The polygenic profile of Russian football players. *J Sports Sci* 32: 1286–1293, 2014.
11. **Ehlert T, Simon P, Moser DA**. Epigenetics in sports. *Sport Med* 43: 93–110, 2013.
12. **Eynon N, Banting LK, Ruiz JR, Cieszczyk P, Dyatlov DA, Maciejewska-Karlowska A, Sawczuk M, Pushkarev VP, Kulikov LM, Pushkarev ED, Femia P, Stepto NK, Bishop DJ, Lucia A**. ACTN3 R577X polymorphism and team-sport performance: a study involving three European cohorts. *J Sci Med Sport* 17: 102–106, 2014.
13. **Eynon N, Duarte JA, Oliveira J, Sagiv M, Yamin C, Meckel Y, Sagiv M, Goldhammer E**. *ACTN3* R577X polymorphism and Israeli top-level athletes. *Int J Sports Med* 30: 695–698, 2009.
14. **Eynon N, Hanson ED, Lucia A, Houweling PJ, Garton F, North KN, Bishop DJ**. Genes for elite power and sprint performance: ACTN3 leads the way. *Sport Med* 43: 803–817, 2013.
15. **Eynon N, Ruiz JR, Femia P, Pushkarev VP, Cieszczyk P, Maciejewska-Karlowska A, Sawczuk M, Dyatlov DA, Lekontsev EV, Kulikov LM, Birk R, Bishop DJ, Lucia A**. The ACTN3 R577X polymorphism across three groups of elite male European athletes. PLoS One 7, 2012.
16. **Eynon N, Ruiz JR, Oliveira J, Duarte JA, Birk R, Lucia A**. Genes and elite athletes: a roadmap for future research. *J Physiol* 589: 3063–3070, 2011.
17. **Fagard R, Bielen E, Amery A**. Heritability of aerobic power and anaerobic energy generation during exercise. *J Appl Physiol* 70: 357–362, 1991.
18. **Garatachea N, Verde Z, Santos-Lozano A, Yvert T, Rodriguez-Romo G, Sarasa FJ, Hernández-Sánchez S, Santiago C, Lucia A**. ACTN3 R577X polymorphism and explosive leg-muscle power in elite basketball players. *Int J Sports Physiol Perform* 9: 226–232, 2014.
19. **Georgiades E, Klissouras V, Baulch J, Wang G, Pitsiladis Y**. Why nature prevails over nurture in the making of the elite athlete. *BMC Genomics* 18: 835, 2017.
20. **Gibson WT**. Core concepts in human genetics: understanding the complex phenotype of sport performance and susceptibility to sport injury. *Med Sport Sci* 61: 1–14, 2016.
21. **Ginevičienė V, Pranculis A**. Genetic variation of the human ACE and ACTN3 genes and their association with functional muscle properties in Lithuanian elite athletes. *Kaunas Lith* 47: 284–90, 2010.

22. **Grealy R, Smith CLE, Chen T, Hiller D, Haseler LJ, Griffiths LR**. The genetics of endurance: frequency of the ACTN3 R577X variant in Ironman World Championship athletes. *J Sci Med Sport* 16: 365–371, 2013.

23. **Jones B, Klissouras V**. Genetic variation in the force-velocity relation of human muscle. In: *Sport and Human Genetics*, edited by Malina RM, Bouchard C. Champaign, IL: Human Kinetics, p. 155–163, 1986.

24. **Kikuchi N, Yoshida S, Min SK, Lee K, Sakamaki-Sunaga M, Okamoto T, Nakazato K**. The ACTN3 R577X genotype is associated with muscle function in a Japanese population. *Appl Physiol Nutr Metab* 322: 1–7, 2014.

25. **Kim H, Song K, Kim C**. The ACTN3 R577X variant in sprint and strength performance. *J Exerc Nutrition Biochem* 18: 347–353, 2014.

26. **Klissouras V**. Heritability of adaptive variation. *J Appl Physiol* 31: 338–344, 1971.

27. **Klissouras V, Casini B, Di Salvo V, Faina M, Marini C, Pigozzi F, Pittaluga M, Spataro A, Taddei F, Parisi P**. Genes and Olympic performance: a co-twin study. *Int J Sports Med* 22: 250–255, 2001.

28. **Komi PV, Klissouras V, Karvinen E**. Genetic variation in neuromuscular performance. *Int Z Angew Physiol* 31: 289–304, 1973.

29. **Komi PV, Viitasalo JH, Havu M, Thorstensson A, Sjodin B, Karlsson J**. Skeletal muscle fibers and muscle enzyme activities in monozygous and dizygous twins of both sexes. *Acta Physiol Scand* 100: 385–392, 1977.

30. **MacArthur DG, North KN**. ACTN3: a genetic influence on muscle function and athletic performance. *Exerc Sport Sci Rev* 35: 30–34, 2007.

31. **Maes HH, Beunen GP, Vlietinck RF, Neale MC, Thomis M, Vanden Eynde B, Lysens R, Simons J, Derom C, Derom R**. Inheritance of physical fitness in 10-yr-old twins and their parents. *Med Sci Sport Exerc* 28: 1479–1491, 1996.

32. **McCarthy MI, MacArthur DG**. Human disease genomics: from variants to biology. *Genome Biol* 18: 18–20, 2017.

33. **Mills M**. Differential expression of the actin-binding proteins, alpha-actinin-2 and -3, in different species: implications for the evolution of functional redundancy. *Hum Mol Genet* 10: 1335–1346, 2001.

34. **Missitzi J, Geladas N, Klissouras V**. Heritability in neuromuscular coordination: implications for motor control strategies. *Med Sci Sports Exerc* 36: 233–240, 2004.

35. **Missitzi J, Gentner R, Misitzi A, Geladas N, Politis P, Klissouras V, Classen J**. Heritability of motor control and motor learning. *Physiol Rep* 1: e00188, 2013.

36. **De Moor MHM, Spector TD, Cherkas LF, Falchi M, Hottenga JJ, Boomsma DI, De Geus EJC**. Genome-wide linkage scan for athlete status in 700 British female DZ twin pairs. *Twin Res Hum Genet* 10: 812–820, 2007.

37. **Moran CN, Vassilopoulos C, Tsiokanos A, Jamurtas AZ, Bailey MES, Montgomery HE, Wilson RH, Pitsiladis YP**. The associations of ACE polymorphisms with physical, physiological and skill parameters in adolescents. *Eur J Hum Genet* 14: 332–339, 2006.

38. **Mustelin L, Latvala A, Pietiläinen KH, Piirilä P, Sovijärvi AR, Kujala UM, Rissanen A, Kaprio J**. Associations between sports participation, cardiorespiratory fitness, and adiposity in young adult twins. *J Appl Physiol* 110: 681–686, 2011.

39. **Naumov VA, Ahmetov II, Larin AK, Generozov EV, Kulemin NA, Ospanova EA, Pavlenko AV, Kostryukova ES, Alexeev DG, Govorun VM**. Genome-wide association analysis identifies a locus on DMD (dystrophin) gene for power athlete status in Russians. *Eur J Hum Genet* 22: 502, 2014.

40. **Niemi A-K, Majamaa K**. Mitochondrial DNA and ACTN3 genotypes in Finnish elite endurance and sprint athletes. *Eur J Hum Genet* 13: 965–969, 2005.

41. **Orysiak J, Busko K, Michalski R, Mazur-Różycka J, Gajewski J, Malczewska-Lenczowska J, Sitkowski D, Pokrywka A**. Relationship between ACTN3 R577X polymorphism and maximal power output in elite Polish athletes. *Medicina (Kaunas)* 50: 303–308, 2014.

42. **Papadimitriou ID, Papadopoulos C, Kouvatsi A, Triantaphyllidis C**. The ACTN3 gene in elite Greek track and field athletes. *Int J Sports Med* 29: 352–5, 2008.

43. **Pasqua LA, Bueno S, Matsuda M, Marquezini MV, Lima-Silva AE, Saldiva PHN, Bertuzzi R**. The genetics of human running: ACTN3 polymorphism as an evolutionary tool improving the energy economy during locomotion. *Ann Hum Biol* 4460: 1–6, 2015.

44. **Pereira A, Costa AM, Izquierdo M, Silva AJ, Bastos E, Marques MC.** ACE I/D and ACTN3 R/X polymorphisms as potential factors in modulating exercise-related phenotypes in older women in response to a muscle power training stimuli. *Age (Omaha)* 35: 1949–1959, 2013.

45. **Pitsiladis YP, Tanaka M, Eynon N, Bouchard C, North KN, Williams AG, Collins M, Moran CN, Britton SL, Fuku N, Ashley EA, Klissouras V, Lucia A, Ahmetov II, de Geus E, Alsayrafi M.** Athlome Project Consortium: a concerted effort to discover genomic and other "omic" markers of athletic performance. *Physiol Genomics* 48: 183–190, 2016.

46. **Puthucheary Z, Skipworth JRA, Rawal J, Loosemore M, Van Someren K, Montgomery HE.** The ACE gene and human performance: 12 years on. *Sports Med* 41: 433–48, 2011.

47. **Rankinen T, Fuku N, Wolfarth B, Wang G, Sarzynski MA, Alexeev DG, Ahmetov II, Boulay MR, Cieszczyk P, Eynon N, Filipenko ML, Garton FC, Generozov EV, Govorun VM, Houweling PJ, Kawahara T, Kostryukova ES, Kulemin NA, Larin AK, Maciejewska-Karlowska A, Miyachi M, Muniesa CA, Murakami H, Ospanova EA, Padmanabhan S, Pavlenko AV, Pyankova ON, Santiago C, Sawczuk M, Scott RA, Uyba VV, Yvert T, Perusse L, Ghosh S, Rauramaa R, North KN, Lucia A, Pitsiladis Y, Bouchard C.** No evidence of a common DNA variant profile specific to world class endurance athletes. *PLoS One* 11: 1–24, 2016.

48. **Rankinen T, Fuku N, Wolfarth B, Wang G, Sarzynski MA, Alexeev DG, Ahmetov II, Boulay MR, Cieszczyk P, Eynon N, Filipenko ML, Garton FC, Generozov EV, Govorun VM, Houweling PJ, Kawahara T, Kostryukova ES, Kulemin NA, Larin AK, Maciejewska-Karlowska A, Miyachi M, Muniesa CA, Murakami H, Ospanova EA, Padmanabhan S, Pavlenko AV, Pyankova ON, Santiago C, Sawczuk M, Scott RA, Uyba VV, Yvert T, Perusse L, Ghosh S, Rauramaa R, North KN, Lucia A, Pitsiladis Y, Bouchard C.** No evidence of a common DNA variant profile specific to world class endurance athletes. *PLoS One* 11: e0147330, 2016.

49. **Roth SM, Walsh S, Liu D, Metter EJ, Ferrucci L, Hurley BF.** The ACTN3 R577X nonsense allele is under-represented in elite-level strength athletes. *Eur J Hum Genet* 16: 391–394, 2008.

50. **Schutte NM, Nederend I, Hudziak JJ, Bartels M, de Geus EJC.** Twin-sibling study and meta-analysis on the heritability of maximal oxygen consumption. *Physiol Genomics* 48: 210–219, 2016.

51. **Scott RA, Moran C, Wilson RH, Onywera V, Boit MK, Goodwin WH, Gohlke P, Payne J, Montgomery H, Pitsiladis YP.** No association between angiotensin converting enzyme (ACE) gene variation and endurance athlete status in Kenyans. *Comp Biochem Physiol A Mol Integr Physiol* 141: 169–175, 2005.

52. **Scott RA, Irving R, Irwin L, Morrison E, Charlton V, Austin K, Tladi D, Deason M, Headley SA, Kolkhorst FW, Yang N, North K, Pitsiladis YP.** ACTN3 and ACE genotypes in elite Jamaican and US sprinters. *Med Sci Sport Exerc* 42: 107–112, 2010.

53. **Sessa F, Chetta M, Petito A, Franzetti M, Bafunno V, Pisanelli D, Sarno M, Iuso S, Margaglione M.** Gene polymorphisms and sport attitude in Italian athletes. *Genet Test Mol Biomarkers* 15: 285–290, 2011.

54. **Seto JT, Quinlan KGR, Lek M, Zheng XF, Garton F, Macarthur DG, Hogarth MW, Houweling PJ, Gregorevic P, Turner N, Cooney GJ, Yang N, North KN.** ACTN3 genotype influences muscle performance through the regulation of calcineurin signaling. *J Clin Invest* 123: 4255–4263, 2013.

55. **Shang X, Zhang F, Zhang L, Huang C.** ACTN3 R577X polymorphism and performance phenotypes in young Chinese male soldiers. *J Sports Sci* 30: 255–260, 2012.

56. **Simonen RL, Rankinen T, Perusse L, Rice T, Rao DC, Chagnon Y, Bouchard C.** Genome-wide linkage scan for physical activity levels in the Quebec Family study. *Med Sci Sports Exerc* 35: 1355–1359, 2003.

57. **Stunkard AJ, Harris JR, Pedersen NL, McClearn GE.** The body-mass index of twins who have been reared apart. *N Engl J Med* 322: 1483–1487, 1990.

58. **Thomis MA, Van Leemputte M, Maes HH, Blimkie CJR, Claessens AL, Marchal G, Willems E, Vlietinck RF, Beunen GP.** Multivariate genetic analysis of maximal isometric muscle force at different elbow angles. *J Appl Physiol* 82: 959–967, 1997.

59. **Venter JC, Adams MD, Myers EW, Li PW, Mural RJ, Sutton GG, Smith HO, Yandell M, Evans CA, Holt RA, Gocayne JD, Amanatides P, Ballew RM, Huson DH, Wortman JR, Zhang Q, Kodira CD, Zheng XH, Chen L, Skupski M, Subramanian G, Thomas PD, Zhang J, Gabor Miklos GL, Nelson C, Broder S, Clark AG, Nadeau J, McKusick VA, Zinder N, Levine AJ, Roberts RJ, Simon M, Slayman C, Hunkapiller M, Bolanos R, Delcher A, Dew**

I, Fasulo D, Flanigan M, Florea L, Halpern A, Hannenhalli S, Kravitz S, Levy S, Mobarry C, Reinert K, Remington K, Abu-Threideh J, Beasley E, Biddick K, Bonazzi V, Brandon R, Cargill M, Chandramouliswaran I, Charlab R, Chaturvedi K, Deng Z, Di Francesco V, Dunn P, Eilbeck K, Evangelista C, Gabrielian AE, Gan W, Ge W, Gong F, Gu Z, Guan P, Heiman TJ, Higgins ME, Ji RR, Ke Z, Ketchum KA, Lai Z, Lei Y, Li Z, Li J, Liang Y, Lin X, Lu F, Merkulov G V, Milshina N, Moore HM, Naik AK, Narayan VA, Neelam B, Nusskern D, Rusch DB, Salzberg S, Shao W, Shue B, Sun J, Wang Z, Wang A, Wang X, Wang J, Wei M, Wides R, Xiao C, Yan C, Yao A, Ye J, Zhan M, Zhang W, Zhang H, Zhao Q, Zheng L, Zhong F, Zhong W, Zhu S, Zhao S, Gilbert D, Baumhueter S, Spier G, Carter C, Cravchik A, Woodage T, Ali F, An H, Awe A, Baldwin D, Baden H, Barnstead M, Barrow I, Beeson K, Busam D, Carver A, Center A, Cheng ML, Curry L, Danaher S, Davenport L, Desilets R, Dietz S, Dodson K, Doup L, Ferriera S, Garg N, Gluecksmann A, Hart B, Haynes J, Haynes C, Heiner C, Hladun S, Hostin D, Houck J, Howland T, Ibegwam C, Johnson J, Kalush F, Kline L, Koduru S, Love A, Mann F, May D, McCawley S, McIntosh T, McMullen I, Moy M, Moy L, Murphy B, Nelson K, Pfannkoch C, Pratts E, Puri V, Qureshi H, Reardon M, Rodriguez R, Rogers YH, Romblad D, Ruhfel B, Scott R, Sitter C, Smallwood M, Stewart E, Strong R, Suh E, Thomas R, Tint NN, Tse S, Vech C, Wang G, Wetter J, Williams S, Williams M, Windsor S, Winn-Deen E, Wolfe K, Zaveri J, Zaveri K, Abril JF, Guigó R, Campbell MJ, Sjolander K V, Karlak B, Kejariwal A, Mi H, Lazareva B, Hatton T, Narechania A, Diemer K, Muruganujan A, Guo N, Sato S, Bafna V, Istrail S, Lippert R, Schwartz R, Walenz B, Yooseph S, Allen D, Basu A, Baxendale J, Blick L, Caminha M, Carnes-Stine J, Caulk P, Chiang YH, Coyne M, Dahlke C, Mays A, Dombroski M, Donnelly M, Ely D, Esparham S, Fosler C, Gire H, Glanowski S, Glasser K, Glodek A, Gorokhov M, Graham K, Gropman B, Harris M, Heil J, Henderson S, Hoover J, Jennings D, Jordan C, Jordan J, Kasha J, Kagan L, Kraft C, Levitsky A, Lewis M, Liu X, Lopez J, Ma D, Majoros W, McDaniel J, Murphy S, Newman M, Nguyen T, Nguyen N, Nodell M, Pan S, Peck J, Peterson M, Rowe W, Sanders R, Scott J, Simpson M, Smith T, Sprague A, Stockwell T, Turner R, Venter E, Wang M, Wen M, Wu D, Wu M, Xia A, Zandieh A, Zhu X. The sequence of the human genome. *Science* 291: 1304–51, 2001.

60. **Voisin S, Eynon N, Yan X, Bishop DJ**. Exercise training and DNA methylation in humans. *Acta Physiol* 213: 39–59, 2015.

61. **Wang G, Padmanabhan S, Wolfarth B, Fuku N, Lucia A, Ahmetov II, Cieszczyk P, Collins M, Eynon N, Klissouras V, Williams A, Pitsiladis Y**. Genomics of elite sporting performance: what little we know and necessary advances. *Adv Genet* 84: 123–149, 2013.

62. **Wang G, Tanaka M, Eynon N, North KN, Williams AG, Collins M, Moran CN, Britton SL, Fuku N, Ashley EA, Klissouras V, Lucia A, Ahmetov II, de Geus E, Alsayrafi M, Pitsiladis YP**. The future of genomic research in athletic performance and adaptation to training. *Med Sport Sci* 61: 55–67, 2016.

63. **Willems SM, Wright DJ, Day FR, Trajanoska K, Joshi PK, Morris JA, Matteini AM, Garton FC, Grarup N, Oskolkov N, Thalamuthu A, Mangino M, Liu J, Demirkan A, Lek M, Xu L, Wang G, Oldmeadow C, Gaulton KJ, Lotta LA, Miyamoto-Mikami E, Rivas MA, White T, Loh P-R, Aadahl M, Amin N, Attia JR, Austin K, Benyamin B, Brage S, Cheng Y-C, Cięszczyk P, Derave W, Eriksson K-F, Eynon N, Linneberg A, Lucia A, Massidda M, Mitchell BD, Miyachi M, Murakami H, Padmanabhan S, Pandey A, Papadimitriou I, Rajpal DK, Sale C, Schnurr TM, Sessa F, Shrine N, Tobin MD, Varley I, Wain LV, Wray NR, Lindgren CM, MacArthur DG, Waterworth DM, McCarthy MI, Pedersen O, Khaw K-T, Kiel DP, Oei L, Zheng H-F, Forgetta V, Leong A, Ahmad OS, Laurin C, Mokry LE, Ross S, Elks CE, Bowden J, Warrington NM, Murray A, Ruth KS, Tsilidis KK, Medina-Gómez C, Estrada K, Bis JC, Chasman DI, Demissie S, Enneman AW, Hsu Y-H, Ingvarsson T, Kähönen M, Kammerer C, Lacroix AZ, Li G, Liu C-T, Liu Y, Lorentzon M, Mägi R, Mihailov E, Milani L, Moayyeri A, Nielson CM, Sham PC, Siggeirsdotir K, Sigurdsson G, Stefansson K, Trompet S, Thorleifsson G, Vandenput L, van der Velde N, Viikari J, Xiao S-M, Zhao JH, Evans DS, Cummings SR, Cauley J, Duncan EL, de Groot LCPGM, Esko T, Gudnason V, Harris TB, Jackson RD, Jukema JW, Ikram AMA, Karasik D, Kaptoge S, Kung AWC, Lehtimäki T, Lyytikäinen L-P, Lips P, Luben R, Metspalu A, van Meurs JBJ, Minster RL, Orwoll E, Oei E, Psaty BM, Raitakari OT, Ralston SW, Ridker PM, Robbins JA, Smith AV, Styrkarsdottir U, Tranah GJ, Thorstensdottir U, Uitterlinden AG, Zmuda J, Zillikens MC, Ntzani EE,

Evangelou E, Ioannidis JPA, Evans DM, Ohlsson C, Pitsiladis Y, Fuku N, Franks PW, North KN, van Duijn CM, Mather KA, Hansen T, Hansson O, Spector T, Murabito JM, Richards JB, Rivadeneira F, Langenberg C, Perry JRB, Wareham NJ, Scott RA. Large-scale GWAS identifies multiple loci for hand grip strength providing biological insights into muscular fitness. *Nat Commun* 8: 16015, 2017.

64. **Williams AG, Day SH, Folland JP, Gohlke P, Dhamrait S, Montgomery HE**. Circulating angiotensin converting enzyme activity is correlated with muscle strength. *Med Sci Sports Exerc* 37: 944–948, 2005.

65. **Wolfarth B, Rankinen T, Hagberg JM, Loos RJF, Pérusse L, Roth SM, Sarzynski MA, Bouchard C**. Advances in exercise, fitness, and performance genomics in 2013. *Med Sci Sports Exerc* 46: 851–859, 2014.

66. **Yang N, MacArthur DG, Gulbin JP, Hahn AG, Beggs AH, Easteal S, North K**. ACTN3 genotype is associated with human elite athletic performance. *Am J Hum Genet* 73: 627–631, 2003.

67. **Yang R, Shen X, Wang Y, Voisin S, Cai G, Fu Y, Xu W, Eynon N, Bishop DJ, Yan X**. ACTN3 R577X gene variant is associated with muscle-related phenotypes in elite Chinese sprit/power athletes. *J Strength Cond Res* 31: 1107–1115, 2016.

25

USING ELITE ATHLETES AS A MODEL FOR GENETIC RESEARCH

Colin N. Moran, Alun G. Williams, and Guan Wang

The general principle behind many human genetic studies is to compare the genetics of a group of individuals with shared characteristics of interest (such as being good at sport) to a control group lacking those characteristics. We would expect that genetic variants related to the production of those characteristics would be more common in the former group. With as much as 66% of athlete status being the result of heritable factors (13), elite athletes must have a genetic profile that predisposes them to being good at sport, responsive to training, and resistant to injury as well as ensuring that they train hard, eat well, and have a skilled team of coaches around them. The more extreme and well-defined this group of athletes is, the more pronounced we would expect any genetic difference to be. Defining that group of individuals well is key to this process.

Defining athletes as elite for genetics research

Elite is defined as "a select group that is superior in terms of abilities or qualities to the rest of a group or society" (37). In terms of athletes, although a consensus definition is not clear, those achieving selection for international teams are often described as elite (50). However, athletes in the Olympic team of any country will come in a variety of shapes and sizes, depending on their sport of choice and particular abilities. Elite distance runners are typically small in stature, with thin limbs, high type I muscle fiber content, and a high maximal oxygen uptake (VO2max) (21, 33, 44) (Figure 25.1). In contrast, elite weightlifters are typically large, with thick limbs, high type II muscle fiber content, and a lower VO2max (25, 49) (Figure 25.1). Many physiological differences can be observed between athletes specializing in different sports. When investigating the genetic components of elite athletes' makeup, it is important to know which sport an athlete is considered to be elite in and what the physiological demands are of that sport.

Grouping together athletes from sports with similar physiological demands is useful. Grouping athletes specializing in strength sports and comparing them to nonathlete controls may tell us something about the genetics that predispose to being good at strength or power events. However, even within one sporting discipline, there are often many different ways to get into the elite group. Typically, athletes will be selected on performance criteria, e.g., what is the fastest time that they have run? However, two elite endurance athletes with identical 10 km performance times may have achieved them quite differently and some of those differences may be

A   B

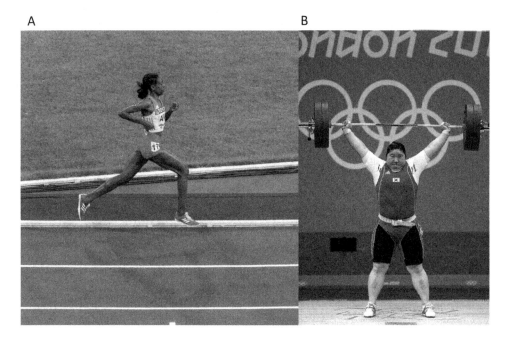

Figure 25.1   Elite distance runner and elite weight lifter: Almaz Ayana (left) and Mi-ran Jang (right). Both are Olympic gold medalists. Ayana pictured at the 2017 world championships in London in the 10,000 m and Jang at the 2012 London Olympics in the women's +75 kg category, respectively. *Source*: Photo of Almaz Ayana by Marco Verch. Photo of Mi-ran Jang by Korean Olympic Committees.

underpinned by genetics. One may have a sprint finish, while the other does not. One may have a phenomenal VO2max and an average running style, while conversely the other has an average VO2max and an exceptional running economy. To understand the genetics of elite athletes, it is important to recognize that athletes achieve elite performance in different ways (11, 23).

Defining elite across multiple sports by a single performance criterion is even more fraught. The combinations of physiological abilities necessary to reach the top echelons are unlikely to be the same in different sports (27) although some common factors exist. Many athletes make use of this and switch sports in search of success. Indeed, if athletes do not quite achieve medal-winning performance in their chosen sport but do have some elite-level physiological characteristics, sports governing bodies now encourage them to switch sports through talent transfer programs (e.g., 52). Of course, the amount of competition may be lower in their new sport, but assuming that it is not and that they achieve success, one could conclude that their combination of genetic predispositions is better suited to their new sport. An athlete could be considered to be elite, or not, in each of several individual characteristics important for performance. However, it is also important to recognize that they will likely achieve elite performance without being elite in every single characteristic that contributes.

Participation rates in many sports differ vastly across borders and sexes as do the standards that would be considered to be elite. Some sports are found in very few countries having barely spread from their country of origin, such as shinty in Scotland (9) (Figure 25.2). Being the best shinty player in Scotland is a different achievement from being the best shinty player in virtually any other country. When participation rates for a sport are low in a country, the individuals with the most suitable genetic profile may not take part in that sport; they may do a different sport

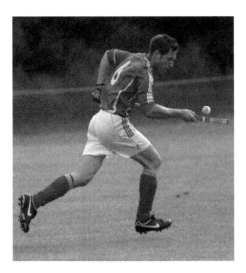

Figure 25.2   Shinty skill from the Kinlochshiel versus Strathglass Balliemore Cup Final (2009).
Source: Photo by Alasdair Middleton.

or they may be inactive. When participation rates are low, there is a higher chance that the best individuals at that sport are there by accident of their involvement and because of their effort in training rather than their genetic predisposition. Devon Harris, Michael White, and brothers Dudley and Chris Stokes were an elite Jamaican bobsleigh crew having competed at the 1988 Calgary Olympics (26), immortalized by the 1993 film Cool Runnings (22). However, they may not be considered truly elite against German or Swiss norms where winter sports are more common. There may even be other Jamaicans with a more suitable genetic profile for bobsleigh who have never had the opportunity to try it. In case–control studies, this can lead to misclassified individuals in the control group, where those with a genetic predisposition to athleticism are included as controls because not everyone with a genetic predisposition gets involved in sport. Since control groups are rarely screened to exclude potential cases, this causes a, typically modest, loss of statistical power (31). Additionally, given the global variation in allele frequencies, controls must be ethnically matched with cases and assessed to avoid confounding by population stratification. Conversely, even when participation rates are high, there are few sports where the top women's achievements would be considered elite compared to the top men in the same sport (51). Or where junior athletes could compete with adults in their prime (6, 24). Nonetheless, they absolutely are elite when compared to the appropriate group norms. When we make use of an elite group, to understand how genetics influences those characteristics, we have to take great care in defining that group and the criteria against which we judge individual achievements.

Within sport there are a variety of ways to define an individual as elite and each comes with its own strengths and weaknesses. Defining elite based on competitive achievements allows rapid and relatively easy identification of appropriate individuals although it may create both athlete and control groups with some mixed physiological abilities. Defining elite based on physiological characteristics is more time-consuming for both researchers and athletes; however, it may allow more appropriate groupings to be identified if a single parameter is of primary interest, e.g., VO2max, because of its known relationships with morbidity and mortality (5, 15). However, if the primary interest is elite performance in a sport per se, then we must know all of those individual characteristics to take this approach and address each one in turn. Restricting a definition of elite to a single phenotype measured in a laboratory instead of success in that sport would be unable to identify the full range of genetic characteristics important for that sporting success. Ideally, we would select athletes from sports with high levels of participation where everyone puts in an equal and large amount of effort in training and we would be careful to compare their achievements to an appropriate set of thresholds for their age or sex group.

Elite athletes can be used to model athletic ability, health, and disease

The central component of any study design is the academic question to be addressed. Clearly elite athletes can be used to model the genetics of being an elite athlete. Depending on which types of athletes have been chosen for study and how elite has been defined, we may ask: Which genetic variants are required to be an elite weightlifter? Or result in a high VO2max? However, while understanding the required components for an elite athlete may motivate many researchers, elite athletes make up only a small proportion of the population and have no specific associated genetic illness that requires attention. There is no imperative to investigate their genetic makeup and such studies are less likely than research into health or disease to attract the necessary grant funding for expensive genetics research. Nonetheless, there is also value in using elite athletes as a model for a number of health and disease research questions less obviously related to athletic performance. Most obvious are the links between exercise and health or all-cause mortality (41, 45). However, elite athletes are extreme, not only in their abilities, but also in the level of stress that they put on their bodies: training over and over again, experiencing muscular, bone, metabolic, and immunological stresses, and pushing themselves daily (4, 10, 47). Diseases often put extreme stresses on similar aspects of our physiology and with severities that vary between individuals partly due to their underlying genetics. For instance, many cancers result in a loss of skeletal muscle mass known as cachexia which correlates with shorter survival in patients (2). Sarcopenia is the age-related decline in skeletal muscle mass, which occurs at different rates in different individuals, and leads to increased risk of falls, fracture, and frailty (43). If we overload our bodies with energy, some individuals develop obesity and diabetes, placing a variety of stresses on our metabolism (54). Understanding what happens to elite athletes and why one copes better with particular stressors than another will give insights into common diseases suffered by individuals all across the population distribution.

Super athletes, lifestyle disease, and ageing

Individuals with noncommunicable diseases may have even more in common with elite athletes. Although genetic variants predispose to athletic ability (46), lifestyle is also a key component and genetic variants that are an advantage in one situation may be neutral or even a disadvantage in another. If the individual with the best genetic profile in the world for elite cycling never gets on a bicycle, she won't be an elite cyclist. In fact, some of the genetic variants that predispose her to being an elite athlete may also predispose her to being unhealthy when there is an absence of the correct lifestyle factors. For example, if part of her genetic predisposition to cycling results from genetic variants making her highly efficient at utilizing the energy she consumes, the lifestyle choices she makes about how to use that energy have particularly significant impacts. If she chooses to cycle, she has an advantage. If instead she is physically inactive, she may be at a higher risk of metabolic disease as she would still be highly efficient with the energy she consumes. This concept is known as the thrifty genotype (35). Many variants can have differing effects depending on the lifestyle or environment in which we chose to consider

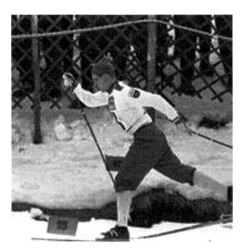

Figure 25.3   Photograph of the Finnish skier Eero Mäntyranta (1937–2013) during the 1964 Winter Olympics in Innsbruck.

them. The multi-Olympic and world championship medal-winning Finnish cross-country skier Eero Mäntyranta (36) (Figure 25.3) had a rare variant (rs121917830) of the erythropoietin receptor gene (*EPOR*), effectively making him hypersensitive to his body's normal erythropoietin levels (34). This condition, known as erythrocytosis, greatly increased his red blood cell count and the oxygen-carrying capacity of his blood giving him a natural advantage as an elite endurance athlete. However, the additional blood cells thicken the blood of carriers of this genetic variant putting them at increased risk of having abnormal blood clots with potential life-threatening complications (8). The consequences of these genetic variants cannot be separated from the environments in which we place them. Investigating how the environment that we control, such as physical activity or dietary choices, interacts with genetic variants in elite athletes pushing themselves to their limits will help us understand how those same genetic variants may interact with lifestyle choices in the general population or unhealthy people.

Additionally, there are clear and important links between components of athlete physiology and many common diseases, such as VO2max and predisposition to chronic disease and longevity (7). Being physically active is thought to be the biological default condition for health, and optimizes the aging process in humans (16). Elite and masters athletes are usually lifelong exercisers, and serve as a unique biological model for studying the fundamental physiological mechanisms underlying health and ageing. It is these relationships that should drive research in this area, and research funding, forward. Elite athletes can be used to improve our understanding of the genetic components of these aspects of physiology. In turn, this will lead to a better understanding of determinants of the long-term health of the general population and what we might do to improve them. The impact of this type of research is likely to be much broader than the elite athletes themselves and ultimately will tell us about genetic aspects of health and disease.

Pluses and minuses of working with elite athletes

Of course, it is possible to investigate the genetics of athletic ability and the genetics of health and disease in less elite individuals: those with disease, the general population, or the recreationally active. However, there are a number of advantages to working with elite athletes. As mentioned above, they are on an extreme part of the phenotypic distribution. This can only be achieved by having both the appropriate genetic profile and the correct environment in terms of nutrition and training. Variation in both genetic predisposition and the appropriateness of the environment is higher in the general population or the recreationally active making it harder to tease out the genetic components. Many performance tasks that we may use in the physiology laboratory are complex or difficult, such as lifting weights, meaning that lack of familiarity can create variation in performance that is unrelated to physiological ability or genetic predisposition (42). Similarly, measuring VO2max requires that individuals push themselves to their physiological limits, something nonathletes may be less able to achieve (28). In essence, elite athletes are more similar to each other, providing a cleaner phenotype and hopefully a cleaner window on to the key aspects of their genetic profile.

Conversely, working with elite athletes presents several problems. Major genetics of common disease initiatives in recent years have recruited increasingly large numbers of participants to allow the detection of small genetic effects using genome-wide association studies (GWAS). This approach has allowed identification of more than 4.3 million common genetic variants as important for the characteristic in question whether we expect that they might be involved or not. Early GWAS experiments had little more than a hundred participants, but the most recent have a few hundred thousand participants with plans for even larger future studies (29). Ideally, we would take a similar approach to elite performance. However, by definition, elite athletes are rare, or they would not be distinguishable from the general population, meaning that this powerful approach is not so straightforwardly applied. Additionally, in laboratory studies we typically control the exercise and nutrition of our participants so that it is uniform. Elite athletes are very unlikely to be willing to deviate from their own personal exercise and nutrition plans. Similarly, no one becomes an elite athlete without spending a great deal of time training, often more than once a day. Consequently, elite athletes are busy. They may not have time or be willing to do detailed physiological testing in the laboratory, unless it can directly inform their training (30).

Although there are pros and cons to working with elite athletes, there is clear value in understanding why they are so good at sport. Understanding how we can accommodate the other demands on their time and ensuring that we provide information useful to them will help create an environment where they are willing to be involved in research. As with any academic research, the place to start when designing a study is by talking to the stakeholders, primarily the athletes and the teams of people around them, so that studies are designed to be mutually beneficial.

Global efforts to investigate elite athletes

There are a number of projects that have set out to understand genetic aspects of elite performance in athletes. They range in size greatly, include varying degrees of elite athletes, and have taken a number of different approaches to study design. Often there is a direct trade-off between the quality and detail of the phenotype data collected and the number of elite athletes willing to take part. The largest cohorts typically are those that simply require information on preferred discipline and a saliva sample for DNA extraction. Some studies include more categorical information, such as highest level of competition or greatest achievements without requiring much more time from the athletes. Some studies make use of existing quantitative information. This may be in the form of personal best competition race times or weights lifted; or it may be testing or biochemical data that at some stage was collected from the athletes to benchmark their performance or improve their training. Again, this requires little more of the athletes' time, although it will require additional ethical permission to access databases and probably more time from someone in the support organization that collected the database. Finally, it may be possible to collect new physiological testing information on the athletes related to their elite performance or the performance of others in the cohort. However, this requires considerable time from athletes and makes it harder to collect large numbers of athletes.

One of the first studies to use elite athletes to investigate the genetics of sporting performance was the *GenAthlete* study (labs.pbrc.edu/humangenomics/#GENATHLETE). This multicenter, case–control study was launched in 1993, primarily to identify genetic variants present at different frequencies in endurance athletes with high VO2max and untrained controls with low to average VO2max. Male endurance athletes of national or international caliber with a VO2max of at least 75 ml/kg/min and male controls were recruited from Canada, Finland, Germany, and the US. The cohort includes 315 elite endurance athletes (mean VO2max of 79 ml/kg/min) and 320 matched controls (mean VO2max of 40 ml/kg/min). Multiple candidate gene studies and a GWAS have been performed using the resources of GenAthlete (40). Further studies are focusing on nuclear and mitochondrial DNA sequencing.

Subsequent studies often took a similar approach, recruiting from national or international teams, although most do not have VO2max cut-offs as inclusion criteria. Nonexhaustive lists of cohorts and consortia known to include elite athletes are given in Tables 25.1 and 25.2 and the following paragraphs.

Despite numerous publications arising from these cohorts advancing our understanding of the genetics of sporting performance, human genetic approaches have moved on to require larger and larger cohorts for research. Researchers in this field now recognize that elite athletes are too rare to allow rapid collection of individual DNA cohorts that are large enough for adequate analysis. Pooling cohorts from different populations presents technical difficulties although these are well understood and can be overcome. One advantage is that the alleles identified will be robust across multiple population groups. Consequently, several collaborative consortia have been set up to allow pooling of precious resources.

The *Athlome Project Consortium* (www.athlomeconsortium.org/) developed from a 2015 symposium in Santorini, Greece, and attempts to bring together all current studies including other consortia and those recently launched into one large collaborative initiative (38). It includes studies on elite athletes, on adaptation to training in both humans and animal models, and on exercise-related injuries. It has four aims: 1) to establish an ethically sound international research consortium and biobank resource systematically across individual centers; 2) to discover genetic variants associated with exercise performance, adaptive response to exercise training and skeletal muscle injuries using the GWAS approach, targeted sequencing, or whole-genome sequencing; 3) to validate and replicate the genetic markers from the discovery phase across sex and ethnicity; and 4) to conduct functional investigations following replicated findings to better understand the associated biology. Athlome includes the *1000 Athlome* sequencing project which aims to sequence 1000 genomes of sprinters and distance runners of West and East African descent, respectively. Major impacts of the consortium include setting a direction for researchers in the field, fostering links between global researchers, and producing a widely read position statement on the direct-to-consumer genetic testing kits for sporting performance (55).

The Exercise at the Limit – Inherited Traits of Endurance (*ELITE*; www.med.stanford.edu/elite.html) consortium involves researchers and athletes from all over the globe with the aim of mapping the role that genetic factors play in determining VO2max. The strategy is to recruit athletes with very extreme VO2max rates, creating a clean phenotype group for comparison to controls. The main inclusion criterion for males is to have a VO2max of ≥75 ml/

Table 25.1 Major study cohorts in the genetics of human elite athletic performance

Study	Primary design	Participants	
GENATHLETE cohort	Case–control association study involving endurance athletes with high VO2max and untrained controls with low to average VO2max	315	Male endurance athletes of national or international caliber with a VO2max of at least 75 ml/kg/min recruited from Canada, Finland, Germany, and the US
		320	Male nonathlete controls matched to athletes
UK cohort (The GENESIS project, including RugbyGene)	Case–control association study involving primarily rugby athletes (RugbyGene) and endurance runners, but also including football and speed/strength/power sports. Phenotype data on some athletes include dual-energy X-ray absorptiometry, vertical jump, isometric mid-thigh pull, independently verified personal best competitive performances, in-game key performance indicators in team sport competitions and certain categories of injury history	800	Rugby athletes (includes some South African), male, elite (compete in top professional leagues)
		675	Endurance runners, male and female, international/national/regional standard including Olympic athletes
		125	Football (soccer), male, international/national/regional standard
		200	Miscellaneous other athletes including sprinters, jumpers, throwers, basketball, field hockey, swimming, cycling, male and female, international/national/regional standard
		1125	Nonathlete controls
Eastern European cohorts (Belarus, Lithuania, Russia, and Ukraine)	Case–control association studies involving 28 different athletic disciplines. The phenotype data on the Lithuanian cohort is comprised of over 20 groups of phenotypic measurements including anthropometrics, isokinetic tests, VO2 max, Wingate, cardiac size and function and blood pressure	9144	Male and female, international/national/regional/local/noncompetitive standard
		4974	Nonathlete controls
Polish cohort	Case–control association study involving 20 different athletic disciplines	660	Male and female, international/national standard
		684	Polish controls
Australian cohort	Case–control association study	125	Endurance runners, male and female, international/national/regional standard
		84	Sprinters, male and female, international/national/regional standard
		258	Australian controls

Table 25.1 (Cont.)

Study	Primary design	Participants	
Spanish cohort	Case–control association study	100	Endurance athletes of world-class status, male
		54	Rowers of world-class status, male
		108	All-time best judo athletes, male
		88	Swimmers, male and female, national standard
		53	Power athletes, male, international/ national standard
		343	Spanish controls
European and Asian swimming cohort	Candidate gene case–control study	200	Caucasian swimmers of world-class status, male and female
		158	Japanese swimmers, male and female, national standard
		649	Japanese controls
		168	Taiwanese swimmers, male and female, international/national standard
		603	Taiwanese controls
Chinese cohort	Candidate gene case–control study	241	Chinese (Han) endurance athletes, male and female, national standard
		504	Chinese (Han) controls
Japanese cohort	Case–control association study	>4000	Endurance and sprint athletes, male and female, international/ national standard including track and field athletes, swimmers and athletes of team sports
		>1000	Japanese controls
Israeli cohort	Candidate gene case–control study	74	Endurance athletes, male and female, international/national standard
		81	Power athletes, male and female, international/national standard
		240	Israeli controls
East African cohort	Case–control association study	291	Kenyan endurance athletes, male and female, international/ national standard
		85	Kenyan controls
		76	Ethiopian endurance athletes, male and female, from junior/senior national athletic teams
		315	Ethiopian controls

(*continued*)

Table 25.1 (Cont.)

Study	Primary design	Participants	
Jamaican and US cohort	Case–control and genome-wide association studies	116	Jamaican sprint athletes, male and female, international/national standard
		311	Jamaican controls
		114	African American sprint athletes, male and female, international/national standard
		191	African American controls

Table 25.2 Major study consortia in the genetics of human elite athletic performance (excluding recently established consortia)

Study	Primary design	Participants	
ATHLOME Consortium	Consortium bringing together many of the individual cohorts and consortia	>19,202 >14,733	Total athletes Total controls Contributing cohorts: GENATHLETE, Eastern European, East African, Japanese, as well as the Netherlands Twin Register, super-athletes, and rat models of exercise and health Contributing consortia: ELITE, GAMES, GENESMART, GENESIS, GOINg, POWERGENE
ELITE Consortium	Case–control association study involving endurance athletes with high VO2max	800 >1000	Male (640) and female (160) endurance athletes with a VO2max of at least 75 ml/kg/min (males) or 63 ml/kg/min (females) Matched controls from databases of samples previously genotyped on same platform Contributing cohorts: GENATHLETE, Eastern European, and Japanese with many individual samples recruited directly from around the globe
GAMES Consortium	Case–control association study involving endurance athletes	1520 2760	Elite endurance athletes Ethnically matched controls Contributing cohorts: GENATHLETE, Australian, Ethiopian, Japanese, Kenyan, Polish, Russian, and Spanish
POWERGENE Consortium	Case–control association study involving elite sprint/power athletes	~500 ~1400	Elite sprint/power athletes Population matched controls Contributing cohorts: Australian, Lithuanian, Russian, Polish, South African, Spanish, UK and US with additional samples from Belgium, Greece, Italy, and Brazil

kg/min; for females it is to have a VO2max of ≥63 ml/kg/min. There are currently no race performance criteria for inclusion in the study to avoid recruiting athletes who win races by being elite in aspects important for endurance performance other than VO2max, although, typically, the athletes are successful in endurance sports. Currently, there are 800 athlete samples (including 160 from females) collected from around the world and the consortium is continuously expanding to include new partners and regions.

GAMES is an international consortium established to compare elite endurance athletes and ethnically matched controls in a case–control study design. It includes 1520 endurance athletes, including Olympic and world champions, and 2760 controls. GWASs identified 45 promising candidate SNPs although the study was underpowered to detect small effect sizes and only one single nucleotide polymorphism (SNP) was successfully replicated in seven additional cohorts (40). Conversely, *POWERGENE* is an ongoing international consortium aiming to investigate the genetic components of elite sprint/power performance. Currently, it includes over 500 sprint/power athletes and 1400 population controls from nine countries.

Other projects leverage unique aspects of the environment in certain specific sports. Rugby players require combinations of both strength and endurance. Nonetheless, there are considerable differences in the anthropometric characteristics, physical demands, and movement patterns of players in different positions on the rugby pitch (39, 48). *RugbyGene*, with a current DNA bank from over 700 elite rugby athletes, makes use of the fact that players specializing in different positions on the rugby pitch require different combinations of these attributes yet train together as a squad making their training intensity, training frequency, and some game demands more similar than when strength and endurance are investigated using separate sports (17–20). Another strength of RugbyGene is a clear definition of eliteness in the context of a team sport, namely regular participation in the top professional league in a major rugby playing country. Similar research efforts in other team sports, e.g., football (soccer), should also prioritize the broader competition for elite status that well-financed competitive leagues provide over international competitive status that requires different performance standards in different countries, as explained earlier.

New projects investigating aspects of elite sporting performance continue to develop, such as *GeneSMART* (genes and the Skeletal Muscle Adaptive Response to Training) and *GENESIS* (Genetics of Elite Status in Sport) that includes over 1700 athletes, mainly endurance runners and the RugbyGene cohort just described, plus selected performance and injury phenotype data for some athletes. The recently established *GOINg* (Genomics Of INjuries) consortium aims to identify genetic variants that modify the risk of anterior cruciate ligament injuries. Additionally, some very large cohorts of nonathletes exist which nonetheless contain quantitative measures related to performance. For instance, the *UK Biobank* (www.ukbiobank.ac.uk/) contains handgrip strength data for over 140,000 participants. One caveat is that typically these very large cohorts only collect simple portable measures of physiological phenotypes rather than gold standard performance-related measurements and the handgrip strength phenotype has several limitations (12). Nevertheless, UK Biobank and other nonelite cohorts may provide insight into the genes that we might expect to contain variants related to elite performance by leveraging substantial statistical power to detect subtle influences of genetic variants.

The future of genetics research into elite athletes

To date, studies into the genetics of human elite performance have identified over 200 gene variants involved in determining the genetic component (46). Perhaps the best known are in alpha-actinin-3 (*ACTN3*) (56) and the angiotensin-converting enzyme (*ACE*) (32). However, missing heritability is as much an issue in the genetics of elite performance as other fields and it is debatable whether many of the variants associated with performance will stand up to the scrutiny of further investigation. Many have been identified in a single, small candidate gene study using only a case–control approach. Undoubtedly, some will be successfully replicated and we will continue to gradually build up a picture of the genetic component of elite athletic performance. However, to move the field forward, we must reach towards the highest standards in human genetics research. Studies must be bigger and should preferably involve both discovery and replication cohorts. Several of the cohorts previously discussed are still collecting samples and continue to grow. The recent formation of consortia, such as Athlome, ELITE, and POWERGENE, is a recognition that the scale of the work needed requires collaboration rather than competition between research groups, to ensure that studies have enough elite athletes involved to provide meaningful insight into their underlying genetics.

In recent years, the techniques involved in capturing genetic variation have been evolving and becoming more effective, comprehensive, and economic. Not only has our ability to detect SNP variation improved, but we now additionally collect information on structural variants such as copy number variation and heritable epigenetic marks such as DNA methylation or noncoding RNAs. Significantly, these epigenetic marks are believed to be both heritable across generations and malleable acutely (1, 3). Thus, in the future it may be important to also consider the time of day and the recent activity and food consumption of elite athletes when collecting samples from them to extract their DNA and RNA. Investigating genetic variations in multiple ethnic groups is also vital to allow assessment of the broader relevance of a finding and identification of any alleles with population-specific effects. This would additionally provide insights into the heritability of a trait across populations. Understanding this diversity will lay the foundation for successful genetics research into a given trait, as well as impact potential applications in precision medicine. Future studies will integrate this complex information into a more complete understanding of the heritable aspects of elite sporting performance.

The interest in this area means that new cohorts will continue to develop. Many sporting bodies hold detailed physiological performance data on current and retired athletes collected to help benchmark and develop the athletes in their care. With appropriate negotiation, these provide an opportunity to quickly develop large study cohorts with the addition of retrospective DNA collection. There are also a number of ongoing studies into the growing area of athlete health, which could have DNA collection added to them. For example, there is a growing recognition of the damage that certain sporting activities may do to aspects of long-term health, such as concussion or mild traumatic brain injury during normal sporting activity that may be linked to later neurodegenerative disease (e.g., 14). Other studies collecting detailed phenotypic information on athletes continue to develop, such as the Retired Athlete Health Project (53). Adding DNA collection to these or other currently nongenetic studies will provide further opportunities to develop our understanding of elite athletes.

Once variants have been conclusively related to performance, it will become important to understand how they could functionally impact phenotypes important for performance. This will require carefully controlled laboratory studies, including some with elite athletes, to better understand the detail of the physiological differences resulting from the genetic differences. It will also involve the creation of appropriate animal or cellular models of key genetic variants for *in vivo* and *ex vivo* experiments. A combination of biological sciences and bioinformatics will provide insights into the biomechanisms underlying health and disease through modeling human elite athletic performance. Perhaps most importantly, they will also allow the development of novel strategies that might mitigate some of these functional differences. Ultimately, this will mean the development of personalized or precision training plans, diets, medical treatments, and lifestyle advice in general and may contribute to the development of novel gene therapy targets for muscular or respiratory conditions.

Conclusion

Investigating the genetic component of human elite athletic performance provides a unique opportunity to tease out the consequences of a variety of rare and common genetic variants for athletic ability as well as health and disease more generally. It will be key to develop cohorts of truly elite individuals large enough in number, and with enough detailed physiological data to provide the necessary resolution, to explore the findings using multidisciplinary approaches and to advance biological and clinical research.

References

1. **Baggish AL, Hale A, Weiner RB, Lewis GD, Systrom D, Wang F, Wang TJ**, and **Chan SY**. Dynamic regulation of circulating microRNA during acute exhaustive exercise and sustained aerobic exercise training. *J Physiol* 589: 3983–3994, 2011.
2. **Baracos VE, Martin L, Korc M, Guttridge DC**, and **Fearon KCH**. Cancer-associated cachexia. *Nat Rev Dis Primers* 4: 17105, 2018.
3. **Barres R, Yan J, Egan B, Treebak JT, Rasmussen M, Fritz T, Caidahl K, Krook A, O'Gorman DJ**, and **Zierath JR**. Acute exercise remodels promoter methylation in human skeletal muscle. *Cell Metab* 15: 405–411, 2012.
4. **Bennell KL** and **Brukner PD**. Epidemiology and site specificity of stress fractures. *Clin Sports Med* 16: 179–196, 1997.
5. **Blair SN**. Physical fitness and all-cause mortality. *JAMA* 262: 1989.
6. **Blythe DA** and **Kiraly FJ**. Prediction and quantification of individual athletic performance of runners. *PLoS One* 11: e0157257, 2016.
7. **Booth FW, Roberts CK**, and **Laye MJ**. Lack of exercise is a major cause of chronic diseases. *Compr Physiol* 2: 1143–1211, 2012.
8. **Braekkan SK, Mathiesen EB, Njolstad I, Wilsgaard T**, and **Hansen JB**. Hematocrit and risk of venous thromboembolism in a general population. The Tromso study. *Haematologica* 95: 270–275, 2010.
9. **Camanachd Association**. History. www.shinty.com/mens/about-us/history. [Accessed February 22, 2018.]
10. **Clark A** and **Mach N**. Exercise-induced stress behavior, gut-microbiota-brain axis and diet: a systematic review for athletes. *J Int Soc Sports Nutr* 13: 43, 2016.
11. **Coh M, Milanovic D**, and **Kampmiller T**. Morphologic and kinematic characteristics of elite sprinters. *Coll Antropol* 25: 605–610, 2001.
12. **Cronin J, Lawton T, Harris N, Kilding A**, and **McMaster DT**. A brief review of handgrip strength and sport performance. *J Strength Cond Res* 31: 3187–3217, 2017.
13. **De Moor MH, Spector TD, Cherkas LF, Falchi M, Hottenga JJ, Boomsma DI**, and **De Geus EJ**. Genome-wide linkage scan for athlete status in 700 British female DZ twin pairs. *Twin Res Hum Genet* 10: 812–820, 2007.
14. **Di Virgilio TG, Hunter A, Wilson L, Stewart W, Goodall S, Howatson G, Donaldson DI**, and **Ietswaart M**. Evidence for acute electrophysiological and cognitive changes following routine soccer heading. *EBioMedicine* 13: 66–71, 2016.
15. **Fogelholm M**. Physical activity, fitness and fatness: relations to mortality, morbidity and disease risk factors. A systematic review. *Obes Rev* 11: 202–221, 2010.
16. **Harridge SD** and **Lazarus NR**. Physical activity, aging, and physiological function. *Physiology (Bethesda)* 32: 152–161, 2017.
17. **Heffernan SM, Kilduff LP, Day SH, Pitsiladis YP**, and **Williams AG**. Genomics in rugby union: a review and future prospects. *Eur J Sport Sci* 15: 460–468, 2015.
18. **Heffernan SM, Kilduff LP, Erskine RM, Day SH, McPhee JS, McMahon GE, Stebbings GK, Neale JP, Lockey SJ, Ribbans WJ, Cook CJ, Vance B, Raleigh SM, Roberts C, Bennett MA, Wang G, Collins M, Pitsiladis YP**, and **Williams AG**. Association of ACTN3 R577X but not

ACE I/D gene variants with elite rugby union player status and playing position. *Physiol Genomics* 48: 196–201, 2016.

19. **Heffernan SM, Kilduff LP, Erskine RM, Day SH, Stebbings GK, Cook CJ, Raleigh SM, Bennett MA, Wang G, Collins M, Pitsiladis YP,** and **Williams AG**. COL5A1 gene variants previously associated with reduced soft tissue injury risk are associated with elite athlete status in rugby. *BMC Genomics* 18: 820, 2017.

20. **Heffernan SM, Stebbings GK, Kilduff LP, Erskine RM, Day SH, Morse CI, McPhee JS, Cook CJ, Vance B, Ribbans WJ, Raleigh SM, Roberts C, Bennett MA, Wang G, Collins M, Pitsiladis YP,** and **Williams AG**. Fat mass and obesity associated (FTO) gene influences skeletal muscle phenotypes in non-resistance trained males and elite rugby playing position. *BMC Genet* 18: 4, 2017.

21. **Holloszy JO** and **Coyle EF**. Adaptations of skeletal muscle to endurance exercise and their metabolic consequences. *J Appl Physiol Respir Environ Exerc Physiol* 56: 831–838, 1984.

22. **IMDb**. Cool Runnings (1993). www.imdb.com/title/tt0106611/. [Accessed February 22, 2018.]

23. **Joyner MJ** and **Coyle EF**. Endurance exercise performance: the physiology of champions. *J Physiol* 586: 35–44, 2008.

24. **Knechtle B, Assadi H, Lepers R, Rosemann T,** and **Rust CA**. Relationship between age and elite marathon race time in world single age records from 5 to 93 years. *BMC Sports Sci Med Rehabil* 6: 31, 2014.

25. **Kraemer WJ, Fleck SJ,** and **Evans WJ**. Strength and power training: physiological mechanisms of adaptation. *Exerc Sport Sci Rev* 24: 363–397, 1996.

26. **Lamont T**. Frozen in time: Jamaica's bobsled team, Calgary Winter Olympics, 13 Feb 1988. In: *The Guardian*. Online: www.theguardian.com, 2010.

27. **Lorenz DS, Reiman MP, Lehecka BJ,** and **Naylor A**. What performance characteristics determine elite versus nonelite athletes in the same sport? *Sports Health* 5: 542–547, 2013.

28. **Magnan RE, Kwan BM, Ciccolo JT, Gurney B, Mermier CM,** and **Bryan AD**. Aerobic capacity testing with inactive individuals: the role of subjective experience. *J Phys Act Health* 10: 271–279, 2013.

29. **Manolio TA**. In retrospect: a decade of shared genomic associations. *Nature* 546: 360–361, 2017.

30. **Martindale R** and **Nash C**. Sport science relevance and application: perceptions of UK coaches. *J Sports Sci* 31: 807–819, 2013.

31. **McCarthy MI, Abecasis GR, Cardon LR, Goldstein DB, Little J, Ioannidis JP,** and **Hirschhorn JN**. Genome-wide association studies for complex traits: consensus, uncertainty and challenges. *Nat Rev Genet* 9: 356–369, 2008.

32. **Montgomery HE, Marshall R, Hemingway H, Myerson S, Clarkson P, Dollery C, Hayward M, Holliman DE, Jubb M, World M, Thomas EL, Brynes AE, Saeed N, Barnard M, Bell JD, Prasad K, Rayson M, Talmud PJ,** and **Humphries SE**. Human gene for physical performance. *Nature* 393: 221–222, 1998.

33. **Mooses M** and **Hackney AC**. Anthropometrics and body composition in East African runners: potential impact on performance. *Int J Sports Physiol Perform* 12: 422–430, 2017.

34. **Moran CN** and **Pitsiladis YP**. Tour de France Champions born or made: where do we take the genetics of performance? *J Sport Sci* 35: 1411–1419, 2017.

35. **Neel JV**. The "thrifty genotype" in 1998. *Nutr Rev* 57: S2–S9, 1999.

36. **Olympic.org**. Eero Mäntyranta. www.olympic.org/eero-mantyranta. [Accessed February 23, 2018.]

37. **Oxford Dictionaries**. Definition of Elite. In: en.oxforddictionariescom/. Oxford: Oxford University Press, 2018.

38. **Pitsiladis YP, Tanaka M, Eynon N, Bouchard C, North KN, Williams AG, Collins M, Moran CN, Britton SL, Fuku N, Ashley EA, Klissouras V, Lucia A, Ahmetov, II, de Geus E, Alsayrafi M,** and **Athlome Project Consortium**. Athlome Project Consortium: a concerted effort to discover genomic and other "omic" markers of athletic performance. *Physiol Genomics* 48: 183–190, 2016.

39. **Quarrie KL, Hopkins WG, Anthony MJ,** and **Gill ND**. Positional demands of international rugby union: evaluation of player actions and movements. *J Sci Med Sport* 16: 353–359, 2013.

40. **Rankinen T, Fuku N, Wolfarth B, Wang G, Sarzynski MA, Alexeev DG, Ahmetov, II, Boulay MR, Cieszczyk P, Eynon N, Filipenko ML, Garton FC, Generozov EV, Govorun VM, Houweling PJ, Kawahara T, Kostryukova ES, Kulemin NA, Larin AK, Maciejewska-Karlowska A, Miyachi M, Muniesa CA, Murakami H, Ospanova EA, Padmanabhan S, Pavlenko AV, Pyankova ON, Santiago C, Sawczuk M, Scott RA, Uyba VV, Yvert T, Perusse L, Ghosh S, Rauramaa R, North KN, Lucia A, Pitsiladis Y,** and **Bouchard C**. No

evidence of a common DNA variant profile specific to world class endurance athletes. *PLoS One* 11: e0147330, 2016.

41. **Reiner M, Niermann C, Jekauc D**, and **Woll A**. Long-term health benefits of physical activity – a systematic review of longitudinal studies. *BMC Public Health* 13: 813, 2013.

42. **Ritti-Dias RM, Avelar A, Salvador EP**, and **Cyrino ES**. Influence of previous experience on resistance training on reliability of one-repetition maximum test. *J Strength Cond Res* 25: 1418–1422, 2011.

43. **Sakuma K, Aoi W**, and **Yamaguchi A**. Current understanding of sarcopenia: possible candidates modulating muscle mass. *Pflugers Arch* 467: 213–229, 2015.

44. **Saltin B, Henriksson J, Nygaard E, Andersen P**, and **Jansson E**. Fiber types and metabolic potentials of skeletal muscles in sedentary man and endurance runners. *Ann N Y Acad Sci* 301: 3–29, 1977.

45. **Samitz G, Egger M**, and **Zwahlen M**. Domains of physical activity and all-cause mortality: systematic review and dose-response meta-analysis of cohort studies. *Int J Epidemiol* 40: 1382–1400, 2011.

46. **Sarzynski MA, Loos RJ, Lucia A, Perusse L, Roth SM, Wolfarth B, Rankinen T**, and **Bouchard C**. Advances in exercise, fitness, and performance genomics in 2015. *Med Sci Sports Exerc* 48: 1906–1916, 2016.

47. **Schwellnus M, Soligard T, Alonso JM, Bahr R, Clarsen B, Dijkstra HP, Gabbett TJ, Gleeson M, Hagglund M, Hutchinson MR, Janse Van Rensburg C, Meeusen R, Orchard JW, Pluim BM, Raftery M, Budgett R**, and **Engebretsen L**. How much is too much? (Part 2) International Olympic Committee consensus statement on load in sport and risk of illness. *Br J Sports Med* 50: 1043–1052, 2016.

48. **Smart DJ, Hopkins WG**, and **Gill ND**. Differences and changes in the physical characteristics of professional and amateur rugby union players. *J Strength Cond Res* 27: 3033–3044, 2013.

49. **Storey A** and **Smith HK**. Unique aspects of competitive weightlifting: performance, training and physiology. *Sports Med* 42: 769–790, 2012.

50. **Swann C, Moran A**, and **Piggott D**. Defining elite athletes: issues in the study of expert performance in sport psychology. *Psychol Sport Exerc* 16: 3–14, 2015.

51. **Thibault V, Guillaume M, Berthelot G, El Helou N, Schaal K, Quinquis L, Nassif H, Tafflet M, Escolano S, Hermine O**, and **Toussaint J**. Women and men in sport performance: the gender gap has not evolved since 1983. *J Sports Sci Med* 9: 214–223, 2010.

52. **UK Sport**. Talent transfer in full swing. www.uksport.gov.uk/news/2007/02/24/talent-transfer-in-full-swing. [Accesssed February 22, 2018.]

53. **University LB**. The Retired Athlete Health Research Project. www.leedsbeckett.ac.uk/ukrugbyhealth/. [Accesssed February 23, 2018.]

54. **Upadhyay J, Farr O, Perakakis N, Ghaly W**, and **Mantzoros C**. Obesity as a Disease. *Med Clin North Am* 102: 13–33, 2018.

55. **Webborn N, Williams A, McNamee M, Bouchard C, Pitsiladis Y, Ahmetov I, Ashley E, Byrne N, Camporesi S, Collins M, Dijkstra P, Eynon N, Fuku N, Garton FC, Hoppe N, Holm S, Kaye J, Klissouras V, Lucia A, Maase K, Moran C, North KN, Pigozzi F**, and **Wang G**. Direct-to-consumer genetic testing for predicting sports performance and talent identification: consensus statement. *Br J Sports Med* 49: 1486–1491, 2015.

56. **Yang N, MacArthur DG, Gulbin JP, Hahn AG, Beggs AH, Easteal S**, and **North K**. ACTN3 genotype is associated with human elite athletic performance. *Am J Hum Genet* 73: 627–631, 2003.

26

TWIN AND FAMILY STUDIES IN SPORT PERFORMANCE

José Maia and Peter T. Katzmarzyk

Introduction and aims

Descriptions of genealogies or the tracing of family lines across the history of mankind are pervasive in many domains. Sometimes, these family histories are related to remarkable men or women whose accomplishments are unparalleled. In a notable book about sport in the ancient world, Kyle (2015) reports that Greek aristocrats "pushed the ideology of ascribed or perceived *arete*, i.e., excellence or virtue, based on pedigree and family status, claiming that athletic excellence came as a birthright in noble families with sporting traditions" (p. 82). For example, Theogenes of Thasos, son of Timosthenes, was one of the most outstanding Greek athletes, winning many victories in *pankration* and in boxing at the Olympian, Pythian, Nemean, and Isthmian games. He was crowned in two Olympiads, in 480 and 476 BC, and impressed by his amazing athletic accomplishments, there was a rumor that he wasn't a mortal, but that he was the son of a priest of Thasion Herakles and that the god impregnated his mother as narrated by the Greek traveler and historian Pausanias.

The most famous family account in classical Greek and Roman mythology is about Hercules, a crossbreed of god and man and a most outstanding hero. His family signature was unique, since he was the son of Zeus, king of the Olympian Gods, and the mortal Alcmene. Through Zeus, he was the grandson of Kronos and Rhea, and was also a great-grandson of Uranus and Gaia. His genetic material most certainly had a unique combination of his earthly mother's mitochondrial DNA to help him perform his incredible 12 labors. Alexander the Great, a mortal, also had an exceptional family line (King Philip II of Macedon and Queen Olympias). Yet, his exposome was unique as we know from history – one of his tutors, Leonidas, taught him math, archery, and horsemanship, whereas Aristotle, the famous Greek philosopher, taught him government, politics, and the sciences.

Perhaps the first systematic inquiry into family lines of outstanding men and women was that of Francis Galton – *Hereditary Genius* – published in 1869 where he tried to demonstrate that genius and greatness runs in families, at least in well-chosen and well-bred British families. He investigated 300 families comprising approximately 1000 eminent members, of whom 450 were illustrious. He presents two examples of sports family lines, one of oarsmen and another of wrestlers. In his own words:

I propose to supplement what I have written about brain by two short chapters on muscle. No one doubts that muscle is hereditary in horses and dogs, but humankind are so blind to facts and so governed by preconceptions, that I have heard it frequently asserted that muscle is not hereditary in men. Oarsmen and wrestlers have maintained that their heroes spring up capriciously, so I have thought it advisable to make inquiries into the matter. The results I have obtained will beat down another place of refuge for those who insist that each man is an independent creation, and not a mere function, physically, morally, and intellectually, of ancestral qualities and external influences.

(Galton, 1869, p. 305)

As far as we know, it was only in the Summer Olympics in Mexico (1968) and in Montreal (1976) that genetic studies were carried out to identify putative genes associated with the superior performance of "*homo olimpicus*" (Bouchard & Malina, 1984; de Garay et al., 1974). Using the best available knowledge of the time, within the Mendelian tradition, about 17 single gene systems (polymorphisms of antigens and enzymes of red cells) were investigated and data obtained from *homo olimpicus* were compared to "normal" humans. These comparisons revealed no relevant differences, even when separating athletes by sport. Of particular note is the book prepared for the Montreal Olympic Games, a resumé of the finest available information of the time concerning *La préparation d'un champion: un essai à la preparation à la performance sportive* (Bouchard et al., 1973). Two chapters are of interest here: *Qu'est qui fait un champion?* (Bouchard et al., 1973), and *La contribution de l'hérédité au plan des determinants physique, physiologique et perceptual de la performance sportive* (Bouchard, 1973). The extent of today's knowledge is vaster and deeper (Ahmetov et al., 2016) when compared to that of sport geneticists in 1973. Nonetheless, we are still struggling with the very same questions that exercised scientists of the last century (Tucker & Collins, 2012), and some suggest that we may still be in the infancy of this extraordinary quest (Pitsiladis et al., 2013). However, major efforts are currently under way, with great expectations (Pitsiladis et al., 2016).

There is a saying, apparently reported by several sport scientists, that runs like this: if you want to be a champion you had better choose your parents wisely. Of course no daughter/son chooses her/his parents. Yet, its meaning is suggestive since belonging to a family of elite athletes increases the odds of also being an elite athlete. Here are two examples separated by more than two millennia: 1) Diagoras of Rhodes, descended from Damagetus, king of Ialysus, and, on his mother's side, from the Messenian hero, Aristomenes. From him, his family dynasty spans through three generations of champions at Olympia, Isthmia and at Nemea games in *Pankration* and boxing from 464 to 424 BCE (Kyle, 2015); his daughter, Kallipáteira, had a son Peisírrhodos as well as a nephew, Euklēs, also winners in the Olympic Games. 2) Anastasia Liukin was born in 1989 in Moscow, and came to the US when she was 2 years old. Her parents, Valeri Liukin and Anna Kotchneva, were Olympic gold medalists in artistic and rhythmic gymnastics, respectively. Later, Anastasia was to become an exceptional gymnast. She won several world and Olympic gymnastics medals in various apparatuses. During the Beijing 2008 Olympic Games she won five medals, especially the highly cherished all-round competition.

In a sense, this will be the motto for this chapter since it will be mostly devoted to summarize available evidence from family lines of athletes. Its aims are to: 1) briefly review available twin and nuclear family data on sport participation; 2) define, as precisely as possible, what is meant by sport performance and/or elite athleticism; 3) review available data on twins associated with sport performance/elite athleticism; 4) investigate family lines of outstanding athletes using historical data as well as a dataset from elite athletes of Colombian origin; and 5) address the issue of intensive deliberate practice and its links to superior performance, together with the idea of athletes' exposome as well as genotype-by-exposome data on families of athletes.

Genetic factors and sports participation

When investigating the relevance of genetic factors in sport participation one finds a wide variety of phenotype definitions (Barbosa et al., 2018; de Vilhena e Santos et al., 2012) that range from very simple questions such as "Do you practice sports?", to "How many hours per week do you practice sport, in a noncompetitive setting, with your friends?", or "Do you in your leisure time practice any of the following sports …?" These phenotypes are then expressed differently in quantitative terms, i.e., from binary data to sport indexes in arbitrary units of different compositions.

As expected, the fraction of the total variance in sports practice that is due to genetic differences among individuals, i.e., the heritability (h^2), also varies substantially. Data on familial resemblance in sport participation from family studies are sparse. Using sport participation data from 2661 Portuguese families, we reported significant familial resemblance; however, the spouse correlation (0.30) was higher than parent–offspring correlations (0.18), and sibling correlations (0.22), suggesting that genetic factors were not playing a major role (Maia et al., 2014). On the other hand, in a review of available twin studies, the h^2 estimates for sport participation ranged from 0% to 85% (de Vilhena e Santos et al. 2012). With the exception of one study in adolescents that reported h^2 estimates of 0% in 13–14- and 15–16-year-olds (Stubbe et al., 2005), the h^2 estimates ranged from 35% to 85% (de Vilhena e Santos et al. 2012). A study of 304 Finnish adult twins reported an h^2 estimate of 56% for sport participation, which falls directly into this range (Mustelin et al., 2011). Thus, overall, there is good evidence of moderate heritability for sport participation from twin studies.

Sport performance and elite athleticism

What exactly is meant by sport performance and elite athleticism? In formulating putative answers to this question, the words of Aylsworth (2006) come to mind: "Morgan and his students understood that accurate phenotype definition is an essential requirement for any scientific inquiry into mechanisms of heredity" (p. 51).

Apart from the general idea that elite athleticism and/or sport performance is a complex phenotype governed by the additive and interactive effects of genes and the environment, seldom do we find formal definitions. For example, Pérusse (2011) used family studies (HERITAGE Family Study, the Quebéc Family Study, and the Canada Fitness Survey) to tackle the issue of genetic factors in sport performance, but families in these studies were not elite sportsman/sportswomen; further, no formal definition of sport performance was provided. Guth and Roth (2013), on the other hand, clearly distinguish physical performance from athletic performance, saying that they are two different phenotypes, but apparently do not provide clear definitions.

Defining our phenotypes is clearly convoluted when considering individual sports or team sports, since in the latter, technical, tactical, and strategic skills contribute to team performance. It has been further suggested that we should view sports teams as micro social systems within dynamic systems/complexity theory, with its manifold units of analysis – the individual player, small sets of players, or the team a whole (Araujo & Davids, 2016). For our purposes we will use suggestions from Druzhevskaya et al. (2008) that classifies levels of athletes: sport performance is that achieved by highly elite (winners of world championships, world cups, or Olympic Games), elite (bronze and silver medalists in world championships, word cups,

European championships, or Olympic Games) and subelite athletes (qualifiers or participants in international championships of world class). Further, by elite athleticism we mean the outstanding display of athletes' attributes like strength, speed, flexibility, coordination, endurance, and agility, for example, as seen in gymnasts, high jumpers, runners, basketball players, javelin throwers, figure skaters, soccer, and team handball payers.

Our general definition of elite athleticism is not to be confused with, for example, the extreme VO_2max cut point (≥75 ml/kg; range: 75.0–92.9 ml/kg) used to define cases in the GENATHLETE study (Wolfarth et al., 2008). In the GENATHLETE study, these cases were compared to sedentary controls to investigate several single nucleotide polymorphisms (SNPs) in candidate genes in relation to this superior phenotype. To date, the results from GENATHLETE have not provided strong evidence for differences in allele and genotype frequencies between the elite endurance athletes and the sedentary controls (Rankinen et al., 2000; Rivera et al., 1997; Wolfarth et al., 2000, 2007, 2008). Further research identified a promising panel of 45 markers in the GAMES consortium (GENATHLETE and Japanese endurance runners), and tested them for replication in seven additional cohorts comprising 1520 endurance athletes and 2760 controls (Rankinen et al., 2016). Unfortunately, the results did not identify a panel of genomic variants common to the elite athlete groups, and the main conclusion was that common genetic variants do not appear to be strong determinants of elite endurance athlete status (Rankinen et al., 2016).

Twin studies

Olympic and international-level twin athletes fascinate sport scientists for they also have the potential to help unravel the influence of their similar genetic endowments and common home environments on how they arrived at the summit of their sports' careers. Here are some examples: José and Ozzie Canseco in baseball, Horace and Harvey Grant in basketball, triplets Leila, Liina, and Lily Luik in marathon running, Katherine and Michelle Plouffe in basketball, Janne and Lieke Wevers in gymnastics, and Frank and Ronald de Boer in soccer.

Although debatable (Rende et al., 1990), Francis Galton was perhaps the first author to suggest, in a landmark paper written in 1875 (Galton, 1875), using the twin method to address the complex issue of disentangling the nature and nurture controversy in the expression of human traits. Although old, and challenging, this issue is still present and pressing in behavioral genetics (Plomin & Asbury, 2005) as well as in the sport sciences (Davids & Baker, 2007).

Most probably the first authors to use the twin method to address the issue of genetics in the performance of *homo sportivus* were Grebe (1955, 1956, 1957) in Germany, and Gedda (1955, 1960) in Italy. This last author presented in his 1960 paper a summary of elite Italian twin athletes. Further, he coined the words *family sportivation*, as well as *isosportivation* (family members practicing the same sport) and *allosportivation* (family members practicing different sports). The main conclusion of this study was: "From the theoretical point of view we may assume that the specific sports genotype, being composed of normal character factors, is transmitted as a dominant. This is what I have been maintaining for some years, and Grebe holds the same opinion" (p. 400). Yet, a review (Klissouras, 2001) on the nature and nurture of human performance did not report on high-elite or elite twin athletes' putative dominant gene(s) vertically transmitted, nor has the TERRY (Casini et al., 2002) or the RITA (Parisi et al., 2001) Italian twin athletes' registers provided information about candidate gene(s) linked to elite sports performance.

In 2013, David Epstein (2013) wrote an amazing book with a thought-provoking title: *The Sports Gene*. One could naively think, along the same lines as in Grebe and Gedda, that some major gene might be the Holy Grail behind the extraordinary performance of elite athletes.

Exactly on the same lines as in the critique of Davids and Baker's (2007) "single gene as a magic bullet." This is probably what happened with the angiotensin-converting enzyme (*ACE*) gene and the alpha-actinin-3 (*ACTN3*) gene and their implications for sports performance, and they showed to be somewhat valid. For example, a meta-analysis and systematic review (Ma et al., 2013) concluded that there was solid evidence for the associations of the *ACE* II genotype and endurance events as well as for *ACTN3* R allele and power events. These conclusions have been supported by Papadimitriou et al. (2016) in elite sprinters from ten countries, although their conclusions were cautionary: "Despite sprint performance relying on many gene variants and environment, the % sprint time variance explained by *ACE* and *ACTN3* is substantial at the elite level and might be the difference between a world record and only making the final" (p. 1). Note that the amount of variance explained by *ACTN3* and *ACE* genotypes was approximately 1–1.5% which could be of paramount importance in winning a gold medal. Yet, it was also stated that a substantial amount of performance variance was not explained and further research with common and rare variants was still needed. Although Santiago et al. (2008) found a higher frequency of the *ACTN3* RR genotype in Spanish soccer players than in controls, Tringali et al. (2014) were not able to replicate these results in high-level Italian gymnasts even for the *ACE* DD genotype. As a concluding note, we concur with Davids and Baker's (2007) "single gene as a magic bullet" in the sense that soccer players' and gymnasts' high-level performance is far more complex than meets the eye with single candidate genes, or that a potential genetic profile of relevant polymorphisms to influence muscular strength that exclusively favors high-level performance is extremely rare to find (Hughes et al., 2011).

Family studies

Some geneticists are apparently favored by the "fire of inspiration" and write remarkable accounts of their daunting quest. Three of these, all *New York Times* book award winners, were written to illuminate the most astonishing accomplishments within the large field of genetics. They all wrote about information, and the gene is but coded information, its copying, transcribing, translation, and also passing it from one generation to the next. The first book was written by Watson and Andrew (2003), narrating the remarkable history of the discovery of the DNA structure. The title is very provocative: *DNA: The Secret of Life*. Also, Ridley (2000) wrote an outstanding account of the genome in 23 chapters. The last in this trilogy was carved by Mukherjee (2016). It is a monumental endeavor concerning the gene and its intimate history. The firing seed of this work erupts from a serious health problem affecting some of his family members, mostly his father's relatives, and he asks poignant questions such as: Is the disease genetic? Why are some of my family members spared from it? What triggers its emergence in some relatives, i.e., what unveiled their predispositions? Who were carriers of the "defected gene(s)?" Am I a carrier? Will these genes be passed on to my progeny? How will we manage the volley between the hands of nature and nurture?

Although framed in a completely different context, sports excellence, also conceived as a marker of a complex "dance" of genes (i.e., additive and epistatic effects), has been historically hunted within family lines, trying to answer some of Mukherjee's questions and rooted inside the tools of medical genetics, namely pedigree analysis. Perhaps the first serious attempts were made by Grebe (1956) and Moser (1960) who examined a series of genealogical diagrams of sportsmen and suggested that sports talent as well as sports abilities were dominant traits within family lines governed by an unknown number of additive gene effects, as well as an intricate set of environmental conditions that mingle with genes to produce outstanding displays of sports performance. Although they suggested a dominant mode of transmission in these reports,

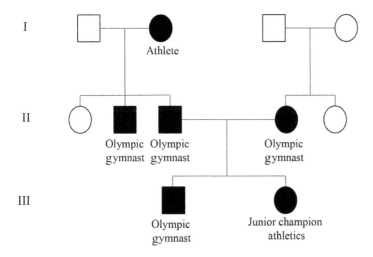

Figure 26.1   A three-generation pedigree of a successful Czech sports family.

one has to bear in mind that no formal segregation analyses were done because at the time no sophisticated statistical techniques, algorithms, and software were available, as we have today (see Sun 2002), to deal with the complexities of data from pedigrees of arbitrary size as well as considering putative environmental covariates, i.e., important events in athletes' sports life histories that in all likelihood push them towards the road of excellence. In any case, Figure 26.1 is an example provided by Kovář (1980) of a pedigree of a high successful sports family mainly with a gymnastics tone.

In 2010, one of the authors (JM), in conjunction with one of his Colombian students (Luis Carlos Muñoz), started collecting information about Colombian families of athletes from individual sports: track-and-field, weightlifting, cycling, wrestling, skating, karate, judo, fencing, swimming, taekwondo, boxing, and diving. Our search started with a reference athlete, i.e., a *proband*, who participated and/or won a medal in at least one international competition (i.e., an elite athlete). From an initial survey of 103 putative families, we only had access to 78 which included 1577 relatives of whom 149 were high elite, elite, and subelite. In order to better understand their family structure, all were divided according to three conditions: 1) families with athletes whose parents, siblings, and progeny also were athletes (*N*=7); 2) families with only siblings as athletes (*N*=30), and 3) families with no parents and siblings as athletes (*N*=41). Yet, before we start presenting aspects of our data it is necessary to inform the reader of the following: 1) today we have several techniques available that address the complex issue of familial aggregation (Keen & Elston, 2003; Mathew et al., 2011; Naj et al., 2002) and we will use them to analyze some of the data; 2) although sophisticated segregation methods of analysis to identify modes of inheritance in families of arbitrary size are available (Sun, 2002), none has been used to study pedigrees of athletes so far as we know, and we also will not use them; 3) finally, there are also techniques to model the genotype–phenotype relationships within pedigrees of arbitrary size (Elston et al., 1992), but because we do not have any genetic information, no such models will be used. Even if we did, using a genome-wide association study approach, or family studies for the optimal detection of rare variants, we would need thousands of subjects, or large-size extended pedigrees (Diego et al., 2015), which are far beyond the scope of this study. We also ask the

Table 26.1 Parameter estimates from the Colombian sports families

Parameters	Estimates	Standard error	P-value
Heritability	0.57	0.06	<0.001
Residual family correlations			
Full sibs	0.59	0.03	<0.001
Half-sibs	0.14	0.01	<0.001
Parent–offspring	0.29	0.03	<0.001
Environmental correlations			
Full sibs	0.72	0.07	<0.001

Note: estimates adjusted for sex and race.

Table 26.2 Information summary of the seven most outstanding Colombian sports families

Family name	Level	# family members in pedigree	# (%) of athletes	Sports practiced		Achievement level		Age at onset of sports practice	
				≠	~	≠	~	≠	~
Tovar Ante	World class	16	7 (44%)		x		x	x	
Howard	World class	15	2 (13%)	x		x		x	
Urrea	World class	21	4 (19%)	x		x		x	
Lozano	Pan American	13	2 (15%)		x		x		x
Garcés Lopez	Pan American	16	5 (31%)		x	x		x	
Osorio	Pan American	21	9 (43%)	x		x		x	
Trujillo	Pan American	13	5 (39%)		x	x		x	

Note: # number; ≠ different; ~ similar.

reader to bear in mind the fact that sport scientists recognize sports performance as a highly complex and multifactorial human trait most often expressed in various quantitative and qualitative ways. Yet, for matters of convenience mainly when investigating a candidate gene marking some aspect of this complexity, sports performance is often dichotomized using some empirical threshold. Consistent with this, as well as with the classification suggested by Druzhevskaya et al. (2008), we also treat sports performance as a discrete trait with three categories (subelite, elite, and high elite) as mentioned above.

Our approach to the Colombian families of athletes will be mainly descriptive. To start with, Table 26.1 contains information regarding the analysis of familial aggregation using a model (Elston & Stewart, 1971) and an algorithm (Elston et al., 1992) implemented in S.A.G.E. genetic epidemiology software (S.A.G.E 64, 2016). Sports performance shows a substantial heritability ($h^2=0.57$), and the residual familial correlations as well as the environmental correlations also reveal the importance of siblings' other shared factors beyond shared genes.

Further, a summary of the data from the available families in condition 1 are in Table 26.2. The number of athletes, within the three-generation pedigrees, belonging to the three sports performance categories varies from 2 (13%) to 7 (44%), and their chosen sport is most often

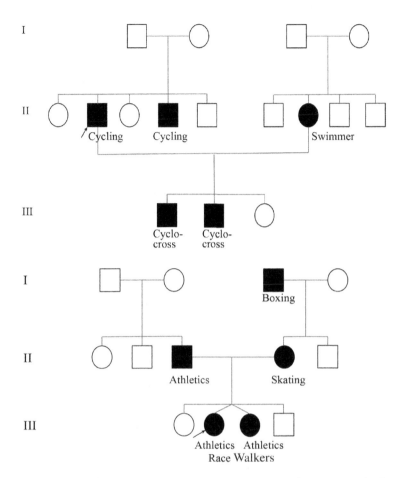

Figure 26.2 Pedigrees of Garcés Lopez (above) and Trujillo (below) sports families. Filled symbols represent elite and subelite athletes.

equal. Additionally, their achievement level varies across the three levels, and the age at onset of sports practice is also different.

In Figure 26.2 we show pedigrees of two representative families. The first one (Garcés Lopez) emphasizes their cycling and cyclo-cross aggregation, whereas the second one (Trujillo) mostly represents a passion for athletics, namely the dizygotic twin sisters' elite and subelite race walking history.

Further, from a pool of 30 three-generation families with only elite and/or subelite siblings' athletes in the third generation, we chose two – the Wilches Tumbia clustering in cycling (above) and the Botero Coy (below) in skating (Figure 26.3).

From families in condition 3, i.e., families with sports "silence" in generations I and II as well as in siblings, we chose two with unique signatures in their outstanding sports performance – Cecília Margarita Baena and Sandra Viviana Roa. Cecília Baena was world champion of in-line skating already at 13 years of age. At 16 years of age she won the 500-meter and 1000-meter gold medals in the 2001 world championship. In her career she won six world titles, and several other first class titles in Central America and Pan American championships.

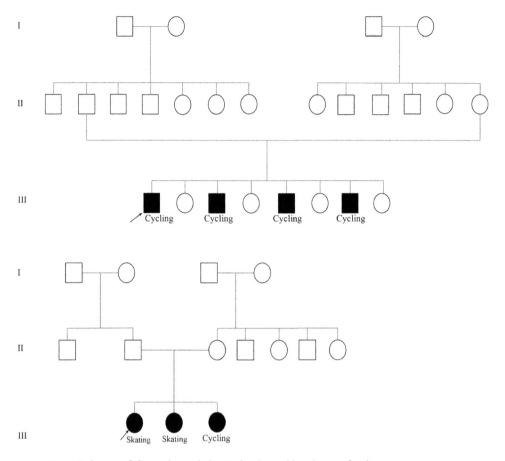

Figure 26.3 Pedigrees of elite and/or subelite Colombian siblings' sports families.

Sandra Viviana Roa is an exceptional wrestler having to her credit bronze and gold medals in several Pan American and Central America championships. At the world level she was several times in the top ten of her weight category.

To finish this very brief description on Colombian sports families, we chose two of them as our case studies – the Tovar Ante and the Urrutia families because they are unique examples. The Tovar Ante family line has a unique signature given that they always have been involved in shooting, pistol class, with the exception of Rafael Tovar Ante whose sports history is rooted in motocross. The family history in pistol class started in the first generation with Bernardo Tovar Paredes who was national champion in Colombia. Then, he transmitted, vertically, his sports passion and his genes to his sons, especially to Bernardo Tovar Ante, who was an outstanding athlete participating in Olympic Games as well as world championships. He is the family member who conquered more medals. He then "contaminated" his wife with his passion since environmental driven conditions were always in place that in all likelihood unveiled her innate predispositions. She was also an elite athlete, and the same applies to their son and daughter, also a unique combination of their genetic endowments and a highly favorable exposome (Figure 28.6).

The Urrutia family is an extreme example of "silence" in sports participation until the fourth generation (Figure 26.7). The most outstanding athlete is Maria Isabel Urrutia. She started in

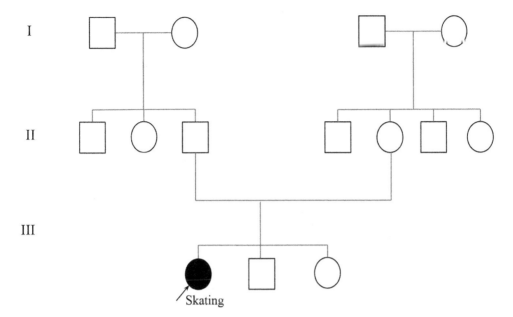

Figure 26.4 Family pedigree of Cecília Margarita Baena.

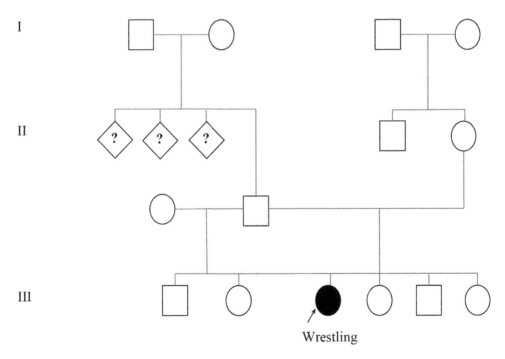

Figure 26.5 Family pedigree of Sandra Viviana Roa.

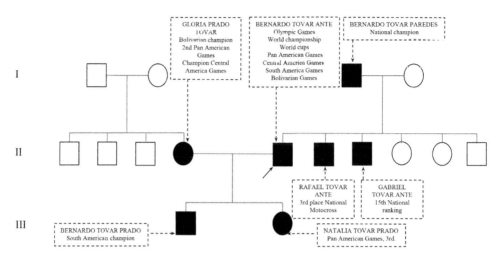

Figure 26.6 Pedigree of the Tovar Ante family.

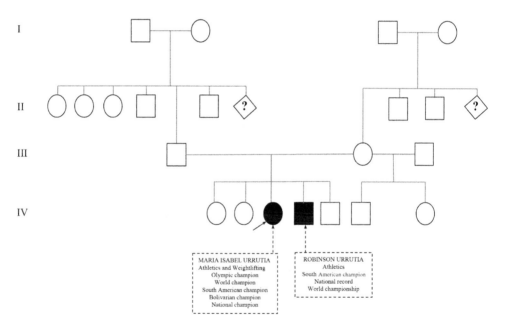

Figure 26.7 Pedigree of the Urrutia family.

track and field, and in 1978 was the youngest national champion of her age category in 100-meter sprint – she was 13 years. She was also fond of discus and shot put, and won several national and international championships. Later she participated in the Seoul Olympics and reached 14th place in the overall ranking in both events. Then, at age 24 years, she also started participating in weightlifting competitions, winning several championships, and a gold medal in the Sidney 2000 Olympics (weight category <75 kg). Her brother Robinson is also an excellent athlete in the 100-meter sprint.

We chose to close this section with three recent stories of successful sports family lines. The first one is about Coco Vandeweghe, a top-class tennis player (ranked 17 by the Women's Tennis Association), and the unique signature of her family. She is the daughter of Tauna Vandeweghe, a US Olympic swimmer; her uncle and grandfather were elite US basketball players and her grandmother was Miss America in 1952. The other two, with apparently similar signatures, are about US athletes participating in the 2018 Peyong Chang Winter Olympics. Nancy Swider-Peltz Jr. participated in the Games with her brother, Jeffrey Swider-Peltz Jr. Their mother is Nancy Swider-Peltz, a four-time US Olympic speed skater who was the first US athlete to compete in four Olympic Winter Games. Cochran-Siegle was also in the 2018 Olympic Games. His mother, Barbara Ann Cochran, won the Olympic gold in the slalom in 1972. His family line also include skiing Olympians, like his aunts Lindy and Marilyn Cochran, uncle Bob Cochran, and cousin Jimmy Cochran.

Deliberate practice, athletes' exposome, and genetic-by-exposome interactions

As far as we know, there is apparently no "long-range" prospective study that investigates the life course to excellence of any high-elite, or elite athletes starting from their youth sport careers, or even as far back as preconception via gametic imprinting (Brutsaert & Parra, 2009). The reason is perceptibly simple – we cannot know where such talented youth are because talent search and identification enterprises have no clear-cut definitions of what "talent" is and we can hardly find an expeditious way of uniquely identifying putative candidates (Johnston et al., 2018; Maia, 1993; Sarmento et al., 2018). We simply do not exactly know what we are looking for because of the complexities of individual development, heterogeneity in responses to sports training and competition, as well as how the same individual will display their manifold attributes across her/his development. Although Guth and Roth (2013) stated that "the drive behind the prediction of athletic performance with genetics is primarily aimed at the early identification of individuals who will become exceptional athletes as adults" (p. 5), to date there is no record about such findings by sports geneticists. Further, the person who first spotted Cristiano Ronaldo, the world's most famous soccer player, did not know about the uniqueness of the pearl he had in his hands. He was a humble soccer coach working with children, but his gaze apparently ranged far.

It is a truism to say that elite athletes are born and then made. Bloom (1985) was probably one of the first that described, in retrospective terms, a few invariant features shared by elite athletes (tennis players and swimmers) during their roads towards outstanding performance: 1) strong interest and emotional involvement in their chosen sport; 2) willingness to devote great amounts of time and efforts towards excellence; 3) great competitiveness with their peers, and firm determination to shine in their sport; and 4) high learning capacity and potential to reach distinctiveness.

Papers by Ericsson et al. (1993, 2009) on intense deliberate practice, where the golden number of 10,000 accumulated hours of training was coined, and its links to exceptional achievements launched a serious debate in the sport science field. Their views were strongly criticized, for example, by Tucker and Collins (2012) namely for inconsistency in their original data, reference model, as well as their insistent call for the nurture aspect (deliberate practice) and removal of the wealthy body of data on genetics of performance in the nature and nurture equation. Additionally, systemic views linking complex synergies of genes and the manifold expressions of family, peers, and training environments to best understand the march towards excellence of any young athlete are now favored instead of the old motto nature versus nurture (see, for example, Davids and Baker (2007); Brutsaert and Parra (2009), or Wai (2014); Plomin et al. (2014)). Yet, to date, there is apparently no longitudinal data linking all the exposome conditions putative talented youth went through interacting with varied sets of genes to express outstanding performance at various stages of their careers. These chronometric time effects of the marriage of young athletes' exposome and genome are simply not known. Even in the exposome, the majority of the available data are retrospective and open to debate (Coutinho et al., 2016). Recently, Rees et al. (2016) reviewed the literature on development of the world's best sporting talent centered on four domains: 1) the performer (birthdate, genetics, anthropometric and physiological factors, psychological skills and motivational orientations, personality traits), 2) the environment (birthplace, support from parents, siblings and coaches, athlete support programs), 3) practice and training (volume of sport-specific practice and training, early specialization versus sampling and play), and 4) other potential factors, and concluded that "in encouraging researchers, we would point to the relative dearth of prospective and multidisciplinary studies that could offer insight regarding the complex interactions that almost certainly exist across domains" (p. 1050).

Conclusion

The world-renowned biologist, E.O.Wilson, wrote the following in his book *On Human Nature* (1978) that won the Pulitzer Prize in 1979:

> Since each individual produced by the sexual process contains a unique set of genes, very exceptional combinations of genes are unlikely to appear twice within the same family. So if genius is to any extent hereditary, it winks on and off through the gene pool in a way that would be difficult to measure or predict. Like Sisyphus rolling his boulder up to the top of the hill only to have it tumble down again, the human gene pool creates hereditary genius in many ways in many places only to have it come apart in the next generation.

Marion Jones and Tim Montgomery, world-renowned track and field athletes had a son. The same happened, for example, to world-ranked tennis players Steffi Graf and Andre Agassi (one son and one daughter), as well as Roger and Mirka Federer (two twin pairs, one of girls and one of boys). Will these children be future champions? Apparently, all odds favor them not only in terms of sharing of genetic material, but also in their highly advantageous environmental conditions, i.e., their exposome. Time will tell.

References

Ahmetov, I. I., Egorova, E. S., Gabdrakhmanova, L. J., & Fedotovskaya, O. N. (2016). Genes and athletic performance: an update. *Med Sport Sci*, 61, 41–54. doi: 10.1159/000445240

Araujo, D. & Davids, K. (2016). Team synergies in sport: theory and measures. *Front Psychol*, 7, 1449. doi: 10.3389/fpsyg.2016.01449

Aylsworth, A. S. (2006). Defining disease phenotypes. In J. L. Haimes & M.A. Pericak-Vance (Eds.), *Genetic Analysis of Complex Disease*. (2nd ed., pp. 51–90). Hoboken, NJ: John Wiley & Sons, Inc.

Barbosa, J., Gomes, T. N., Forjaz, C. L. M., & Maia, J. (2018). Correlational analysis of Physical activity levels and sport participation. Research in twins and in families. RPEFE, 31, 505.

Bloom, B. S. (1985). *Developing Talent in Young People*. New York: Ballantine Publishing Books.

Bouchard, C. (1973). Qu'est-ce qui fait un champion? In C. Bouchard, J. Brunelle & P. Godbout (Eds.), *La preparation d'un Champion. Un essai à la performance sportive*. (pp. 75–106). Québec: Éditions du Pélican.

Bouchard, C., Brunelle, J., & Godbout, P. (1973). *La preparation d'un Champion. Un essai à la performance sportive*. Québec: Éditions du Pélican.

Bouchard, C. & Malina, R. M. (1984). Genetics of Olympic athletes: a discussion of methods and issues. In J. E. L. Carter (Ed.), *Physical Structure of Olympic athletes. Part II Kinanthropometry of Olympic athletes* (pp. 28–38). Basel: Karger.

Brutsaert, T. D. & Parra, E. J. (2009). Nature versus nurture in determining athletic ability. *Med Sport Sci*, 54, 11–27. doi: 10.1159/000235694

Casini, B., Pittaluga, M., & Parisi, P. (2002). Two Italian twin registers for research in human biology and sport science. *Twin Res*, 5(5), 376–381. doi: 10.1375/136905202320906129

Coutinho, P., Mesquita, I., & Fonseca, A. M. (2016). Talent development in sport: a critical review of pathways to expert performance. *Int J Sports Sci Coach*, 11(2), 279–293.

Davids, K. & Baker, J. (2007). Genes, environment and sport performance: why the nature-nurture dualism is no longer relevant. *Sports Med*, 37(11), 961–980.

de Garay, A. L., Levine, L., & Carter, J. E. L. (1974). *Genetic and Anthropological Studies of Olympic Athletes.* New York: Academic Press.

de Vilhena e Santos, D. M., Katzmarzyk, P. T., Seabra, A. F., & Maia, J. A. (2012). Genetics of physical activity and physical inactivity in humans. *Behav Genet*, 42(4), 559–578. doi: 10.1007/s10519-012-9534-1

Diego, V. P., Kent, J. W., & Blangero, J. (2015). Familial studies: genetic inferences. In J. D. Wright (Ed.), *International Encyclopedia of the Social & Behavioral Sciences* (2nd ed.) (pp. 715–724). Oxford: Elsevier.

Druzhevskaya, A. M., Ahmetov, I. I., Astratenkova, I.V., & Rogozkin, V.A. (2008). Association of the ACTN3 R577X polymorphism with power athlete status in Russians. *Eur J Appl Physiol*, 103(6), 631–634. doi: 10.1007/s00421-008-0763-1

Elston, R. C., George, V.T., & Severtson, F. (1992). The Elston-Stewart algorithm for continuous genotypes and environmental factors. *Hum Hered*, 42(1), 16–27. doi: 10.1159/000154043

Elston, R. C. & Stewart, J. (1971). A general model for the genetic analysis of pedigree data. *Hum Hered*, 21(6), 523–542. doi: 10.1159/000152448

Epstein, D. (2013). *The Sports Gene: Inside the Science of Extraordinary Athletic Performance.* New York: Penguim Book.

Ericsson, K.A., Krampe, R.T., & Tesch-Römer, C. (1993). The role of deliberate practice in the acquisition of expert performance. *Psychol Rev*, 100(3), 363–406.

Ericsson, K. A., Nandagopal, K., & Roring, R. W. (2009). Toward a science of exceptional achievement: attaining superior performance through deliberate practice. *Ann N Y Acad Sci*, 1172, 199–217. doi: 10.1196/annals.1393.001

Galton, F. (1869). *Hereditary Genius: An Inquiry into its Laws and Consequences.* London: Macmillan.

Galton, F. (1875). The history of twins, as a criterion of the relative powers of nature and nurture. *Fraser's Magazine*, 566–576.

Gedda, L. (1955). La valutazione genética dell'atleta. *Acta Genet Med Gemellol (Roma)*, 4, 249–260.

Gedda, L. (1960). Sport and genetics. A study on twins (312) pairs. *Acta Genet Med Gemellol (Roma)*, 9, 387–405.

Grebe, H. (1955). Sport bei zwillingen. *Acta Genet Med Gemellol (Roma)*, 4, 275–295.

Grebe, H. (1956). Sportfamilien. *Acta Genet Med Gemellol (Roma)*, 5, 318–326.

Grebe, H. (1957). Genotypus und konstitution im sport. *Sportmedizin*, 10, 269–274.

Guth, L. M. & Roth, S. M. (2013). Genetic influence on athletic performance. *Curr Opin Pediatr*, 25(6), 653–658. doi: 10.1097/MOP.0b013e3283659087

Hughes, D. C., Day, S. H., Ahmetov, I. I., & Williams, A. G. (2011). Genetics of muscle strength and power: polygenic profile similarity limits skeletal muscle performance. *J Sports Sci*, 29(13), 1425–1434. doi: 10.1080/02640414.2011.597773

Johnston, K., Wattie, N., Schorer, J., & Baker, J. (2018). Talent identification in sport: a systematic review. *Sports Med*, 48(1), 97–109. doi: 10.1007/s40279-017-0803-2

Keen, K. J. & Elston, R. C. (2003). Robust asymptotic sampling theory for correlations in pedigrees. *Stat Med*, 22(20), 3229–3247. doi: 10.1002/sim.1559

Klissouras, C. (2001). The nature and nurture of human performance. *Eur J Sport Sci* 1(1), 1–10. doi: 10.1080/17461390100071207

Kovář, R. (1980). *Human Variation in Motor Abilities and its Genetic Analysis.* Prague: Charles University Prague.

Kyle, D. G. (2015). *Sport and Spectacle in the Ancient World.* (2nd ed.). Chichester, West Sussex: Wiley Blackwell.

Ma, F., Yang, Y., Li, X., Zhou, F., Gao, C., Li, M., & Gao, L. (2013). The association of sport performance with ACE and ACTN3 genetic polymorphisms: a systematic review and meta-analysis. *PLoS One*, 8(1), e54685. doi: 10.1371/journal.pone.0054685

Maia, J., Gomes, T. N., Tregouet, D. A., & Katzmarzyk, P. T. (2014). Familial resemblance of physical activity levels in the Portuguese population. *J Sci Med Sport*, 17(4), 381–386. doi: 10.1016/j.jsams.2013.09.004

Maia, J. A. R. (1993). *Anthropobiological Approach to Selection in Sport. A Multivariate Study of Biosocial Selection Markers in Team Handball Players Aged 13 to 16 Years*. (PhD), Faculty of Sport Sciences and Physical Education, Porto, Portugal.

Mathew, G., Song, Y., & Elston, R. (2011). Interval estimation of familial correlations from pedigrees. *Stat Appl Genet Mol Biol*, 10, Article 11.

Moser, H. (1960). *Uber die vererbung der sportlichen fähigkeiten*. (1st ed.). München.

Mukherjee, S. (2016). *The Gene: An Intimate History*. New York: Scribner.

Mustelin, L., Latvala, A., Pietilainen, K. H., Piirila, P., Sovijarvi, A. R., Kujala, U. M., Rissanen, A., & Kaprio, J. (2011). Associations between sports participation, cardiorespiratory fitness, and adiposity in young adult twins. *J Appl Physiol (1985)*, 110(3), 681–686. doi: 10.1152/japplphysiol.00753.2010

Naj, A. C., Park, Y. S., & Beaty, T. H. (2002). Detecting familial aggregation. In R. C. Elston, J. M. Satagopan & S. Sun (Eds.), *Statistical Human Genetics: Methods and Protocols*. (pp. 119–150). New York: Humana Press.

Papadimitriou, I. D., Lucia, A., Pitsiladis, Y. P., Pushkarev, V. P., Dyatlov, D. A., Orekhov, E. F., Artioli, G. G., Guilherme, J. P., Lancha, A. H., Jr., Gineviciene, V., Cieszczyk, P., Maciejewska-Karlowska, A., Sawczuk, M., Muniesa, C. A., Kouvatsi, A., Massidda, M., Calo, C. M., Garton, F., Houweling, P. J., Wang, G., Austin, K., Druzhevskaya, A. M., Astratenkova, I. V., Ahmetov, I. I., Bishop, D. J., North, K. N., & Eynon, N. (2016). ACTN3 R577X and ACE I/D gene variants influence performance in elite sprinters: a multi-cohort study. *BMC Genomics*, 17, 285. doi: 10.1186/s12864-016-2462-3

Parisi, P., Casini, B., Di Salvo, V., Pigozzi, F., Pittaluga, M., Prinzi, G., & Klissouras, V. (2001). The Registry of Italian Twin Athletes (RITA): Background, design, and procedures, and twin data analysis on sport participation—an application to twin swimmers. *Eur J Sport Sci*, 1(2), 1–12. doi: 10.1080/17461390100071208

Pérusse, L. (2011). Role of genetics factors in sport performance: evidence from family studies. In C. Bouchard and E. Hoffman (Eds.) *Genetic and Molecular Aspects of Sport Performance* (pp. 90–100). Chichester, West Sussex: Wiley-Blackwell.

Pitsiladis, Y., Wang, G., Wolfarth, B., Scott, R., Fuku, N., Mikami, E., He, Z., Fiuza-Luces, C., Eynon, N., & Lucia, A. (2013). Genomics of elite sporting performance: what little we know and necessary advances. *Br J Sports Med*, 47(9), 550–555.

Pitsiladis, Y. P., Tanaka, M., Eynon, N., Bouchard, C., North, K. N., Williams, A. G., Collins, M., Moran, C. N., Britton, S. L., Fuku, N., Ashley, E. A., Klissouras, V., Lucia, A., Ahmetov, I. I., de Geus, E., & Alsayrafi, M. (2016). Athlome Project Consortium: a concerted effort to discover genomic and other "omic" markers of athletic performance. *Physiol Genomics*, 48(3), 183–190. doi: 10.1152/physiolgenomics.00105.2015

Plomin, R. & Asbury, K. (2005). Nature and nurture: genetic and environmental influences on behavior. *Ann Am Acad Pol Soc Sci*, 600, 86–98.

Plomin, R., Shakeshaft, N. G., McMillan, A., & Trzaskowski, M. (2014). Nature, nurture, and expertise. *Intelligence*, 45, 46–59. doi: 10.1016/j.intell.2013.06.008

Rankinen, T., Fuku, N., Wolfarth, B., Wang, G., Sarzynski, M. A., Alexeev, D. G., Ahmetov, I. I., Boulay, M. R., Cieszczyk, P., Eynon, N., Filipenko, M. L., Garton, F. C., Generozov, E. V., Govorun, V. M., Houweling, P. J., Kawahara, T., Kostryukova, E. S., Kulemin, N. A., Larin, A. K., Maciejewska-Karlowska, A., Miyachi, M., Muniesa, C. A., Murakami, H., Ospanova, E. A., Padmanabhan, S., Pavlenko, A. V., Pyankova, O. N., Santiago, C., Sawczuk, M., Scott, R. A., Uyba, V. V., Yvert, T., Perusse, L., Ghosh, S., Rauramaa, R., North, K. N., Lucia, A., Pitsiladis, Y., & Bouchard, C. (2016). No evidence of a common DNA variant profile specific to world class endurance athletes. *PLoS One*, 11(1), e0147330. doi: 10.1371/journal.pone.0147330

Rankinen, T., Wolfarth, B., Simoneau, J. A., Maier-Lenz, D., Rauramaa, R., Rivera, M. A., Boulay, M. R., Chagnon, Y. C., Perusse, L., Keul, J., & Bouchard, C. (2000). No association between the angiotensin-converting enzyme ID polymorphism and elite endurance athlete status. *J Appl Physiol (1985)*, 88(5), 1571–1575. doi: 10.1152/jappl.2000.88.5.1571

Rees, T., Hardy, L., Gullich, A., Abernethy, B., Cote, J., Woodman, T., Montgomery, H., Laing, S., & Warr, C. (2016). The Great British Medalists Project: a review of current knowledge on the development of the world's best sporting talent. *Sports Med*, 46(8), 1041–1058. doi: 10.1007/s40279-016-0476-2

Rende, R. D., Plomin, R., & Vandenberg, S. G. (1990). Who discovered the twin method? *Behav Genet*, 20(2), 277–285.

Ridley, M. (2000). *Genome: The autobiography of a species in 23 chapters*. New York: Perennial.

Rivera, M. A., Dionne, F. T., Wolfarth, B., Chagnon, M., Simoneau, J. A., Perusse, L., Boulay, M. R., Gagnon, J., Song, T. M., Keul, J., & Bouchard, C. (1997). Muscle-specific creatine kinase gene polymorphisms in elite endurance athletes and sedentary controls. *Med Sci Sports Exerc*, 29(11), 1444–1447.

S.A.G.E 64. (2016). Statistical analysis for genetic epidemiology. http://darwin.cwru.edu/sage/.

Santiago, C., Gonzalez-Freire, M., Serratosa, L., Morate, F. J., Meyer, T., Gomez-Gallego, F., & Lucia, A. (2008). ACTN3 genotype in professional soccer players. *Br J Sports Med*, 42(1), 71–73. doi: 10.1136/bjsm.2007.039172

Sarmento, H., Anguera, M. T., Pereira, A., & Araujo, D. (2018). Talent identification and development in male football: a systematic review. *Sports Med*, 48(4), 907–931. doi: 10.1007/s40279-017-0851-7

Stubbe, J. H., Boomsma, D. I., & De Geus, E. J. (2005). Sports participation during adolescence: a shift from environmental to genetic factors. *Med Sci Sports Exerc*, 37(4), 563–570.

Sun, X. (2002). Segregation analysis using a unified model. In R. C. Elston, J. M. Satagopan & S. Sun (Eds.), *Statistical Human Genetics: Methods and Protocols* (pp. 211–236). New York: Humana Press.

Tringali, C., Brivio, I., Stucchi, B., Silvestri, I., Scurati, R., Michielon, G., Alberti, G., & Venerando, B. (2014). Prevalence of a characteristic gene profile in high-level rhythmic gymnasts. *J Sports Sci*, 32(14), 1409–1415. doi: 10.1080/02640414.2014.893371

Tucker, R. & Collins, M. (2012). What makes champions? A review of the relative contribution of genes and training to sporting success. *Br J Sports Med*, 46(8), 555–561. doi: 10.1136/bjsports-2011–090548

Wai, J. (2014). Experts are born, then made: Combining prospective and retrospective longitudinal data shows that cognitive ability matters. *Intelligence*, 45, 74–80. doi: 10.1016/j.intell.2013.08.009

Watson, J. D. & Andrew, B. (2003). *DNA: The Secret of Life*. New York: Alfred A. Knopf.

Wilson, E. O. (1978). *On Human Nature*. Cambridge, MA: Harvard University Press.

Wolfarth, B., Rankinen, T., Muhlbauer, S., Ducke, M., Rauramaa, R., Boulay, M. R., Perusse, L., & Bouchard, C. (2008). Endothelial nitric oxide synthase gene polymorphism and elite endurance athlete status: the Genathlete study. *Scand J Med Sci Sports*, 18(4), 485–490. doi: 10.1111/j.1600-0838.2007.00717.x

Wolfarth, B., Rankinen, T., Muhlbauer, S., Scherr, J., Boulay, M. R., Perusse, L., Rauramaa, R., & Bouchard, C. (2007). Association between a beta2-adrenergic receptor polymorphism and elite endurance performance. *Metabolism*, 56(12), 1649–1651. doi: 10.1016/j.metabol.2007.07.006

Wolfarth, B., Rivera, M. A., Oppert, J. M., Boulay, M. R., Dionne, F. T., Chagnon, M., Gagnon, J., Chagnon, Y., Perusse, L., Keul, J., & Bouchard, C. (2000). A polymorphism in the alpha2a-adrenoceptor gene and endurance athlete status. *Med Sci Sports Exerc*, 32(10), 1709–1712.

27

SPORT CONCUSSION GENETICS

Ryan T. Tierney and Jane K. McDevitt

Reading news headlines could lead someone to believe that playing contact sports such as football will lead to a degenerative neurological condition in early adulthood. Indeed, participation in sports such as high school football has declined as the number of news reports of concussion in sports has increased (11). However, research indicates that although higher than the normal population, only a low percentage of former athletes such as NFL players are reporting such problems (20). Since most of these players were likely exposed to thousands of subconcussive (and some concussive) impacts over a career, why are only some athletes exhibiting problems? The answer may lie in intrinsic factors such as genetics in combination with their environment (repetitive head impacts). Thus, risk of poor mental or cognitive health may not come from playing contact sports alone, but playing them in addition to having a specific genetic predisposition. In this chapter, we will explore genes and polymorphisms potentially associated with sport concussion.

Concussion pathomechanics and pathophysiology

Traumatic brain injury (TBI) can be viewed along a continuum (Figure 27.1) with high head-impact acceleration events (e.g., high-speed car accident) yielding severe TBI and low head accelerations (e.g., soccer heading) eliciting seemingly no injury (i.e., subconcussion). Concussion and subconcussion are on the low end of the continuum and are the most common impact types encountered in sports. The level of injury is determined through clinical assessment and, when appropriate, includes diagnostic imaging assessment. Subconcussion is a head impact (or head acceleration event) that does not result in any outward signs (e.g., unsteadiness) or subjective reporting of symptoms (e.g., headache) (4). A concussion is a head impact (or head acceleration event) that does result in signs and symptoms (37). A concussion would not yield any remarkable signs on diagnostic imaging (e.g., magnetic resonance imaging), which helps differentiate concussion from a moderate or severe brain injury.

To understand the role genetics may play in predisposing someone to a concussion, it is important to further understand concussion injury pathomechanics and pathophysiology. A concussion is an injury to the brain caused by acceleration forces (15). These forces can occur from something hitting the head, the head hitting something, or an indirect blow to the

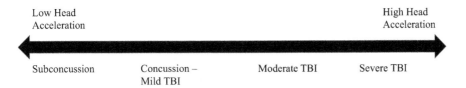

Low Head
Acceleration

High Head
Acceleration

Subconcussion   Concussion –   Moderate TBI   Severe TBI
                   Mild TBI

Figure 27.1   Traumatic brain injury pathomechanics spectrum.

body causing whiplash (3). The brain, which is floating in cerebrospinal fluid, moves rapidly within the skull creating tensile, compressive, or shear forces on the brain tissue producing cell deformation (i.e., pathomechanics) (45). The two main cell types in the brain are neurons, the conducting cells, and glia, the supporting cells. Identifying structures that manage stress and strain within these cells is important to finding a possible genetic predisposition to concussion (Figure 27.2).

A number of neuronal structures can help manage mechanical stress including the cell membrane, microtubules, and intermediate filaments. The cell membrane is stabilized by cholesterol embedded, in part, by the function of apolipoprotein. Neuronal microtubules give cells form and help transport cellular material, and are stabilized by the protein tau. Neuronal intermediate filaments are composed of proteins such as neurofilament heavy (NEFH) and light (NEFL), and form an internal cell scaffolding that helps create form and resist changes in cell shape. In astrocytes, the predominant glial cell comprising a large percentage of brain volume, a main component of intermediate filaments is glial fibrillary acidic protein (GFAP). These structures help resist cell deformation in response to mechanical stress. If deformation is large enough (e.g., > 5% of resting length), this axonal stretch can lead to neurometabolic events and cell dysfunction (i.e., concussion pathophysiology) (13).

Concussion pathophysiology involves a neurometabolic cascade of cellular events that occur post insult and trigger neuron dysfunction. These events have been described previously (16) and can include ion flux (e.g., Na^+, Ca^+) and glutamate release, cytoskeletal damage to microtubules and neurofilaments, altered neurotransmission due to glutamate and calcium channel disruption, inflammation, and potential cell death. Therefore, proteins involved in cytoskeleton stabilization (e.g., tau), cell membrane channel function, and glutamate regulation may play key roles in attenuating concussion pathophysiology. The ability of the proteins mentioned above to function properly to help withstand mechanical stress and restore proper neuronal function is largely due to their structure. In the next sections, we will review some of the genes that code for these proteins (see Tables 27.1 and 27.2), in particular distinguishing studies that have focused on pathomechanical and pathphysiological outcomes.

Pathomechanical genetic associations

Apolipoprotein E

Apolipoprotein E (*APOE*) is one of the most studied genes associated with concussion and manifests multiple genetic polymorphisms. The *APOE* gene is located on chromosome 19 and produces the apolipoprotein E (ApoE) glycoprotein. This protein is involved in the redistribution of lipids to maintain and restore the neuronal membrane after an injury (7). ApoE exists in three isoforms, ApoE2, ApoE3, and ApoE4 encoded by three common alleles ε2, ε3, and ε4, respectively, and result in changes in different single amino acid changes (34). The three allelic variants

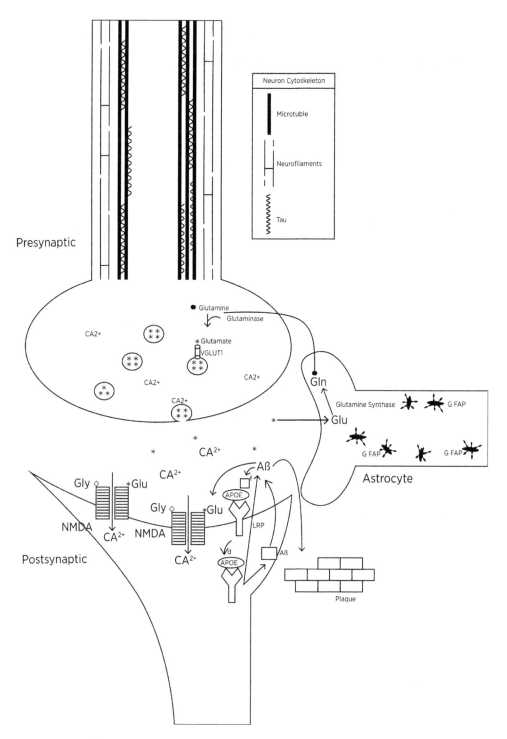

Figure 27.2 Cellular structures involved in concussion pathomechanics and pathophysiology.

Table 27.1 Concussion pathomechanical genetic associations

Protein	Gene (abbreviation)	Variant	Findings
Apolipoprotein E	Apolipoprotein E (*APOE*)	ε4	30 professional boxers (23–76 years of age) underwent neurological examination using the chronic brain injury scale. Authors found the ε4 allele was associated with worse cognition scores in high-exposure boxers (22)
		ε4	318 collegiate athletes (~52% male) were prospectively followed after a concussion. Authors found after adjusting for sex, weight, height, and team type that there was no association with ε4 and concussion risk (28)
		ε4	195 collegiate athletes (163 football and 33 female soccer players) self-reported the number of previous concussions (72 with concussion, 123 with no concussion). After adjusting for age, school, and years of sport experience, carrying the ε4 allele was not associated with concussion history (49)
		ε2, ε3, ε4, G(−219) T-promoter SNP	196 collegiate athletes (163 football and 33 female soccer players) self-reported the number of previous concussions (48 with concussion, 148 with no concussion). Authors found carrying the T promoter allele and X alleles were associated with history of concussion (52)
Apolipoprotein E	Apolipoprotein E (*APOE*)	G(−219)T-promoter SNP	196 collegiate athletes (163 football and 33 female soccer players) self-reported the number of previous concussions (48 with concussion, 148 with no concussion). Authors found an increased risk of two or more concussions when carrying the minor T allele (52)
		G(−219)T-promoter SNP	195 collegiate football and female soccer athletes self-reported previous history of concussion (72 with concussion, 123 with no concussion). After adjusting for age, school, and years of sport experience, carrying the *APOE* promoter TT was associated with increased concussion risk (49)

(*continued*)

Table 27.1 (Cont.)

Protein	Gene (abbreviation)	Variant	Findings
Tau	Microtubule-associated protein tau (*MAPT*)	Tau E6 variants	195 collegiate football and female soccer athletes self-reported previous history of concussion (72 with concussion, 123 with no concussion). After adjusting for age, school, and years of sport experience there was no association between increased concussion risk and the Ser53Pro tau polymorphism (49)
Neurofilament heavy polypeptide	Neurofilament heavy (*NEFH*)	rs165602, glutamic acid to an alanine at amino acid sequence 805, E805A	48 athletes with a reported history of concussion were matched by age, height, sport, and position to 48 athletes with no history of concussion (~19 years of age). Authors found no association between concussion history or risk and carrying the rare C allele (38)

Table 27.2 Concussion pathophysiological genetic associations

Protein	Gene (abbreviation)	Variant	Findings
Glutamate receptor inotropic NMDA type subunit 2A	Glutamate receptor inotropic NMDA type subunit 2A (*GRIN2A*)	GT(n)-promoter repeat polymorphism	87 concussed athletes (~19 years of age; 74% male) were followed prospectively. Authors found an association with prolonged recovery (greater than 60 days) from concussion and carrying 25 or more GT repeats (39)
Solute carrier family 17 member 7; vesicle glutamate transporters (VGLUT 1)	Solute carrier family 17 member 7 (*SLC17A7*)	rs74174284	40 concussed athletes (72% male; ~20 years of age) were followed prospectively. Authors found an association with prolonged recovery (greater than 20 days) from concussion and carrying the G allele (33)

are distinguished by single nucleotide polymorphisms (SNPs) in exon 4 of the *APOE* gene. SNP rs7412C>T is present in alleles ε3 and ε4. SNP rs429358T>C is present in allele ε4. The most common allele is ε3 (65–70% frequency), with two others being rarer variants (ε2, 5–10%, and ε4, 15–20%;) (35). The rs7412C>T SNP that causes a change of an amino acid in ApoE2 effects binding to the low-density lipoprotein receptor, while the rs429358T>C SNP that produces the ApoE4 polypeptide results in preferential binding of very low density lipoprotein particles and reduced ApoE4 stability (35). Previous studies attributed these effects to altered interactions between two functional domains within the ApoE polypeptide chain (35,54).

The effect of ApoE allelic variants on TBI outcome are likely modulated by mechanical force, age, or time post TBI. Several studies have indicated an association between *APOE* genotype and moderate/severe TBI poor outcome. Several studies have also demonstrated that the rare *APOE* variants are associated with greater risk of concussion, greater severity of symptoms, or poor outcomes following a concussion injury.

Recent meta-analyses of studies investigating the role of ApoE4 on moderate and TBI indicate an association with an increased risk of poor outcome in pediatric carriers of at least one ApoE4 allele (29). Such an association presents differently depending on trauma severity. In mild concussion, ApoE4 was not associated with post-concussion outcomes in 58.3% of the studies, while in more severe TBI, the role of ApoE4 was hazardous in 63.6% of the studies. Another meta-analysis of six studies including a total of 358 cases of pediatric TBIs revealed that at 6 months, there was over two times higher odds of poor outcome following TBI in children with at least one *APOE* ε4 allele, compared with children without an ε4 allele (26). In a meta-analysis of 12 studies on ApoE and functional outcome after TBI revealed an association with increased risk of unfavorable long-term functional outcome (≥6 months) (30). Due to the wide spectrum of brain injury severity, it is difficult to ascertain if TBI is different from concussion or repeated head impacts. Several studies are trying to bridge this gap; however, there are controversial findings.

For example, carrying the ε4 allele has been associated with poor outcome following TBI. Within a small sample of 30 boxers, including high-exposure boxers (12 or more professional matches; 23–76 years of age), researchers examined the relationship between carrying the ε4 allele and their Chronic Brain Injury Scale scores. The Chronic Brain Injury Scale assesses motor function (gait), cognitive deficits, and behavioral abnormalities, where 0 is normal and above 4 is severely impaired. The authors found that carriers of the ε4 allele had worse Chronic Brain Injury Scale scores (37% had normal scores). Within the same study, all boxers with severe impairment were found to carry at least one ε4 allele, and had high exposure to boxing (60% participated in 12 or more professional bouts) (22). Other studies, which examined self-reported concussion history and *APOE* genotype, reported no association with carrying the ε4 allele or other *APOE* variants were significantly associated with poor outcomes (28, 49, 50, 52).

In a large cohort of 318 collegiate athletes (~20 years of age; 51% male; eight different sports) authors evaluated the association between *APOE* ε4 and concussion risk. The authors measured time to first concussion and calculated athletic exposures. The mean number of athletic exposures was approximately 100. Approximately 25% of the athletes carried the ε4 allele and 8% suffered a concussion during the course of the research study. The authors found no association between carrying the *APOE* ε4 allele and sustaining a concussion (28). In a multicenter study that included 195 college athletes (~19 years of age; male football, female soccer players) authors assessed self-reported concussion over an 8-year time period obtained via a questionnaire. The athletes reported a total of 97 documented concussions. None of the athletes with reported concussion carried the homozygous ε4 genotype; however, approximately 40% of the concussed cohort carried the G(−219)T SNP in the *APOE* promoter region. Therefore the authors demonstrated that homozygous carriers of the promoter G(−219)T SNP in the *APOE* promoter region were at increased risk for having a history of concussion, but did not find any difference between ε2, ε3, and ε4 allele carriers (49, 50).

In a similar multicenter study, the authors evaluated the self-reported history of documented concussions within a cohort of 196 collegiate athletes (163 football and 33 female soccer players). Twenty-five percent of the athletes suffered a concussion, of whom 32% carried the ε4 allele, and 50% carried the promoter allele. The authors found a significant association was reported between college athletes who carried all three alleles and history of concussion (i.e., heterozygous ε2/ε4 and carried the rare promoter allele G) (52). In the same study Tierney et al. also found a significant association between homozygous carriers of G(−219)T SNP and athletes reporting two or more concussions. With only limited evidence suggesting the important role *APOE* allelic variants play in concussion incidence and recovery, conflicting results do not allow us to make a formal confirmation of this hypothesis at this time. The ultimate confirmation would require prospective, multicenter studies with sufficient power and carefully selected inclusion/exclusion criteria (18, 51). For example, a genome-wide association study would be beneficial to identify if *APOE* is a significant genetic marker for brain injury. For this type of research design, thousands of athletes' genomes with a concussion history would be compared to thousands of those with no concussion history.

One of the reasons *APOE* is targeted as a genetic marker is due to the fact that head injury is reported to trigger amyloid B protein deposition, which is also a key factor in the progression of Alzheimer's disease (AD) (44). Similar to TBI, AD displays as a cognitive decline. A recent review found this cognitive decline seems to be accelerated in patients carrying the *APOE* ε4 allele (31). This was attributed to the APOE4 protein being not as efficient in delivering cholesterol to maintain synaptic transmission. Additionally, the authors of the review found that APOE4 protein promotes proinflammatory processes that further exacerbate the disease progression. Similar to genetic associations to brain injury, not everyone carrying the rare allele/genotype has poor outcomes. Approximately 34–65% of patients with AD carry the *APOE* ε4 allele, while it is present in about 20–30% of the nonaffected adult population (43).

Tau

Tau is a microtubule-associated protein that stabilizes microtubules. The human tau gene (*MAPT*) is located on chromosome 17 and contains 16 exons (coding regions of the gene). Two different tau gene haplotypes have been identified (H1 and H2), consisting of eight common SNPs. H1 is the most common, and it is overexpressed in disorders such as progressive neurological disorders. In the central nervous system, alternative splicing of exons 2, 3, and 10 result in the appearance of six tau isoforms (2).

There is a paucity of research examining tau genotype and concussion. Terrell et al. (details of study reported above) (49, 50) reported that tau variants in exon 6 (Ser53Pro (TauSer), Hist47Tyr (TauHis)) were not associated with acute concussion. In spite of this, tau does seem to be an important protein to focus on for genetic predisposition to brain injury due to its association with chronic traumatic encephalopathy (CTE) and AD. CTE is a neurodegeneration characterized by the abnormal accumulation of hyperphosphorylated tau protein within the brain; however, CTE can only be definitively diagnosed postmortem (40). CTE is also thought to be associated with subconcussive blows to the head (14). Therefore, it is plausible that tau genetic polymorphisms may be key in determining the risk of CTE or AD in relation to contact sport participation. Currently, there are no genetic studies involving tau, contact sport participation, and CTE. In a postmortem study, authors examined numerous genes in 17 military personnel and football athletes with a history of repetitive brain injury and found that *MAP2* is upregulated in brains with late-stage CTE (42). Similar to *MAPT*, *MAP2* codes for microtubule-associated proteins involved in stabilizing the dendrite shape during neurodevelopment. The authors did not evaluate *MAPT*. Currently, many of the studies examining tau focus on cerebral spinal fluid and plasma tau protein concentrations following acute brain injury (56).

Neurofilament

The neuronal cytoskeleton is composed of 50% neurofilaments including light (NEFL), medium (NEFM) and heavy neurofilament (NEFH) (17, 53). These neurofilaments are composed of proteins that determine the quality of the cytoskeleton. The *NEFH* gene resides on chromosome 22, and several variants within this gene have been associated with neurodegenerative conditions, such as amyotrophic lateral sclerosis (1).

Only the NEFH has been examined to date in association with concussion outcomes. The authors of one study sought to determine an association between a SNP within a gene coding for a neuronal structural protein (i.e., neurofilament heavy) and previous occurrence and severity of concussions in college athletes (38). Using a case–control study design, 48 athletes with a reported history of concussion were matched by age, height, sport, and position to 48 athletes with no history of concussion (~19 years of age). The authors reported that 24% of the athletic cohort carried the *NEFH* rare allele, but there was no significant association between carrying the rare allele and concussion history or severity. Although the rare allele alters the NEFH protein sequence, this SNP does not seem to influence an athlete's susceptibility to concussion (38).

Pathophysiological genetic associations

Glutamate receptor ionotropic NMDA receptor 2A (GRIN2A)

The primary function of the *N*-methyl-D-aspartate (NMDA) receptor is to act as synaptic connectivity between two neurons as well as to trigger postsynaptic potentials and dendritic spikes, where action potentials are formed. Mechanical stress activates NMDA receptors via overstimulation by the increased glutamate concentration within the synaptic cleft, and causes excitotoxicity (injury to the nerve due to excessive stimulation by glutamate). Ionotropic NMDA receptors are recognized as the major source of glutamate excitotoxicity dependent on the influx of Ca^{2+} when glutamate binds to NMDA receptors. NMDA receptors are composed of four subunits forming a ligand–gated cation (e.g., Ca^{2+}) channel in which the NR1–NR2A heterodimer is the functional unit. The main NR2 subunits are NR2A and NR2B encoded by the *GRIN2A* and *GRIN2B* genes, respectively. *GRIN2A* is located on chromosome 16 and contains multiple SNPs in the coding, intronic, and promoter regions, and has been implicated in several cognitive brain diseases including dementia, AD, depression, and schizophrenia (21).

Functional involvement of NMDA receptors in the concussion stress response is supported by several lines of evidence (25, 41). An important role of polypeptide components of the NMDA receptor was demonstrated in experiments with genetically manipulated mice. Less brain ischemia was detected in *NR2A* or *NR2A/NR2B* knockout mice, after they were subjected to focal cerebral ischemia. The lack of NR2A is likely to alleviate glutamate excitotoxicity due to the decreased amount of blood volume, which could be explained by decreased NMDA channel activity (41). The reduced functionality of the NMDA receptors results in less Ca^{2+} entering the cell (25). Taken together, the above data support the premise that variability in NMDA receptor expression could be a risk factor for concussion outcome. Therefore, variants of the genes coding for the components of the NMDA receptor complex are attractive candidates for association with concussion incidence or recovery.

One important type of genetic variability is the number of tandem repeats (i.e., GT) in the promoter region of the *GRIN2A* gene. GRIN2A expression is modulated by (GT)n VNTR in the promoter region. The (GT)n VNTR in the promoter region had been earlier associated with altered expression level of *GRIN2A* (23, 25). The length of (GT)n repeat modulates

GRIN2A expression level, with longer alleles (≥25 repeats) associated with lower transcription of *GRIN2A* mRNA. In a study of 87 athletes (~19 years of age; 74% male) suffering with a concussion, homozygous carriers of the longer alleles (>25 repeats) were found to be six times more likely to recover in 60 or more days, compared with homozygous carriers of the shorter (<25 repeats) alleles (39). With athletes categorized to one of two groups (prolonged recovery vs. normal recovery), significant variation between the frequencies of longer alleles and shorter alleles was detected, where the carriers of longer alleles were two times more likely to be in the prolonged recovery group than those carrying shorter alleles. Moreover, homozygous carriers of longer alleles demonstrated a significant association with prolonged recovery when compared with homozygous carriers of shorter alleles (39).

Vesicle glutamate transporters

Uptake of glutamate at the synapse following a mechanical insult (e.g., concussion) is important for the restoration of normal neuron function. The synaptic uptake of glutamate is facilitated by vesicular transporters (i.e., vesicle glutamate transporter (VGLUT)-1, VGLUT2, and VGLUT3) encoded by the solute carrier subfamily of genes located on chromosomes 19 (*SLC17A7*), 11 (*SLC17A6*), and 12 (*SLC17A8*), correspondingly. VGLUT1 performs synaptic uptake of glutamate and deposits it into neurosecretory vesicles and is expressed in cerebrum, cerebellum, and hippocampus. Downregulation of VGLUT1 vesicular transport production was shown to cause severe changes in the neurological phenotype of experimental animals (12). Knockout studies demonstrated reduction of vesicle pool size accompanied by residually high concentrations of glutamate within the synaptic cleft (55). Another piece of evidence indicating that VGLUT activity could modulate synaptic efficacy came from the clinical studies of VGLUT expression in schizophrenic patients. VGLUT expression in the hippocampus and the dorsolateral prefrontal cortex was reduced in the brains of schizophrenic patients (9).

If the expression level of a protein responsible for reducing the amount of glutamate (e.g., VGLUT1) within the synaptic cleft is altered due to genetic variation, this may affect the severity of the concussive injury, and the recovery time. A study in 40 athletes (~20 years of age; 73% male) demonstrated that carriers of the rs74174284:G allele in the *SLC17A7* promoter were five times more likely to exceed 20 days to recover from a concussion (33). These results are in parallel with the hypothesis that low expression of *SLC17A7* encoding VGLUT1 probably reduces glutamate transport in the carriers of G allele (55).

Future directions

Sport concussion is its own entity within TBI science. Concussion is not severe TBI or a neurodegenerative disease. As we learn more about how these injuries and diseases overlap, it provides an opportunity to explore new genetic associations. Table 29.3 provides a summary of some genes (and proteins) studied in other conditions or that have a hypothetical role in the pathomechanics and/or pathophysiology of sport concussion. Genetic associations studied in other neurological conditions, in addition to our ever-growing understanding of concussion, are the key to enlightening the science of sport concussion genetics.

This type of genetics research can be challenging for many reasons. For example, there are multiple outcomes with variable responses that could have genetic associations such as the acute and long-term response to repetitive subconcussion, acute concussion, or severe TBI. Further complicating matters is that each of these injuries are based on clinical decision-making and management. For example, a researcher studying concussion response (e.g., return to play

Table 27.3 Potential concussion genetic associations

Protein	Gene (abbreviation)	Variant	Findings
Glial fibrillary acidic protein	Glial fibrillary acidic protein (*GFAP*)	10 different isoforms within exons 6, 7 and the 5′ UTR	A literature review revealed isoforms α, β, γ, δ, and ε were associated with a greater risk of Alexander's disease (46)
S100 calcium binding protein B	S100 calcium binding B (*S100B*)	rs9722	794 participants (396 ischemic stroke patients and 398 controls; ~58 years of age; ~61% male). Authors found carriers of the A allele had an increased S100B serum, which increased risk for ischemic stroke (32)
Calcium voltage-gated channel subunit alpha-1A	Calcium voltage-gated channel subunit alpha-1A (*CACNA1A*)	rs121908225	Within 3 participants with delayed severe edema and 152 nonaffected family members and controls, authors found that carriers of the T allele had increased brain swelling and coma after TBI (27) In a review of literature, authors found an increased risk of hemiplegic migraine and cerebral edema after minor head injury in carriers of the S218L mutation in exon 5 (48)
Calcium voltage-gated channel subunit alpha-1E	Calcium voltage-gated channel subunit alpha-1E (*CACNA1E*)	rs704326	1q31 and 1q32 provide genes that code for proteins such as ATPase, and proteins integral for active transport of sodium ions. This SNP within exon 43 lies within this region of the gene that is associated with migraines (10)
Glutamate receptor ionotropic NMDA type subunit 2B	Glutamate receptor ionotropic NMDA type subunit 2B (*GRIN2B*)	rs228411	Using the FBAT program, the authors found the C allele carriers had greater symptoms scored and were associated with attention deficit disorder (8)
Glutamate ionotropic receptor AMPA type subunit 1–4	Glutamate ionotropic receptor AMPA type subunit 1–4 (*GRIA1–4*)	Tandem repeats in exons 4, 5, and 12	Associated with autism and intellectual disability (5, 6, 19)

(continued)

Table 27.3 (Cont.)

Protein	Gene (abbreviation)	Variant	Findings
Brain-derived neurotrophic factor	Brain-derived neurotrophic factor (BDNF)	rs6562	113 participants (75 with mild TBI and 38 healthy; ~33 years of age; 61% male) were assessed using five different cognitive assessments. The authors found that the Met allele was associated with slower processing speed in the entire group, but not within the mild TBI group specifically. Other SNPS in linkage disequilibrium may increase risk of slower processing speeds after mild traumatic brain injury (36)

time) should consider factors such as: When was injury identified? Who identified the injury? What assessments were perfomed? Was rehabilitation implemented? What was the return to play protocol? and When was it initiated? Due to the number of factors affecting outcomes, large multicentered prospective studies involving a large number of particpants are needed.

The largest study of sport concussion ever conducted began in 2015 by the Care Consortium (www.careconsotium.net). The Care Consortium is a joint effort by the National Collegiate Athletic Association (NCAA) and the US Department of Defense involving 30 NCAA institutions as data collection sites. The consortium aims to conduct prospective, longitudinal research to study the natural history of concussion and conduct advanced studies integrating biomechanics, neuroimaging, and neurobologic and genetic markers of injury. Over the initial 3-year period, more than 39,000 baseline and 2800 postinjury assessments have been performed. Additionally, researchers are looking to examine athletes over the long term, making this one of the most important research endeavors ever conducted. Projects such as this are the key to advancing the science of sport concussion genetics.

References

1. **Al-Chalabi A, Andersen PM, Nilsson P, Chioza B, Andersson JL, Russ C, Shaw CE, Powell JF**, and **Leigh PN**. Deletions of the heavy neurofilament subunit tail in amyotrophic lateral sclerosis. *Human Molecular Genetics* 8: 157–164, 1999.
2. **Andreadis A, Brown WM**, and **Kosik KS**. Structure and novel exons of the human tau gene. *Biochemistry* 31: 10626–10633, 1992.
3. **Aubry M, Cantu R, Dvorak J, Graf-Baumann T, Johnston K, Kelly J, Lovell M, McCrory P, Meeuwisse W**, and **Schamasch P**. Summary and agreement statement of the first international conference on concussion in sport, Vienna. *British Journal of Sports Medicine* 36: 6–10, 2002.
4. **Bailes JE, Petraglia AL, Omalu BI, Nauman E, Talavage T**. Role of subconcussion in repetitive mild traumatic brain injury. *Journal of Neurosurgery* 119: 1235–1245, 2013.
5. **Bonnet C, Leheup B, Béri M, Philippe C, Grégoire M-J**, and **Jonveaux P**. Aberrant GRIA3 transcripts with multi-exon duplications in a family with X-linked mental retardation. *American Journal of Medical Genetics Part A* 149A: 1280–1289, 2009.
6. **Chiyonobu T, Hayashi S, Kobayashi K, Morimoto M, Miyanomae Y, Nishimura A, Nishimoto A, Ito C, Imoto I, Sugimoto T, Jia Z, Inazawa J**, and **Toda T**. Partial tandem duplication of GRIA3 in a male with mental retardation. *American Journal of Medical Genetics Part A* 143A: 1448–1455, 2007.

7. **Dardiotis E, Fountas KN, Dardioti M, Xiromerisiou G, Kapsalaki E, Tasiou A**, and **Hadjigeorgiou GM**. Genetic association studies in patients with traumatic brain injury. *Neurosurgical Focus* 28: 1–12, 2010.

0. **Duval KM, Wigg KG, Crosbie J, Tannock R, Kennedy JL, Ickowicz A, Pathare T, Malone M, Schachar R**, and **Barr CL**. Association of the glutamate receptor subunit gene *GRIN2B* with attention-deficit/hyperactivity disorder. *Genes, Brain and Behavior* 6: 444–452, 2007.

9. **Eastwood SL** and **Harrison PJ**. Decreased expression of vesicular glutamate transporter 1 and complexin II mRNAs in schizophrenia: further evidence for a synaptic pathology affecting glutamate neurons. *Schizophrenia Research* 73: 159–172, 2005.

10. **Fernandez F, Curtain RP, Colson NJ, Ovcaric M, MacMillan J**, and **Griffiths LR**. Association analysis of chromosome 1 migraine candidate genes. *BMC Medical Genetics* 8: 57, 2007.

11. **Feudtner C** and **Miles SH**. Traumatic brain injury news reports and participation in high school tackle football. *JAMA Pediatrics* 172: 492–494, 2018

12. **Fremeau RT, Kam K, Qureshi T, Johnson J, Copenhagen DR, Storm-Mathisen J, Chaudhry FA, Nicoll RA**, and **Edwards RH**. Vesicular glutamate transporters 1 and 2 target to functionally distinct synaptic release sites. *Science* 304: 1815–1819, 2004.

13. **Gaetz, M.** The neurophysiology of brain injury. *Clinical Neurophysiology* 115: 4–18, 2004.

14. **Gavett BE, Stern RA, Cantu RC, Nowinski CJ**, and **McKee AC**. Mild traumatic brain injury: a risk factor for neurodegeneration. *Alzheimer's Research and Therapy* 2: 18, 2010.

15. **Gennarelli TA, Segawa H, Wald U, Czernicki Z, Marsh K**, and **Thompson C**. Physiological response to angular acceleration of the head. In: *Head injury: Basic and Clinical Aspects*, edited by Grossman RG, Gildenberg PL. New York: P. L. Ravens Press, 1982, p. 129–140.

16. **Giza CC** and **Hovda DA**. The new neurometabolic cascade of concussion. *Neurosurgery* 75: S24–S33, 2014.

17. **Godsel LM, Hobbs RP**, and **Green KJ**. Intermediate filament assembly and dynamics of disease. *Cell* 18: 28–37, 2007.

18. **Gordon KE**. Apolipoprotein E genotyping and concussion: time to fish or cut bait. *Clinical Journal of Sports Medicine* 20: 405–406, 2010.

19. **Guilmatre A, Dubourg C, Mosca AL, Legallic S, Goldenberg A, Drouin-Garraud V, Layet V, Rosier A, Briault S, Bonnet-Brilhault F, Laumonnier F, Odent S, Le Vacon G, Joly-Helas G, David V, Bendavid C, Pinoit JM, Henry C, Impallomeni C, Germano E, Tortorella G, Di Rosa G, Barthelemy C, Andres C, Faivre L, Frébourg T, Saugier Veber P**, and **Campion D**. Recurrent rearrangements in synaptic and neurodevelopmental genes and shared biologic pathways in schizophrenia, autism, and mental retardation. *Archives in General Psychiatry* 66: 947–956, 2009.

20. **Guskiewicz KM, Marshall SW, Bailes J, McCrea M, Cantu RC, Randolph C**, and **Jordan BD**. Association between recurrent concussion and late-life cognitive impairment in retired professional football players. *Neurosurgery* 57: 719–726, 2005.

21. **Huang YJ, Lin CH, Lane HY**, and **Tsai GE**. NMDA neurotransmission dysfunction in behavioral and psychological symptoms of Alzheimer's disease. *Current Neuropharmacology* 10: 272–285, 2012.

22. **Jordan BD, Relkin NR, Ravdin LD, Jacobs AR, Bennett A**, and **Gandy S**. Apolipoprotein E epsilon4 associated with chronic traumatic brain injury in boxing. *Journal of the American Medical Association* 278: 136–140, 1997.

23. **Inoue H, Yamasue H, Tochigi M, Suga M, Iwayama Y, Abe O, Yamada H, Rogers MA, Aoki S, Kato T, Sasaki T, Yoshikawa T**, and **Kasai K**. Functional (GT)n polymorphisms in promoter region of N-methly-D-aspartate receptor 2A subunit (GRIN2A) gene affect hippocampal and amygdala volumes. *Genes, Brain and Behavior* 9: 269–275, 2010.

24. **Itokawa M, Yamada K, Yoshitsugu K, Toyota T, Suga T, Ohba A, Watanabe A, Hattori E, Shimizu H, Kumakura T, Ebihara M, Meerabux JM, Toru M**, and **Yoshikawa T**. A microsatellite repeat in the promoter of the N-methyl-D-Aspartate receptor 2A subunit (GRIN2A) gene suppresses transcriptional activity and correlates with chronic outcome in schizophrenia. *Pharmacogenetics* 13: 271–278, 2003.

25. **Iwayama-Shigeno Y, Yamada K, Itokawa M, Toyota T, Meerabux J**. Extended analyses support the association of a functional (GT)n polymorphism in the GRIN2A promoter with Japanese schizophrenia. *Neuroscience Letters* 378: 102–105, 2005.

26. **Kassam I, Gagnon F**, and **Cusimano MD**. Association of the APOE-epsilon4 allele with outcome of traumatic brain injury in children and youth: a meta-analysis and meta-regression. *Journal of Neurology, Neurosurgery, and Psychiatry* 87: 433–440, 2016.

27. Kors EE, Terwindt GM, Vermeulen FL, Fitzsimons RB, Jardine PE, Heywood P, Love S, van den Maagdenberg AM, Haan J, Frants RR, and Ferrari MD. Delayed cerebral edema and fatal coma after minor head trauma. role of the *CACNA1A* calcium channel subunit gene and relationship with familial hemiplegic migraine. *Annals of Neurology* 49: 753–760, 2001.

28. Kristman VL, Tator CH, Kreiger N, Richards D, Mainwaring L, Jaglal S, Tomlinson G, and Comper P. Does the apolipoprotein epsilon 4 allele predispose varsity athletes to concussion? A prospective cohort study. *Clinical Journal of Sports Medicine* 18: 322–328, 2008.

29. Lawrence DW, Comper P, Hutchison MG, and Sharma B. The role of apolipoprotein E epsilon (epsilon)-4 allele on outcome following traumatic brain injury: a systematic review. *Brain Injury* 29: 1018–1031, 2015.

30. Li L, Bao Y, He S, Wang G, Guan Y, Ma D, Wu R, Wang P, Huang X, Tao S, Liu Q, Wang Y, and Yang J. The association between apolipoprotein E and functional outcome after traumatic brain injury: a meta-analysis. *Medicine (Baltimore)* 94: e2028, 2015.

31. Liu C, Kanekiyo T, Xu H and Bu1 G. Apolipoprotein E and Alzheimer disease: risk, mechanisms, and therapy. *Nature Reviews Neurology* 9: 106–118, 2013.

32. Lu Y, Wang R, Huang H, Qin H, Liu C, Xiang Y, Wang C, Luo H, Wang J, Lan Y, and Wei Y. Association of S100B polymorphisms and serum S100B with risk of ischemic stroke in a Chinese population. *Scientific Reports* 8: 971, 2018.

33. Madura SA, McDevitt JK, Tierney RT, Mansell JL, Hayes DJ, Gaughan JP, and Krynetskiy E. Genetic variation in SLC17A7 promoter associated with response to sport-related concussions. *Brain Injury* 30: 908–913, 2016.

34. Mahley RW. Apolipoprotein E: cholesterol transport protein with expanding role in cell biology. *Science* 240: 622–630, 1988.

35. Mahley RW. Apolipoprotein E: From cardiovascular disease to neurodegenerative disorders. *Journal of Molecular Medicine (Berlin)* 94: 739–746, 2016.

36. McAllister TW, Tyler AL, Flashman LA, Rhodes H, McDonald BC, Saykin AJ, Tosteson TD, Tsongalis GJ, and Moore JH. Polymorphisms in the brain-derived neurotrophic factor gene influence memory and processing speed one month after brain injury. *Journal of Neurotrauma* 29: 1111–1118, 2012.

37. McCrory P, Meeuwisse W, Dvorak J, Aubry M, Bailes J, Broglio S, Cantu RC, Cassidy D, Echemendia RJ, Castellani RJ, Davis GA, Ellenbogen R, Emery C, Engebretsen L, Feddermann-Demont N, Giza CC, Guskiewicz KM, Herring S, Iverson GL, Johnston KM, Kissick J, Kutcher J, Leddy JJ, Maddocks D, Makdissi M, Manley GT, McCrea M, Meehan WP, Nagahiro S, Patricios J, Putukian M, Schneider KJ, Sills A, Tator CH, Turner M, and Vos PE. Consensus statement on concussion in sport- The 5th international conference on concussion in sport held in Berlin, October 2016. *British Journal of Sports Medicine* 51: 838–847, 2017.

38. McDevitt JK, Tierney RT, Mansell JL, Driban JB, Higgins M, Toone N, Mishra A, and Krynetskiy E. Neuronal structural protein polymorphism and concussion in college athletes. *Brain Injury* 25: 1108–1113, 2011.

39. McDevitt J, Tierney RT, Phillips J, Gaughan JP, Torg JS, and Krynetskiy E. Association between *GRIN2A* promoter polymorphism and recovery from concussion. *Brain Injury* 29: 1674–1681, 2015.

40. McKee AC, Cairns NJ, Dickson DW, Folkerth RD, Keene CD, Litvan I, Perl DP, Stein TD, Vonsattel J, Stewart W, Tripodis Y, Crary JF, Bieniek KF, Dams-O'Connor K, Alvarez VE, Gordon WA, and TBI/CTE group. The first NINDS/NIBIB consensus meeting to define neuropathological criteria for the diagnosis of chronic traumatic encephalopathy. *Acta Neuropathology* 131: 75–86, 2016.

41. Morikawa E, Mori H, Kiyama Y, Mishina M, Asano T, and Kirino T. Attenuation of focal ischemic brain injury in mice deficient in the epsilon1 (NR2A) subunit of NMDA receptor. *Journal of Neuroscience* 18: 9727–9732, 1998.

42. Mufson EJ, He B, Ginsberg SD, Carper BA, Bieler GS, Crawford F, E. Alvarez VE, Huber BR, Stein TD, McKee AC, and Perez SE. Gene profiling of nucleus basalis tau containing neurons in chronic traumatic encephalopathy: a Chronic Effects of Neurotrauma Consortium Study. *Journal of Neurotrauma* 35: 1260–1271, 2018.

43. Myers RH, Schaefer EJ, Wilson PW, D'Agostino R, Ordovas JM, Espino A, Au R, White RF, Knoefel JE, Cobb JL, McNulty KA, Beiser A, and Wolf PA. Apolipoprotein E epsilon4 association with dementia in a population-based study: The Framingham study. *Neurology* 46:673–677, 1996.

44. **Nathoo N, Chetty R, van Dellen JR**, and **Barnett GH**. Genetic vulnerability following traumatic brain injury: the role of apolipoprotein E. *Molecular Pathology*. 56: 132–136, 2003.

45. **Ommaya AK** and **Gennarelli TA**. Cerebral concussion and traumatic unconsciousness: correlation of experimental and clinical observations on blunt head injuries. *Brain* 97: 633–654, 1974.

46. **Quinlan RA, Brenner M, Goldman JE**, and **Messing A**. GFAP and its role in Alexander disease. *Experimental Cellular Research* 313: 2077–2087, 2007.

47. **Single FN, Rozov A, Burnashev N, Zimmermann F, Hanley DF, Forrest D, Curran T, Jensen V, Hvalby O, Sprengel R**, and **Seeburg PH**. Dysfunctions in mice by NMDA receptor point mutations NR1(N598Q) and NR1(N598R). *Journal of Neuroscience* 20: 2558–2566, 2000.

48. **Stam AH, Luijckx GJ, Poll-Thé BT, Ginjaar IB, Frants RR, Haan J, Ferrari MD, Terwindt GM**, and **van den Maagdenberg AM**. Early seizures and cerebral oedema after trivial head trauma associated with the CACNA1A S218L mutation. *Journal of Neurology, Neurosurgery, and Psychiatry* 80: 1125–1129, 2009.

49. **Terrell TR, Bostick RM, Abramson R, Xie D, Barfield W, Cantu R, Stanek M**, and **Ewing T**. APOE, APOE promoter, and Tau genotypes and risk for concussion in college athletes. *Clinical Journal of Sports Medicine* 18: 10–17, 2008.

50. **Terrell TR, Bostick RM, Barth J, McKeag D, Cantu RC, Sloane R, Galloway L, Erlanger D, Valentine V**, and **Bielak K**. Genetic polymorphisms, concussion risk, and post concussion neurocognitive deficits in college and high school athletes. *British Journal of Sports Medicine* 47: e1, 2013.

51. **Terrell TR, Bostick R, Barth J, Sloane R, Cantu RC, Bennett E, Galloway L, Laskowitz D, Erlanger D, McKeag D, Valentine V**, and **Nichols G**. Multicenter cohort study on association of genotypes with prospective sports concussion: methods, lessons learned, and recommendations. *The Journal of Sports Medicine and Physical Fitness* 57: 77–89, 2017.

52. **Tierney RT, Mansell JL, Higgins M, McDevitt JK, Toone N, Gaughan JP, Mishra A**, and **Krynetskiy E**. Apolipoprotein E genotype and concussion in college athletes. *Clinical Journal of Sports Medicine* 20: 464–468, 2010.

53. **Wagner OI, Rammensee S, Korde N, Wen Q, Leterrier JF**, and **Janmey PA**. Softness, strength and self-repair in intermediate filament networks. *Experimental Cell Research* 313: 2228–2235, 2007.

54. **Wintjens R, Bozon D, Belabbas K, MBou F, Girardet JP, Tounian P, Jolly M, Boccara F, Cohen A, Karsenty A, Dubern B, Carel JC, Azar-Kolakez A, Feillet F, Labarthe F, Gorsky AM, Horovitz A, Tamarindi C, Kieffer P, Lienhardt A, Lascols O, Di Filippo M**, and **Dufernez F**. Global molecular analysis and APOE mutations in a cohort of autosomal dominant hypercholesterolemia patients in France. *The Journal of Lipid Research* 57: 482–491, 2016.

55. **Wojcik SM, Rhee JS, Herzog E, Sigler A, Jahn R, Takamori S, Brose N**, and **Rosenmund C**. An essential role for vesicular glutamate transporter 1 (VGLUT1) in postnatal development and control of quantal size. *Proceedings of the National Academy of Science USA* 101: 7158–7163, 2004.

56. **Zetterberg H, Morris HR, Hardy J**, and **Blennow K**. Update on fluid biomarkers for concussion. *Concussion* 1: 3, 2016.

28

SYSTEMS GENETIC FACTORS UNDERLYING SOFT TISSUE INJURY

Masouda Rahim, Alison V. September, and Malcolm Collins

Introduction

Although there are numerous benefits to participating in regular physical activity (7, 59), the risk of acute and chronic musculoskeletal soft tissue injuries has risen (44), with approximately 30–50% of all sporting injuries affecting tendons (23). Over the last few decades, the incidence of these sport-associated injuries has escalated in both elite and recreational athletes due to increased participation, and intensity and duration of sporting activities (44). The exact etiology underlying soft tissue injuries remains to be elucidated though they are recognized as complex phenotypes with both intrinsic and extrinsic factors contributing to injury risk (4).

Genetics, in particular, is increasingly recognized as a key intrinsic risk factor predisposing individuals; with over 80 polymorphisms implicated in the profiles of several musculoskeletal soft tissue injuries, such as anterior cruciate ligament (ACL) ruptures, tennis elbow, tendinopathy of the posterior tibialis tendon, Achilles tendinopathy, and rotator cuff injuries, to date (53, 65, 72). These genetic loci encode an array of proteins essential for maintaining the structural and functional integrity of musculoskeletal soft tissues and were primarily uncovered through case–control genetic association studies following a candidate gene approach (19). With the advancement of genomics techniques in recent years, there has been a transition towards employing a hypothesis-free approach, using genome-wide association studies (GWAS) and next-generation sequencing (NGS) technologies. These methods have the added advantage of potentially identifying novel candidates and providing researchers with new insight into the underlying pathophysiological processes (32).

This chapter will review our current understanding and examine the latest findings on the genetic contribution to musculoskeletal soft tissue injuries. Additionally, the clinical significance of this research area will be discussed and future directions proposed.

Genetic risk factors underlying musculoskeletal soft tissue injuries

Candidate gene studies

Through the application of molecular genetics techniques, aided by molecular and cellular biology techniques, researchers have begun exploring and highlighting functional biological pathways and molecular mechanisms contributing to the pathogenesis of sporting injuries. The genes implicated thus far include structural proteins, such as the collagens and fibrillins, as well as regulators of the extracellular matrix, such as proteoglycans, matrix metalloproteinases (MMPs), growth factors, cytokines and caspases (Tables 28.1–28.3). Collectively, these proteins function to maintain the integrity of the extracellular matrix (ECM) allowing the tissue to respond and ideally appropriately adapt to loading. Keeping in mind the intricacies of the ECM remodeling pathway, it is not surprising that alongside the independent genetic associations, several gene–gene interactions have also been reported implicating proteins functioning in common biological pathways (57, 63, 67). For the purpose of this review, several of the main findings will be presented together with the proposed biological mechanisms.

Structurally, tendons and ligaments are collagenous tissues predominantly composed of heterotrimeric type I collagen fibrils. The *COL1A1* gene encoding the α1(I) chain of type I collagen contains a functional Sp1 binding site polymorphism (rs1800012 G/T) within its first intron. The rare T allele was reported to have increased binding affinity for the Sp1 transcription factor leading to increased production of α1(I) chains and by implication increased type I collagen homotrimers in the tissue (40). The rs1800012 polymorphism has been associated with risk of cruciate ligament ruptures (25, 50, 68), shoulder dislocations (25), and acute soft tissue ruptures in a combined analysis (15); with all except one of the studies (68) reporting an underrepresentation of the TT genotype in the cases compared to the controls (Table 28.1). However, the contrasting results may be attributable to differences in the mechanism of ACL injuries in skiers (8). A later study by Ficek et al. (2013) reported the association of a second functional single nucleotide polymorphism (SNP) (rs1107946 G/T) within the promoter region of *COL1A1*, which is in linkage disequilibrium with the Sp1 polymorphism (17). Together, the two form a functional haplotype that regulates *COL1A1* transcription (24) and the combination of the two polymorphisms was associated with a reduced risk of ACL rupture (17).

Type V collagen is a minor fibrillar collagen implicated in regulating the collagen fibril diameter and its lateral growth during fibrillogenesis, with the α1(V) chain encoded by the *COL5A1* gene. A number of polymorphisms (rs13946 T/C, rs14776422 C/T, rs5574880 G/A, rs12722 T/C, rs3196378 C/A, rs71746744 −/AGGG, rs16399 −/ATCT, rs1134170 A/T) within the 3′-untranslated region (UTR) of *COL5A1* have been investigated to date (Table 28.1). Specifically, several independent and haplotype associations were reported with Achilles tendinopathy (10, 43, 66), Achilles tendon ruptures (10), tennis elbow (2), ACL ruptures in females (38, 46, 51), and carpal tunnel syndrome – an occupational injury in which tendon involvement was previously proposed (11). The 3′-UTR of genes usually contains important regulatory elements and therefore it is not surprising that several of these polymorphisms were reported to affect *COL5A1* mRNA secondary structure (1). Laguette et al. (2011) identified two major allelic forms of the *COL5A1* 3′-UTR with functional consequences. Specifically, the "T functional form," generally identified in tendinopathic patients, demonstrated increased mRNA stability compared to the "C functional form" (35). Moreover, the microRNA, Hsa-miR-608 (*MIR608*) binds to the 3′-UTR and regulates *COL5A1* mRNA stability and the CC genotype of the functional rs4919510 (C/G) polymorphism was associated with increased Achilles tendinopathy risk (1). In light of these findings, a functional hypothesis for the *COL5A1* 3′-UTR was proposed wherein altered *COL5A1* mRNA stability may alter type V collagen production with potential implications on collagen fibril diameter and, as a result, the biomechanical properties of the tissue (14). In addition to these findings, genetic associations have also been noted for the *COL3A1*, *COL11A1*, *COL11A2*, *COL12A1*, and *COL27A1* genes (Table 28.1).

The structural integrity of tendons and ligaments is tightly regulated by myriad proteoglycans, MMPs, caspases, cytokines, growth factors and signaling factors. Collectively these regulatory

Table 28.1 Genetic variants within the collagen genes and the associated musculoskeletal soft tissue injuries in which they were implicated

Gene and chromosomal location	Encoded protein	Protein function	Polymorphism	Location	Soft tissue injury	Reference
COL1A1 (17q21)	α1 (I) collagen chain	Major fibrillar collagen	rs1107946 (G/T)	Promoter	ACL[a]	17
			rs1800012 (G/T)	Intron 1	ACL[b], shoulder dislocations, acute soft tissue ruptures	15, 17, 25, 50, 68
COL3A1 (2q31)	α1 (III) collagen chain	Major fibrillar collagen	rs1800255 (G/A)	Exon 30	ACL	46, 69
COL5A1 (9q34)	α1 (V) collagen chain	Minor fibrillar collagen	rs13946 (C/T)	3'-UTR	LE	2
			rs12722 (T/C)		ACL, AT, LE	2, 10, 38, 43, 46, 51, 66
			rs3196378 (C/A)		ATP[b]	10, 66
			rs71746744 (−/AGGG)		AT	1
			rs16399 (ATCT/−)			
			rs1134170 (A/T)			
COL11A1 (1p21)	α1 (XI) collagen chain	Minor fibrillar collagen	rs3753841 (T/C)	Exon 52	AT[a]	22
			rs1676486 (C/T)	Exon 62	AT[a]	22
COL11A2 (6p21)	α2 (XI) collagen chain		rs1799907 (T/A)	Intron 6	AT[a]	22
COL12A1 (6q12–q13)	α1 (XII) collagen chain	FACIT collagen	rs970547 (A/G)	Exon 65	ACL	46, 52
COL27A1 (9q32)	α1 (XXVII) collagen chain	Minor fibrillar collagen	rs946053 (G/T)	Intron 41	AT[a]	64

Associations denoted with an [a] indicate the variant was associated as part of an inferred haplotype or an inferred allele combination. Associations denoted with a [b] indicate the variant was independently associated with the musculoskeletal soft tissue injury, as well as part of an inferred haplotype or an inferred allele combination. ACL=anterior cruciate ligament ruptures; AT=Achilles tendinopathy; ATP=Achilles tendon pathology; FACIT=fibril-associated collagens with interrupted triple helices; LE=lateral epicondylitis (tennis elbow); PTT=tendinopathy of the posterior tibialis tendon.

elements function within the broader matrix remodeling pathway and are activated in response to mechanical loading to allow the tissue to remodel, heal, and adapt. It is hypothesized that dysregulation of this pathway may negatively impact the tissue thereby increasing the likelihood of injury.

The ECM glycoprotein tenascin-C (*TNC*) is abundantly expressed in tissues experiencing high tensile and compressive loads and plays a role in regulating cell–matrix interactions (33). Mokone et al. (2005) reported a GT dinucleotide repeat polymorphism in intron 17 of the gene modulated the risk of Achilles tendon injuries (42) (Table 28.2). Following on from this, Saunders et al. (2013) identified the G-C-A inferred haplotype of two *TNC* SNPs (rs13321 G/C and rs2104772 T/A) and the neighboring *COL27A1* rs946053 (G/T) SNP to increase risk of Achilles tendinopathy in two independent study groups (64). More recently, Kluger and colleagues (2016) found the rs13321 and rs2104772 polymorphisms were also associated with degenerative rotator cuff tendinopathy (RCT) (33). In total, the authors identified 15 SNPs, within a region of the *TNC* gene, which were associated with susceptibility to RCT, of which six polymorphisms remained significantly associated after Bonferroni correction: rs1138545 (C/T), rs3789870 (C/T), rs10759753 (T/C), rs72758637 (G/C), rs7021589 (A/G), and rs7035322 (G/T) (33). Subsequent analysis of the same variants identified the novel C-A-G (rs1138545 C/T, rs2104772 A/T, rs10759752 A/G) haplotype to be associated with a failure to heal after RCT (34). These results are therefore highlighting a genomic interval within the *TNC* gene which requires a more comprehensive examination.

Proteoglycans are structurally and functionally integral to tendon and ligament tissues by providing resistance to compressive forces, regulating fibrillogenesis, and contributing to matrix remodeling through various interactions with ECM components (76). Up until now, the genes encoding aggrecan (*ACAN*), biglycan (*BGN*), decorin (*DCN*), and lumican (*LUM*) have only been investigated with susceptibility to ACL ruptures (41) (Table 28.2). Independent associations were observed for the *ACAN* rs1516797 (T/G) (13, 41) and *DCN* rs516115 (T/G) SNPs with the rs1516797 T allele and the rs516115 GG genotype decreasing susceptibility to ACL ruptures. Interestingly, the association with *DCN* was limited to female participants and several other studies have also reported sex-specific associations (46, 51, 54). In addition, the authors also highlighted several genomic regions for further interrogation across the *ACAN*, *BGN*, and the *LUM-DCN* genes, through inferred haplotype analysis (41).

The MMPs are a family of endopeptidases catalyzing a broad spectrum of matrix components. Functional polymorphisms within the *MMP1* and *MMP8* promoters were implicated in tendinopathy of the posterior tibialis tendon (PTT) (21) (Table 28.2). Specifically, the rs1799750 (1G/2G) 2G and rs1144393 (A/G) G alleles, as well as a haplotype of the two SNPs, conferred an increased risk of PTT tendinopathy (6, 21). The rs1799750 2G allele was also associated with a risk of rotator cuff tears (3). Additionally, the *MMP8* rs11225395 (C/T) TT genotype and T allele were significantly associated with an increased risk of developing PTT tendinopathy (20).

Several variants within the *MMP3* gene (rs679620 A/G, rs591058 T/C and rs650108 A/G) have been implicated in injury phenotypes. Raleigh et al. (2009) reported the rs679620 GG, rs591058 CC, and rs650108 AA genotypes were associated with an increased risk of Achilles tendinopathy while the inferred A-T-G haplotype, comprising the alternate alleles, was associated with decreased risk (58). The functional rs3025058 (5A/6A) polymorphism has also been implicated in Achilles tendinopathy (18), rotator cuff tears (3), and ACL ruptures (39). Additionally, an inferred haplotype spanning the *MMP10–MMP1–MMP3–MMP12* gene cluster, localized to chromosome 11q22, was associated with a decreased risk of ACL ruptures (49). There is currently limited research on the role of the ADAMs (a disintegrin

Table 28.2 Genetic variants within genes encoding regulatory components of the extracellular matrix and the associated musculoskeletal soft tissue injuries in which they were implicated

Gene and chromosomal location	Encoded protein	Protein function	Polymorphism	Location	Soft tissue injury	Reference
TNC (9q33)	Tenascin-C glycoprotein	Regulates cell–matrix interactions	G–T tandem repeat	Intron 17	AT	42
			rs1330363 (G/A)	Intron 15	AT[a]	64
			rs2104772 (T/A)	Exon 17		
			rs13321 (G/C)	Exon 24		
			rs1138545 (G/A)	Exon 10	RCT[b]	33
			rs3789870 (C/T)	Intron 10		
			rs7021589 (A/G)	Intron 17		
			rs10759753 (T/C)	Intron 19		
			rs72758637 (G/C)	Intron 19		
			rs7035322 (G/T)	Intron 28		
FBN2 (5q23–q31)	Fibrillin-2	Component of connective tissue microfibrils	rs331079 (G/T)	Intron 7	ACL, AT	27
MIR608 (10q24)	MicroRNA 608	Regulation of COL5A1 mRNA stability	rs4919510 (C/G)	3'-UTR	ATP	1, 10
ACAN (15q26)	Aggrecan	Major proteoglycan of articular cartilage – contributes to load-bearing properties of cartilage	rs2351491 (C/T)	Exon 11	ACL[a]	41
			rs1042631 (C/T)			
			rs1516797 (T/G)	Intron 12	ACL[b]	
BGN (Xq28)	Biglycan	Involved in collagen fibrillogenesis	rs1126499 (C/T)	Exon 4	ACL[a]	41
			rs1042103 (G/A)	Exon 8		
DCN (12q21)	Decorin		rs13312816 (C/T)	Intron 1	ACL[a]	41
			rs516115 (T/G)	Intron 3	ACL[b]	
LUM (12q21)	Lumican		rs2268578 (T/C)	Intron 3	ACL[a]	41

Gene	Description	Variant	Location	Associations	References
MMP1 (11q22)	Degradation of collagenous and noncollagenous ECM components	rs1799750 (1G/2G)	Promoter	ACL[a], PTT[b], RCT	3, 6, 21, 49
		rs1144393 (A/G)		PTT[b]	6
MMP3 (11q22)		rs3025058 (5A/6A)	Promoter	ACL, AT[b]	18, 39
		rs679620 (A/G)	Exon 2	ACL[a], ATP[b]	18, 28, 45, 58
		rs591058 (T/C)	Intron 4	ATP[b]	18, 58
		rs650108 (A/G)	Intron 8		
MMP8 (11q22)	Matrix metalloproteinase 8	rs11225395 (C/T)	Promoter	PTT	20
MMP10 (11q22)	Matrix metalloproteinase 10	rs486055 (C/T)	Exon 1	ACL[a]	49
MMP12 (11q22)	Matrix metalloproteinase 12	rs2276109 (A/G)	Promoter	ACL[b]	49
TIMP2 (17q25)	Metalloproteinase inhibitor 2	Essential regulator of ECM turnover and remodeling	rs4789932 (C/T)	Promoter	ATP	26, 28

Associations denoted with an [a] indicate the variant was associated as part of an inferred haplotype or an inferred allele combination. Associations denoted with [a b] indicate the variant was independently associated with the musculoskeletal soft tissue injury, as well as part of an inferred haplotype or an inferred allele combination. ACL=anterior cruciate ligament ruptures; AT=Achilles tendinopathy; ATP=Achilles tendon pathology; ECM=extracellular matrix; PTT=tendinopathy of the posterior tibialis tendon; RCT=rotator cuff tendinopathy.

and metalloproteinase), ADAMTS (ADAM with thrombospondin motifs), and TIMPs (tissue inhibitors of metalloproteinases) in injury risk (26, 28).

September et al. (2011) investigated the interleukin genes (interleukin-1β (*IL-1B*), interleukin-1 receptor antagonist (*IL-1RN*) and interleukin-6 (*IL-6*)) with risk of Achilles tendinopathy (Table 28.3). Although no independent associations were noted, the variants were observed to collectively modulate the risk of Achilles tendinopathy in combination with the previously associated *COL5A1* rs12722 SNP (67). Similarly, a subsequent study collectively implicated polymorphisms within the *IL-1B*, *IL-6*, *IL-6R*, and *COL5A1* genes with risk of ACL ruptures (57). These two inferred haplotypes are therefore very similar and only differ at the A2 allele implicated for the *IL-1RN* rs2234663 VNTR locus. Although both studies only investigated relatively small sample sizes, the similarities between the associations are highlighting a potentially important biological interacting network underpinning both acute and chronic musculoskeletal soft tissue injuries which needs exploration (57). Several independent and haplotype associations have been reported for the *VEGFA* and *KDR* genes (54–56, 61) functioning in the angiogenesis pathway, the *CASP8* gene involved in apoptosis (10, 45, 57), and the *GDF5* gene involved in regulating cell growth and differentiation (48) (Table 28.3). Additional research is necessary to understand the full spectrum of signaling molecules and the manner in which they may potentially impact ECM remodeling.

Hypothesis-free approach

Traditionally, genetics research in the field of musculoskeletal soft tissue injuries has followed a candidate gene approach (19). However, it is necessary to consider the limitations of such an approach (37). For example, the majority of these studies are conducted in relatively small cohorts and therefore, the reported associations are not always reproducible or able to detect genetic contributions of small effect sizes (odds ratio <2.0) (37). It should, however, be noted that in many of these studies careful attention was given to include well-defined cases and controls. As a result, these studies have been able to add to the body of knowledge in understanding risk and are advantageous in locating genomic intervals of interest, especially when the effect sizes have been relatively large, allowing subsequent research to follow a more directed approach.

A novel approach to explore tendinopathy, employed by Saunders et al. (2016), was the application of bioinformatics tools to data-mine existing databases for interactions and biological relationships to increase the probability of identifying novel and unobvious candidate genes. The authors used the BioOntological Relationship Graph database (BORG) to integrate multiple sources of genomic and biomedical knowledge, including human, mouse, and rat orthologs, and following further prioritization were able to identify four strong candidate genes for investigation (62).

More recently, studies are now opting for an unbiased, hypothesis-free approach employing GWAS or NGS methods such as whole-exome and whole-genome sequencing (WES/WGS). Although this research is still in its infancy and the detection and interpretation of these loci may not be as straightforward, these studies can lead to new discoveries on the genetic and biological contributions to complex phenotypes (73). Moreover, the findings may deliver new insight into previously reported associations. However, the main disadvantage to these studies, at present, is the lack of large, well-defined cohorts for investigation of soft tissue injuries (74). Consequently, public databases are often utilized and due to the inclusion of these heterogeneous cohorts, particularly for the controls, these studies can still produce negative results.

The first GWAS investigating susceptibility to soft tissue injuries was undertaken in a canine ACL rupture model which identified 99 loci as risk variants for ACL ruptures (5). The

Table 28.3 Genetic variants within genes encoding cell signaling molecules and the associated musculoskeletal soft tissue injuries in which they were implicated

Gene and chromosomal location	Encoded protein	Protein function	Polymorphism	Location	Soft tissue injury	Reference
IL-1B (2q14)	Interleukin-1β	Role in the inflammatory pathway and ECM degradation	rs16944 (T/C) rs1143627 (C/T)	Promoter	ACL[b], AT[a],	57, 67
IL-1RN (2q14)	Interleukin-1 receptor antagonist	Antagonist for IL-1α and IL-1β	rs2234663 VNTR	Intron 2	ACL[a], AT[a]	57, 67
IL-6 (1q21)	Interleukin-6	Role in apoptosis and the inflammatory pathway	rs1800795 (G/C)	Promoter	ACL[a], AT[a]	57, 67
IL-6R (1q21)	Interleukin-6 receptor	Receptor for IL-6	rs2228145 (A/C)	Exon 9	ACL[a]	57
VEGFA (6p21)	VEGF-A isoform	Essential regulator of angiogenesis	rs699947 (C/A) rs1570360 (G/A) rs2010963 (G/C)	Promoter Promoter 3'-UTR	ACL[b], ATP[b]	54, 56
KDR (4q11–4q12)	Kinase insert-domain receptor	Receptor for VEGF and mediates VEGF signaling	rs2071559 (G/A) rs2305948 (G/A) rs1870377 (T/A)	Promoter Exon 7 Exon 11	ACL[b], AT[a] AT[b] ACL[b], AT[a]	54–56, 61
GDF5 (20q11)	Growth differentiation factor 5	Regulates cell growth and differentiation	rs143383 (T/C)	5'-UTR	ATP	48
CASP8 (2q33–q34)	Caspase 8	Initiator caspase	rs3834129 (ins/del) rs1045485 (G/C)	Promoter Exon 9	ACL[b], AT[b]	10, 45, 57

Associations denoted with an [a] indicate the variant was associated as part of an inferred haplotype or an inferred allele combination. Associations denoted with a [b] indicate the variant was independently associated with the musculoskeletal soft tissue injury, as well as part of an inferred haplotype or an inferred allele combination. ACL: anterior cruciate ligament ruptures; AT: Achilles tendinopathy; ATP: Achilles tendon pathology; ECM: extracellular matrix; VEGF: vascular endothelial growth factor.

highlighted variants implicated biological networks regulating aggrecan signaling, cellular proliferation, and membrane transport proteins involved in functions such as signal transduction and pH regulation for further investigation (5). Subsequently, Kim et al. (2017) conducted a genome-wide screen for ACL ruptures, Achilles tendinopathy, and Achilles tendon ruptures in a human model (31). In contrast to the canine model, no significant associations were observed though this may be attributable to a poor study design. For instance, care was not taken to ensure well-defined cases and controls. Specifically, the GWAS cohort included patients irrespective of physical activity level whereas the candidate gene studies typically include physically active individuals with no history of previous tendon or ligament injury. Three independent studies investigating shoulder dislocations identified a total of five genetic markers for risk using a GWAS approach (29, 60, 70). A genome-wide screen for ankle injuries, including sprains, strains, and other joint derangements, reported two loci as contributors (30). These studies also share the same limitations due to study design.

NGS technologies have revolutionized genomic research for complex phenotypes but, to date, only one paper has been published employing NGS technologies to explore susceptibility to musculoskeletal soft tissue injuries. Caso et al. (2016) used WES analysis on twin sibling males surgically diagnosed with ACL ruptures and their nonaffected progenitors (12). The authors reported a set of 11 new variants shared by the family members which were associated with noncontact ACL ruptures and which they hypothesized may contribute to homeostatic imbalance of the ECM (12). As evidenced from the literature, considerable research is still needed in this sphere to decode the genetic architecture of musculoskeletal soft tissue injuries. Collectively, the results of the candidate gene, bioinformatics, GWAS, and WES studies add to the evidence recognizing musculoskeletal soft tissue injuries as complex, polygenic conditions. Additional studies are necessary to understand and validate the biological significance of these loci. Nevertheless, these findings are an important first step in unravelling the genetic contribution to soft tissue injury risk.

Researchers also need to consider applying a broader approach incorporating genomics, transcriptomics, epigenomics, and proteomics to provide a more complete understanding of injury predisposition. Li et al. (2017) identified 39 differentially expressed microRNAs in ACL tissues from patients with osteoarthritis (36). The dysregulated microRNAs were predicted to interact with target genes involved in several essential biological processes including cartilage development and remodeling, collagen biosynthesis and degradation, and ECM homeostasis. Trancriptome-wide gene expression analysis of ACL tissue from time of injury identified numerous differentially expressed transcripts representing important biological processes (9). Studies such as these provide insight into the healing capacity of ruptured ACLs and may be particularly relevant to the development of effective ACL repair and reconstruction techniques (9).

Clinical relevance

The precise mechanisms culminating in injury are yet to be elucidated and therefore any predictive or diagnostic, as well as injury-risk tests available at present are largely premature (16). Despite this, there are a growing number of direct-to-consumer genetic tests available on the market without offering the appropriate counseling or clarification on the results (75). Moreover, these tests do not take into consideration the multifactorial nature of sporting injuries and are therefore more than likely to interpret the results incorrectly (16, 65). In fact, the primary objective in elucidating the genetic contribution to musculoskeletal soft tissue injuries is to identify the biological pathways and molecular mechanisms contributing to pathogenesis warranting subsequent in-depth exploration. Only upon validation of these genetic and molecular markers in larger samples within independent studies will it be meaningful to design possible genetic tests examining an individual's injury susceptibility. In particular, insight into how the fine balance between matrix synthesis and degradation is regulated and dysregulated is required to inform new therapeutic interventions and identify potential biological targets.

Although predictive genetic testing is not possible for these injuries, a genetic test included in a holistic risk assessment tool may have future applications in the design of prehabilitation strategies for genetically predisposed individuals or in analyzing how an individual is likely to respond to load. Moreover, one's genetic makeup may aid in the prescription of appropriate treatment strategies after injury and to inform decision-making on operative versus nonoperative injury management.

Future work

The main limitations to the current evidence are that: 1) the majority of studies have investigated relatively small samples, 2) the findings have not been replicated in independent populations, and 3) the studies were primarily conducted in Caucasian populations and therefore the results are not necessarily representative of populations across the world. As a result, additional research in large, independent sample sets is ultimately required to confirm the reported genetic associations. The establishment of international consortia is therefore essential to achieving this goal by pooling knowledge and resources to overcome the current barriers (47, 74). In doing so, researchers will be also able to undertake GWAS and NGS approaches in large, carefully phenotyped cohorts of cases and controls which may aid in the discovery of rare variants with large effect sizes on modulating injury risk, and assist in refining the genomic regions to which these variants cluster.

At present, there is limited functional evidence to support the current genetic associations (24, 35). The results from genetic studies cannot be understood in isolation. Rather these results need to pave the direction of future research, with the proposed markers interrogated using a multidisciplinary approach, including omics technologies, RNA sequencing analysis, differential gene expression, and protein studies to establish their role in injury susceptibility (12, 65). In addition, the clinical relevance of these biological markers also needs investigation (9, 14, 33, 71).

Conclusion

Today, genetics is increasingly recognized as a key risk factor predisposing individuals to an increased risk of ligament and tendon injuries. The genes implicated thus far encode an array of proteins essential to maintaining tissue homeostasis including collagens, noncollagenous structural proteins, and regulators of the ECM. Musculoskeletal soft tissue injuries are likely a result of disturbance to biological networks and not isolated proteins and genes and therefore the interactions between proteins functioning in common biological pathways are intriguing and should also be explored (5). In addition, recent research from bioinformatics analysis, GWAS and WES analysis are proposing novel candidates and biological pathways for examination. Research in this domain will continue to provide insight into the genetic, molecular, and cellular mechanisms that may potentially serve as therapeutic targets. Thus, it is critical that large data sets are collected and international consortia are established to effectively pool resources and a multidisciplinary approach utilized to understand the biological significance of these genetic loci in contributing to musculoskeletal soft tissue injury risk susceptibility.

References

1. **Abrahams Y, Laguette M-J, Prince S, Collins M.** Polymorphisms within the COL5A1 3'-UTR that alters mRNA structure and the MIR608 gene are associated with Achilles tendinopathy. *Ann Hum Genet* 77: 204–214, 2013.

2. **Altinisik J, Meric G, Erduran M, Ates O, Ulusal AE, Akseki D.** The BstUI and DpnII variants of the COL5A1 gene are associated with tennis elbow. *Am J Sports Med* 43: 1784–1789, 2015.

3. **Assunção JH, Godoy-Santos AL, dos Santos MCLG, Malavolta EA, Gracitelli MEC, Ferreira Neto AA.** Matrix metalloproteases 1 and 3 promoter gene polymorphism is associated with rotator cuff tear. *Clin Orthop Relat Res* 475: 1904–1910, 2017.

4. **Bahr R, Krosshaug T.** Understanding injury mechanisms: a key component of preventing injuries in sport. *Br J Sports Med* 39: 324–329, 2005.

5. **Baker LA, Kirkpatrick B, Rosa GJM, Gianola D, Valente B, Sumner JP, Baltzer W, Hao Z, Binversie EE, Volstad N, Piazza A, Sample SJ, Muir P.** Genome-wide association analysis in dogs implicates 99 loci as risk variants for anterior cruciate ligament rupture. *PLoS One* 12: e0173810, 2017.

6. **Baroneza JE, Godoy-Santos A, Ferreira Massa B, Boçon de Araujo Munhoz F, Diniz Fernandes T, Leme Godoy Dos Santos MC.** *MMP-1* promoter genotype and haplotype association with posterior tibial tendinopathy. *Gene* 547: 334–337, 2014.

7. **Behrens G, Fischer B, Kohler S, Park Y, Hollenbeck AR, Leitzmann MF.** Healthy lifestyle behaviors and decreased risk of mortality in a large prospective study of U.S. women and men. *Eur J Epidemiol* 28: 361–372, 2013.

8. **Bere T, Flørenes TW, Krosshaug T, Koga H, Nordsletten L, Irving C, Muller E, Reid RC, Senner V, Bahr R.** Mechanisms of anterior cruciate ligament injury in World Cup alpine skiing: a systematic video analysis of 20 cases. *Am J Sports Med* 39: 1421–1429, 2011.

9. **Brophy RH, Tycksen ED, Sandell LJ, Rai MF.** Changes in transcriptome-wide gene expression of anterior cruciate ligament tears based on time from injury. *Am J Sports Med* 44: 2064–2075, 2016.

10. **Brown KL, Seale KB, El Khoury LY, Posthumus M, Ribbans WJ, Raleigh SM, Collins M, September AV.** Polymorphisms within the COL5A1 gene and regulators of the extracellular matrix modify the risk of Achilles tendon pathology in a British case-control study. *J Sports Sci* 35: 1475–1483, 2017.

11. **Burger M, de Wet H, Collins M.** The *COL5A1* gene is associated with increased risk of carpal tunnel syndrome. *Clin Rheumatol* 34: 767–774, 2015.

12. **Caso E, Maestro A, Sabiers CC, Godino M, Caracuel Z, Pons J, Gonzalez FJ, Bautista R, Claros MG, Caso-Onzain J, Viejo-Allende E, Giannoudis P V, Alvarez S, Maietta P, Guerado E.** Whole-exome sequencing analysis in twin sibling males with an anterior cruciate ligament rupture. *Injury* 47: S41–S50, 2016.

13. **Cięszczyk P, Willard K, Gronek P, Zmijewski P, Trybek G, Gronek J, Weber-Rajek M, Stastny P, Petr M, Lulińska-Kuklik E, Ficek K, Kemeryte-Riaubiene E, Maculewicz E, September AV.** Are genes encoding proteoglycans really associated with the risk of anterior cruciate ligament rupture? *Biol Sport* 2: 97–103, 2017.

14. **Collins M, Posthumus M.** Type V collagen genotype and exercise-related phenotype relationships. *Exerc Sport Sci Rev* 39: 191–198, 2011.

15. **Collins M, Posthumus M, Schwellnus MP.** The *COL1A1* gene and acute soft tissue ruptures. *Br J Sports Med* 44: 1063–1064, 2010.

16. **Collins M, September AV, Posthumus M.** Biological variation in musculoskeletal injuries: current knowledge, future research and practical implications. *Br J Sports Med* 49: 1497–1503, 2015.

17. **Ficek K, Cieszczyk P, Kaczmarczyk M, Maciejewska-Karłowska A, Sawczuk M, Cholewinski J, Leonska-Duniec A, Stepien-Slodkowska M, Zarebska A, Stepto NK, Bishop DJ, Eynon N.** Gene variants within the *COL1A1* gene are associated with reduced anterior cruciate ligament injury in professional soccer players. *J Sci Med Sport* 16: 396–400, 2013.

18. **Gibbon A, Hobbs H, van der Merwe W, Raleigh SM, Cook J, Handley CJ, Posthumus M, Collins M, September AV.** The *MMP3* gene in musculoskeletal soft tissue injury risk profiling: a study in two independent sample groups. *J Sports Sci* 35: 655–662, 2017.

19. **Gibson WT.** Genetic association studies for complex traits: relevance for the sports medicine practitioner. *Br J Sports Med* 43: 314–316, 2009.

20. **Godoy-Santos, A, Ortiz RT, Junior RM, Fernandes TD, Santos MCLG.** *MMP-8* polymorphism is genetic marker to tendinopathy primary posterior tibial tendon. *Scand J Med Sci Sport* 24: 220–223, 2014.

21. **Godoy-Santos A, Cunha M V, Ortiz RT, Fernandes TD, Mattar R, dos Santos MCLG.** *MMP-1* promoter polymorphism is associated with primary tendinopathy of the posterior tibial tendon. *J Orthop Res* 31: 1103–1107, 2013.

22. **Hay M, Patricios J, Collins R, Branfield A, Cook J, Handley CJ, September AV, Posthumus M, Collins M.** Association of type XI collagen genes with chronic Achilles tendinopathy in independent populations from South Africa and Australia. *Br J Sports Med* 47: 569–574, 2013.

23. **Järvinen TAH, Kannus P, Maffulli N, Khan KM.** Achilles tendon disorders: etiology and epidemiology. *Foot Ankle Clin* 10: 255–266, 2005.

24. **Jin H, van't Hof RJ, Albagha OME, Ralston SH.** Promoter and intron 1 polymorphisms of *COL1A1* interact to regulate transcription and susceptibility to osteoporosis. *Hum Mol Genet* 18: 2729–2738, 2009.

25. **Khoschnau S, Melhus H, Jacobson A, Rahme H, Bengtsson H, Ribom E, Grundberg E, Mallmin H, Michaëlsson K.** Type I collagen alpha1 Sp1 polymorphism and the risk of cruciate ligament ruptures or shoulder dislocations. *Am J Sports Med* 36: 2432–2436, 2008.

26. **El Khoury L, Posthumus M, Collins M, Handley CJ, Cook J, Raleigh SM.** Polymorphic variation within the *ADAMTS2, ADAMTS14, ADAMTS5, ADAM12* and *TIMP2* genes and the risk of Achilles tendon pathology: a genetic association study. *J Sci Med Sport* 16: 493–498, 2013.

27. **El Khoury L, Posthumus M, Collins M, van der Merwe W, Handley C, Cook J, Raleigh S.** *ELN* and *FBN2* gene variants as risk factors for two sports-related musculoskeletal injuries. *Int J Sports Med* 36: 333–337, 2014.

28. **El Khoury L, Ribbans WJ, Raleigh SM.** *MMP3* and *TIMP2* gene variants as predisposing factors for Achilles tendon pathologies: attempted replication study in a British case-control cohort. *Meta Gene* 9: 52–55, 2016.

29. **Kim S, Kleimeyer J, Ahmed M, Avins A, Fredericson M, Dragoo J, Ioannidis J.** A genetic marker associated with shoulder dislocation. *Int J Sports Med* 38: 508–514, 2017.

30. **Kim SK, Kleimeyer JP, Ahmed MA, Avins AL, Fredericson M, Dragoo JL, Ioannidis JPA.** Two genetic loci associated with ankle injury. *PLoS One* 12: e0185355, 2017.

31. **Kim SK, Roos TR, Roos AK, Kleimeyer JP, Ahmed MA, Goodlin GT, Fredericson M, Ioannidis JPA, Avins AL, Dragoo JL.** Genome-wide association screens for Achilles tendon and ACL tears and tendinopathy. *PLoS One* 12: e0170422, 2017.

32. **Kitsios GD, Zintzaras E.** Genome-wide association studies: hypothesis-"free" or "engaged"? *Transl Res* 154: 161–164, 2009.

33. **Kluger R, Burgstaller J, Vogl C, Brem G, Skultety M, Mueller S.** Candidate gene approach identifies six SNPs in tenascin-C (TNC) associated with degenerative rotator cuff tears. *J Orthop Res* 35: 894–901, 2017.

34. **Kluger R, Huber KR, Seely PG, Berger CE, Frommlet F.** Novel tenascin-C haplotype modifies the risk for a failure to heal after rotator cuff repair. *Am J Sports Med* 45: 2955–2964, 2017.

35. **Laguette M-J, Abrahams Y, Prince S, Collins M.** Sequence variants within the 3'-UTR of the *COL5A1* gene alters mRNA stability: implications for musculoskeletal soft tissue injuries. *Matrix Biol* 30: 338–345, 2011.

36. **Li B, Bai L, Shen P, Sun Y, Chen Z, Wen Y.** Identification of differentially expressed micrornas in knee anterior cruciate ligament tissues surgically removed from patients with osteoarthritis. *Int J Mol Med* 40: 1105–1113, 2017.

37. **Little J, Higgins JPT, Ioannidis JP a., Moher D, Gagnon F, von Elm E, Khoury MJ, Cohen B, Davey-Smith G, Grimshaw J, Scheet P, Gwinn M, Williamson RE, Zou GY, Hutchings K, Johnson CY, Tait V, Wiens M, Golding J, van Duijn C, McLaughlin J, Paterson A, Wells G, Fortier I, Freedman M, Zecevic M, King R, Infante-Rivard C, Stewart A, Birkett N.** STrengthening the REporting of Genetic Association studies (STREGA) – an extension of the STROBE statement. *Eur J Clin Invest* 39: 247–266, 2009.

38. **Lulińska-Kuklik E, Rahim M, Domańska-Senderowska D, Ficek K, Michałowska-Sawczyn M, Moska W, Kaczmarczyk M, Brzeziański M, Brzeziańska-Lasota E, Cieszczyk P,** September AV. Interactions between *COL5A1* gene and risk of the anterior cruciate ligament rupture. *J Hum Kinet* 62: 65–71, 2017.

39. **Malila S, Yuktanandana P, Saowaprut S, Jiamjarasrangsi W, Honsawek S.** Association between matrix metalloproteinase-3 polymorphism and anterior cruciate ligament ruptures. *Genet Mol Res* 10: 4158–4165, 2011.

40. **Mann V, Hobson EE, Li B, Stewart TL, Grant SFA, Robins SP, Aspden RM, Ralston SH.** A *COL1A1* Sp1 binding site polymorphism predisposes to osteoporotic fracture by affecting bone density and quality. *J Clin Invest* 107: 899–907, 2001.

41. **Mannion S, Mtintsilana A, Posthumus M, van der Merwe W, Hobbs H, Collins M, September AV.** Genes encoding proteoglycans are associated with the risk of anterior cruciate ligament ruptures. *Br J Sports Med* 48: 1640–1646, 2014.

42. **Mokone GG, Gajjar M, September A V, Schwellnus MP, Greenberg J, Noakes TD, Collins M.** The guanine-thymine dinucleotide repeat polymorphism within the tenascin-C gene is associated with Achilles tendon injuries. *Am J Sports Med* 33: 1016–1021, 2005.

43. **Mokone GG, Schwellnus MP, Noakes TD, Collins M.** The *COL5A1* gene and Achilles tendon pathology. *Scand J Med Sci Sports* 16: 19–26, 2006.

44. **Morrow JR, Defina LF, Leonard D, Trudelle-Jackson E, Custodio MA.** Meeting physical activity guidelines and musculoskeletal injury: the WIN study. *Med Sci Sports Exerc* 44: 1986–1992, 2012.

45. **Nell E-M, van der Merwe L, Cook J, Handley CJ, Collins M, September AV.** The apoptosis pathway and the genetic predisposition to Achilles tendinopathy. *J Orthop Res* 30: 1719–1724, 2012.

46. **O'Connell K, Knight H, Ficek K, Leonska-Duniec A, Maciejewska-Karlowska A, Sawczuk M, Stepien-Slodkowska M, O'Cuinneagain D, van der Merwe W, Posthumus M, Cieszczyk P, Collins M.** Interactions between collagen gene variants and risk of anterior cruciate ligament rupture. *Eur J Sport Sci* 15: 341–350, 2015.

47. **Pitsiladis YP, Tanaka M, Eynon N, Bouchard C, North KN, Williams AG, Collins M, Moran CN, Britton SL, Fuku N, Ashley EA, Klissouras V, Lucia A, Ahmetov II, de Geus E, Alsayrafi M.** Athlome Project Consortium: a concerted effort to discover genomic and other "omic" markers of athletic performance. *Physiol Genomics* 48: 183–190, 2016.

48. **Posthumus M, Collins M, Cook J, Handley CJ, Ribbans WJ, Smith RKW, Schwellnus MP, Raleigh SM.** Components of the transforming growth factor-beta family and the pathogenesis of human Achilles tendon pathology – a genetic association study. *Rheumatology (Oxford)* 49: 2090–2097, 2010.

49. **Posthumus M, Collins M, van der Merwe L, O'Cuinneagain D, van der Merwe W, Ribbans WJ, Schwellnus MP, Raleigh SM.** Matrix metalloproteinase genes on chromosome 11q22 and the risk of anterior cruciate ligament (ACL) rupture. *Scand J Med Sci Sport* 22: 523–533, 2012.

50. **Posthumus M, September AV, Keegan M, O'Cuinneagain D, Van der Merwe W, Schwellnus MP, Collins M.** Genetic risk factors for anterior cruciate ligament ruptures: *COL1A1* gene variant. *Br J Sports Med* 43: 352–356, 2009.

51. **Posthumus M, September AV, O'Cuinneagain D, van der Merwe W, Schwellnus MP, Collins M.** The *COL5A1* gene is associated with increased risk of anterior cruciate ligament ruptures in female participants. *Am J Sports Med* 37: 2234–2240, 2009.

52. **Posthumus M, September AV, O'Cuinneagain D, van der Merwe W, Schwellnus MP, Collins M.** The association between the *COL12A1* gene and anterior cruciate ligament ruptures. *Br J Sports Med* 44: 1160–1165, 2010.

53. **Rahim M, Collins M, September AV.** Genes and musculoskeletal soft-tissue injuries. In: *Medicine and Sport Science*, edited by Posthumus M, Collins M. Basel: Karger, p. 68–91, 2016.

54. **Rahim M, Gibbon A, Hobbs H, van der Merwe W, Posthumus M, Collins M, September AV.** The association of genes involved in the angiogenesis-associated signaling pathway with risk of anterior cruciate ligament rupture. *J Orthop Res* 32: 1612–1618, 2014.

55. **Rahim M, Hobbs H, van der Merwe W, Posthumus M, Collins M, September AV.** Investigation of angiogenesis genes with anterior cruciate ligament rupture risk in a South African population. *J Sports Sci* 36: 551–557, 2018.

56. **Rahim M, El Khoury LY, Raleigh SM, Ribbans WJ, Posthumus M, Collins M, September AV.** Human genetic variation, sport and exercise medicine, and Achilles tendinopathy: role for angiogenesis-associated genes. *Omi A J Integr Biol* 20: 520–527, 2016.

57. **Rahim M, Mannion S, Klug B, Hobbs H, van der Merwe W, Posthumus M, Collins M, September AV.** Modulators of the extracellular matrix and risk of anterior cruciate ligament ruptures. *J Sci Med Sport* 20: 152–158, 2017.

58. **Raleigh SM, van der Merwe L, Ribbans WJ, Smith RKW, Schwellnus MP, Collins M.** Variants within the *MMP3* gene are associated with Achilles tendinopathy: possible interaction with the *COL5A1* gene. *Br J Sports Med* 43: 514–520, 2009.

59. **Reiner M, Niermann C, Jekauc D, Woll A.** Long-term health benefits of physical activity – a systematic review of longitudinal studies. *BMC Public Health* 13: 813, 2013.

60. **Roos TR, Roos AK, Avins AL, Ahmed MA, Kleimeyer JP, Fredericson M, Ioannidis JPA, Dragoo JL, Kim SK.** Genome-wide association study identifies a locus associated with rotator cuff injury. *PLoS One* 12: e0189317, 2017.

61. **Salles JI, Duarte MEL, Guimarães JM, Lopes LR, Vilarinho Cardoso J, Aguiar DP, Machado Neto JO, Machado DE, Perini JA.** Vascular endothelial growth factor receptor-2 polymorphisms have protective effect against the development of tendinopathy in volleyball athletes. *PLoS One* 11: e0167717, 2016.

62. **Saunders CJ, Jalali Sefid Dashti M, Gamieldien J.** Semantic interrogation of a multi knowledge domain ontological model of tendinopathy identifies four strong candidate risk genes. *Sci Rep* 6: 19820, 2016.

63. **Saunders CJ, van der Merwe L, Cook J, Handley CJ, Collins M, September AV.** Extracellular matrix proteins interact with cell-signaling pathways in modifying risk of Achilles tendinopathy. *J Orthop Res* 33: 898–903, 2015.

64. **Saunders CJ, van der Merwe L, Posthumus M, Cook J, Handley CJ, Collins M, September AV.** Investigation of variants within the *COL27A1* and *TNC* genes and Achilles tendinopathy in two populations. *J Orthop Res* 31: 632–637, 2013.

65. **September AV, Rahim M, Collins M.** Towards an understanding of the genetics of tendinopathy. In: *Advances in Experimental Medicine and Biology*, edited by Ackermann PW, Hart DA. New York: Springer, p. 109–116, 2016.

66. **September AV, Cook J, Handley CJ, van der Merwe L, Schwellnus MP, Collins M.** Variants within the *COL5A1* gene are associated with Achilles tendinopathy in two populations. *Br J Sports Med* 43: 357–365, 2009.

67. **September AV, Nell E-M, O'Connell K, Cook J, Handley CJ, van der Merwe L, Schwellnus M, Collins M.** A pathway-based approach investigating the genes encoding interleukin-1β, interleukin-6 and the interleukin-1 receptor antagonist provides new insight into the genetic susceptibility of Achilles tendinopathy. *Br J Sports Med* 45: 1040–1047, 2011.

68. **Stępień-Słodkowska M, Ficek K, Eider J, Leońska-Duniec A, MacIejewska-Karłowska A, Sawczuk M, Zarębska A, Jastrzębski Z, Grenda A, Kotarska K, Cięszczyk P.** The +1245G/T polymorphisms in the collagen type I alpha 1 (*COL1A1*) gene in polish skiers with anterior cruciate ligament injury. *Biol Sport* 30: 57–60, 2013.

69. **Stępień-Słodkowska M, Ficek K, Maciejewska-Karłowska A, Sawczuk M, Ziętek P, Król P, Zmijewski P, Pokrywka A, Cięszczyk P.** Overrepresentation of the *COL3A1* AA genotype in Polish skiers with anterior cruciate ligament injury. *Biol Sport* 32: 143–147, 2014.

70. **Tashjian RZ, Granger EK, Farnham JM, Cannon-Albright LA, Teerlink CC.** Genome-wide association study for rotator cuff tears identifies two significant single-nucleotide polymorphisms. *J Shoulder Elb Surg* 25: 174–179, 2016.

71. **Tashjian RZ, Granger EK, Zhang Y, Teerlink CC, Cannon-Albright LA.** Identification of a genetic variant associated with rotator cuff repair healing. *J Shoulder Elb Surg* 25: 865–872, 2016.

72. **Vaughn NH, Stepanyan H, Gallo RA, Dhawan A.** Genetic factors in tendon injury: a systematic review of the literature. *Orthop J Sport Med* 5: 2325967117724416, 2017.

73. **Visscher PM, Brown MA, McCarthy MI, Yang J.** Five years of GWAS discovery. *Am J Hum Genet* 90: 7–24, 2012.

74. **Wang G, Tanaka M, Eynon N, North KN, Williams AG, Collins M, Moran CN, Britton SL, Fuku N, Ashley EA, Klissouras V, Lucia A, Ahmetov II, de Geus E, Alsayrafi M, Pitsiladis YP.** The future of genomic research in athletic performance and adaptation to training. In: *Medicine and Sport Science*, edited by Posthumus M, Collins M. Basel: Karger, p. 55–67, 2016.

75. **Williams AG, Wackerhage H, Day SH.** Genetic testing for sports performance, responses to training and injury risk: practical and ethical considerations. In: *Medicine and Sport Science*, edited by Posthumus M, Collins M. Basel: Karger, p. 105–119, 2016.

76. **Yanagishita M.** Function of proteoglycans in the extracellular matrix. *Acta Pathol Jpn* 43: 283–293, 1993.

29

SEX AND PERFORMANCE: NATURE VERSUS NURTURE

Mindy Millard-Stafford and Matthew T. Wittbrodt

Ever since the first Olympiad in the modern era (1896), sport is recognized to play a relevant societal role to promote education, health, intercultural dialogue, and the development of individuals – regardless of sex, race, age, gender orientation, and socioeconomic background (5). Conversely, sport performance is also affected by societal influences as one of many factors that ultimately coalesce and contribute to athletic success. These factors could generally be categorized as either predominantly inherent (i.e., nature) and/or environmental (i.e., nurture). It is well accepted that elite athletes are endowed with exceptional genetic potential but require the appropriate deliberate sport-specific practice/training and environment to develop these talents (14, 55). The relative contribution of nature to sport performance is likely above 50% but less than 100% (14). Figure 29.1 presents a general theoretical model that considers many of these factors influencing sport performance without basis for the relative weighting of each. Regarding those of primarily genetic origin, sex is clearly one fundamental genetic factor that dictates performance, particularly in sports objectively measured by time, distance, or weight.

The term "sex" differences relative to the discussion in this chapter is based upon the biological genetic difference between men and women rather than the term "gender" differences. A far wider concept than biological sex, "gender" implies life conditions, cultural and societal expectations about femininity/masculinity, and fundamentally one's own sense of self. As will be discussed elsewhere (Chapter 34), sex is recognized as not a true binary classification due to rare conditions of sexual development (30), which present increasingly complex challenges in the contemporary world of sport competition.

Considered as the "weaker sex," creating an equal and level competitive playing field has been the basis for classifying most sports by sex. In fact, there are few sports today (equestrian, sailing) where men directly compete against women in the same classification. There are separate divisions (and length of matches) at Wimbledon, and distinct competitions held for bicycle stage races and FIFA World Cups. EA Sports only started to provide female soccer players for girls (and boys) to select from when playing video games in 2015. The "fairer" sex has been segregated from most sport competitions for a long time. Is this basis solely due to biological and/or cultural advantages for men? Historical traditions? A quote from the famous marathoner, Grete Waitz (world record holder 1979–1983) epitomizes this concept: "As long as women are women, I don't think they will surpass men." Some of these complex issues affecting

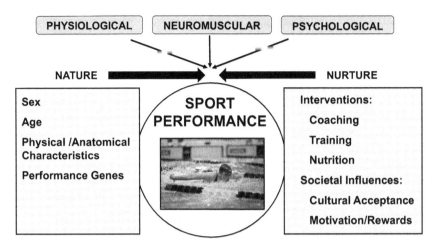

Figure 29.1 A theoretical model for contributing factors impacting sport performance.

our understanding of "sex differences" in sport performance must also be considered when discussing the tension between the biological versus environmental factors influencing the sex difference in sports performance.

Historical perspectives

Since the modern era of the Olympic Games, women have been playing "catch-up" to men in terms of societal acceptance for female participation and the available opportunities for sport competition. The first Olympiad (1896) was open only to men. However, at the 1900 Paris Olympics, 22 women participated out of a total 997 athletes, representing approximately 2% of all athletes. Women competed alongside their male counterparts in sailing, croquet, and equestrian. Only two sports were segregated by sex: tennis and golf. Over time, more Olympic sports were gradually added: archery, swimming, and athletics (track and field) by 1928. Yet, in the inaugural Olympic 800-meter track event for women, several runners "reportedly" collapsed during competition although the veracity of this report is debated (41). Officials subsequently deemed the distance too great a call on feminine strength with grave concerns physical exhaustion would "harm a women's reproductive organs." The 800 meters for women did not return to the Olympic Games program for another 30 years! Ironically, this same rationale by male officials in the International Olympic Committee continued for sports such as the women's ski jump until Sochi 2014.

Unfortunately, the persistent notion labeling certain athletic events as "inappropriate" for women during most of the 20th century prevailed (e.g., women were considered "too frail" to compete in demanding events lasting more than 1–2 minutes). The 1500-meter run was not a permanent event to the Olympic Games until 1972, 76 years later than was available for men. In the US, women were banned from *official* competition in the Boston marathon until 1972. Prior to 1972, race officials would physically remove women from the course if entered under an assumed "male" name. The women's marathon has an even shorter Olympic history than the 1500 meters, as it was not included until the 1984 Los Angeles Games. Ironically, in that first Olympic marathon for women (won by American Joan Benoit Samuelson), another top woman Gabriela Andersen-Scheiss also collapsed in front of TV cameras on the final track leg due to heat stroke. Fortunately, sport governing bodies did not repeat the mistake of eliminating the women's marathon based upon presumed "risk."

In the United States, a federal law – Title IX legislation – passed in 1972 requiring equal funding for federally sponsored educational programs, including sports. To date, the influence of this policy continues to spur girls' participation in sports (34). Yet, not until 40 years later, in the 2012 London Summer Olympic Games, would every country include a female athlete as part of their delegation (comprising 44% of all competitors). However, coaching staffs and the upper echelons of sports administrative bodies have not caught up (46). Prior to 2004, no female coach had *ever* been a part of the US Olympic swimming staff. Furthermore, less than 14% of Division I National Collegiate Athletic Association (NCAA) women's swimming programs have a female head coach as of 2015. Moreover, the International Olympic Committee has stated the goal of women holding 20% of all administrative and decision-making positions within national organizing committees and international federations.

Thus, across many sport disciplines, women had few role models in sport and started competing chronologically later than their male counterparts. The hammer throw, pole vault, and 3000-meter steeplechase were the last athletics events introduced into the Olympics, while women still do not compete in the 50 km racewalk (only recently recognized by the IAAF and held for the first time in the London 2017 World Athletics Championships). Even in the 2016 Rio Olympics, the 1500 meters freestyle, the longest pool event in Olympic swimming for men, was not a competitive distance for women (only up to 800 meters). However, this inequality is finally slated to be rectified with the addition of the 1500 meters freestyle for women in Tokyo 2020 (and 800 meters for men), nearly a century since swimming has been in the Olympic Games!

In summary, over the past 40 years in the US, the environment or nurture factor for women to pursue and compete in sport has clearly changed to level the playing field. Equal access to training and coaching has widened (e.g., in many sports such as swimming, boys and girls even train together up past the age group through college ranks). When a *culture* is acceptable for girls to play a particular sport starting in their youth, girls are more likely to be encouraged to pursue their interest through parents, friends, and environment to develop their skills. This factor increases young girls' motivation and confidence in their ability to pursue sport at the highest level. The global impact of one country's federal legislation, however, remains difficult to measure. In terms of sport performance, opportunities for sport participation clearly have an important influence on the motivation for women to devote their lives to sport, since the Olympic Games results in financial incentives for winning medals and other "rewards" both intrinsic and extrinsic in nature often follow (5).

Other nurture influences on the performance gap

Age is also an inherent factor contributing to sport performance (Figure 29.1). In some women's sports such as figure skating or gymnastics, a delay in maturation has biomechanical advantages for younger-aged female competitors that are not necessarily similar for men in the same sport (3). However, not long ago, assumptions regarding the "peak" age for sprint/power or team sports was believed to be in the early 20s, especially for women, due solely to the fact that women did not continue to compete beyond high school. For example in 1968, Debbie Meyer, at 16 years of age, became the first female swimmer to win three individual gold medals in one Olympics (200-, 400-, and 800-meter freestyles), a feat not repeated until Rio 2016 by 19-year-old Katie Ledecky (already appearing in her second Olympiad). Debbie Meyer seemed to be at the "peak" of her career, but did not defend her titles and "retired" in 1972. In that era, strict amateurism rules prevailed and few college swimming programs, let alone athletic scholarships, were available to continue the rigorous training required to be successful in the sport.

In terms of contributing factors that might underlie the sex differences, motivation for athletes to stay in the sport are reflected by an increased age of elite athletes over time. An analysis of the change in US Olympic swimming and track competitors' average age is depicted in Figure 29.2. Male and female swimmers (combined) increased in age significantly from 1972 (18.5 ± 2.7 years) to 1992 (21.9 ± 3.0 years) and became progressively higher in 2012 (23.6 ± 3.9 years). After 2000, the age for female Olympians (21 years) remained similar but males increased (from 21 to 24.5 years) over this same period of time (Figure 29.2A). These data indicate elite US male swimmers are consistently older than females but that over the past 40+ years, age has increased for both men (to >24 years) and women (>21 years). In the track running events (Figure 29.2B), there is no clear sex difference in the age of US Olympians although the increased age over time remains consistent to that observed in swimming. Track competitors (up through the marathon) also appear to be older overall compared to swimmers. Recent reports comparing the top five places in key marathon competitions over the years indicate men and women physiologically peak at a similar age (29–30 years) in running performance (24). This differs somewhat from the 2015 report (1) that 20 years old is the peak age for international swimming in both sprint and distance events, with "little sex difference" in estimates of peak age. However, there are increasingly more "outlier" older athletes defying published trends by competing longer in their sport due to professional opportunities available and returning after childbirth (e.g., 41-year-old 2008 Olympic silver medalist Dara Torres). Thus, a current change in this nurture variable is reflected in the older ages of contemporary elite athletes, which have advanced past the 1972 statistic when 17 years old was the average age for an elite female swimmer.

When does the performance gap appear?

National youth surveys indicate girls are overall less physically active than boys, particularly striking around adolescence (53). It would also seem logical that since girls tend to mature earlier than boys, there would be little physical differences in sport performance prior to sexual maturation (with biological differences gradually more pronounced due to increasing testosterone in boys). If a "gap" in sports performance is related primarily to biology (i.e., hormonal changes throughout growth and maturation), then this should occur progressively in sports where it is common for boys and girls to train together and have access to similar coaching and league competition. In swimming, boys and girls train together in the same pool practices from youth through adulthood with the same access to coaching often through the college ranks, although they compete separately. In Figure 29.3, the sex difference is plotted based upon US national age-group records. For each age group of interest, performance time(s) were recorded by sex classification across each event. The percentage sex difference in performance time was then calculated using a pairwise comparison by rank using the following equation:

$$\% \text{Difference} = \frac{\text{Female time} - \text{Male time}}{\text{Male time}} \times 100$$

Each dot represents the difference between matched pairs of boys and girls from 1st to 16th place across history in USA Swimming (as of 2015), thus reducing selection bias. Any points above zero represent a case where similarly ranked boys' times were faster than the corresponding girls' times. As early as 9–10 years old (and likely prior to puberty for boys), in more cases than

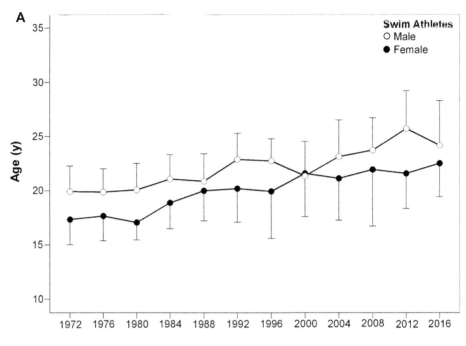

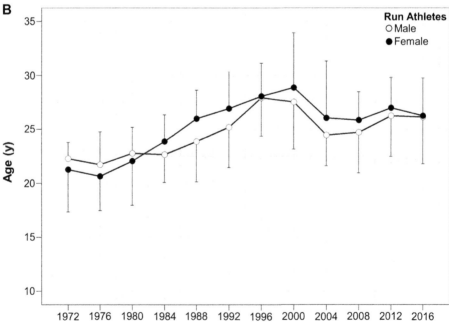

Figure 29.2 Mean (± standard deviation) age for US Olympic team members in swimming (top) and running events in track (bottom) over time.

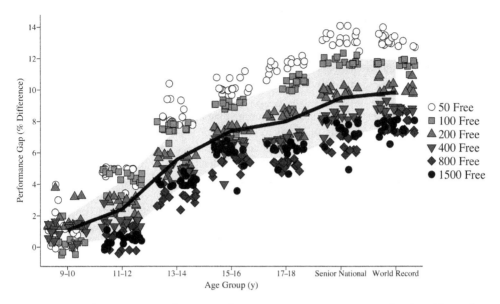

Figure 29.3 Performance gap in elite top-16 all-time US age group, senior national and world record swimmers. Differences were significant across each age group (except for 15–16 vs. 17–18 years and senior national vs. world record) with progressively increasing performance gaps between boys and girls.

not, the boys seem to be somewhat faster (~1.1%), which progressively increases with each successive 2-year age group category. Moving to 11–12-year-olds, only in the longer distances (1500 meters) are girls sometimes faster and with each successive age group thereafter, the performance gap widens significantly between boys and girls with the greatest discrepancy observed in the sprints (50 meters). On average, across all events at the highest level of senior national competition (no age limitations), the performance gap averages remarkably close to approximately 10%. It is impossible to know the maturity of the respective boys and girls within each chronological age bracket in this cross-sectional data set, but typically early maturing boys dominate the national top times at early ages (9, 10) but often those individuals do not remain in the national ranking lists in later years. In contrast, national record holders for girls in 11–12 years age groups often remain in the nationally ranked lists in later age groups. Finally, unlike the relatively similar sex difference observed across the spectrum of Olympic running events (49), the sex difference in sprints (50 meters) was nearly double that of endurance pool events (400 meters and above), and this inverse relationship between sex difference and swim distance is observed as early as 11–12 years and remains throughout growth and maturity.

Sports participation and opportunity as a nurture factor

Using data on elite athletes' performances to understand the sex difference may be challenging when attempting to tease out the influence of environmental or "nurture" factors. In older master athletes, Hunter and Stevens (23) indicate greater than one-third of the sex difference is based on differential participation. The potential number of competitors (i.e., depth of field) impacts record performances worldwide (9); thus, if opportunities are not equal for men and women, the utility of using performances from isolated races or databases may be limited by fewer females competing.

Most sport governing bodies track their membership by sex and age group. In USA Swimming, participation numbers for girls equal and, in many age groups, exceed that of boys (56). In 2013 and 2014, male and female swimmers comprised 43% and 57% of year-round USA Swimming athlete membership, respectively (147,180 vs. 193,388 athletes). The only age group (from <8 to >19 years) in which there were more males than females was over 19 years old (4785 females, 5961 males representing 1.5% and 1.8% of all swimmers, respectively); otherwise, more girls participate year round in swimming than boys beginning at 8 years of age. Youth boys have a slightly wider array of sports to select from (e.g., football), and therefore, youth swimming for boys may be less popular compared to other team sports.

Educational institutions in the US that require federal funding (high schools and universities) are also required to provide participation data. However, in contrast to club participation, NCAA statistics (35) indicate that since the early 1980s in Division I swimming (which can offer athletic scholarships), the number of intercollegiate women athletes (and teams) has increased from 3038 (161 teams) to 5393 (195 teams) while men swimmers have dropped from 4109 (181 teams) to 3839 (134 teams). This greater female participation rate in swimming is likely attributed not only to Title IX legislation which increased opportunities for girls, but also the long-standing historical "social acceptability" of swimming and somewhat fewer popular sport options for girls to participate in as a youth. The reason for slightly greater American men currently remaining in USA Swimming (club and collegiate) beyond 19 years old is unclear, but may reflect greater professional opportunities for men and/or other challenges for women to devote sufficient time towards training in their child-bearing years. Therefore, the parity in participation rates across most of the age groups for US swimmers suggests that the sex difference in performing this sport is not likely due to a smaller pipeline of female athletes, although other sociological factors cannot be ruled out.

Quantifying the performance gap

Why discuss the aforementioned contextual historical events and sociological factors? In order to fully appreciate the "science" of sex differences, the social environment must be considered when examining research that compares phenotypes and performances of men and women. Two different approaches used to "quantify" the sex difference have been to either examine physiological responses (i.e., aerobic capacity, muscular strength) in groups of men and women or calculate the performance difference or "gap" (e.g., in world records) from similarly trained elite athletes representing the extreme tail of the population distribution. With a plethora of publications over the past two decades, scientists have weighed in on both sides of the argument: either the performance gap is predetermined and will remain (19, 25, 43, 44, 53) or that it will eventually close (4, 10, 12, 25, 29, 42, 51, 52, 60) and perhaps remain in only select events.

The first study to examine this question, "Will women soon outrun men?", was published in the highly respected journal, *Nature*, in 1992 (60). Brian Whipp and Susan Ward plotted the historical progression of mean running velocity in world records over time for the 200 meters up through the marathon. Since the slope for women's improvement was far steeper over time (due to the relatively "late start" in distance running competitions and compressed time scale), the model predicted that female marathon performance would intersect with men's in 1998 at a time under 2 hours and 2 minutes. Based on their statistical models for all running events, this suggested the performance gap between men and women would eventually disappear, prompting much media interest. However, those knowledgeable about distance running understood this was an incorrect assumption based on the rapid positive societal change rather than an emerging biological advantage for women. To illustrate this miscalculation of the "opportunities bias," as of 2017, the marathon world record was 2:02:57 for men but 2:15:25 for women (set by Paula Radcliffe in 2003).

As sport opportunities for women have improved over time, the performance gap appears to have stabilized in the last couple of decades, particularly in objectively measured sports (in centimeters, seconds, or kilograms) where the human body is the motor. Recent analyses of world record performances indicate a stability in the performance gap (43, 61) across a number of sports and event distances (53) since the early 1980s. However, there have been circumstances (e.g., anaerobic/power events after more controlled drug testing was implemented to screen for anabolic steroids) in which the gap has actually widened (44). In 1998, the magnitude of the performance gap was roughly 11% slower for women in running events from the 1500 meters through the marathon distance (49). Sparling et al. (49) stated the biological differences between men and women provide men with an advantage in distance running and recent data have not altered this conclusion regarding these competitive running distances (18, 22, 25), although a lower depth of field (i.e., fewer elite competitors) and participation are still acknowledged as factors (23). Thus, one major limitation in using world records to examine sex differences include the fact that participation and opportunity may still not be universal around the globe (5) and records are set under different conditions and competition venues.

The impact of Title IX on the performance gap in the US was recently assessed (33). As observed in Figure 29.4, computing male–female differences in time by rank (1st through 8th place at the Olympic Trials) by distance and event, the performance gap closed by approximately 2% and 5% in Olympic trial swimming (top) and running (bottom), respectively, from 1972 to 1980 (with no meaningful change thereafter over nearly 40 years). Performance gaps of 13% in elite mid-distance running and 8% in swimming (of similar ~4-minute duration) have remained steady for four decades, the 5% differential between sports indicative of load carriage disadvantages of higher female body fatness in running. Conversely, sprint swimming exhibits a greater sex difference than sprint running suggesting height and anthropometric advantages unique to swim block starts compared to overcoming height disadvantages in track block starts (57).

Based on world records, what is the range overall for the performance gap? Sandbakk et al. (43) have recently summarized the performance gap of 8–12% between the sexes as stable with two notable exceptions: >12% for "upper body power" events and <8% in "ultra"-endurance swimming – although this point remains somewhat controversial if controlling for representative population sampling (58). Vogt et al. (58) reported performance gaps of 6.6% in 25 km open water events during the 2008 and 2012 Olympic Games and 7.8% for world championships. These values contrast with other selected open water ultra-distance races (42) reporting sex differences varying from 14.4% to as low as 3.7%. Moreover, some (29) reported women were actually 12–14% faster than men in a 46 km event held in <20°C water. In contrast, a stable sex difference of approximately 11.5% has been reported in a 26 km Lake Zurich, Switzerland, swim event (11). An "advantage" for women during prolonged open water swimming (no turns or block starts) is postulated to be the enhanced buoyancy of additional body fat. However, "ultra"-endurance open water swimming has only recently been added to elite competition (Olympics, world championships); thus, the lack of an equivalent depth of field in selected events likely also contributes to these differential findings (9, 45, 46). Moreover, any potential female metabolic advantage for fat utilization during ultra-endurance running (events longer than marathon distance) has limited supporting evidence (43), particularly when coupled with drastically lower recreational participation rates (20%) in female ultra-marathoners (28). In addition to sampling bias, the variable duration of ultra-running events (6 hours up to 10 days) complicates the female–male performance comparison.

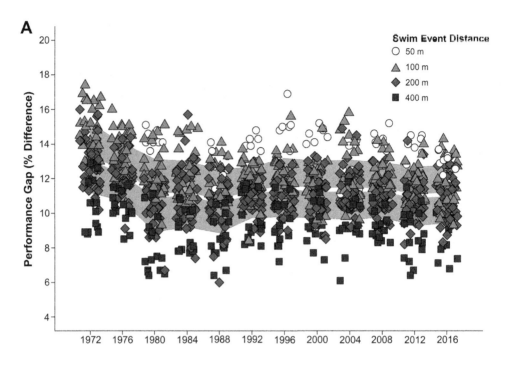

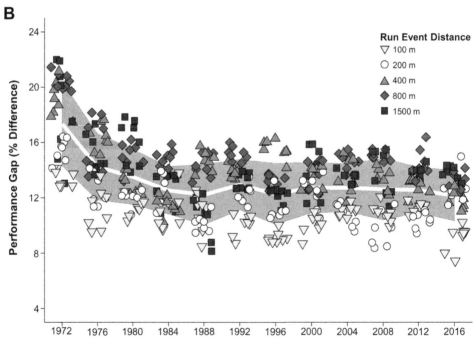

Figure 29.4 Performance gap in US Olympic trials (1972–2016) for top eight finalists by event. Scatter plot for male/female computed comparisons for (A) swimming and (B) running events with mean ± standard deviation denoted by the white line and grey shaded region. The performance gap was higher in 1972 and 1976 compared to all other subsequent years (1980–2016).

Source: Modified from Millard-Stafford et al. (33).

Sex differences due to biology

Why are men faster and stronger than women? The most plausible answer is a biological one based on XX and XY chromosomes, and specifically the testis-determining factor or sex-determining region (SRY) on the Y chromosome that dictates development of male sexual characteristics (27). SRY induces a cascade of events involving other genes (e.g., *SOX9*) to promote development of the testes and suppress development of the ovaries (2, 27). The physical characteristics under the influence of testosterone are fairly well documented (31) and appear to provide biological advantages in sport ranging from musculoskeletal morphology to neurocognitive influences on behavior. Only selected key physiological characteristics are presented in this section, based upon the prevailing evidence on sport performance when comparing representative cross-sections of the population (which in itself is a scientific challenge when examining the published literature on sex differences). Rarely are elite male and female athletes (of similar world ranking) brought into the same laboratory for assessment of their physical characteristics and physiological responses during exercise. Historically, such descriptive studies have been cross-sectional, occurring at different historical time points and laboratories (37, 38), often relying upon different techniques and methods for measurement.

Female hormones have important influences on physiology beyond reproduction but biomedical studies still lag in this regard (50). Although the effects of fluctuating levels of female sex steroid hormones (e.g., estrogens, progestins) during the menstrual cycle on women's sport performance have been a topic of interest, firm conclusions have yet to be reached (7, 13). Mechanisms linked to altered substrate (e.g., fat) metabolism (36), thermoregulatory (6), cardiorespiratory, and psychological changes have all been implicated more or less to some degree as to whether these interact to enhance or detract from performance. However, reaching a consensus is unlikely due to an overall lack of studies and inherent individual variability among the women examined (7), in addition to the fact that few studies are performed on elite athletes.

Body composition is clearly a differentiating factor between the sexes, specifically when compared in the leanest elite athletes such as world-class marathoners (15, 40). Although assessment methods change over time and have inherent known error and variability, women (due to estrogen effects) have greater essential (sex-specific) fat compared to men. Even an elite female distance runner has a body fatness 8–10% greater compared to her male counterpart. This excess fat acts as added load to carry during weight-bearing exercise since it does not contribute to propulsive force. Thus, in weight-bearing sports (e.g., distance running, jumping), the sex difference may be more pronounced due to the penalty of added load carriage (e.g., sex-specific fat) relative to muscle mass. Excess load carriage explained roughly one-third of the endurance running performance gap in both experimental models (8) and in population comparisons of elite athlete performances for running versus swimming (33). Moreover, greater relative fat mass was a stronger predictor of the sex difference in running performance compared to either running economy or cardiorespiratory capacity (48).

Distance running performance is related to maximal aerobic capacity ($\dot{V}O_2$max), which is greater in elite male versus female marathoners (37, 39). This sex difference in $\dot{V}O_2$max has been attributed to greater male relative heart/lung size, muscle mass, and hemoglobin concentration (47) in addition to body composition differences. However, at an elite level, the highest sustainable work rate and running economy are better predictors of performance (26) than $\dot{V}O_2$max; yet, sex-based differences in running economy are not observed (16). Therefore, the current world record in the women's marathon (2:15.25 by Paula Radcliffe in 2003) has been deemed "equivalent" to a 2-hour marathon time projected in the future for men (22).

Muscle cross-sectional area is generally regarded to be directly proportional to muscular strength and on average, men have greater overall muscle mass than women although this varies by sport (32). However, does testosterone enhance the anabolic response to increase muscle mass following training? Lower testosterone concentrations in women presumably limits protein synthesis and muscle hypertrophy, although this direct relationship is not consistently observed in experimental studies examining the acute resistance training-induced responses in men and women (59). Although peak strength is greater for men than women (particularly in the upper body), women may have greater ability to sustain the same relative maximal force (sustained or intermittent isometric contractions) compared to men (17, 20), although this is not universal across all tasks. Dr. Sandra Hunter has summarized (21) this body of scientific literature, acknowledging challenges such as limited comparable biomedical data on women and future research is needed before definitive sex differences in physiology or response to training can be determined.

Summary

Although sport opportunities for women have improved, the performance gap between men and women has stabilized within recent decades. Over this period, the average age of elite running and swimming athletes has increased, suggesting greater opportunities to pursue sport as a professional. Despite these changes in the sociocultural landscape, significant performance differences in comparable elite male and female athletes remain. These performance gaps are not uniform across different sports or within the sprint-endurance domain in a single sport. Although the performance gap narrows as swimming distance increases from the pool sprints to open water endurance events, this is not consistent with weight-bearing events such as running, likely due to the differential impact of load carriage (e.g., added sex-specific fat mass in women). Other biological factors also contribute, such as lower maximal aerobic capacity, peak muscular forces, and anthropometrical differences. The performance gap between boys and girls occurs early (prior to adolescence) and progresses with maturity (and presumably testosterone influences) past the teenage years. Current evidence from world record databases suggests women will not close the performance gap with men in sports where the human body acts as the motor. Recent stability in historical trends of elite athletes suggest the current performance gap is due primarily to underlying biological/genetic differences rather than sociocultural disparities in sports participation, but challenges are inherent by relying upon a cross-sectional approach to answer the question: Are sex differences due to nature versus nurture?

References

1. **Allen SV** and **Hopkins WG**. Age of peak competitive performance of elite athletes: a systematic review. *Sports Medicine* 45: 1431–1441, 2015.
2. **Arboleda VA** and **Vilain E**. The evolution of the search for novel genes in mammalian sex determination: from mice to men. *Molecular Genetics and Metabolism* 104: 67–71, 2011.
3. **Baxter-Jones ADG, Thompson AM**, and **Malina RM**. Growth and maturation in elite young female athletes. *Sports Medicine and Arthroscopy Review* 10: 42–49, 2002.
4. **Beneke R, Leithauser RM**, and **Doppelmayr M**. Women will do it in the long run. *British Journal of Sports Medicine* 39: 410, 2005.
5. **Capranica L, Piacentini MF, Halson S, Myburgh KH, Ogasawara E**, and **Millard-Stafford M**. The gender gap in sport performance: equity influences equality. *International Journal of Sports Physiology and Performance* 8: 99–103, 2013.
6. **Charkoudian N** and **Stachenfeld N**. Sex hormone effects on autonomic mechanisms of thermoregulation in humans. *Autonomic Neuroscience: Basic and Clinical* 196: 75–80, 2016.
7. **Constantini NW, Dubnov G**, and **Lebrun CM**. The menstrual cycle and sport performance. *Clinics in Sports Medicine* 24: e51–82, xiii–xiv, 2005.

8. **Cureton KJ** and **Sparling PB**. Distance running performance and metabolic responses to running in men and women with excess weight experimentally equated. *Medicine and Science in Sports and Exercise* 12: 288–294, 1980.

9. **Deaner RO**. Physiology does not explain all sex differences in running performance. *Medicine and Science in Sports and Exercise* 45: 146–147, 2013.

10. **Deaner RO**, **Carter RE**, **Joyner MJ**, and **Hunter SK**. Men are more likely than women to slow in the marathon. *Medicine and Science in Sports and Exercise* 47: 607–616, 2015.

11. **Eichenberger E**, **Knechtle B**, **Knechtle P**, **Rust CA**, **Rosemann T**, **Lepers R**, and **Senn O**. Sex difference in open-water ultra-swim performance in the longest freshwater lake swim in Europe. *Journal of Strength and Conditioning Research* 27: 1362–1369, 2013.

12. **Eichenberger E**, **Knechtle B**, **Rust CA**, **Knechtle P**, **Lepers R**, and **Rosemann T**. No gender difference in peak performance in ultra-endurance swimming performance – analysis of the "Zurich 12-h Swim" from 1996 to 2010. *Chinese Journal of Physiology* 55: 346–351, 2012.

13. **Friden C**, **Hirschberg AL**, and **Saartok T**. Muscle strength and endurance do not significantly vary across 3 phases of the menstrual cycle in moderately active premenopausal women. *Clinical Journal of Sport Medicine* 13: 238–241, 2003.

14. **Georgiades E**, **Klissouras V**, **Baulch J**, **Wang G**, and **Pitsiladis Y**. Why nature prevails over nurture in the making of the elite athlete. *BMC Genomics* 18: 835, 2017.

15. **Graves JE**, **Pollock ML**, and **Sparling PB**. Body composition of elite female distance runners. *International Journal of Sports Medicine* 8 (Suppl 2): 96–102, 1987.

16. **Helgerud J**. Maximal oxygen uptake, anaerobic threshold and running economy in women and men with similar performances level in marathons. *European Journal of Applied Physiology and Occupational Physiology* 68: 155–161, 1994.

17. **Hicks AL**, **Kent-Braun J**, and **Ditor DS**. Sex differences in human skeletal muscle fatigue. *Exercise and Sport Science Reviews* 29: 109–112, 2001.

18. **Hoffman MD**. Performance trends in 161-km ultramarathons. *International Journal of Sports Medicine* 31: 31–37, 2010.

19. **Holden C**. An everlasting gender gap? *Science* 305: 639–640, 2004.

20. **Hunter SK**. The relevance of sex differences in performance fatigability. *Medicine and Science in Sports and Exercise* 48: 2247–2256, 2016.

21. **Hunter SK**. Sex differences in human fatigability: mechanisms and insight to physiological responses. *Acta Physiologica* 210: 768–789, 2014.

22. **Hunter SK**, **Joyner MJ**, and **Jones AM**. The two-hour marathon: what's the equivalent for women? *Journal of Applied Physiology* 118: 1321–1323, 2015.

23. **Hunter SK** and **Stevens AA**. Sex differences in marathon running with advanced age: physiology or participation? *Medicine and Science in Sports and Exercise* 45: 148–156, 2013.

24. **Hunter SK**, **Stevens AA**, **Magennis K**, **Skelton KW**, and **Fauth M**. Is there a sex difference in the age of elite marathon runners? *Medicine and Science in Sports and Exercise* 43: 656–664, 2011.

25. **Joyner MJ**. Physiological limits to endurance exercise performance: influence of sex. *The Journal of Physiology* 595: 2949–2954, 2017.

26. **Joyner MJ**, **Ruiz JR**, and **Lucia A**. The two-hour marathon: who and when? *Journal of Applied Physiology* 110: 275–277, 2011.

27. **Kashimada K** and **Koopman P**. Sry: the master switch in mammalian sex determination. *Development (Cambridge, England)* 137: 3921–3930, 2010.

28. **Knechtle B**. Ultramarathon runners: nature or nurture? *International Journal of Sports Physiology and Performance* 7: 310–312, 2012.

29. **Knechtle B**, **Rosemann T**, **Lepers R**, and **Rust CA**. Women outperform men in ultradistance swimming: the Manhattan Island Marathon Swim from 1983 to 2013. *International Journal of Sports Physiology and Performance* 9: 913–924, 2014.

30. **Kousta E**, **Papathanasiou A**, and **Skordis N**. Sex determination and disorders of sex development according to the revised nomenclature and classification in 46,XX individuals. *Hormones (Athens, Greece)* 9: 218–131, 2010.

31. **Lamb DR**. Androgens and exercise. *Medicine and Science in Sports* 7: 1–5, 1975.

32. **Maughan RJ**, **Watson JS**, and **Weir J**. Relationships between muscle strength and muscle cross-sectional area in male sprinters and endurance runners. *European Journal of Applied Physiology and Occupational Physiology* 50: 309–318, 1983.

33. **Millard-Stafford M, Swanson AE**, and **Wittbrodt MT**. Nature vs. nurture: have performance gaps between men and women reached an asymptote? *International Journal of Sports Physiology and Performance*: 13: 1–19, 2018.

34. **National Federation of State High School Associations** (**NFHS**). High school participation increases for 28th consecutive year. *NFHSnewscom* www.nfhs.org/articles/high-school-sports-participation-increases-for-28th-straight-year-nears-8-million-mark/, 2017.

35. **National Collegiate Athletic Association**. NCAA sports sponsorship and participation rates report 1981–82 – 2014–15. www.ncaa.org, 2016.

36. **Oosthuyse T** and **Bosch AN**. The effect of the menstrual cycle on exercise metabolism: implications for exercise performance in eumenorrhoeic women. *Sports Medicine* 40: 207–227, 2010.

37. **Pate RR, Sparling PB, Wilson GE, Cureton KJ**, and **Miller BJ**. Cardiorespiratory and metabolic responses to submaximal and maximal exercise in elite women distance runners. *International Journal of Sports Medicine* 8 (Suppl 2): 91–95, 1987.

38. **Pollock ML**. Characteristics of elite class distance runners-overview. *Annals of the New York Academy of Sciences* 301: 278–282, 1977.

39. **Pollock ML**. Submaximal and maximal working capacity of elite distance runners. Part I: Cardiorespiratory aspects. *Annals of the New York Academy of Sciences* 301: 310–322, 1977.

40. **Pollock ML, Gettman LR, Jackson A, Ayres J, Ward A**, and **Linnerud AC**. Body composition of elite class distance runners. *Annals of the New York Academy of Sciences* 301: 361–370, 1977.

41. **Robinson R**. "Eleven Wretched Women": what really happened in the first Olympic women's 800 m. *Runner's World*, May 14, 2012.

42. **Rust CA, Knechtle B, Rosemann T**, and **Lepers R.** Women reduced the sex difference in open-water ultra-distance swimming La Traversee Internationale du Lac St-Jean, 1955–2012. *Applied Physiology Nutrition and Metabolism* 39: 270–273, 2014.

43. **Sandbakk O, Solli GS**, and **Holmberg HC**. Sex differences in world-record performance: the influence of sport discipline and competition duration. *International Journal of Sports Physiology and Performance* 13: 2–8, 2018.

44. **Seiler S, De Koning JJ**, and **Foster C.** The fall and rise of the gender difference in elite anaerobic performance 1952–2006. *Medicine and Science in Sports and Exercise* 39: 534–540, 2007.

45. **Senefeld J, Smith C**, and **Hunter SK**. Sex differences in participation, performance, and age of ultramarathon runners. *International Journal of Sports Physiology and Performance* 11: 635–642, 2016.

46. **Smith M** and **Wrynn A**. *Women in the 2012 Olympic and Paralympic Games: An Analysis of Participation and Leadership Opportunities*. Ann Arbor, MI: SHARP Center for Women and Girls, 2013.

47. **Sparling PB**. A meta-analysis of studies comparing maximal oxygen uptake in men and women. *Research Quarterly for Exercise and Sport* 51: 542–552, 1980.

48. **Sparling PB** and **Cureton KJ**. Biological determinants of the sex difference in 12-min run performance. *Medicine and Science in Sports and Exercise* 15: 218–223, 1983.

49. **Sparling PB, O'Donnell EM**, and **Snow TK**. The gender difference in distance running performance has plateaued: an analysis of world rankings from 1980 to 1996. *Medicine and Science in Sports and Exercise* 30: 1725–1729, 1998.

50. **Stachenfeld NS** and **Taylor HS**. Challenges and methodology for testing young healthy women in physiological studies. *American Journal of Physiology Endocrinology and Metabolism* 306: E849–E853, 2014.

51. **Tanaka H**. The battle of the sexes in sports. *Lancet* 360: 92, 2002.

52. **Tatem AJ, Guerra CA, Atkinson PM**, and **Hay SI**. Athletics: momentous sprint at the 2156 Olympics? *Nature* 431: 525, 2004.

53. **Thibault V, Guillaume M, Berthelot G, Helou NE, Schaal K, Quinquis L, Nassif H, Tafflet M, Escolano S, Hermine O**, and **Toussaint JF**. Women and men in sport performance: the gender gap has not evolved since 1983. *Journal of Sports Science & Medicine* 9: 214–223, 2010.

54. **Troiano RP, Berrigan D, Dodd KW, Masse LC, Tilert T**, and **McDowell M**. Physical activity in the United States measured by accelerometer. *Medicine and Science in Sports and Exercise* 40: 181–188, 2008.

55. **Tucker R** and **Collins M**. What makes champions? A review of the relative contribution of genes and training to sporting success. *British Journal of Sports Medicine* 46: 555–561, 2012.

56. **USA Swimming**. Statistics 2014. www.usaswimming.org/_Rainbow/Documents/a31bc239-b31f-4834-87bf-accb09e8a834/Statistics-2014.pdf. 2014.

57. **Uth N**. Anthropometric comparison of world-class sprinters and normal populations. *Journal of Sports Science & Medicine* 4: 608–616, 2005.

58. **Vogt P**, **Rüst CA**, **Rosemann T**, **Lepers R**, and **Knechtle B**. Analysis of 10 km swimming performance of elite male and female open-water swimmers. *SpringerPlus* 2: 603, 2013.

59. **West DW**, **Burd NA**, **Churchward-Venne TA**, **Camera DM**, **Mitchell CJ**, **Baker SK**, **Hawley JA**, **Coffey VG**, and **Phillips SM**. Sex-based comparisons of myofibrillar protein synthesis after resistance exercise in the fed state. *Journal of Applied Physiology* 112: 1805–1813, 2012.

60. **Whipp BJ** and **Ward SA**. Will women soon outrun men? *Nature* 355: 25, 1992.

61. **Wild S**, **Rust CA**, **Rosemann T**, and **Knechtle B**. Changes in sex difference in swimming speed in finalists at FINA World Championships and the Olympic Games from 1992 to 2013. *BMC Sports Science, Medicine and Rehabilitation* 6: 25, 2014.

SECTION 6

The ethics of systems genetics in exercise and sport

In Section 6 we come to the end of our endeavor to provide both breadth and depth in our analysis of the systems genetics of sport and exercise. Unlike previous chapters, with their in-depth examination of research studies and tables and figures of genes and outcomes, the authors in Section 6 cause us to pause and reflect on how this knowledge is being used, and is anticipated to be used, by athletes, coaches, and other stakeholders.

We start with a discussion of the controversial topic of race and sport performance, examining whether genetic advantage in sport is based on geographic ancestry. Are East Africans genetically endowed to be better distance runners, while West Africans better sprinters? Would Jamaican bobsledders beat German bobsledders if only for more opportunities to pursue this winter sport and perfect their technique in the tropics? Or is race simply a proxy for cultural differences and environmental and economic opportunities that mirror race differences in other aspects of our lives? Drs. Nauright and Wiggins in Chapter 30 focus on these themes and provide unique insights into these questions.

Tying back to the preceding sections, Chapter 31, by Drs. Andrew Venezia and Stephen Roth, examines the explosion of genetic testing for a variety of traits now available to anyone with an Internet connection and a credit card. Genetic testing technology is robust and becoming relatively inexpensive, allowing companies to develop tests and sell them online to a variety of consumers. Whether the science backing the results or conclusions of those tests is high-quality or inconclusive is another question altogether. With genetic testing comes a variety of interesting and challenging ethical questions around talent identification and performance prediction, especially appropriate to consider for children.

Beyond genetic testing is the realm of gene therapy, the direct manipulation of genetic sequences to alter our biology. Gene therapy has had mixed success in the realm of disease therapy, but progress is being made. The potential for athletes to misuse gene therapy for performance enhancement, otherwise known as gene doping, has been anticipated for over a decade, with the World Anti-Doping Agency holding its first scientific workshop on gene doping in 2002. How should we view gene therapy in sport? Should it be completely banned or used only for injury treatment in rare cases? Or, should we embrace this new technology and the performance enhancements that are sure to be generated with its careful use? Drs. Verner Møller and Rasmus Bysted Møller of Aarhus University in Denmark outline their views on the ethics of gene doping in Chapter 32, while Dr. Andy Miah of the University of Salford in the UK counters with a transhumanist perspective in Chapter 33.

While gene therapy in sport and gene doping remained mostly hypothetical concerns as this book was coming to conclusion, an area of very real controversy is the subject of the final chapter in this section. Chapter 34, contributed by Dr. Jaime Schultz of Pennsylvania State University in the US, examines the ethics of sex and gender testing in sport competition. As outlined in Section 5, we know that sex differences result in very real differences in performance in many sports, resulting in sex-specific leagues and competitions. But how is sex determined for the purpose of distinguishing the members of those competitions? And is sex truly a binary of male and female that fits neatly into the structure of our sport leagues? This final chapter shows the difficult history of sex and gender testing and outlines the challenges of present-day approaches to ensuring "fair" competition between the sexes.

The chapters in Section 6 are meant to open readers' eyes to the consequences of this growing knowledge of systems genetics in sport. While researchers may have the best of intentions, and in fact may not be focused on sport at all in their conceptions of their work, knowledge of the genetic underpinnings of traits relevant to sport performance will be used, misused, and abused by athletes, much as we have seen with drug-related doping for many decades. As leaders in our respective fields, we must be aware of the indirect implications of our work and not shy away from helping to inform and educate the public about the consequences of both genetic testing and gene therapy in the world of sport.

30

RACE AND SPORTS PERFORMANCE

John Nauright and David K. Wiggins

From the 19th century and the emergence of modern sports competitions, athletes and scientists sought ways to enhance and improve performance relative to other athletes, countries, and races. While much of performance science was initially applied to race horses, increasingly understanding of the moving body, its capabilities and its limits engaged scientists internationally (12). While modern science was being applied to the body, anthropologists and ethnologists were attempting to understand differences between races and cultures. Ideas about temperament were applied to cultures and sports. For example, many English observers believed that the sport of cricket did not translate well outside of upper levels of society in the English-speaking world because the French, other Europeans, and native peoples did not have the patience or temperament to master the psychological aspects of the sport. Additionally, urbanization and the spread of disease, which led to sanitation movements and sewage systems for cities, raised alarm bells for European and North American observers by 1900 as they became more and more obsessed with the fear that the "white race" was in decline. After the South African (or Boer) War of 1899–1902, numerous commissions in Britain examined the state of working class British men and determined, in publications such as the *Report of the Inter-departmental Committee on Physical Deterioration* (1904), that the average health of British men had declined as a result of urbanization. Following on from this, defeats of British Isles national and regional rugby teams by New Zealand (1905), South Africa (1906, 1912), and Australia (1908), whose troops had been deemed to be more healthy than English ones, provided further "evidence" that it was only in colonial settings (Australia, New Zealand, Canada, the American West in the US) where a rugged and rural lifestyle was thought to abound where the white race was potentially improving (20, 21).

The emergence of black athletes particularly in boxing (Peter Jackson, Jack Johnson), American football (Paul Robeson and others), cycling (Marshall "Major" Taylor), and athletics (Sol Butler) between 1890 and 1920 added to fears that white athletes might not be as able to compete in the long run. The world championship victory by Jack Johnson over white Canadian Tommy Burns in Sydney, Australia in 1908, coupled with Johnson's interaction with white women, raised racial concerns to extreme levels (27). The response was to harden the color line and segregation became the norm in American baseball and basketball, though a small number of black athletes were able to compete through to the 1930s in American football and in Olympic sports.

We should remember the emergence of black athletic success in the US occurred against hardening racial lines as promoted in popular culture through Thomas Dixon's novel *The Clansman* (1905) which was later turned into the movie *Birth of a Nation* (1915). Dixon's book was an argument against desegregation and he argued black men would turn towards savage behavior if allowed too much freedom (24).

The first attempt at a scientific examination of physical abilities of races appeared in Joseph-Marie Degerano's *The Observation of Savage Peoples* which was published in 1800. The use of dynamometers during the 19th century was common and used in several widely publicized studies to substantiate claims that English or French men were the strongest and Australian Aborigines the weakest among groups of peoples. Many of these early experiments were shown to lack scientific validity and merely served to legitimate the ideologies of hierarchy of races which always placed northern European or North American white men at the top of the scales of civilization as well as in physical capacity. Athletic challenges by black athletes, however, placed a strain on this dominant ideology and so analyses began to link athleticism with savagery and physicality became increasingly juxtaposed against mental capabilities (12).

In 1936, W. Montague Cobb, a prominent black medical doctor and physical anthropologist from Howard University, Washington DC, published the well-known essay "Race and Runners" in *The Journal of Health and Physical Education* that attempted to refute the claims by popular writers and others both in and outside of sport that black people were endowed with innate anatomical and physiological gifts that accounted for their great athletic performances. Based on anthropometric measurements he had taken from track and field star Jesse Owens and other black athletes, Cobb made clear his view that it was erroneous to argue that black people possessed a musculature and genes unique to their race that allowed them to shatter athletic records and achieve unparalleled success on America's playing fields. Instead, noted Cobb, the success of black individuals in sport, albeit in only a select number of sports, resulted from a combination of great physical talent and opportunities as well as hard work, desire, dedication, and a host of other character traits so admired in American culture (6, 34).

Cobb's refutation of the concept of biological determinism did not put an end to the debate regarding the impact of race on sport performance that had been waged since the latter part of the 19th century and continues, in one form or another, to this very day. It was merely one of the most explicit and logical denunciations of the persistent belief that race predisposed black people to superior athletic performances made by a prestigious scientist with a national profile by virtue not only of his academic work but his civil rights activism and leadership in national organizations. Importantly, it was also a denunciation of the notion of biological determinism made during a period of time that the athletic accomplishments of black athletes were becoming far more visible at both the national and international levels of competition. Notable examples of this fact were the increasing number of black athletes distinguishing themselves in sport at prestigious predominantly white universities in the US and in both the 1932 Olympic Games in Los Angeles and 1936 Olympic Games in Berlin (11, 34).

The public debate regarding race and sport performance lost some of its steam during World War II as athletic programs at all levels of competition lost some of their best performers to the war effort and with the cancellation or alteration of games and leagues and organizations. Once the war to defend Franklin Roosevelt's "Four Freedoms" was complete, the debate would heat up as ordinary fans, popular writers, coaches, academicians, and others from various walks of life would offer their views as to what accounted for the great performances of black athletes. Not unexpectedly, the debate always seemed to gain momentum during the summer Olympic Games as black athletes, particularly in track and field, displayed their speed and jumping abilities against other countries' best athletes in front of a worldwide audience. This was certainly the case regarding the 1948 Olympic Games in London, 1952 Olympic Games in Helsinki, and 1956 Olympic Games in Melbourne, as the outstanding accomplishments of such great black athletes from the US as Harrison Dillard, Mal Whitfield, Milt Campbell, Barney Ewell, and William Steele would attest (11, 18).

Two essays published in 1952 point to the decidedly different views that would continue to exist regarding the debate over race and sports performance. G.P. Meade, manager of the Colonial Sugars Company in Gramercy, Louisiana, and a man who had a fascination with records and sports accomplishments, proffered in his essay "The Negro in Track Athletics" in the *Scientific Monthly* that why African Americans had provided such a large proportion of extremely high class performances could not be accounted for by innate natural differences, "but probably because of sociologic reasons" (18). British medical doctor Adolph Abrahams, on the other hand, took a decidedly different position in his article "Race and Athletics" in the *Eugenics Review*. He came down on the side of innate physiological differences to account for the outstanding performances of black athletes. "I think there is some special quality in his [African American] muscles" wrote Abrahams. "A more rapid contractibility or reduced viscosity. Alternatively, there may be a superior co-ordination related to his nervous system" (18). The pattern of the debate during the 1950s continued unabated during the following decade as every Summer Olympic Games brought more individuals into the discussion. If there is one distinguishing feature of the debate during the 1960s it is the increasing attention given to the topic in newspapers and popular journals, an indication perhaps more than anything else of the ever-expanding visibility of the Olympic Games resulting from television coverage and other media forms. The decade began with British medical doctor James M. Tanner publishing the results of the anthropometric measurements he completed on 137 athletes from the Rome Olympics of 1960. Included in his text, *The Physique of the Olympic Athlete*, Tanner conceded that economic and social factors undoubtedly played a part in the number of blacks participating in highly organized sport, but noted that the different body types of black track and field athletes is perhaps what accounted for their outstanding performances in particular events (30). In 1964, writer Marshall Smith, in his provocatively titled *Life* magazine article "Giving the Olympics an Anthropological Once-Over" echoed some of what Tanner had expressed in his study (29). Smith relied to a great extent on the views of well-known anthropologists Carleton S. Coon and Edward E. Hunt, Jr., both of whom were solidly in the camp of biological determinists by stressing the importance of "inherited physical adaptations" and contending that the unique body type of black athletes gave them a distinct advantage in certain sporting events (7). Finally, in 1968, sportswriter Charles Mahar summed up the various arguments given up to that time about the connection between race and sports performance in two articles in a five-part series on the black athlete in the *Los Angeles Times*. As the titles of his two articles suggest, "Blacks Physically Superior? Some Say They're Hungrier" and "Do Blacks Have a Physical Advantage? Scientists Differ" Mahar essentially categorizes the arguments into those that took a biological determinist approach to the debate and those that viewed the success of black athletes as resulting from a combination of finely tuned physical skills, hard work, dedication, opportunities, and a host of other social and economic factors (17).

Certainly a watershed episode in the debate regarding race and sport performance involved an article written by sportswriter Martin Kane and the pointed and strongly worded responses to that article by Harry Edwards, a professor of sociology at the University of California, Berkeley, and architect of the proposed boycott of the 1968 Mexico City Olympic Games (9). In 1971, Kane penned a detailed account of the debate in *Sports Illustrated*, a highly popular journal in which he served as senior editor. Depending on the expertise of various individuals, including coaches, medical doctors, and sport researchers, Kane made the case in the article

"An Assessment of Black is Best" that the dominance of black athletes resulted from race-based psychological, historical, and physiological factors (15). Kane relied to a great extent on the expertise of famous University of Indiana and US Olympic swimming coach James Councilman who contended that the large number of white muscle fibers in black athletes was responsible for their outstanding performances in sports that put a premium on speed and power (8). Conversely, the preponderance of red muscle fibers in white athletes made them ideally suited for those sports requiring endurance. Oddly, Councilman turns to socioeconomic reasons to explain the few number of blacks in his sport, contending that blacks lacked the money and access to facilities that were essential to participating and realizing success in swimming. For whatever reason, he does not state in the Kane piece like he did in the previously mentioned Marshall Smith essay in *Life* magazine of 1964 that it was difficult for black people to learn how to swim because of their "lack of buoyancy," one of several long-held racial stereotypes used to explain away the lack of black participants in the sport (8).

Edwards, obviously deeply troubled by the *Sports Illustrated* piece, quickly responded to the article with a serious article of his own that countered in great detail Kane's assertions. Edwards was highly critical of Kane's generalizations about the supposed special aptitudes and abilities of a particular racial group, especially when considering, as W. Montague Cobb had postulated years before, the fact that there were "more differences between individual members of any one racial group than between any two groups as a whole." This obviously precluded any arguments that certain racial groups were uniquely built and destined to achieve success in certain sports. Edwards asserted that Kane's notion that black people possessed a unique psychological disposition in being able to relax under pressure was ludicrous, a deep-seated stereotypical notion that had no basis in fact. Edwards vehemently disputed Kane's claim that hereditarily weaker black individuals had been separated out during slavery and what was left was a physically superior group uniquely predisposed to athletic success. Implied in Edward's comment is that Kane's assertion regarding biological determinism and connection to superior athleticism was the same racialist thinking that had been used for years to claim black intellectual inferiority. In the end, Edwards asserted that a number of interrelated societal conditions and circumstances accounted for the outstanding performances of black athletes as well as their commitment to the institution of sport that had traditionally been perceived to be open to them (9).

Kane's article and Edwards' response to it seems particularly important for at least three different reasons. First of all, it took place during a period of time in which the lives and careers of black athletes were receiving increased attention from scholars and the academic community more generally. The involvement of black athletes in the larger civil rights struggle, including the protests they waged during Olympic competitions and on predominantly white university campuses, combined with a new-found interest in the life and culture of black Americans, expanded their public profile and resulted in a plethora of academic studies that not only addressed questions about their excellence in certain sports but also such issues as inequality in salaries and inability to secure coaching and upper level administrative positions. Second, Edwards' claim that the same racialist thinking used to account for black dominance in sport was used to explain supposed black intellectual inferiority was certainly correct and not proffered in a vacuum as the US was in the midst of a controversial debate about race, IQ scores, and academic achievement (9). In 1969, just 2 years before the publication of Kane's article, Arthur R. Jensen, a professor of psychology at the University of California, Berkeley, published a lengthy study in the *Harvard Educational Review* that reenergized the long-standing debate regarding the impact of race on the supposed differences between black and white intelligence. "Genetic differences are manifested" noted Jensen, "in virtually every anatomical, physiological, and biological comparison one can make between representative samples of identifiable racial groups. There is no reason why the brain should be exempt from this generalization" (13). Jensen's views, along with others that took the same position like Stanford University physicist and Nobel Laureate William B. Shockley, drew volatile responses from both black and white people appalled by such racialist thinking and the disregard for the social, economic, and environmental factors that play extraordinarily important roles in any differences between and among men and women (28). Third, but certainly not least, Kane's article and Edwards' response to it makes patently clear an important fact about the debate over the impact of race on sport performance that is not always acknowledged and that is almost the entire focus of the discussions on black male rather than black female athletes. One simple reason for this, as sport management scholar Jennifer Bruening and others have pointed out, is that black women are largely invisible, never fully recognized for their singular experiences, regularly marginalized by either being categorized in the same group as white women or black men (4).

The ensuing debate regarding race and sport performance would certainly have practical implications and potentially deleterious effects. One prime example would be the impact it would have on black athletes themselves. Although not responding uniformly to issues surrounding the debate, some black athletes have bought into the notion that their race is innately gifted physically and that it has resulted in superior sporting accomplishments. In a 1977 *Time* magazine article titled "Sport: The Black Dominance," football's infamous O.J. Simpson and baseball Hall of Famer Joe Morgan expressed such views. "We are built a little differently" said Simpson, "built for speed—skinny calves, long legs, high asses are all characteristic of blacks." Morgan was just as explicit as his football counterpart by noting: "I think blacks, for physiological reasons, have better speed, quickness, and ability. Baseball, football, and basketball put a premium on those skills" (31). More recently, in 2012 to be exact, multiple Olympic gold medal-winning track and field athlete Michael Johnson weighed in on the matter with obvious conviction by talking about the impact of slavery on him and other members of his race. "All my life," said Johnson, "I believed I became an athlete through my own determination, but it's impossible to think that being descended from slaves hasn't left an imprint through the generations. Difficult as it was to hear, slavery has benefited descendants like me—I believe there is a superior athletic gene in us" (14).

Holding on to the belief they had genes that predisposed them to great sporting feats would certainly give Simpson, Morgan, Johnson, and other black athletes a psychological advantage, while having the opposite effect for white athletes who held the same views. Believing in "biological cultural destiny" could certainly provide a psychological edge for black athletes in an activity where the margins of victory are often very slim and usually determined by participants with high confidence levels as well as finely tuned bodies and carefully honed athletic skills. Conversely, believing in such a faulty supposition was of little help, in fact it could be a devastating blow, to those black athletes that did not have the requisite physical skills to reach the highest levels of sport that everyone expected of them. In addition, whether black athletes were cognizant of the fact or not, the racialist thinking that undergird the debate regarding race and sport performance was also used to discriminate against them, limit them to particular playing positions, and deny them opportunities to freely compete for coaching, managerial, and upper-level administrative positions. Perhaps there was no more famous example of this then Los Angeles Dodger Vice President Al Campanis attempting to explain to host Ted Kopell of *Nightline* in 1987 on the 40th anniversary of Jackie Robinson's shattering of the color line in Major League Baseball why there were still so few black managers and upper level administrators in the sport. When Kopell specifically asked Campanis "Is there still that much prejudice in baseball today?" the Dodger Vice President responded by saying "No, I don't believe it's prejudice. I truly believe that they may not have some of the necessities to be, let's say, a field manager, or perhaps a general manager." When Kopell pressed him further on the matter, Campanis continued spouting illogical racialist theories, noting for instance at one point that "So, it might be—why are black men, or black people, not good swimmers? Because they don't have the buoyancy." Not unexpectedly, Campanis was forced to resign from his position with Dodger owner Peter O'Malley noting that "Campanis' statements on the ABC *Nightline* show Monday night were so far removed from the belief of the Dodger organization that it was impossible for him to continue in his duties" (32, 33).

Unfortunately, the belief on the part of people, obviously both black and white and from every stratum of society, that black people were endowed with special physical talents was slow to fade away as evidenced by the periodic spewing of such beliefs throughout the latter stages of the 20th century. The pattern would become clear. Someone who took the view that race was a biological phenomenon would make the assertion that black people had unique anatomical and physiological gifts that accounted for their outstanding performances in particular activities and this would then be countered by those who recognized the erroneous nature of this argument and that a combination of physical, sociological, economic, and cultural factors accounted for the success of athletes irrespective of the race in which they identified. This would happen with some regularity with those in the public eye who espoused the view that black athletes achieved success in certain activities because of anatomical and physiological abilities unique to their race, sometimes actually losing their jobs because of the racialist position they took. The examples are many, but two that garnered much attention and controversy were the infamous 1988 interview conducted by Ed Hotaling with CBS prognosticator and sports broadcaster Jimmy "The Greek" Snyder and Jon Entine's attention-grabbing 2000 book *Taboo: Why Black Athletes Dominate Sports and Why We're Afraid to Talk About It* (10, 26).

On Martin Luther King Day (January 15) in 1988 at a restaurant in Washington, DC, local newscaster Hotaling asked Snyder his opinion as to the progress being made by black athletes. The response that Snyder gave to Hotaling's question, a response he must have regretted until the day he died, was laced with illogical assumptions, deep-seated stereotypical notions about race, and generalizations that were decidedly ahistorical in nature. He noted that black people were far better athletes than white people since they had been "bred to be that way since the days of slavery" and that if more black people found their way into coaching positions "there's not going to be anything left for the white people." The origin of black dominance in sport took place during the period of the Civil War when "the slave owner would breed his big black with his big woman so that he could have a big black kid." It is a fact, said Snyder, that black athletes "jump higher and run faster" as a result of their "thigh size and big size." In an apparent sign of regret, he argued that white athletes would never be able to overcome these physical disadvantages and achieve the same level of accomplishments as their black counterparts, particularly because they were lazy and less motivated to realize success in sport (26).

Not unexpectedly, Snyder's comments drew harsh criticism from those in the popular press. The editors of *Sports Illustrated* wrote that Snyder obviously had no understanding of history or the institution of sport and that his broad generalizations were exactly the way in "which racial stereotypes and prejudices are built." *Washington Post* writer Carl Rowan compared Snyder to Joseph Goebbels, Adolph Hitler's cruel Minister of Public Enlightenment and Propaganda (25). A cartoon in the *Boston Globe* showed Snyder being comforted by a hooded Ku Klux Klan member. After just 2 days of intense and far-reaching public condemnation of Snyder, CBS had no choice but to fire him. Apparently, Snyder learned nothing from the Al Campanis debacle that took place some 9 months earlier.

Snyder's disturbing and offensive remarks also brought sport studies scholars, particularly from sociology, even more squarely into the debate regarding race and sport performance. Harry

Edwards, for instance, did not mince words, calling Snyder ignorant and incompetent and regularly spoke of the fallacy of the broadcaster's statements in written form and through interviews and other public forums. Jay Coakley, primarily through the multiple editions of his text *Sport in Society: Issues and Controversies*, stepped up his already vehement denunciation of racial science, arguing that the preponderance of black athletes in particular sports had to do with a combination of racial discrimination, characteristics of certain sports, and the motivation of individual athletes. It also has to do, says Coakley, with how black athletes defined their chances for success and those sports participated in by those successful athletes who served as role models during their youth (5).

Beyond the US, discussions continued to either try and legitimate strong performance or explain poor performance in certain sports by African and other black athletes. As late as 1996, British Prime Minister John Major suggested Britain send "athletic missionaries" to Africa in search of talent while in South Africa, white rugby officials tried to explain away the low numbers of black rugby players at top levels by arguing they did not have experience playing the sport. These assertions went counter to the more than 100-year history of black rugby in South Africa which developed alongside that of white rugby, though mostly in segregated environments (22).

In 2000, Jon Entine raised the level of debate regarding race and sport performance to an even more feverish pitch internationally with the publication of his controversial book *Taboo: Why Black Athletes Dominate Sports and Why We're Afraid to Talk About It*. Entine, a journalist and author who had helped produce, with the iconic American broadcaster Tom Brokow, a 1989 1-hour documentary on the topic, put together a book of over 300 pages that largely sums up the many issues long associated with the debate. Perhaps most importantly, however, Entine's arguments and interpretations helped revive the bitter disputes that had always placed in opposition the biological determinists and cultural theorists who had broached the topic. Although asserting he was only concerned with acknowledging human diversity, not interested in spewing racialist beliefs, and distancing himself from "The Bell Curve" that connected intelligence and race, Entine's belief in race as a biological phenomenon and his undying faith in the objective and value-neutral nature of science ultimately precluded him from seriously considering the myriad sociological and cultural factors that largely accounted for those sports in which they participated and, in some cases, dominated. Very troubling is Entine's decision to lump Africans and African Americans into one group and attempting to explain the differences between sprinters and long-distance runners based on such anatomical and physiological factors as muscle fibers, muscle mass, lung capacity, body size, centers of gravity, and enzymes. Just as disturbing is Entine's claim that white athletes have been marginalized, false statements that black athletes have achieved relatively much success in most sports, and inexplicable commitment to racial science while at once disparaging the racist eugenics studies of the late 19th and early 20th centuries, which he details in the book as being misplaced and without thorough vetting (10).

Like Al Campanis and Jimmy "The Greek" Snyder some 12 years earlier, Entine received a rash of criticism for the arguments he put forward in *Taboo*. In spite of the criticism, however, it did not put an end to the efforts of biological determinists to locate the genes that accounted for the success of black athletes. The insistence on searching for unique athletic genes among black athletes has not been an innocent endeavor, but evidence of the continual need to rank people based on skin color so as to rationalize inequitable treatment and confirm the supposed superiority of one race over another. There has been no comparable search for anatomical and physiological differences among white athletes that could explain their domination of golf, tennis, ice hockey, swimming, skating, skiing, field hockey, volleyball, and so many other sports. No need to explain the overrepresentation of white participants in these sports by virtue of the fact that many people gloss over this reality, viewing the overwhelming success of individual black athletes in a few selected sports as emblematic of the entire race.

Tellingly, much of the scholarly focus on the topic beginning with the publication of Entine's book has been on Kenyan distance runners. The extraordinary success of these athletes in the recent past has generated much interest from scientists, an interesting but not surprising juxtaposition in the debate regarding race and sports performance considering that for years the focus was on finding the anatomical and physiological reasons for the seeming dominance of African American sprinters and assumptions that the modest performances by African American distance runners was merely the result of a lack of stamina and, by extension, the heart. Examples of the thrust of the studies on Kenyon distance runners can be gleaned from their titles, including headings ranging from "Kenyan and Ethiopian Distance Runners: What Makes Them So Good" (35) and "Demographic Characteristics of Elite Kenyan Endurance Runners" (23) to "Kenyan Dominance in Distance Running" (16) and "Dissociation Between Running Economy and Running Performance in Elite Kenyan Distance Runners" (19).

John Bale and Joe Sang, writing in 1996, clearly outlined a multifaceted rationale for Kenyan running success which scientists obsessed with racial explanations have largely ignored. Bale and Sang demonstrate that nearly all top runners from Kenya are Kalenjin. The Maasai, who the British originally thought would be more successful as athletes, live in similar environmental conditions, yet very few have achieved success in distance running. The Kalenjin do live at altitude, but, uniquely have a very high achievement principle in their culture. Bale and Sang also demonstrate that many other African countries are underrepresented as are non-African countries where many people live at altitude, thus neither race nor geography can fully explain successes. Furthermore, Bale and Sang show that Kenya was one of the first places where Finnish methods of running coaching were taught such that by their first major international competition at the 1954 Empire Games, Kenyan runners were competitive (3).

Despite no real evidence of a "magic racial gene," scientists and observers continue to search for explanation of success by black athletes in any sport where they are overrepresented or achieve disproportionate success. The converse, as we stated, is never applied to white athletes or the sports where they are overrepresented. Professor Yannis Pitsiladis, director of the Sub2hrs marathon project and expert on genomics and sport performance, has argued there is no magic gene thus agreeing with the assessment of Montague Cobb from the 1930s. Pitsiladis does argue, however, that genetics matter in that athletes who have successful athletic parents and grandparents are more likely to succeed than those who do not. Importantly though, there is no skin color correlation. Scientists would do better to eliminate skin color from experimentation and deracialize the science of human performance.

References

1. **Anthony, A.** White men can't run. *The Observer* June 4, 2000. www.jonentine.com/reviews/observer. htm. [Accessed April 17, 2018.]
2. **Ashe, A.R.** *A Hard Road to Glory: A History of the African-American Athlete Since 1946.* New York: Amistad Press, 1993.
3. **Bale, J.** and **Sang, J.** *Kenyan Running.* London: Frank Cass, 1996.
4. **Bruening, J.** Gender and racial analysis in sport: are all the women white and all the blacks men? *Quest* 57: 330–349, 2005.
5. **Coakley, J.** *Sports in Society: Issues and Controversies.* 12th edition. New York: The McGraw-Hill Companies, 2017.
6. **Cobb, W.M.** Race and runners. *The Journal of Health and Physical Education* 7: 3–7, 52–56, 1936.
7. Quoted in **Smith, M.** Giving the Olympics an anthropological once over. *Life Magazine*, October 23, 83, 1964.

8. Quoted in **Kane, M.** An assessment of black is best. *Sports Illustrated*, January 18, 72–73, 1971.

9. **Edwards, H.** The sources of the black athletes superiority. *The Black Scholar* 3: 32–41, 1971.

10. **Entine, J.** *Taboo: Why Black Athletes Dominate Sports and Why We're Afraid to Talk About It.* New York: Public Affairs, 2000.

11. **Gleaves, J.** and **Dyreson, M.** The Black Auxiliaries in American Memories: Sport, Race And Politics in the Construction of Modern Legacies. *The International Journal of the History of Sport* 27: 2893–2924, 2010.

12. **Hoberman, J.** *Mortal Engines: The Science of Human Performance and the Dehumanization of Sport.* New York: The Free Press, 1992.

13. **Jensen, A.R.** How much can we boost I.Q. and scholastic achievement? *Harvard Educational Review* 39: 1–123, 1969.

14. Quoted in **Chase, C.** Michael Johnson says slavery descendants run faster because of "superior athletic gene". *Yahoo Sports*, July 5, 2012. sports.yahoo.com/blogs/olympics-fourth-place-medal/ michaeljohnson-says-slavery-descendents. [Accessed September 14, 2018.]

15. **Kane, M.** An assessment of black is best. *Sports Illustrated*, January 18, 72–83, 1971.

16. **Larsen, H.B.** Kenyan dominance in distance running. *Comparative Biochemistry And Physiology- Part A: Molecular & Integrative Physiology* 136: 161–170, 2003.

17. **Maher, C.** Blacks physically superior? Some say they're hungrier. *Los Angeles Times*, March 24, 1968; **Maher, C.** Do blacks have a physical advantage? scientists differ. *Los Angeles Times*, March 29, 1968.

18. **Meade, G.P.** The Negro in track athletics. *Scientific Monthly* 75: 366–371, 1952; **Abrahams, A.** *Race and Athletics* 44: 143–145, 1952.

19. **Mooses, M., Mooses, K., Haile, D.W., Durussel, J., Kaasik, P.** and **Pitsiladis, Y.P.** Dissociation between running economy and running performance in elite Kenyan distance runners. *Journal of Sports Sciences* 33: 136–144, 2014.

20. **Nauright, J.** Sport and the image of colonial manhood in the British mind: British physical deterioration debates and colonial sporting tours, 1878–1906. *Canadian Journal of History of Sport* 23: 54–71, 1992.

21. **Nauright, J.** Colonial manhood and imperial race virility: British responses to colonial rugby tours. In: Nauright J and Chandler TJL (Eds.), *Making Men* (pp. 121–139). London: Routledge, 1996.

22. **Nauright, J.** *Long Run to Freedom: Sport Cultures and Identities in South Africa.* Morgantown, WV: Fitness Information Technology, 2010.

23. **Onywera, V.O, Scott, R.A, Boit, M.K** and **Pitsiladis, Y.P.** Demographic characteristics of elite Kenyan endurance runners. *Journal of Sports Sciences* 24: 415–422, 2006.

24. **Robinson, C.** *Forgeries of Memory and Meaning: Blacks and the Regimes of Race in American Theater and Film before World War II.* New Edition. Chapel Hill, NC: The University of North Carolina Press, 2007.

25. **Rowan, C.** It didn't start with Jimmy the Greek. *Washington Post* January 21, 1988; **Range, P.R.** What we say, what we think. *U.S. News & World Report* 104: 27–28, 1988.

26. **Rowe, J.** The Greek chorus: Jimmy the Greek got it wrong but so did his critics. *The Washington Monthly* 20: 31–34, 1988.

27. **Runstedtler, T.** *Jack Johnson, Rebel Sojourner: Boxing in the Shadow of the Global Color Line.* Berkeley & Los Angeles, CA: University of California Press, 2013.

28. **Pearson, R.** *Shockey on Eugenics and Race.* Washington, DC: Townsend Publishers, 1992.

29. **Smith, M.** Giving the Olympics an anthropological once-over. *Life* 57: 80–84, 1964.

30. **Tanner, J.M.** *The Physique of the Olympic Athlete: A Study of 137 Track and Field Athletes at The XVII Olympic Games, Rome, 1960.* London: G. Allen and Unwin, 1964.

31. **Time.** Sport: the black dominance. *Time* 109: 57–60, 1977.

32. **Uhlig, M.** Racial remarks cause furor. *New York Times*, January 16, 1988.

33. **Weinbaum, W.** The legacy of Al Campanis. *ESPN.com* April 1, 2012.

34. **Wiggins, D.K.** Black athletes in white men's games: race, sport, and American national pastimes. *The International Journal of the History of Sport* 31: 181–202, 2014.

35. **Wilber, R.L** and **Pitsiladis, Y.P.** Kenyan and Ethiopian distance runners: what makes them so good? *International Journal of Sports Performance* 7: 92–102, 2012.

31

THE SCIENTIFIC AND ETHICAL CHALLENGES OF USING GENETIC INFORMATION TO PREDICT SPORT PERFORMANCE

Andrew C. Venezia and Stephen M. Roth

Introduction

Children and adolescents are encouraged to participate in athletic competition for several reasons. For many, the participation is simply an opportunity to engage in activities that are fun, social, and healthy for mind and body. For others, whether internally or externally driven, their goals and aspirations reach a much higher level, namely that of becoming an elite athlete with the hope of securing a position on a professional or Olympic team. Behind these young athletes are numerous stakeholders, including family members, coaches, and sponsors, who can be intimately involved in the development of athletic potential, all with similar hopes of greatness for the athlete, though perhaps for more self-serving reasons. The culture and economy surrounding athletic excellence has produced a demand for early talent identification, the process of recognizing a propensity for athletic excellence, to streamline the process of talent development ensuring that resources are efficiently utilized and future stars have a chance to develop. But the efficacy of talent identification strategies is limited due to the complexity of physical and psychological development in children, as well as numerous other factors, including the sport, types of evaluations, and interpretation of data (3, 6). Because the financial and social consequences for helping to develop an elite athlete are so high, talent identification remains an area of great interest for many in the world of sports.

Ideally, stakeholders would be able to predict future athletic performance using physiological, psychological, and genetic characteristics, which would be measurable well before adulthood with both high validity and predictive value. While the intricate balance between nature (genetic predisposition) and nurture (environmental factors) is open to debate, it is generally recognized that not all young athletes have the potential to progress to elite status, whether due to limited innate talent or simply lack of training opportunities (time, access to facilities, etc.). Coaches and sport organizations must therefore carefully select the targets for enhanced training opportunities, hoping to focus the best of training resources on those athletes most likely to have the innate traits needed for success. Early talent identification is an especially more efficient approach to talent development compared to treating all young athletes equally until a few athletes separate themselves from the pack in young adulthood. Instead of including all young athletes in a talent development program, only the best young athletes are included, which allows those athletes with presumably the most potential for elite status in adulthood to be exposed to the highest level of training opportunities (3). While exceptions may exist, in most athletic endeavors a certain level of genetic advantage is required to reach elite status (17). Similarly, having a genetic advantage alone is not sufficient to become a champion unless combined with an optimal training environment (17). With this in mind, one can see the utility in identifying the youth athlete with the ideal genetic makeup and placing them in the ideal environment to have the best chance of developing an elite athlete.

Although the entire process of developing an elite athlete is challenging, the talent identification process itself presents a unique set of challenges. By necessity, talent identification models will vary by sport, yet most will contain a combination of tests that assess anthropometric, physiological, and cognitive/psychological variables, as well as certain sport-related technical skills (29). Beyond the difficulties of testing the complex combination of skills and abilities required in certain sports, there are several major obstacles to identifying youth athletes with the potential for success. For example, the physical and psychological development of children does not follow a uniform trajectory. Biological age and chronological age can differ dramatically, giving some precocious youth an advantage over later-developing peers, though those differences tend to minimize over time (29). As such, testing in children will necessarily provide advantage to those who are more physically or mentally developed at that chronological age, regardless of the predictive value of those traits later in life. Because many youth sports are separated by age groups, talent development programs tend to select athletes that are born early in the selection year, resulting in more mature youth athletes being identified as "talented" (47), a concept known as the relative age effect. Although biobanding, the process of grouping youth athletes based on physical and psychological maturation instead of chronological age alone, is currently being explored and utilized by certain sporting organizations, this concept is not fully optimized and requires more investigation to best determine its usefulness in different sports (12). Obstacles such as these increase the likelihood of traditional talent identification models resulting in tremendous error in the form of false positives and false negatives. In contrast to most physiological and psychological traits, the DNA sequence does not change over time or experience day-to-day variability depending on the health, training status, or mental state of the athlete, and therefore potentially offers a steadfast glimpse at athletic potential. Rather than relying on a snapshot of a child's performance at age 9 years, for example, a genetic analysis could provide insights into physical and mental traits that are likely to be present in the fully developed young adult, regardless of the developmental trajectory those traits take during childhood. Advances in genetic testing have now made it relatively cheap and easy to evaluate gene sequence variation in individuals; the challenge is knowing which gene sequences to examine and how to incorporate these into talent identification programs. Of note, the fast-developing field of epigenetics represents a unique complexity to this idea, as epigenetic modification of the DNA sequence may impart influences on gene expression not observable with a traditional genetic test. We will save discussion of this emerging field for the future when additional evidence of the importance of epigenetics in this context becomes available.

At any one time during the 2017 National Basketball Association (NBA) Finals, up to 40% of players on the court had a father that also played in the NBA. With this information alone, we cannot separate the influence of nature versus nurture in these athletes, yet this remarkably high percentage certainly indicates a familial contribution of some kind. Indeed, twin and family studies have shown that key sport-related traits are heritable, such as height (38), somatotype (30), aerobic capacity and trainability (4, 5), strength, power (10), muscle fiber type (22), and even elite athletic status (13). Yet despite knowing the heritability of many athletic traits and the considerable research dedicated to finding genetic markers relevant to sport performance (and, thus, talent identification), identifying specific genetic predictors of elite athletic performance has been exceedingly challenging. This is especially true in sports such as basketball or soccer that require a unique combination of aerobic and anaerobic endurance, anaerobic power, sport-specific skills, and cognitive abilities such as game understanding and decision-making, in addition to team dynamics.

As earlier chapters in the present book have discussed, several innovative, large-scale genetic investigations of sport-related traits are currently underway and have the potential to elucidate some of the current unknowns in the genetics of elite athletic potential (43). With these and future studies utilizing new genetic tools, it seems possible that one day evidence-based genetic analysis during childhood or even prenatally could be efficacious and perhaps even ubiquitous in talent identification programs. The incorporation of evidence-based genetic analysis into talent identification and development processes would likely improve outcomes compared to current programs, and may even improve prediction of athletes predisposed to serious injury or activity-related mortality (41). However, this ability to make such predictions presents a set of ethical issues that must be considered and directly addressed. In the remaining sections of the present chapter, we aim to address these ethical issues, many of which are relevant beyond sport, as the direct-to-consumer (DTC) genetic testing market is rapidly expanding in numerous health- and medicine-related areas.

Potential for using genetic testing for talent identification

Although research over the past several decades has been devoted to identifying the heritability and genetic factors underlying traits related to athletic performance (19, 25, 31, 34, 36, 37, 46), we are still in the infancy of the field as new tools and large-scale collaborative projects are being developed. The intense focus on genetic predictors of athletic performance has led to the identification of several genetic markers and polygenic profiles associated with athletic performance; however, the field is rife with underpowered studies and unreplicated findings. A recent investigation of available literature found 155 genetic markers associated with elite sport performance (1), yet even the most consistent of associated genetic markers account for only a small variance (e.g., 1–2% at most) in athletic performance and are limited to determining likelihood of success in endurance or sprint/power activities (27) rather than sport performance itself. For example, the R allele of the alpha-actinin-3 (*ACTN3*) R577X variant is advantageous for power-oriented events (see Chapter 23). While this does not exclude the possibility of an individual with the X allele from participating in power-oriented events (26), there is certainly an association between the R allele and elite power performance (28). A child with this allele is hypothetically more likely to excel in events such as powerlifting and sprinting. Similarly, the angiotensin-converting enzyme (*ACE*) I/I genotype is associated with greater endurance performance while the *ACE* D/D genotype is associated with strength and power performance (27) and this genotype could be similarly used for prediction in young athletes (see Chapter 17). Importantly, sports like basketball, boxing, soccer, rugby, and American football are characterized by a combination of aerobic and anaerobic qualities, along with numerous other physical and psychological characteristics. Using genetic profiling to predict success in sports with complex physical and psychological requirements is a daunting task. The number of possible polygenic profiles contributing to an elite boxer or soccer player is likely enormous. To add to the difficulties of identifying polygenic profiles in elite athletes, we are limited by the number of "elite" athletes on the planet, with even fewer available or willing to participate in genetic research.

Add to this limitation that sex and race are also important considerations, and the sample pool is reduced even more. Breitbach et al. (6) suggest that utilizing the GWAS approach roughly 100,000 elite athletes from a defined discipline would be necessary to explain 15% of variance in elite performance in that specific sport discipline. Even if there were 100,000 elite athletes in any specific sport discipline, 85% of the variance in elite performance would remain undefined. Chapter 25 of this volume outlines some of the efforts of the field to improve the ability to study elite athletes and more effectively identify contributing genetic factors.

Considering the above information, we do not believe that the available evidence is strong enough to responsibly favor, or especially exclude, young athletes from participating in specific sports based on their genetic makeup. This opinion is shared by several researchers in the field (8, 18, 24, 33, 41, 44, 45). In a 2015 consensus statement, Webborn et al. (44) argue against the use of genetic testing for talent identification by stating "in the current state of knowledge, no child or young athlete should be exposed to direct-to-consumer genetic testing to define or alter training or for talent identification aimed at selecting gifted children or adolescents." Similarly, a position statement from the Australian Institute of Sport in 2017 (40) indicated that "despite the correlation between some genes and elite athletic performance, there is no scientific evidence for the predictive value of genetic profiling in sports performance." Despite this general consensus on the present inadequacies of genetic prediction in talent identification, the next decades of collaborative high-quality investigations with large populations of elite-level athletes may ultimately provide the ability to use polygenic prediction models to identify potential for success. Moreover, advances in genetic technologies are leading to remarkable prenatal and preimplantation screening tools to identify potential genetic disorders and select embryos for certain traits (39). This preimplantation genetic diagnosis is primarily used to identify embryos with genetic disorders to avoid transmission to offspring; however, this same technology could be used to select specific advantageous polygenic profiles for athletic excellence. As such, discussion of the ethical issues surrounding such predictive tests is important.

Potential benefits of using genetic testing for talent identification

Assuming the scientific evidence advances to the point where talent can be predicted using genetic techniques, there are several benefits to this approach. As with other talent identification methods, early identification of athletes with potential for greatness provides young athletes with the opportunity to dedicate years to sport-specific deliberate practice. The volume of 10,000 hours of dedicated training is often referenced and some have indicated that at least 10 years of dedicated practice is necessary to achieve peak performance in various endeavors, including sports (14). Considering the age at which many athletes enter professional or Olympic competition, the 10,000 hours and/or 10 years of dedicated training needs to begin at a young age. It is also recognized that family support is necessary for reaching the highest levels of athletic competition (11). Parents may face several obstacles (financial, geographic, time limitations, etc.) to providing resources necessary for success (coaching, equipment, etc.). Therefore, parents interested in supporting an elite-level athlete need to carefully select the activity with the most likelihood for success. Stakeholders want to make certain that they are devoting their limited resources to the activity that will prove to be most fruitful. If genetic screening identifies that a child may be uniquely capable for success in a specific sport domain, parents may be more likely to make sacrifices for the child to succeed in that domain.

Unlike traditional methods of talent identification, genetic approaches could allow for selection of athletic superiority well before any special physical attributes present themselves. As outlined above, determining the potential for success in children is difficult given different developmental patterns. Genetic talent identification could avoid the relative age effect, where more physically mature athletes are selected for talent development programs, since the genetic code is not sensitive to the developmental variation of physical and psychological phenotypes. Using heritability of traits to predict athletic potential most certainly already occurs without the use of sophisticated genetic analytic tools. For example, height and arm span are important contributors to success in basketball (20). Suppose we compare two young basketball players who are equal in stature and skill, yet one has two parents with above-average height and wing-span, while the other has two parents with below-average height and wingspan. A coach would be wise to presume that the player with the "ideal" parents will develop into a more basketball-appropriate body type and will have more potential for future success. That is not to say that the young athlete with the shorter parents cannot develop into an outstanding basketball player, but they will likely not develop the ideal body type for optimal success in basketball and would likely have to make up for the limitation with other physical, psychological, and skill-related qualities. This is an ideal scenario with each athlete having two parents with similar statures and a sport with a certain body type associated with success. Other sports may not align so clearly with a specific body type. For example, soccer, wrestling, judo, sprinting, and other sports are not so clearly associated with a specific body type and the use of genetic screening along with nongenetic talent identification techniques could prove useful for talent selection.

Another considerable benefit of genetic testing of young athletes is the identification of individuals who are at increased risk of injury, since time lost to injury can derail the trajectory of athletic development. Consider how losing months or years of deliberate practice due to a major ligament injury during the teen years could significantly affect the necessary 10 years of dedicated practice to the specific sport discipline. Moreover, time lost to injury can interfere with success in team sports, making this a major concern for coaches and other stakeholders in collegiate, professional, and Olympic team events. Some of these polymorphisms have been described in Chapters 27 and 28. By identifying genetic determinants of soft tissue injuries, for example, adequate focus on preventative training strategies can be provided for predisposed individuals. However, while such testing may offer a valuable tool for reducing risks associated with sporting activities, it certainly presents several ethical considerations. For one, how this information is shared and used can be challenging. For example, can a third party (e.g., coaches or team owners) request this genetic information and use it in recruiting or contract negoti-ations? Parents and coaches likely lack the expertise and/or training to fully understand the genetic information and may not recognize the limitations of the test results. Suppose an ath-lete has a 10% increased risk for developing a concussion or soft tissue injury. What does a 10% increased risk mean in the context of sport and injury and is this worth specific attention (40) or possible exclusion? Equally important is ensuring confidentiality and procedures for secondary findings, a concern that will be addressed later in this chapter. What today is associated with increased soft tissue injuries may be found to be associated with other conditions unrelated to sport performance in the future.

Other conditions with more dire consequences may also be identified by genetic screening and this may be a more appropriate use of the tool. In cases such as hypertrophic cardiomyop-athy and other inherited cardiac conditions, genetic screening has the potential to save lives by identifying individuals with an increased risk of sudden cardiac death. Other conditions such as Marfan syndrome, which is associated with the tall, slender build and long limbs generally associated with success in basketball and volleyball, is a genetic condition that increases the risk of sudden cardiac death during high-intensity exercise. Importantly, if genetic screenings are to be used for identifying inherited life-threatening cardiac conditions and Marfan syndrome, they should be ordered by a medical professional upon symptoms or a family history of the disease (41). In cases such as these, the medical professional can provide the necessary genetic counseling to help the individual and/or family understand the results of the genetic testing. Increasing safety in sports is paramount and genetic screenings have the potential to help in the prevention of injuries and sudden events that threaten the life of the athlete. However, the available evidence is still insufficient to rely on genetic screening for determining injury predisposition (41) and it is not likely that many sports medicine practitioners will have the necessary level of expertise in medical genetics to fully understand and interpret the findings of a genetic test (40). Moreover, mandating any type of health-related screening of heritable traits carries ethical concerns. As an example, the mandate by the National Collegiate Athletic Association in the US that all student athletes need to be screened for sickle cell trait, provide evidence of their sickle cell trait status, or sign a waiver to avoid screening has been met with controversy and disapproval from several organizations, even though the goal of the program was designed to enhance student athlete safety (15). This mandate, in particular, is complicated by the considerably higher fraction of individuals of African descent carrying the sickle cell trait, thus potentially opening doors for racial discrimination in the testing process.

Potential drawbacks of using genetic testing for talent identification

Despite some positive aspects of including genetic testing in talent identification programs, there are a number of potential negatives to such use. For genetic talent identification strategies to be successful, sampling and determination of the genetic profile needs to occur at a young enough age to reap the benefits of targeted resources and training, which means such testing necessarily occurs in children. In fact, prenatal or preimplantation (if *in vitro* fertilization) genetic profiling is arguably optimal for predicting future likelihood of success, injury, or disease, and although this tool is unlikely to be used for athletics anytime soon, it is currently feasible and will likely become more commonplace for diagnosis of genetic disorders (39). Whether genetic profiling occurs during childhood or prenatally, the identified "prodigy" can receive the familial support, coaching, and resources necessary for elite proficiency. Because this determination is made in childhood, however, the decisions made by parents and coaches may result in the loss of the child's autonomy and right to an open future (9). This is a complex issue concerning genetic testing for elite performance and is not restricted to the competitive sports world. Early identification of genetic predisposition for elite proficiency in any specific domain will certainly allow for mentors/instructors/coaches and parents to promote and encourage the development of that talent. Coaches and parents are fundamental in the cultivation of talent since a young child does not have the experience or maturity to carry the responsibility of knowing what is best for them. Indeed, talent must be nurtured, and parents must do most of this nurturing, yet children depend on parents to provide them with a wide breadth of experiences to develop into a well-rounded individual with the capacity to make their own life choices (9). The potential for aggressive parental control over a child's activities may be increased if genetic screening indicates that the child is "uniquely" capable of achieving excellence, especially if the parents do not recognize the limitations of these genetic predictions. The aggressive control of athletic endeavors may not only come at the expense of other sporting activities but also at the expense of other childhood experiences. According to Camporesi (9), it is perfectly reasonable for parents to expose children to sporting activities within their own financial situation and personal preferences but unreasonable to actively discourage other sporting opportunities. Although early specialization is becoming more commonplace, research suggests that participating in several sports at a young age is the best strategy to develop athletic ability (11, 16, 21). Early specialization has the potential to lead to overuse injuries and burnout (7, 21). Importantly, if the child achieves the ultimate goal of professional or Olympic status, the sacrifices made *may* have been worth it; however, consider the enormous percentage of athletes who do not achieve that level of success. For this large percentage of young athletes, they will have missed out on several childhood experiences, potentially with little to show for their dedication.

Another challenge is the issue of consent in genetic testing. It can be argued that every individual has the right to know their genetic profile since it belongs to them (23); however, this is a complex issue, especially when considering talent identification in young athletes. For one, youth athletes under 18 years of age do not have the capacity to provide informed consent. Indeed, a recent position statement from the Australian Institute of Sport suggests that genetic testing for sport is only appropriate if the individual being tested is 18 years of age (40). In fact, due to the complexities and technical nature of genetic testing, it might be difficult for adults to provide adequate informed assent for their child without a certain level of genetic counseling prior to the genetic screening. Whether a legal adult or young athlete, all genetic screening should be voluntary, requested by the individual to be tested (or medical professional in the patient–provider relationship), and free from any form of coercion. This may be difficult in the case of young athletes who are at a significant power disparity and may feel pressured to submit to a genetic test if requested by a coach, team owner, or parent. If genetic testing is included in the process of talent identification for entry into talent development programs, young athletes that decline participation in the testing may be discriminated against. Athletes should be allowed to decline genetic testing and have no penalties or negative consequences as a result of that decision.

If young athletes are undergoing medically supervised genetic screenings, parents, coaches, and athletes *should* have access to experts and trained professionals who can sufficiently and accurately explain the results as well as provide necessary genetic counseling. In fact, prior to any genetic screening, individuals should undergo genetic counseling (40), which should include information about the purposes and consequences of testing, limitations, potential harms, etc. (35). Prescreening genetic counseling is helpful for providing enough information for the potential subject to provide informed consent. Concerning genetic screening for risks of sports injury, a trained professional can provide interpretation of the results and potential courses of action based on the findings. Similarly, if testing for athletic potential, the trained professional can provide facts and details concerning the relevance and limitations of the genetic profile. Considering the status of the field at the time of writing this chapter, the role of the genetic counselor would likely be to advise against this type of screening or thoroughly explain the limitations of the results.

Although sport and exercise genetics researchers generally agree that the evidence is insufficient for using genetic tests for talent identification, several companies sell the promise of using this technology to determine potential for athletic success and for designing individualized exercise training programs. This promise comes in the form of DTC genetic testing. These products can be ordered online and delivered to the home, providing the capacity to sidestep the medical supervision of a physician or trained professional. The regulations for DTC tests vary from country to country and, while the quality and regulation of these tests have generally improved over the past several years (2), the quality control of tests for sporting potential is currently lacking. Although there is considerable turnover of companies in this industry, an investigation in 2015 identified 39 companies selling DTC genetic tests for sport, fitness, or injury risk (44). The majority of these tests did not indicate the specific DNA markers being tested. If we consider the proposition that everyone has the right to know their own genetic code (23), tests that do not report the specific genetic markers being tested do not provide the ability to know. These tests only provide the buyer with an interpretation of findings, which cannot be verified by an expert in the field. The 2015 investigation also found that the two most commonly tested variants were *ACE* I/D and *ACTN3* R557X (44). While these two genetic markers do have scientific support (as outlined in previous chapters), they are certainly not strong enough inform life-plans for young athletes. Because sport and exercise genetic screens do not qualify as medical advice or disease risk assessment, these DTC tests may avoid the regulation that limits the use of other health-related genetic screenings. Therefore, the claims made concerning predictive potential of sport performance, response to training, and/or injury risk are not under the same scrutiny as tests for genetic risk of breast cancer or Alzheimer's disease, for example. Without such regulation, companies continue to market the ability to predict sport performance and training adaptations even though the scientific evidence does not support such conclusive claims. Although not all companies advertise to parents and coaches (42), the ability of parents to purchase these tests and obtain a buccal cell sample from their child is uncomplicated. Informed consent and genetic counseling can easily be avoided and the results of these screens may be used to influence the sport participation and training decisions for a child even though the tests have virtually no predictive capacity.

The potential for inappropriate discrimination and exclusion is a major concern in the era of DTC genetic testing for sport performance. With the two most common markers for athletic potential being *ACTN3* R577X and *ACE* I/D, which indicate some propensity for success in endurance and power activities, one can imagine the number of children who could be eliminated from participating in certain sports due to having the "wrong" genotype. Interestingly, a case report from 2007 indicated that an Olympic long jumper carried the *ACTN3* XX genotype (26), which should indicate limited potential for success in sprint and power-related sports (e.g., long jump). If this individual had underwent a genetic screening to predict athletic potential as a child, he likely would have missed out on winning a gold medal in the under-17 category of the world championships and the opportunity to represent his country in two Olympic Games. This athlete is an excellent case study to highlight the importance of recognizing the limitations of using single genetic markers to guide sport participation choices, the importance of genetic counseling, and the inappropriate marketing techniques of some DTC genetic testing companies in the sport arena.

Another issue of concern with genetic testing is the shared nature of DNA in families. A genetic test can provide information about family members who did not assent to obtaining or to sharing genetic information with others. This is particularly true for parents and siblings, especially monozygotic twins. These individuals may not have been involved in the consent and genetic counseling process, nor would they have undergone a careful evaluation of the implications of the testing. This is a mostly unavoidable consequence of genetic screening in general and certainly extends to genetic testing for sport. And while the genetic test results for sport performance may not appear inherently meaningful for family members, secondary findings from genetic testing are a concern. We can use the example of the gene apolipoprotein E (*APOE*) as a case in point for both unintended secondary findings and familial-shared information risks. The *APOE* ε4 allele has consistently been shown as a genetic risk factor for late-onset Alzheimer's disease (AD), while the *APOE* ε2 allele is generally considered protective against AD. Unfortunately, some DTC companies have provided *APOE* genotyping to inform individuals about their likelihood of suffering and recovering from a concussion, which is an association that is far from being scientifically confirmed, with only limited investigations focused on this question to date (see Chapter 27). In this case, a DTC test result focused on a person's risk for sport-related injury is in fact far more informative for AD risk, and a quick Internet search would show the linkage of *APOE* genotype with disease risk. There are considerable psychological consequences to such an unintended discovery. Moreover, now the athlete who likely does not have the necessary training to understanding the full consequences of the association of *APOE* genotype with AD also has information concerning AD risk of parents, siblings, and future children. Could this change the individual's behavior toward family members? Will those family members want to know this information? Thus, both secondary findings and shared genetic information are both potential hazards in any form of genetic testing. *APOE* is an ideal and arguably extreme example, but even recent research on *ACTN3* is finding that it is associated with exercise recovery and risk of injury (32). An individual may provide consent for genetic testing to understand their propensity for success in a speed-related event but then find out that they are at increased risk for injury, information they may not have been anticipating.

Conclusion

In this chapter, we have outlined a variety of scientific and ethical challenges to genetic testing for sport performance prediction. While the present scientific evidence for such testing is highly limited and numerous position stands argue against the use of genetic testing in talent identification programs, the expansion of DTC genetic tests and lack of regulation over such testing in the area of sport performance mean that athletes and/or their parents and other stakeholders will have the option of pursuing such information with the potential for considerable negative consequences. And while we can envision a day when the scientific evidence is strengthened and the inclusion of genetic testing for talent identification is arguably justified, significant ethical issues will remain in the use of such testing, particularly in young (or unborn) children. While these are important conversations to have with parents, and some medical professionals may be informed enough to have such conversations, the likelihood that parents will be informed participants generally is unlikely. Ultimately, it will be the organizations that oversee talent identification and sport development that will need to provide oversight and protect young athletes by preventing or carefully limiting the use of such genetic screening. As a field, we must push for position stands and chapters like these to be provided to the leadership within these sport organizations and federations to better ensure the safety and autonomy of young athletes, which will ultimately benefit both the athletes and sport more generally by emphasizing an informed and evidence-based approach for talent identification.

References

1. **Ahmetov II, Egorova ES, Gabdrakhmanova LJ** and **Fedotovskaya ON**. Genes and Athletic Performance: An Update. *Medicine and Sport Science* 61: 41–54, 2016.
2. **Allyse MA, Robinson DH, Ferber MJ** and **Sharp RR**. Direct-to-Consumer Testing 2.0: Emerging Models of Direct-to-Consumer Genetic Testing. *Mayo Clinic Proceedings* 93: 113–120, 2018.
3. Bergeron MF, Mountjoy M, Armstrong N, Chia M, Côté J, Emery CA, Faigenbaum A, Hall G, Kriemler S, Léglise M, Malina RM, Pensgaard AM, Sanchez A, Soligard T, Sundgot-Borgen J, van Mechelen W, Weissensteiner JR and Engebretsen L. International Olympic Committee Consensus Statement on Youth Athletic Development. *British Journal of Sports Medicine* 49: 843–851, 2015.
4. **Bouchard C, An P, Rice T** and **Skinner JS**. Familial Aggregation of VO$_{2max}$ Response to Exercise Training: Results from the HERITAGE Family Study. *Journal of Applied Physiology* 87: 1003–1008, 1999.
5. **Bouchard C, Daw EW, Rice T**, Pérusse L, **Gagnon J, Province MA, Leon AS, Rao DC, Skinner JS** and **Wilmore JH**. Familial Resemblance for VO$_{2max}$ in the Sedentary State: The HERITAGE Family Study. *Medicine & Science in Sports & Exercise* 30: 252–258, 1998.
6. **Breitbach S, Tug S** and **Simon P**. Conventional and Genetic Talent Identification in Sports: Will Recent Developments Trace Talent? *Sports Medicine* 44: 1489–1503, 2014.

7. **Brenner JS** and **AAP Council on Sports Medicine and Fitness**. Sports Specialization and Intensive Training in Young Athletes. *Pediatrics* 138: e20162148, 2016.

8. **Camporesi S** and **McNamee MJ.** Ethics, Genetic Testing, and Athletic Talent: Children's Best Interests, and the Right to an Open (Athletic) Future. *Physiological Genomics* 48: 191–195, 2016.

9. **Camporesi S.** Bend it like Beckham! The Ethics of Genetically Testing Children for Athletic Potential. *Sport, Ethics and Philosophy* 7: 175–185, 2013.

10. **Costa AM**, **Breitenfeld L**, **Silva AJ**, **Pereira A**, **Izquierdo M** and **Marques MC.** Genetic Inheritance Effects on Endurance and Muscle Strength: An Update. *Sports Medicine* 42: 449–458, 2012.

11. **Côté J.** The Influence of the Family in the Development of Talent in Sport. *The Sport Psychologist* 13: 395–417, 2009.

12. **Cumming SP**, **Lloyd RS**, **Oliver JL**, **Eisenmann JC** and **Malina RM.** Bio-banding in Sport: Applications to Competition, Talent Identification, and Strength and Conditioning of Youth Athletes. *Strength and Conditioning Journal* 39: 34–47, 2017.

13. **De Moor MHM**, **Spector TD**, **Cherkas LF**, **Falchi M**, **Hottenga J-J**, **Boomsma DI** and **De Geus EJC.** Genome-Wide Linkage Scan for Athlete Status in 700 British Female DZ Twin Pairs. *Twin Research and Human Genetics* 10: 812–820, 2007.

14. **Ericsson KA.** Deliberate Practice and Acquisition of Expert Performance: A General Overview. *Academic Emergency Medicine* 15: 988–994, 2008.

15. **Ferrari R**, **Parker LS**, **Grubs RE** and **Krishnamurti L.** Sickle Cell Trait Screening of Collegiate Athletes: Ethical Reasons for Program Reform. *Journal of Genetic Counseling* 24: 873–877, 2015.

16. **Fransen J**, **Pion J**, **Vandendriessche J**, **Vandorpe B**, **Vaeyens R**, **Lenoir M** and **Philippaerts RM.** Differences in Physical Fitness and Gross Motor Coordination in Boys Aged 6–12 Years Specializing in One Versus Sampling More Than One Sport. *Journal of Sports Sciences* 30: 379–386, 2012.

17. **Georgiades E**, **Klissouras V**, **Baulch J**, **Wang G** and **Pitsiladis Y.** Why Nature Prevails Over Nurture in the Making of the Elite Athlete. *BMC Genomics* 18: 835, 2017.

18. **Guth LM** and **Roth SM.** Genetic Influence on Athletic Performance. *Current Opinion in Pediatrics* 25: 653–658, 2013.

19. **Hagberg JM**, **Rankinen T**, **Loos RJF**, **Pérusse L**, **Roth SM**, **Wolfarth B** and **Bouchard C.** Advances in Exercise, Fitness, and Performance Genomics in 2010. *Medicine & Science in Sports & Exercise* 43: 743–752, 2011.

20. **Hoare DG.** Predicting Success in Junior Elite Basketball Players – The Contribution of Anthropometric and Physiological Attributes. *Journal of Science and Medicine in Sport* 3: 391–405, 2000.

21. **Jayanthi N**, **Pinkham C**, **Dugas L**, **Patrick B** and **Labella C.** Sports Specialization in Young Athletes: Evidence-Based Recommendations. *Sports Health* 5: 251–257, 2013.

22. **Komi PV**, **Viitasalo JH**, **Havu M**, **Thorstensson A**, **Sjödin B** and **Karlsson J.** Skeletal Muscle Fibres and Muscle Enzyme Activities in Monozygous and Dizygous Twins of Both Sexes. *Acta Physiologica Scandinavica* 100: 385–392, 1977.

23. **Loi M.** Direct to Consumer Genetic Testing and the Libertarian Right to Test. *Journal of Medical Ethics* 42: 574–577, 2016.

24. **Loland S.** Against Genetic Tests for Athletic Talent: The Primacy of the Phenotype. *Sports Medicine* 45: 1229–1233, 2015.

25. **Loos RJF**, **Hagberg JM**, **Pérusse L**, **Roth SM**, **Sarzynski MA**, **Wolfarth B**, **Rankinen T** and **Bouchard C.** Advances in Exercise, Fitness, and Performance Genomics in 2014. *Medicine & Science in Sports & Exercise* 47: 1105–1112, 2015

26. **Lucia A**, **Oliván J**, **Gómez-Gallego F**, **Santiago C**, **Montil M** and **Foster C.** Citius and Longius (Faster and Longer) with no Alpha-Actinin-3 in Skeletal Muscles? *British Journal of Sports Medicine* 41: 616–617, 2007.

27. **Ma F**, **Yang Y**, **Li X**, **Zhou F**, **Gao C**, **Li M** and **Gao L.** The Association of Sport Performance with ACE and ACTN3 Genetic Polymorphisms: A Systematic Review and Meta-Analysis. *PLoS ONE* 8: e54685, 2013.

28. **Papadimitriou ID**, **Lucia A**, **Pitsiladis YP**, **Pushkarev VP**, **Dyatlov DA**, **Orekhov EF**, **Artioli GG**, **Guilherme JPLF**, **Lancha AH**, **Ginevičienė V**, **Cieszczyk P**, **Maciejewska-Karlowska A**, **Sawczuk M**, **Muniesa CA**, **Kouvatsi A**, **Massidda M**, **Calò CM**, **Garton F**, **Houweling PJ**, **Wang G**, **Austin K**, **Druzhevskaya AM**, **Astratenkova IV**, **Ahmetov II**, **Bishop DJ**, **North KN** and **Eynon N.** ACTN3 R577X and ACE I/D Gene Variants Influence Performance in Elite Sprinters: A Multi-Cohort Study. *BMC Genomics* 17: 285, 2016.

29. **Pearson DT, Naughton GA** and **Torode M**. Predictability of Physiological Testing and the Role of Maturation in Talent Identification for Adolescent Team Sports. *Journal of Science and Medicine in Sport* 9: 277–287, 2006.

30. **Peeters MW, Thomis MA, Loos RJF, Derom CA, Fagard R, Claessens AL, Vlietinck RF** and **Beunen GP.** Heritability of Somatotype Components: A Multivariate Analysis. *International Journal of Obessity* 31: 1295–1301, 2007.

31. **Pérusse L, Rankinen T, Hagberg JM, Loos RJF, Roth SM, Sarzynski MA, Wolfarth B** and **Bouchard C.** Advances in Exercise, Fitness, and Performance Genomics in 2012. *Medicine & Science in Sports & Exercise* 45: 824–831, 2013.

32. **Pickering C** and **Kiely J.** ACTN3: More than Just a Gene for Speed. *Frontiers in Physiology* 8: 1080, 2017.

33. **Pitsiladis Y, Wang G, Wolfarth B, Scott R, Fuku N, Mikami E, He Z, Fiuza-Luces C, Eynon N** and **Lucia A.** Genomics of Elite Sporting Performance: What Little We Know and Necessary Advances. *British Journal of Sports Medicine* 47: 550–555, 2013.

34. **Rankinen T, Roth SM, Bray MS, Loos R, Pérusse L, Wolfarth B, Hagberg JM** and **Bouchard C.** Advances in Exercise, Fitness, and Performance Genomics. *Medicine & Science in Sports & Exercise* 42: 835–846, 2010.

35. **Rantanen E, Hietala M, Kristoffersson U, Nippert I, Schmidtke J, Sequeiros J** and **Kääriäinen H.** What is Ideal Genetic Counselling? A Survey of Current International Guidelines. *European Journal of Human Genetics* 16: 445–452, 2008.

36. **Roth SM, Rankinen T, Hagberg JM, Loos RJF, Pérusse L, Sarzynski MA, Wolfarth B** and **Bouchard C.** Advances in Exercise, Fitness, and Performance Genomics in 2011. *Medicine & Science in Sports & Exercise* 44: 809–817, 2012.

37. **Sarzynski MA, Loos RJF, Lucia A, Pérusse L, Roth SM, Wolfarth B, Rankinen T** and **Bouchard C.** Advances in Exercise, Fitness, and Performance Genomics in 2015. *Medicine & Science in Sports & Exercise* 48: 1906–1916, 2016.

38. **Silventoinen K, Magnusson PKE, Tynelius P, Kaprio J** and **Rasmussen F.** Heritability of Body Size and Muscle Strength in Young Adulthood: A Study of One Million Swedish Men. *Genetic Epidemiology* 32: 341–349, 2008.

39. **Vermeesch JR, Voet T** and **Devriendt K.** Prenatal and Pre-Implantation Genetic Diagnosis. *Nature Reviews Genetics* 17: 643–656, 2016.

40. **Vlahovich N, Fricker PA, Brown MA** and **Hughes D.** Ethics of Genetic Testing and Research in Sport: A Position Statement from the Australian Institute of Sport. *British Journal of Sports Medicine* 51: 5–11, 2017.

41. **Vlahovich N, Hughes DC, Griffiths LR, Wang G, Pitsiladis YP, Pigozzi F, Bachl N** and **Eynon N.** Genetic Testing for Exercise Prescription and Injury Prevention: AIS-Athlome Consortium-FIMS Joint Statement. *BMC Genomics* 18: 818, 2017.

42. **Wagner JK** and **Royal CD.** Field of Genes: An Investigation of Sports-Related Genetic Testing. *Journal of Personalized Medicine* 2: 119–137, 2012.

43. **Wang G, Tanaka M, Eynon N, North KN, Williams AG, Collins M, Moran CN, Britton SL, Fuku N, Ashley EA, Klissouras V, Lucia A, Ahmetov II, De Geus E, Alsayrafi M** and **Pitsiladis YP.** The Future of Genomic Research in Athletic Performance and Adaptation to Training. *Medicine and Sport Science* 61: 55–67, 2016.

44. **Webborn N, Williams A, McNamee M, Bouchard C, Pitsiladis Y, Ahmetov I, Ashley E, Byrne N, Camporesi S, Collins M, Dijkstra P, Eynon N, Fuku N, Garton FC, Hoppe N, Holm S, Kaye J, Klissouras V, Lucia A, Maase K, Moran C, North KN, Pigozzi F** and **Wang G.** Direct-to-Consumer Genetic Testing for Predicting Sports Performance and Talent Identification: Consensus Statement. *British Journal of Sports Medicine* 49: 1486–1491, 2015.

45. **Williams AG, Wackerhage H** and **Day SH.** Genetic Testing for Sports Performance, Responses to Training and Injury Risk: Practical and Ethical Considerations. *Medicine and Sport Science* 61: 105–119, 2016.

46. **Wolfarth B, Rankinen T, Hagberg JM, Loos RJF, Pérusse L, Roth SM, Sarzynski MA** and **Bouchard C.** Advances in Exercise, Fitness, and Performance Genomics in 2013. *Medicine & Science in Sports & Exercise* 46: 851–859, 2014.

47. **Yan X, Papadimitriou I, Lidor R** and **Eynon N.** Nature versus Nurture in Determining Athletic Ability. *Medicine and Sport Science* 61: 15–28, 2016.

32

GENE DOPING: ETHICAL PERSPECTIVES

Verner Møller and Rasmus Bysted Møller

Since the turn of the 21st century, concerns about the impact of gene therapy on sports have gathered speed and a number of thought-provoking books have been produced. Andy Miah's ground-breaking work, *Genetically Modified Athletes: Biomedical Ethics, Gene Doping and Sport* (2004) drew attention to many problems and prospects that potentially would make anti-doping impotent if the ethically laden endeavour should not become unethical. For instance, he mentions "that muscle biopsy may be the only way to detect some forms of genetic modification in sport, which would be a significant challenge for anti-doping policy given the invasiveness of such a procedure" (Miah, 2004, p. 34). If Miah's assertion is correct that muscle biopsies are needed to detect gene doping this would certainly, as he implies, pose a huge threat to the integrity of anti-doping.

Miah offers a thorough analysis of the implication of gene therapy for the human future. Money is not invested in gene technology with a view to develop Frankenstein monsters but because it has medical potential. It is hoped that it can result in medical breakthroughs leading to remedies for currently incurable diseases. If gene technology makes it possible to speed up injured athletes' recovery as well, should athletes then be forbidden to take advantage of that? Such scenarios make it clear that "genetic enhancement cannot be characterized in the same way as other ways of doping" he rightly maintains (Miah, 2004, p. 178). The magnitude of the ethical dilemmas that occurs with gene technology is such that one easily understands why Miah does not take upon himself to search for an ethically viable way for sport to negotiate the future he foresees. Instead he ends his book by proposing a tentative solution which, as provocative as it appears, leaves the ethical problem unresolved. "Perhaps one solution to this ethical dilemma," he professes, "is to create distinct, genetically enhanced competitions and to continue voluntary submission to anti-doping testing procedures" (Miah, 2004, p. 178).

Rather than solving the ethical dilemma, splitting sports into two distinctly different types of sport amplifies the ethical problem. First, accepting a category of genetically enhanced competition is to accept that this category of sport in effect is transformed into a gene-tech laboratory where elite sport's competitive nature, pursuit of perfection, and will to win, tempts ambitious athletes to accept the role as willing guinea pigs for medical and other companies interested in human enhancement. The only way this "solves" the ethical dilemma is by throwing ethics out of the window. Second, having an alternative category of sport for athletes who want to compete without having their bodies genetically modified only accessible for individuals who consent to having regular biopsies taken is equally indefensible. It implies that athletes who do not want to have their bodies tampered with in order to be competitive in the gene-doping category are forced to accept to have their bodies tampered with by a doping control officer's muscle fiber-cutting needle.

The profoundness of the ethical problems left unresolved by Miah's proposed solution was reflected in Claudio Tamburrini and Torbjörn Tännsjö's edited book *Genetic Technology and Sport: Ethical Questions* (2005). This collection written by scholars and scientists from various disciplines and with disparate attitudes to the prospects of genetic enhancement is an excellent introduction to the field. It is beyond the scope of this chapter to present the breadth and depth of the themes the book comprises but it is worthwhile quoting Christian Munthe's contribution about the ethics of controlling gene doping because it so clearly illustrates why a gene doping-free sports category with consensual testing is unjustifiable:

> Due to the apparent need for quite extensive and repeated sample-taking, health risks due to the repeated application of biopsy procedures to various parts of the body have to be taken quite seriously. The same goes, of course, for the direct and rather obvious inconvenience of the athlete who has to be subjected to such procedures. Any programme for controlling gene doping would therefore have to consider the risks and problems created by the sample-taking alone as an ethically highly relevant factor that needs to be balanced against the reasons for enforcing and upholding the ban on gene doping.
>
> (Munthe, 2005, p. 114)

The ethical challenges Munthe highlights were not foreign to the World Anti-Doping Agency (WADA). The agency, established in 1999 in the wake of the 1998 revelations of organized and vast doping used at the Tour de France, understood that the fast expansion of scientific research in gene therapy around the world meant that a spillover to sport might be on the horizon. Acknowledging that pre-WADA anti-doping efforts had been reactive with the unfortunate consequence that regulations and test procedures and methods were playing a frustrating game of catch-up, the agency understood it had to be proactive if it should not be caught off guard by this new threat to sport. So, no more than 3 years after its foundation, the year before the first World Anti-Doping Code was drafted, WADA organized a meeting in New York where representatives from the athletic community were brought together with scientists and scholars to discuss the various aspects of the gene doping issue. Among the participants were Angela Schneider and Theodore Friedmann who subsequently wrote an introductory book *Gene Doping in Sports: The Science and Ethics of Genetically Modified Athletes* (2006). Here they explain the basics of gene therapy and the potential applications of this emerging science to sports and offer some ethical considerations related to the issue. What is particularly laudable about this book is its sobering approach. It does not entertain the reader with exciting *Brave New World* scenarios. On the contrary, it shows how embryonic this field of science is, and presents some of the severe setbacks it has faced in the form of unexpected fatal side effects in experiments carried out on patients suffering from severe genetic diseases. There are still many miles to go before promising experiments on mice will translate to successful clinical treatment in humans. As Friedmann and Schneider explain, "A great deal of additional basic and applied medical research will be required before anyone can say with comfort that gene transfer, even for such dire diseases [as Parkinson's, Alzheimer's and Lou Gehring's] is safe and effective" (Schneider & Friedmann, 2006, p. 35). Gene doping is in all likelihood even farther away because the present state of the technology of gene transfer for application in therapy is not sufficiently advanced "to conduct a gene transfer application for athletic performance that would meet the requirements for ethical research in human research subjects" (Schneider & Friedmann, 2006, p. 39f). However, this does not rule out hazardous experiments the authors warn. "To do a scientifically poor and dangerous study in humans would be far less difficult, probably less successful, and certainly perilous for the athlete" (Schneider & Friedmann, 2006, p. 41).

For readers who wants a broader introduction than this chapter offers to the field of gene doping – and the ethical issues that evolve with it – the abovementioned books are commendable.

Gene doping unthinkable – but not *that* unthinkable

Schneider and Friedmann's understanding resonates with our own opinion. We share the view that gene doping is not around the corner. In fact, as late as 2018 one of the authors of this chapter published a book which preface announced that:

> we should note that the future of sport might be revolutionised if the spectre of gene doping becomes a reality, though for the moment we have no evidence that it will. Should new undetectable gene-based technologies emerge then anti-doping will become obsolete. Since we have not yet reached that point, we shall explore the state of the system in its current form.
>
> (Dimeo & Møller, 2018, p. viii)

When this was written, we were of course aware that research in gene technology is progressing and reckon that in a more or less distant future it will probably bless humankind with marvelous cures for severe diseases. However, in the late 1990s we listened to scientific lectures in which experiments on mice were introduced that showed the effect of inactivation of the myostatin gene. It was fascinating to see on slides the huge difference in muscle growth between a normal mouse and the so-called Schwarzenegger mouse. The problem with blocking the myostatin gene, we learned, was that muscle growth continued and that it was not yet possible to reactivate the myostatin gene when the desired muscle size had been reached. This convinced us that gene doping was of scientific interest for futurists, but that gene doping at present was still too speculative to be relevant to consider in a book dealing with the current anti-doping crisis. Our conviction was based on two things. First, there is a big difference between learning to inject oneself with anabolic steroids, erythropoietin, cortisone etc. and to perform genetic engineering safely. Second, if scientists with knowledge about gene technology offered to help athletes with the process we thought it unlikely that athletes would accept the offer so long as the procedure was not tried and tested, the outcome uncertain, and the risk immense. But these may well have been too conservative assumptions based on too much faith in human ethics and rationality.

The state-run doping program in the former East Germany exposed in the wake of the German reunion in 1989 proved that some regimes can be reckless enough to sacrifice their own citizens in pursuit of international fame and glory in the sports arena (Franke & Berendonk, 1997). Despite the collapse of the Iron Curtain and the former Eastern bloc countries' closed regimes being replaced by democracies, the 2015 revelations of organized doping in Russia, which resulted in Russia's exclusion from the 2018 Winter Olympics in PyeongChang, indicates that states' willingness to exploit their athletes for propaganda purposes is not a thing of the past and may include willingness to work towards the creation of genetically modified super-athletes. The difference between doping in the East German dictatorship and post-Soviet Russia is the extent to which the enhancement measures transformed the athletes', particularly the females', bodies. In the former East Germany, children and adolescents were unknowingly administered potent steroids such as Oral Turinabol in quantities that resulted in visible masculinization. This practice was coined "coerced doping" (Zwangsdoping) by the German sports historian Giselher Spitzer (1998).

The doping practice that was revealed in Russia was different. According to whistle-blower Yuliya Stepanova, the state assisted athletes' doping but she was informed what she was injected with. Hence, she could reveal that she was given testosterone and other anabolic steroids, plus erythropoietin (Ash, 2016). She might at the time have felt it difficult to refuse the injections because if she did she might be expelled from the national team. But in case she had experienced negative side effects such as visible signs of masculinization she could have walked away, which is probably the reason why we do not see female athletes as bulky and masculine as we did during the Cold War. We considered that so long as athletes' agency was not suppressed by state coercion, athletes would only (accept to) use doping up to the point where their health would be at significant risk. Accordingly, we reasoned that gene doping, the outcome of which is uncertain and the results irreversible, will put athletes off regardless of potential gains. However, a 2017 article in the magazine *New Scientist* gave reason to reconsider our confidence in reason.

Gene hacking

New Scientist is a popular science magazine established to inform laypeople of advances in science. Its articles sometimes appear simplistic and sensationalist and has on occasion been criticized by scientists. Some have even called for a boycott of the magazine and encouraged scientists to stop working and writing for it in order to prevent the public from being misled by its catchy covers and headlines (Whyevolutionistrue, 2009). Having said that, *New Scientist* is generally sufficiently accurate and true to the science it covers which is why esteemed scientists like Richard Dawkins consider it worthwhile to voice their criticism when they find the magazine guilty of misrepresentation of a topic. Thus, we hold that its 2017 article about biohacking cannot immediately be discarded as science fiction even though it may sound as such and give cause for concern.

The article introduces clustered regularly interspaced short palindromic repeats (CRISPR), which is a new and cheap technique to make changes to DNA sequence. It is considered a big leap forward in medical science's attempt to find remedies for incurable diseases. But the CRISPR technology is not confined to medical laboratories. The article's main character is Josiah Zayner, a biochemist and former NASA employee who was the first person to edit his own DNA by the use of this new method to genetic engineering. Livestreamed on Facebook, he explained the technique and showed how to perform it on himself. He simply took out a vial that contained a CRISPR-edited copy of his own DNA where the myostatin gene had been removed and injected himself. His intention was to increase muscle growth. Another aim was to promote a do-it-yourself kit he sells through his private company, The Odin, by which others can replicate his work. The author of the article quotes other so-called biohackers who embrace this advance in science. One wants to use Zayner's kit to remedy his color blindness, another wants to use genetic engineering to inject an extra copy of the gene follistatin, which increases muscle growth much like myostatin does. So, Schneider and Friedmann's prediction that whereas gene doping based on authorized sciences that meets the requirements for ethical research in human subjects may be far away, to carry out uncontrolled experiments is far less difficult. In fact, the first movers have already begun. Whether it still holds true after the invention of CRISPR that genetic modification is a perilous practice, as Schneider and Friedmann presume, is an open question. Robin Lovell-Badge a leading CRISPR researcher at the Francis Crick Institute in London, UK, is quoted as saying: "Zayner's experiment was 'foolish' and could have unintended consequences, including tissue damage, cell death, or an immune response that attacks his own muscle" (Pearlman, 2017, p. 22). Bioethicist John Harris from the University of Manchester, UK, holds a different view similar to Miah's bioscience optimism. According to Harris, biohackers could help to accelerate the safe use of CRISPR in humans, pointing out that there is "a long and noble history of both doctors and scientists experimenting on themselves [that] has proven tremendously valuable in the public interest" (Pearlman, 2017, p. 23). Günes Taylor at the Francis Crick Institute in London who also work with CRISPR takes the middle ground. "Part of me is, like, 'that is so awesome'… but it won't work." In her opinion it will be more difficult than the biohackers think. "CRISPR has been sold as a cure all, but actually getting it to do the thing that you want it to do successfully is more complicated" she says, echoing Schneider and Friedmann (Pearlman, 2017).

For better or worse, the possibility of having one's body changed by genetic manipulation has become a reality and because the kit made for it is not technically a drug, "the FDA will not yet regulate at-home genome editing." As a result, self-experimentation is not illegal in the US. Zayner is living evidence that there are dedicated persons who without the guarantee of a positive outcome, are willing to jeopardize their health in the hope they can break natural limits to muscle growth. He is also proof that there are unauthorized experts willing to make the necessary tools available for unauthorized people who may not be aware of the risks involved. The combination of unscrupulous persons with sufficient knowledge about gene manipulation and people dedicated to a cause who are willing to take risk are all that is needed for gene doping to evolve. Hence it is understandable that WADA has taken a proactive approach to the issue and in October 2017 announced that from 2018:

The following with the potential to enhance sports performance are prohibited:

1. The use of polymers of nucleic acids or nucleic analogues.
2. The use of gene editing agents designed to alter genome sequences and/or the transcriptional or epigenetic regulation of gene expression.
3. The use of normal or genetically modified cells.

(WADA, 2017, p. 6)

This means in effect that all forms of gene therapy or gene doping are banned from international competitive sport. The immediate problem for WADA in this regard is that it is much easier to introduce a ban than find effective measures to enforce it. However, in what follows we will argue that a blanket ban on gene therapy will be ethically indefensible in case gene therapy actually becomes so potent, safe, and successful as the most optimistic futurists foresee, and why such a scenario will spell and end to the meaning of anti-doping.

The controversial case of Lionel Messi

As a child, Lionel Messi, one of the world's best ever football players, was diagnosed with growth hormone deficiency (GHD). Fortunately for him, growth hormone (GH) therapy for that condition had been developed. Human growth hormone (hGH) was first isolated from the human pituitary gland in 1956. This hormone had to be extracted from humans, so availability was limited and expensive. Only the most severe cases were offered treatment. In 1960, the American National Pituitary Agency was established with the purpose to coordinate collection and extraction of the hormone. From 1963 to 1985, the agency registered no more than 7700 children in the US who were treated with GH extracted from humans. The number of children treated worldwide was 27,000 (Ayyar, 2011). In 1972, the biochemical structure of hGH was identified. This paved the way for the invention of recombinant human growth hormone (rhGH). The first time the gene was successfully cloned was in 1979 and the American company Genentech developed rhGH in 1981 by a biosynthetic process (Ayyar, 2011). Hence treatment was no longer limited by availability of hGH. When diagnosed, Messi was only 4 feet 3 inches tall (127 centimetres). Doctors predicted his final height would be 4 feet 3 inches (140 centimetres) (Cooney, 2016). Thanks to the advances in medicine, Messi's GHD could be treated. For 3 years from 1998 at the age of 11, he had injections of rhGH. However, treatment was still expensive. It cost more than his family could afford. His luck was that he was such an outstanding talent that FC Barcelona agreed to pay for his treatment. It proved to be a fabulous investment. Messi now stands 5 feet 7 inches tall (170 centimetres) and he has been instrumental to the success of the club since his debut in 2004, winning nine Spanish Championships and four UEFA Champions Leagues among a host of other trophies (FC Barcelona, 2017). It is unlikely he would have become an equally successful footballer without treatment for his GHD.

At first glance, the Messi case is uncontroversial from an anti-doping perspective because the World Anti-Doping Code allows use of banned substances for medical purposes. If an athlete is diagnosed with a condition that needs medical treatment the person in question can be granted a Therapeutic Use Exemption (TUE). The justification for this is the claim that necessary medical treatment is not performance enhancing but performance enabling. The TUE system does not allow athletes a competitive advantage, only sufficient treatment without which it would be impossible for the athlete to participate in sports. The review process is rigorous. Four criteria must be met for a TUE to be granted including that the "therapeutic use of the substance would not produce significant enhancement of performance" (WADA, 2016). If clean sport is the ideal, ideally the TUE system should be repealed. However, according to WADA it is not possible to preclude athletes who suffer from various illnesses and conditions because it "would undermine a fundamental value of sport that is the right of access and participation to sport and play, which has long been recognized by numerous international conventions" (WADA, 2016, p. 4).

The problem for WADA is of course that the criterion, that treatment would not produce any significant enhancement of performance, is impossible to determine. The reason why there is zero tolerance for the vast majority of substances on the banned list is that ever so small amounts found in a test may be residues of larger dosages taken in order to gain performance-enhancing effect. That is, allowance of small quantities can be exploited for doping purposes. Moreover, it is impossible to establish that a performance-enhancing substance administered for health reasons does not have a significant performance-enhancing effect on the person who is treated. Obviously, if an athlete cannot breathe properly because he or she suffers from asthma and thus would perform significantly below the level needed to be competitive in elite sport, asthma medication has a significant performance enhancing effect on this person. So what WADA has in mind must be that if, hypothetically, the athlete was not an asthmatic he would perform at a higher or exact same level as he does with asthma medication but not on a slightly lower level. However, since the introduction of the Code and the TUE system, some asthma medications have proven so effective that athletes who have been granted a TUE due to confirmed asthma/airway hyper-responsiveness have outperformed their nonasthmatic rivals (Fitch, 2016).

If it is true that asthma medication is so effective that treatment unintentionally provides the athlete patients a slight advantage, gene therapy that could once and for all remedy the condition seems a fairer solution should such therapy become available. But with the new WADA policy banning all kinds of gene doping and therapy, this fairer solution is ruled out. For example, athletes with asthma who want to exercise their fundamental right to participate in sport and play will paradoxically be forced to live with their disease and fight its symptoms by an inhaler, which has the side effect that it boosts their performance capacity.

One of WADA's main concerns in relation to gene doping and the TUE system is that it will continue to benefit the athlete when the medication is no longer needed for medical treatment. Hence they emphasize that "TUEs are granted for a specific method or a substance with a defied dosage and route of administration. They are also granted for a specific period of time and do expire" (WADA, 2016, p. 3).

If we now return to the case of Messi, what immediately appeared uncontroversial seems at closer inspection less clear cut. The treatment he received as a child did not prevent him from playing football. He was playing football and identified as a rare talent so if he had been denied a TUE this would not have violated his rights of access and participation to sport and play. Moreover, it is hard to argue that his treatment did not significantly improve his perform-ance ability when considering there is not a single player in world elite football nearly as short as 4 feet 7 inches. The shortest is Élton José Xavier Gomes who was signed by Romanian side Steaua Bucuresti in 2007 who stands 5 feet 0.63 inches (154 centimetres) tall (FootyFan, 2013). In addition to this, it does not seem that Messi's condition met the first of the four criteria that all must be met for granting a TUE namely that the "athlete would experience significant health problems without taking the prohibited substance or method" (WADA, 2016). It is true that adults who suffer from GHD can experience symptoms such as reduced bone density, insulin resistance, and heart problems, but these symptoms do not appear in childhood so it is unlikely that Messi had experienced significant health problems when he began treatment (Toft, 2014).

If in the future it will be possible to treat GHD by gene therapy rather than by injections with rhGH, a "new Messi" could not benefit from that according to WADA's abovementioned announcement. On the other hand, it would not make much sense to grant an athlete a TUE for use of rhGH to treat GHD in the old-fashioned style if another more efficient treatment became available. And the problem is bigger than that.

Height is recognized as a general advantage in life and positively related to socioeconomic status. A British study that evaluated genetic data of 396 genetic variants associated with height from 120,000 persons aged between 40 and 70 found that tallness on average led to higher levels of education, higher job status, and better income (Tyrrell et al., 2016). Most parents wish the best for their children. Height is determined by genes, so it is predictable that if one day it becomes possible for parents to safely boost their children's growth by genetic modifica-tion such therapy will be in demand. This has already been the case with rhGH. In 2003, the US Food and Drug Administration (FDA) approved treatment with rhGH for children with idiopathic short stature. That is, kids who are short without suffering from GHD. However, shortness is a relative concept. In an interview with ABC News, pediatric endocrinologist Paul Desroiers explains that since the FDA's approval, ambitious parents with healthy kids regularly turn up in the hope that he will give GH to their child. Desroiers gives a striking example: "Just last week, the father of a young baseball player – a 14-year-old who was already 5 feet 6 inches (167 centimetres) tall – expected [me] to prescribe recombinant growth hormone to add height to his budding athlete." The father wanted to make his kid big in the vain hope that he thereby could turn him into a baseball star. "He was willing to pay more than $45,000 a year and didn't even bat an eyelash" (James, 2009).

When parents successfully begin to make their children grow taller by gene therapy, other parents may be afraid their children will fall behind. Consequently, demand for this kind of therapy will likely grow to the extent it becomes mainstream as we have seen with other body improvement services such as botox injections, breast implants, and facelifts etc. However, when it comes to height, the decision must be made by the parents before their child is of legal age. Most of these hypothetical children will become taller than their parents and may benefit from the therapy by getting better-paid jobs than their shorter parents had. An infinitesimal number of these children will be gifted by a unique talent for sport, whether it be football or something else. It does not seem just to exclude these children from exercising their right to participate in sport because of the decision their parents made to prevent them from being disadvantaged in life in general without the intention to increase their ability to succeed in sport. It will also be hard to find a valid argument for exclusion of a person who is standing 5 feet 7 inches tall thanks to gene therapy decided by his or her parents from competing in sports with people who are of similar size.

If WADA will indeed stand firm on their ban on all forms of gene therapy as the 2018 *Prohibited List* announces, they would have to develop ways to measure all international athletes' genetic makeup to exclude the ones who have reached a certain height, strength, or stamina by genetic modification. One should be forgiven for thinking that subjecting all international athletes to gene testing raises serious questions about privacy rights. However, based on the development of anti-doping so far, there is nothing to suggest that respect for athletes' privacy rights will represent an obstacle for the introduction of this additional measure.

There is a general consensus that the fight against doping is in the public interest. It is backed almost universally by the international sports federations. Almost all nations have signed the WADA Code. The commitment to anti-doping is further established by the United Nations via UNESCO's International Convention against Doping in Sport and by the Council of Europa via its Anti-Doping Convention. Based on this consensus, the European Court of Human Rights has hitherto accepted every obligation forced upon athletes including the requirement to provide urine and blood samples and whereabouts information 24/7 all year round. Because, as the Court reasons, any "reduction or removal of the relevant obligations on athletes would inevitably lead to an increase in doping and would be at odds with the consensus on the need for unannounced testing as part of doping control" (WADA, 2018). In light of this, if WADA argues that gene doping poses a threat to the integrity of sport, the introduction of gene testing, even if it necessitated athletes' submission to regular biopsies, would in all likelihood be condoned by legal authorities no matter how unethical this would appear to ordinary people. So, it is not because of judicial objections that advances in gene technology will spell an end to anti-doping, nor is it because gene modification may be undetectable. Since the formation of WADA there is no indication that a doping substance or method has *not* been banned because of the fact that there was no detection method in place. Gene doping does not represent anything novel in this regard (Franks, 2014). The core of the problem for WADA is that the ban on gene therapy is not anti-doping. It is anti-progress. The concept of gene doping is misleading. If this is not immediately clear from the Messi example, let us conclude this chapter with a thought experiment.

Health protection and longevity

According to the World Health Organization, ischemic heart disease and stroke are the world's most common causes of death accounting for 15 million deaths globally in 2015 (World Health Organization, 2017). There is a hereditary, that is, genetic, component to heart and circulatory diseases. So, imagine that it became possible to reduce the risk of developing heart diseases by gene-editing human embryos with the only side effect being that heart strength and circulation capacity improves significantly. Parents with a family history of heart failure and early deaths would be eligible for treatment. However, children whose parents had accepted the treatment would not be eligible for international sports participation under the remit of WADA-compliant international sports federations. In effect, parents who would choose the protection of their children's health long term would thereby preclude them from competing in sports at elite level should they be gifted with the required sports talent.

If children's life expectancy can be increased by embryo editing it is predictable that the practice will follow the same trend as has been the case with *in vitro* fertilization. The demand for this treatment will grow. As a consequence, more and more athletes from the affluent world will be excluded from elite sports due to their genetic makeup. And this without having done anything wrong, being negligent, or even consented to the health prevention therapy that has simply been forced upon them. Under such circumstances, their exclusion will be ethically indefensible because it is discriminatory and punishes individuals for a condition that in no way is their own fault.

At first glance, a TUE-like acceptance of athletes who have been genetically modified as embryos looks like a solution that would not compromise the ban on gene therapy performed after birth. But if athletes modified as embryos shall be accepted in sport because they were not responsible for the editing of their genes, children whose parents have subjected them to gene therapy while they were under legal age should also be given exemption regardless that their parents subjected them to gene therapy due to concerns about their height, strength, or stamina. Otherwise these unfortunate children, whose parents did not edit their embryos but waited till their babies were born and proved to be at a disadvantage in comparison with other children, would be discriminated against and punished for something they were not legally able to consent to.

If WADA in this future scenario would resist sports participation of involuntarily genetically modified athletes based on the premise that these modified individuals would undermine the integrity of sport, the long-term consequence will be that elite sport becomes a museum. A spectacle of the past. Those who will be allowed to compete will be the natural bodied, relatively weak with a below-average life expectancy. The men and women whose parents secured them strong physiques will, if they bother at all, watch in pity the unfortunates who struggle unimpressively in the sports arenas for glory and fame, before they go out to do their own sports at a much higher level, recreationally.

References

Ash, L. (2016, December 30). Yuliya Stepanova: what do Russians think of doping whistleblower? www.bbc.com/news/magazine-38406627.

Ayyar, V.S. (2011). History of growth hormone therapy. *Indian Journal of Endocrinology and Metabolism* 15(3), 162–165.

Cooney, G. (2016, April 4). After yesterday's revelations, it's worth asking again: would Messi be Messi without HGH? www.balls.ie/football/after-yesterdays-revelations-its-worth-asking-again-would-messi-be-messi-without-hgh-329558.

Dimeo, P. & Møller, V. (2018). *The Crisis of Anti-Doping: Causes, Consequences, Solutions*. London: Routledge.

FC Barcelona. (2017). Honours. www.fcbarcelona.com/football/card/honours-football.

Fitch, K. (2016). The World Anti-Doping Code: can you have asthma and still be an elite athlete? *Breathe* 12(2), 148–158.

FootyFan. (2013). Top 10 shortest football players in the world. www.sportskeeda.com/football/top-10-shortest-players-in-football/4.

Franke, W.W. & Berendonk, B. (1997). Hormonal doping and androgenization of athletes: a secret program of the German Democratic Republic government. *Clinical Chemistry* 43(7), 1262–1279.

Franks, T. (2014, January 14). Gene doping: sport's biggest battle? www.bbc.com/news/magazine-25687002.

James, S.D. (2009, September 15). Growth hormones on rise in healthy kids. http://abcnews.go.com/Health/growth-hormones-healthy-kids-increase/story?id=8571628.

Miah, A. (2004). *Genetically Modified Athletes: Biomedical Ethics, Gene Doping and Sport.* London: Routledge.

Munthe, C. (2005). Ethics of controlling genetic doping. In C. Tamburrini & T. Tännsjö (Eds.), *Genetic Technology and Sport: Ethical questions* (pp. 107–125). London: Routledge.

Pearlman, A. (2017). My body, my genes. *New Scientist* 236, 22–23.

Schneider, A. & Friedmann, T. (2006). *Gene Doping in Sport: The Science and Ethics of Genetically Modified Athletes.* San Diego, CA: Elsevier.

Spitzer, G. (1998). *Doping in der DDR: Ein historischer Überblick zu einer konspirativen Praxis: Genese – Verantwortung – Gefahren.* Köln: Sport und Buch Strauss.

Toft, D.J. (2014, May 12). Growth hormone deficiency symptoms. www.endocrineweb.com/conditions/growth-disorders/growth-hormone-deficiency-symptoms.

Tyrrell, J., Jones, S.E., Beaumont, R., Astley, C.M., Lovell, R., Yaghootkar, H., et al. (2016). Height, body mass index, and socioeconomic status: mendelian randomisation study in UK Biobank. *BMJ* 352.

World Anti-Doping Agency. (2016, September 27). WADA releases frequently asked questions (FAQs) on Therapeutic Use Exemptions (TUEs). www.wada-ama.org/en/media/news/2016-09/wada-releases-frequently-asked-questions-faqs-on-therapeutic-use-exemptions-tues.

World Anti-Doping Agency. (2017, September 29). The World Anti-Doping Code International Standard Prohibited List 2018. www.wada-ama.org/en/media/news/2017-09/wada-publishes-2018-list-of-prohibited-substances-and-methods.

World Anti-Doping Agency. (2018, January 18). WADA welcomes ECHR decision to back Whereabouts rules. Retrieved from www.wada-ama.org/en/media/news/2018-01/wada-welcomes-echr-decision-to-back-whereabouts-rules.

World Health Organization. (2017, January 2). The top 10 causes of death. www.who.int/mediacentre/factsheets/fs310/en/.

Why Evolution is True. (2009, March 21). The New Scientist has no shame – again. whyevolutionistrue.wordpress.com/2009/03/21/the-new-scientist-has-no-shame-again/.

33

ENHANCING EVOLUTION: THE TRANSHUMAN CASE FOR GENE DOPING

Andy Miah

Introduction

The conventional view on gene doping is that it should be treated like other forms of doping, both in scientific and ethical terms, as evidenced by its inclusion within the World Anti-Doping Code back in 2003 (World Anti-Doping Agency (WADA), 2003). The basis for this position is that, like other forms of doping, gene doping involves the use of medical technologies for nontherapeutic biological modifications, as described in WADA's initial terminology banning gene doping, which described it as:

> M3: Gene Doping
> The non-therapeutic use of cells, genes, genetic elements, or the modulation of gene expression, having the capacity to enhance athlete performance.
>
> (WADA, 2003)

Over the years, this terminology has been extended and clarified towards the following definition of gene doping, which removes the term "non-therapeutic," due to the term "enhance" providing adequate determination of unacceptable use:

> M3: Gene Doping
> The following, with the potential to enhance sport performance, are prohibited:
>
> 1. The use of polymers of nucleic acids or nucleic acid analogues.
> 2. The use of gene editing agents designed to alter genome sequences and/or the transcriptional or epigenetic regulation of gene expression.
> 3. The use of normal or genetically modified cells.
>
> (WADA, 2018, p. 6)

In this respect, gene doping violates crucial characteristics of scientific and medical ethics, which at best, will permit the use of experimental techniques in service of a therapeutic need, but which would not be allowed merely to enhance an athlete's performance. The argument underpinning this stance is that medical interventions are inherently risky and taking such risks can only be justified when there are no other means of treating a person who suffers from some illness, injury, or disease. In this sense, medical treatment is a practice of necessity rather than a practice of preference. It is the only means by which we have the potential to alleviate biological suffering.

This principal concern about medicine being misused is articulated at the beginning of the World Anti-Doping Agency's *Prohibited List*, which states:

> Any pharmacological substance which is not addressed by any of the subsequent sections of the List and with no current approval by any governmental regulatory health authority for human therapeutic use (e.g. drugs under pre-clinical or clinical development or discontinued, designer drugs, substances approved only for veterinary use) is prohibited at all times.
>
> (WADA, 2011)

This stipulation means that, for the sports world to endorse gene doping, it would need to advocate a position that contradicts worldwide codes of conduct in scientific research and medical care. This is especially challenging when the sports industries rely heavily on the endorsements of medical professionals to ensure that their events remain sufficiently safe. In many sports, athletes must pass a medical, physical examination to demonstrate that they are fit for competition, before they are allowed to compete. Indeed, in sports where this does not happen, it is due to lack of resources, but an ideal system is one where the health risks an athlete encounters can be monitored continuously and where medical interventions can occur as soon as possible, once a risk becomes apparent. These characteristics of elite sport's medicalized infrastructure are reinforced when considering that those working within sports governance are often people involved with the medical professions. For example, the former International Olympic Committee (IOC) President, Dr. Jacques Rogge and many celebrated athletes who have gone on to be involved in the administration of sport have medical or scientific expertise. The history of anti-doping may even be described as a movement progressed by key individuals within the medical professions.

In this respect, sports – especially elite sports competitions – should be understood sociologically and culturally as industries that are regulated, not just by medical concerns pertinent to the practice of sport, but industries that are engaged with wider healthcare priorities. Indeed, the pursuit of IOC member and long-term anti-doping advocate Arne Ljungqvist to ensure all Olympic bidding nations have a criminal law against doping speaks to the manner in which many doping substances derive from an illegal black trade and where such use coheres with wider concerns about drug abuse within society at large.

As such, advocating doping – or promoting gene doping – is incompatible with the duty of care taken by medical professionals towards athletes, a commitment which is central to the execution of a sports event. These circumstances are made all the more complicated because elite adult sport is intimately connected with the development of sporting experiences in childhood. While there are reasonable distinctions to be made between these two stages of life, their continuity through sport makes it all the more challenging to hold a position on gene doping – or doping generally – that is anything other than supportive of prohibition or deterrence.

This position is made manifest in the deliberations of sport authorities explicitly via the WADA Code, which identifies three areas of interest when determining whether or not a substance, method, or technology should be considered a doping practice. Thus, a new candidate for inclusion within the list must engage two of three conditions to be worthy of consideration:

- 4.3.1 A substance or method shall be considered for inclusion on the Prohibited List
      if WADA, in its sole discretion, determines that the substance or method meets
      any two of the following three criteria:
  - 4.3.1.1 Medical or other scientific evidence, pharmacological effect or experi-
         ence that the substance or method, alone or in combination with other
         substances or methods, has the potential to enhance or enhances sport
         performance;
  - 4.3.1.2 Medical or other scientific evidence, pharmacological effect or experi-
         ence that the Use of the substance or method represents an actual or
         potential health risk to the Athlete;
  - 4.3.1.3 WADA's determination that the Use of the substance or method violates
         the spirit of sport described in the introduction to the Code.

(WADA Code, 2015)

When confronted with a new means of altering an athlete's biological circumstances, WADA tests against these parameters to determine its degree of concern. Together, the three criteria provide scope for a range of performance enhancements to be acceptable, but are sufficiently broad to address a range of examples, from hypobaric chambers to the use of gene doping or steroid use.

Aside from the third criteria, the emphasis on medical and scientific evidence reinforces the points outlined above, which explain how the problem with the sports world endorsing any form of performance enhancement that involves medical substances or method has to do with the ethical commitments made by – and thus, legal restrictions upon – health professions allied to the practice of sports. In this respect, it is a general conclusion that sports are incompatible with the pursuit of human enhancement, where this involves the use of scientific and medical techniques, substances, or methods, which aim to provide a performance effect that exceeds therapy. Indeed, even therapeutic use of such things requires special approval, if an athlete expects to use them while competing.

However, there is an alternative view, which provides scope for sports to embrace gene doping, while maintaining a hard line on other forms of doping, and this article outlines the basis of that position. The argument requires sports – and society more widely – to embrace a nontherapeutic model of health, whereby the role of medicine is not just to treat patients towards the achievement and maintenance of a biostatistical norm of health, but where it embraces a definition of health that is epitomized by the transhumanist conviction that our biology must evolve alongside technology, not independent of it. By implication, this commitment also involves foregoing the idea that healthcare should be focused just on repair, arguing instead that a healthier population would emerge from circumstances where human enhancement is central to health maintenance. This aspect of enhancing evolution also allows us to endorse gene doping, without needing to embrace all other forms of doping. In this respect, gene doping is valued partly for its capacity to take evolution to a new level of functioning. We can call this the *germ line proposition* and, while somatic cell line modifications would not have any evolutionary impact, there are also reasons to endorse these kinds of enhancements, particularly where research can lead to safer forms of performance enhancement than current methods which we call doping.

The starting point for this position derives from what may be described as the western model of healthcare, although I offer some caution when using such terminology. In this case, I use the term *western model* to describe a system of approaching medicine and healthcare as leading inexorably to the pursuit of immortality and indefinite health span, where aging is, increasingly, treated as a disease to be resisted, rather than an inevitable consequence of life (Gladyshev & Gladyshev, 2016; Janaca et al., 2017). While such notions may seem to be located in the realm of science fiction, there are credible, tangible examples of scientific research and healthcare policy, which expose these aspirations (Bulterjs et al., 2016).

In so doing, this paper questions the scientific and ethical basis for anti-doping work; arguing that the pursuit of human enhancement – through sport or other means – ought not be described as medicine at all, but as some new category of human intervention, which consists of our intervening with or disrupting the course of evolution. At the very least, the implications of these circumstances should lead WADA and sports organizations to rearticulate their approach to gene doping specifically and human enhancement generally. Such repositioning would involve reorienting itself around the changing circumstances within our society and embracing the wider commitment that this implies to support the principle that humanity embraces the pursuit of perfecting technology, in order to optimize our capacity to evolve.

In making this case, I recognize that many anti-doping advocates will not take these terms as being the starting point for a debate about the ethics of doping. Instead, discussions often focus on what kinds of practices sports are, from which we may then ascertain whether enhancements are consistent with such criteria. Consequently, before returning to the medical model as the basis for my reasoning, I will outline why it is that I think that the ethics of sport do not matter to resolving the doping dilemma.

Why appeals to the "spirit of sport" don't resolve the doping dilemma

The World Anti-Doping Code outlines that its mandate is interwoven within a range of critical concerns that seek to protect the "intrinsic value of sports" (WADA, 2015), which it collectively describes as the "spirit of sport." It states:

> Anti-doping programs seek to preserve what is intrinsically valuable about sport. This intrinsic value is often referred to as "the spirit of sport." It is the essence of Olympism, the pursuit of human excellence through the dedicated perfection of each person's natural talents. It is how we play true. The spirit of sport is the celebration of the human spirit, body and mind, and is reflected in values we find in and through sport, including:

- Ethics, fair play and honesty
- Health
- Excellence in performance
- Character and education
- Fun and joy
- Teamwork
- Dedication and commitment
- Respect for rules and laws
- Respect for self and other Participants
- Courage
- Community and solidarity

> Doping is fundamentally contrary to the spirit of sport.

(WADA, 2015)

While each of these elements resonates with what one may conventionally think of as the values of sports, taken individually, they do not make a compelling case against doping, nor are uniquely characteristic of sport at all. For instance, one could envisage a system of pro-doping which preserves fair play – even enhances it. Thus, the sports world may just allow all athletes to use whatever enhancements they wish (or even just the ones currently prohibited by WADA). If every athlete operates by the same rule that stipulates they are free to use any such means, then all will be competing by the same rules and fairness will prevail. While there may still be athletes who seek to find other means as yet unimagined by the scope of the WADA *Prohibited List*, this would not be dramatically different from the present circumstances. Indeed, it may be far better as there may be far fewer alternatives by which an athlete could try to cheat.

Similarly, "excellence in performance" need not be jeopardized by doping, as, for instance, the use of blood doping, would still require an athlete to train their body and minds to a comparable degree as an athlete who does not use blood doping. The gain in their performance would not lead to a situation where the pursuit of excellence is diminished, especially if one characterizes this pursuit as the perfection of athletic skills, where this is evidenced by being the most proficient athlete. While this may be too narrow a characterization of sporting excellence, Berg (2015) notes that the definition of excellence is malleable and changes depending on the social context. While Berg also goes on to note that there may be a deeper characterization of excellence which has to do with integrity, this does not help us terribly in resolving the doping dilemma as, if doping were made legal, there would be no loss of integrity in using such means.

One could also easily imagine athletes working as a "team" while also doping. Indeed, one might even find a reasonable articulation of how being able to dope effectively involves being part of a highly sophisticated team of pro-doping scientists, with whom they would have to work carefully to achieve the optimal form of enhancement. Such endeavours may even involve significant sacrifice or "courage" and "character" to achieve these goals.

In sum, any one of these characteristics may be supported in a climate where doping is allowed, but the most challenging one to uphold is "health." I am skeptical that health promotion can be argued as intrinsic to the value of sport – at an elite level so many players are injured either through incident or over-training/competing – and even the IOC Medical Commission recognized that there is greater prevalence of some health risks resulting from elite sports participation, compared to regular citizenship (IOC, 2009). Nevertheless, the incompatibility of health promotion with nontherapeutic interventions makes pro-doping untenable, which is why my focus in presenting an alternative response to gene doping relies heavily on this dimension of the problem. In short, determining that doping would be acceptable requires approaching health from a very different perspective than is conventionally held, but this is a perspective which I will argue to be intrinsic to the logic of medicine, though we often do not acknowledge this. Essentially, this is to say that the end goal of healthcare is the eradication of the need for medicine or the medical services that we utilize across our lives. When healthcare reaches this endpoint, then it will cease to be necessary. At most, it will become something else other than direct care.

The purpose of healthcare is changing

In 2001, the Human Genome Project published the first draft of its findings in *Nature*, showcasing 90% of the genome map. It was quickly accompanied by many discussions about what may become of our world if we are able to intervene genetically in either the eradication of disease and illness or through our ability to pick, choose, or enhance our genetic characteristics. At the time – and still – the excitement was broadly focused on the gains that could be made towards diagnostic discoveries or therapeutic interventions, though even here there have been controversies over the eradication of illness or disease. For example, disability scholars have argued against "ableism" (Wolbring, 2008), which is the unjustified presumption that disability is something that needs fixing – through genetic means or otherwise – as opposed to something that societies should seek to accommodate. Even stronger concerns are found in how the eradication of biological dysfunction could lead to a eugenic ideology becoming reinforced within society, whereby unintelligent and socially damaging views may become commonplace, such as determining a person's worth on the basis of their genome. Some have even argued that removing genetic dysfunctions by tinkering with our genes could have a negative evolutionary impact, just because we do not yet fully comprehend our genes (Kozubek, 2017).

In any case, since the publication of the Human Genome Project, full genome sequencing has changed dramatically in terms of cost and the methods by which altering the genome would take place. Whereas the first human genome map cost around $2.5 billion and 20 years to produce, it now costs less than $1000 and takes just a few weeks to process (Ray, 2016). A future where every citizen has their own genome mapped continually across their lifetime to minimize health risks and costs seems a highly likely scenario. While the number of therapeutic interventions has been limited to date, scientists are optimistic that more successes will follow. However, these limitations in present application are not really the crucial detail in this discussion. Rather, the more relevant aspect of this story to our present discussion about what to do with gene doping in sport has to do with the purpose of science, medicine, and healthcare, namely, the complete alleviation of biological suffering.

Whether it is mental or physical, the logic of the western model of health is to drive humanity towards circumstances where, across our entire lives, we actually have no need for medicine whatsoever. The end goal of healthcare is for us to get to a point where there is no need to see a doctor, nurse, or to enter a hospital. No need for medication, for treatment, or rehabilitation; where we are healthy and where this good health persists over our entire lives. These characteristics describe the ideal healthcare system, but in a world where this is achieved, the parameters by which we judge the worth of scientific experimentation are also different. It will cease to be necessary to focus just on repair or maintenance, leaving open the possibility that biology may be modified to transcend such limits and norms.

Of course, for anybody working within science or medicine, these circumstances are a long way off. For many years to come, healthcare will be far more focused on health maintenance than human enhancement. Yet, it is crucial that the goals of medicine are clear before we can then consider how best to achieve them. As such, I argue that the end point of healthcare is for nobody to need healthcare at all. This claim is central to my argument, as it frames how one later approaches what society wants from biology and what is sought from its modification through technology, which is an intermediary step towards embracing gene doping in sport. However, before imagining a range of radical new transhumanist interventions, it is helpful to consider something more familiar, such as vaccinations. Such medical interventions are consistent with the ideas outlined above. Thus, a vaccination should be regarded in a similar manner as a way of supplementing inadequacies within our genomes to cope with exposure to viruses that would be catastrophic to our survival. People vaccinate themselves against such vulnerabilities to prevent the possibility of becoming ill, even if the chances of this occurring are remote. In this sense, healthcare works in a pre-emptive way responding to the risks within our environment. For sport – and life more generally – such risks require a more radical enhancement of our biology to ensure such aims are met.

The specifics of these changes are characterized neatly in Buchanan et al. (2000), who describe how science is moving humanity from circumstances where biological characteristics are defined mostly by chance to circumstances where they are defined by choice. Choices to enhance humanity are made all the more critical because people make prior decisions to put themselves in positions of high biological risk, whether that is through the pursuit of sport or any number of other lifestyle choices, which are made in order to live the kind of life that people deem to make life worth living. Whether our activities involve deciding to go to space or going deep underwater, the extremities of these experiences require people to seek enhancements in order to be fit for purpose. Equally, humanity's desire to evolve or transcend its biological limits – typified by the pursuit of elite sports – provides a foundation for pursuing radical biological interventions, such as gene doping. Admittedly, I am mindful of the fact that this argument may lead a critic to ask why this position does not simply open the door to all forms of doping. My response to this has to do with the characteristics of the technology and how it compares to all other doping methods. Gene doping's capacity to modify us in a more precise manner, but also because of its impact on our evolutionary trajectory, justifies it being treated differently ethically.

Humanity's interest in pursuing such alterations is evidenced by the many ways in which people pursue aesthetic or functional enhancements throughout their lives – choices made just because they consider that such changes will permit the enjoyment of the kind of life that they seek to live. The specifics of those choices may be worthy of vigorous debate, but then so too might one debate the merit of dedicating a life to elite sport, which some would argue to be mostly in the service of a capitalist economy which exploits the many (those athletes who struggle to make ends meet) in order to benefit the few (those athletes and institutions who are winners economically).

There may be further reasons to question such choices, especially where they may lead to a range of health risks. For instance, one would want to ensure that such decisions are not made under unreasonable duress or in the context of an excessively coercive environment (recognizing that many choices occur within climates where such behaviors are reasonably coercive, such as the coercive environment of sports training which requires athletes to train full time in order to be competitive). To feel reassured about such choices, one must acknowledge that they are not made in isolation, but that our choices are always shaped by a range of societal influences. While one should always interrogate the value of such influence, our determination of values *always* operates within such conditions. There is no sense of self or interests outside of our social circumstances, no choices that operate outside of a social context. There is no inherent value to a new mobile phone, car, house, or even having a child, which can be explained in and of itself, without recourse to some wider framework of values which is located within a social network. In this sense, questioning the legitimacy of human enhancement, or the value of leading a transhumanist existence, on the basis of concerns about being pressured to make limiting decisions has only limited force.

What transhumanism means for gene doping

The arguments outlined above explain how humanity's pursuit of a long and healthy life is interwoven with the fabric of modern society and how this commitment drives us towards the transhumanist aspiration to continually remake the species through means arising from intellectual discoveries. Indeed, it recognizes that the proliferation of the human species is explicable in large part due to technological innovation. Humanity's evolutionary course has been shaped by its utilization of technology. Whether it is the discovery of penicillin, an understanding of hygiene, the development of artificial intelligence, or indeed, bikes, bakelite (the first synthetic plastic), and bulbs (Bijker 1995), humanity has sought such means to redefine its existence through technological advancement. On these terms, technology is defined in a very broad sense to describe the application of humanity's ideas to the natural world in a way which transforms its characteristics. The breeding of animals, agriculture, tool development, science, industry, medicine, and cartography, among many other examples, are all manifestations of this journey.

Indeed, sports themselves are manifestations of this transhumanist trajectory. The present value system that operates around elite sports elevates the importance of competition, winning, and transcendence through the recording of results, world records, personal bests, and using science to remove inhibitors to performance. These dimensions of modern sport are not simply unintended consequences of the intrinsic values of sports, but have become sport's intrinsic values. Loland (2002, 2003) describes this view of sport's value as the thin theory of sport, which elevates the quantitative evaluation of performance. However, Loland argues that this is an impoverished characterization of sport's value, arguing instead on behalf of a thick theory, which champions the development of a wider range of sporting virtues, such as effort or personal development. Yet, Loland overlooks the fact that the pursuit of thinner priorities does not jeopardize the enjoyment of his thicker values. The thick theory is not incompatible with the thin theory. Indeed, it is apparent in the exhibition of contemporary elite sports that athletes are able to apply both sets of values simultaneously in their conduct of competition.

What should sports do about gene doping right now?

Based on the current state of policy discourse in elite sports, it is highly unlikely that, any time soon, the world of sport will embrace the transhumanist aspiration to use technology to continually expand the potential of our biology, and so bring about an age of precautionary pro-doping. Even preparing for gene doping remains somewhat contested, with the WADA Health, Medical and Research Committee working group in Gene and Cell Doping determining in August 2017 that "gene doping did not appear to represent an immediate threat" (WADA, 2017). This view is hard to understand given the volume of research, commentaries, and discussion that have taken place about the imminent prospects of gene doping in sport, which have surrounded each Olympic Games at least since Athens 2004. Nevertheless, the present limited success of novel therapeutic genetic interventions means that it is not likely any time in the next 10 years to create a situation where either therapeutic interventions translate into enhanced humans, or where specific selective or editing choices could permit a new kind of superhuman athlete to emerge.

Thus, many of the ideas expressed in this chapter will seem somewhat removed from the present-day complexity of dealing with doping. After all, the present-day reality that faces anti-doping has to do with maintaining a level playing field when competitors try to cheat by means of doping. This chapter does not propose a solution to that problem. Indeed, I rather think that this is an inherent feature of competitive, rule-bound environments and it makes no sense to complain about such characteristics, or to expect them to be absent within some imagined, ideal scenario. For as long as we permit free will, we are likely to be stuck with behavior that deviates from rule keeping.

Yet, the world of sport does need to get its thinking right on the future of genetic interventions and their impact on the state of humanity. Part of this process involves moving on from theoretical philosophy and precautionary policymaking – namely, the prohibition of things that are not yet here – towards scenario planning and differentiating between forms of gene doping challenges. Many of the discussions so far have been theoretical. They involve the world of sport – or philosophers – trying to establish sound principles by which sport can be governed to protect its so-called intrinsic value (WADA, 2015). Yet, this theoretical work must be accompanied by some realistic expectations about how genetic technology may find its way into society. For instance, there are at least four kinds of gene doping, which we are likely to see impact upon the world of sport:

1) The conventional doping athlete.
2) The genetically identified athlete.
3) The genetically pre-selected athlete.
4) The genetically enhanced descendent athlete.

Getting sport policy right means getting it right for society at large, and not just for the short term. For years, various theorists have been developing legal definitions that take into account the imminent biological complexity of future humans. For example, Miah (2003) considers the rights of the genetically modified athlete, arguing that sport policy on the use of gene doping would need to be consistent with wider societal entitlements to genetic modification, even if the consequence of such changes is enhancement. Alternatively, UNESCO even adopted a Universal Declaration on the Human Genome and Human Rights (1997) to prepare for an era where genetically modified persons may find their rights curtailed were it not for an expanded definition of what is recognized as genetically human. To this end, sports must plan for these future humans, to ensure it creates a climate of inclusion for people who are genetically enhanced and to ensure humanity can take advantage of technology in order to preserve and enrich the species and maximize its chances of survival.

Of course there is an alternative to the value system I describe above. Indeed, it is likely that many people would consider humanity's pursuit of transhumanism to be misguided where, instead, our focus should be simply on enabling people to live a reasonably healthy life, where one accepts the natural consequences of our biology's fallibility, vulnerability, and eventual degradation. Parens (1995) redescribes Martha Nussbaum's characterization of the "fragility of goodness" (1986) when talking about the "goodness of fragility" as a basis for determining which kinds of things we should seek to modify versus the kinds of things we should seek to leave and accept as being part of the natural circumstances of our existence. Indeed, Parens goes on to suggest that life may be more impoverished by this loss of fragility.

While I accept that it is prudent to ready oneself for a life that will involve some degree of biological suffering brought about by our imperfect genomes, or by the inevitability of our decline and eventual death, we should not mistake our need to prepare psychologically for such circumstances for a willful desire for them to exist. Understood on this level, one must look to a broader sense of humanity's aspirations beyond simply the needs of individuals to find a way to get through life, in order to derive a more comprehensive and prudential view of what things matter to us. In this manner, one can draw on the evidence of humanity's pursuit of eradicating disease, or of trying to pursue a longer healthier life through scientific discovery and medical intervention, as the basis for determining our wider interests in ideas that we currently regard to be unrealistic, improbable, or utopian.

A further caveat to this conversation is to note that the circumstances I have described would be mistakenly characterized as utopian. The shift from chance to choice brings with it a number of new burdens, not least of which is the fact that people will have many more decisions to make about their existence within these circumstances. For example, people may need to consider which types of characteristics they design into the genomes of their progeny and, equally, which characteristics they seek to remove. These are both highly burdensome and highly controversial choices to make and it may be preferable to leave things to chance, rather than be confronted with the division that will likely arise from having the capacity to make such choices. Yet, I am optimistic that, with the fullness of time, humanity will find a way to make sensible and effective decisions in this regard and further consider that this predicament is precisely what distinguishes humanity as a species.

Of course, among any population there will be those who make choices that are ill conceived or based upon some dubious logic, which will surely bring about the exact opposite conditions they seek to promote. This is especially worrisome in cases where people are modifying genes in such a way that might affect the human gene pool. Indeed, at this point in our history, it is apparent that we have no good system for thinking through the basis on which we should make such decisions, or even where such decisions should be made as individuals or where they should be determined by a wider governing authority, which restricts elements of that freedom. There are some examples already where this has been considered. For instance, various countries permit genetic sex selection so as not to pass on a debilitating genetic disease, but not all countries are yet comfortable with permitting such choices for family balancing, or because prospective parents might prefer to have a boy or a girl. Indeed, one of the reasons for not allowing this is that there is some understanding how this may create a climate in which people are allowed to impose their own gendered prejudices onto future generations in a way that is challenging both in terms of population balance, but also because it reinforces unintelligent stereotypes about the worth of either sex.

On this matter alone there are already words of caution for how we may think about something like gene doping. Prospective parents who might seek to modify or select an embryo on the basis of its being able to pursue some kind of athletic ability, would likely misconstrue the potential of our genes to determine our abilities. Such freedom would also – if indeed it were possible – promote a particular range of abilities, which is so narrow in function as to undermine the agency of the life that is created through such choices. One could quite reasonably envisage that a person born from such choices and subject to their limitations would feel that their chances to flourish in life had been hampered due to their having been modified for a specific purpose in mind, rather than for a broader sense of what might be a life where a range of choices are available to them. This critique of gene doping would be particularly important in cases where one choice may mean that another choice is frustrated. While a child could hardly blame their parents for being very tall when the parents themselves are very tall, there may be more foundation for complaint when their phenotype has been chosen, regardless of those parental characteristics.

In pursuing these elements of the conversation, I am especially mindful of how far removed this will seem from the present-day realities of anti-doping authorities whose challenges focus mostly on trying to determine whether there are effective tests by which the sports industries could even discover evidence of gene doping. Instead of attending to this immediate challenge, my discourse has focused on the wider questions that surround the pursuit of testing at all and the questions that enhancement more generally create. These parallel conversations are brought together when thinking about the underpinning rationale and interests of anti-doping.

What I want from anti-doping authorities is for their codes to recognize that the rules are incompatible with the wider pursuit of health that we see operating within society at large today, which encompasses investment into finding safer forms of human enhancement. The rules also must make provision for addressing the prospect of there being people within our society who have been born with genetic modification within their ancestry or having been born themselves as a result of genetic modification or selection. The fundamental values of anti-doping should expand to recognize and acknowledge that there would be no discrimination towards such people, so as to ensure that sports remain open to how such technologies may become inextricable from what we think of as the means by which good health is possible.

These would be quite minor modifications to the World Anti-Doping Code, but would allow it to maintain its pursuit of anti-doping as it presently is, while also ensuring that it recognizes its mission to be subject to wider trends in human society, where the pursuit of health beyond our species' typical functioning has become a valued pursuit of humanity.

Alongside this is the further commitment to seek safer forms of performance enhancement within sport and to ensure athletes have access to and information about such means. In this sense, there are also implications for how anti-doping authorities approach education which is, presently, entirely predicated on the idea that athletes must be educated in order to ensure they do not dope. Yet, instead of framing the value of an education program as merely a means towards fostering "anti-doping behaviors," as the WADA Education program describes its purpose, it should seek to nurture a critical awareness of the complexities of performance enhancement and their wider context, as described within this chapter. It should seek to engage athletes on matters wider than sport, not least because many athletes who go through the elite sports system end up in some form within health promotion industries. Pedagogically, education should never be about indoctrination; it should never begin with a narrowly prescribed outcome as its consequence. Rather, education programs within anti-doping should seek to foster critical thinking, not just about performance enhancement, but also its governance. This is of urgent need, especially given the controversies that surround the administration of sports that we have seen in recent years. This more critical approach to anti-doping education would not just work towards a great achievement for the present anti-doping system and its priorities, it would also be of much greater service to humanity more widely.

References

Berg, A. (2015). The ethos of excellence. *Journal of the Philosophy of Sport*, 42, 233–249.

Bijker, W.E. (1995). *Of Bicycles, Bakelites, and Bulbs: Toward a Theory of Sociotechnical Change*. London: MIT Press.

Buchanan, A., Brock, D.W., Daniels, N., & **Wikler, D.** (2000). *From Chance to Choice: Genetics & Justice*. Cambridge: Cambridge University Press.

Bulterijs, S., Hull, R.S., Björk, V.C.E., and **Roy, A.G.** (2015). It is time to classify biological aging as a disease, *Frontiers in Genetics*, 6, 205.

Gladyshev, T.V. & **Gladyshev, V.N.** (2016). A disease or not a disease? Aging as a pathology. *Trends Mol Med*, 22, 995–996.

International Olympic Committee (2009). The International Olympic Committee (IOC) Consensus Statement on Periodic Health Evaluation of Elite Athletes. https://stillmed.olympic.org/media/Document%20Library/OlympicOrg/News/20090716-The-IOC-Consensus-Statement-on-Periodic-Health-Evaluation-of-Elite-Athletes/EN-Health-Evaluation-of-Elite-Athletes-2009-report-1448.pdf#_ga=2.261766285.1075817988.1529839491-1215944620.1528100467.

Janaca, S., Clarke, B., and **Gems, D.** (2017). Aging: natural or disease? A view from medical textbooks, in Vaiserman, A.M. (Ed) *Anti-aging Drugs: From Basic Research to Clinical Practice.*, pp. 11–34. London: The Royal Society of Chemistry.

Kozubek, J. (2017, January 9). How gene editing could ruin human evolution. *Time*. http://time.com/4626571/crispr-gene-modification-evolution/.

Loland, S. (2002). *Fair Play in Sport: A Moral Norm System*. London: Routledge.

Loland, S. (2003). Technology in sport: three ideal-typical views and their implications. Idrotts-Forum. www.idrottsforum.org/articles/loland/loland_2.html [Accessed June 23, 2018]

Miah, A. (2003). Genetic modification (GM) in sport: legal implications. *Contemporary Issues in Law*, 6, 207–226.

Nussbaum, M. (1986). *The Fragility of Goodness*. New York: Cambridge University Press.

Parens, E. (1995). The goodness of fragility: on the prospect of genetic technologies aimed at the enhancement of human capacities. *Kennedy Institute of Ethics Journal*, 5, 141–153.

Ray, T. (2016). With $999 whole-genome sequencing service, Veritas embarks on goal to democratize DNA information. Genome Web. www.genomeweb.com/sequencing-technology/999-whole-genome-sequencing-service-veritas-embarks-goal-democratize-dna#.WzJm7RMbPOS. [Accessed June 23, 2018.]

UNESCO. (1997). The Universal Declaration on the Human Genome and Human Rights. http://unesdoc.unesco.org/images/0012/001229/122990eo.pdf. [Accessed June 23, 2018.]

Wolbring, G. (2008). Why NBIC? Why human performance enhancement? *Innovation: The European Journal of Social Science Research*, 21, 25–40. https://doi.org/10.1080/13511610802002189.

World Anti-Doping Agency. (2003). *Prohibited List*. Montreal: WADA.

World Anti-Doping Agency. (2011). *Prohibited List*. Montreal: WADA.

World Anti-Doping Agency. (2015). *World Anti-Doping Code*. Montreal: WADA.

World Anti-Doping Agency. (2017). *Minutes of the Health, Medical and Research Committee.* Montreal: WADA. www.wada-ama.org/sites/default/files/resources/files/minutes_hmr_committee_august_29-30_2017_final.pdf. [Accessed June 23, 2018.]

World Anti-Doping Agency. (2018). *Prohibited List*. Montreal: WADA.

34

THE ETHICS OF SEX TESTING IN SPORT

Jaime Schultz

Sport is one of the few remaining institutions to mandate sex segregation, but defining sex is not as clear cut as it may seem. Since at least the 1930s, athletic authorities have been consumed with the problem of how to distinguish between women and men. More accurately, they have been consumed with which characteristics best determine femaleness. In the process, they have relied on a range of "sex tests": physical examinations, sex chromatin tests, genetic analyses, and hormonal assessments, all of which have disqualified women with differences of sex development (DSD) that may or may not relate to athletic potential (48).[1] In their efforts to level the playing field for women athletes, sport policymakers have generated more questions than answers when it comes to solving the riddles of sex.

An early history of sex verification, 1936–1966

In the late 18th and early 19th centuries, men established elite sports organizations, including the International Olympic Committee (IOC) and the International Amateur Athletic Federation (IAAF, now the International Association of Athletic Federations), to govern male athletes and their competitions. Early organizers were not interested in providing opportunities to women. Their general attitude was that women were too weak or frail to engage in the rigors of highly competitive sport. Those women who proved otherwise, the logic continued, must not be "real" women.

In the 1920s, the IOC and the IAAF grudgingly relented to pressures to add events for women, but progress was slow and limited. Track and field, one of only four Olympic disciplines open to women at the 1928 Games in Amsterdam, The Netherlands, especially troubled organizers who argued that the events were "profoundly unnatural" for female competitors and would cause them to "develop wholly masculine physiques and behavior traits" (39). Critics openly disputed the sex/gender of several women in the early days of athletics and in 1936, IOC member Avery Brundage "roundly recommended that all women athletes entered in the Olympics be subjected to a thorough physical examination to make sure they were really 100% female" (34). That same year, at the Olympic Games in Berlin, Germany, officials reportedly demanded that American Helen Stephens prove her sex after her superlative performance in the 100-meter race. Stephens's biographer writes that the athlete's response was that reporters

475

could "check the facts with the Olympic committee physician who sex-tested all athletes prior to competition" (14).

The story of Heinrich Ratjen makes it unlikely that physicians tested "all athletes" before the Games. At age 17, Ratjen, who competed under his given name Dora, took fourth in the 1936 Olympic women's high jump. Ratjen was not a "gender fraud," as many accounts have unjustly characterized him. Rather, he was someone who did not fit neatly into the sex/gender binary (18). The details of his life are murky and were only made public in 2009 after the Department for Sexual Medicine at Kiel University Hospital posthumously released Ratjen's file to a German newspaper. The records revealed that a midwife declared Ratjen female at birth and his parents raised him as such. Two years after the 1936 Berlin Games, a German police officer questioned Ratjen's sex – judging his feminine clothing incongruent with his masculine features. A subsequent medical examination reclassified Ratjen as male, and he lived the remainder of his life as a man (1).

Ratjen would have likely failed an Olympic Games sex check in 1936, yet there is no evidence to suggest that any of his contemporaries doubted his eligibility to compete as a woman. However, several athletes in the 1930s and 1940s underwent female-to-male gender confirmation surgeries (6). Their stories further stoked anxieties about the "femininity" of women athletes and authorities escalated their discussions about the need for compulsory sex verification (37).

Although World War II halted most major international sports competitions, the conflict did little to quell apprehensions about the sex of women athletes. To the contrary, in the post-war era, the outstanding achievements of women "from Communist countries" who, were "of questionable femininity" (according to Western journalists) only intensified those concerns (46). In 1946, the IAAF required all women who competed in women-only events to present a physician's letter confirming their sex. The IOC instituted the same requirement at the 1948 Olympic Games in London, though neither organization defined the parameters of femaleness. Soon, the growing significance of sport in the Cold War era made it clear that affidavits from team and family physicians could no longer suffice – the documents were too easily falsified in the quest for athletic supremacy.

In the 1960s, sports authorities grew increasingly concerned with two issues – doping and sex – and experimented with different ways to test for both (29). In 1966, the IAAF initiated its first standardized, precompetition sex test by requiring female athletes at the British Empire and Commonwealth Games in Kingston, Jamaica, to undergo gynecological examinations. IAAF officials did not tell the women what to expect, as pentathlete Mary Peters described in her autobiography. Just before the competition, officials forced her to undergo what she called "the most crude and degrading experience I have ever known in my life. I was ordered to lie on the couch and pull my knees up … Presumably they were searching for hidden testes" (36).

Perhaps sympathetic to the distress the exams caused competitors, the IAAF changed its procedures later that year at the European Athletics Championships in Budapest, Hungary. There, female athletes went through a visual inspection or "nude parade." As *Time* reported, "The examination, as it turned out, was perfunctory. Lined up in single file, the 234 female athletes paraded past three female gynecologists. 'They let you walk by,' said one competitor afterward. 'Then they asked you to turn and face them, and that was it'" (38). All participants passed the survey, although there were five women who did not attend the competition. Italy's Maria Vittoria Tria declared that her religious convictions did not allow her "to undress in front of unknown people" (38). The other athletes, one from Romania and three from Russia, did not explain their absences and abrupt retirements from sport, which all but validated speculations about their "manly" appearance and skills (52).[2]

The chromosome formula, 1967–1988

Athletic officials next turned to the buccal smear, which was, at the time, a relatively new cytological test. Specifically, technicians looked for the presence of the second inactive X chromosome or Barr body. Women who tested "positive" for the Barr body earned their "certificate of femininity" or "GV [gender verification] card," a license they could submit at future competitions to avoid retesting (16). Women who tested "negative" for the Barr body could opt for additional examinations – a full chromosome analysis and, if necessary, a gynecologic exam, after which authorities ruled on their eligibility. More often, though, athletes who failed at the first stage withdrew from competition to avoid additional humiliation (8).

The IAAF first introduced the sex chromatin test at the 1967 European Cup in Kiev, Ukraine – the "Sex-Check Track Meet," as the press called it (42). Polish sprinter Ewa Kłobukowska, who passed the visual inspection the previous year, became the buccal smear's first athletic casualty when authorities determined she had "one chromosome too many" (presumed to be 46,XY/ 47,XXY mosaicism) (46, 47). At 21 years old, Kłobukowska could no longer compete in the sport to which she had devoted her life. "It's a dirty and stupid thing to do to me," she said at the time. "I know what I am and how I feel" (40).

Despite a brief protest from Kłobukowska and her compatriots, members of the IOC's newly established Medical Commission lauded the laboratory-based assessment as "simpler, objective and more dignified" than earlier verification procedures (16). The commission experimented with "the chromosome formula" at the 1968 Winter Games in Grenoble, France, and officially introduced it for all female participants competing in women's sports at the 1968 Mexico City Summer Games (35). As Eduardo Hay, chief of testing for the IOC's Medical Commission explained, "The investigation for femininity of the athletes participating in the Olympic Games verifies that the athletes are competing on an equal basis considering their physical status. In the cases of intersexuality or hermaphroditism, the athlete must be barred from competition in order to insure fair play" (16). In telling language, a 1968 issue of the IOC's newsletter proclaimed that from that point on, "All women athletes participating in the Games will be controlled" (25).

From the beginning, members of the international medical community denounced sex testing as "grossly unfair," arguing that "no single index or criterion can signify the appropriate sex for an individual." The sex chromatin test, anatomist Keith L. Moore stressed in 1968, "should not be used as absolute criteria of sexual identity" (33). As early as 1969, specialists refused to administer the exam on the grounds that it was scientifically unreliable and ethically unsound (13). Danish researchers issued a memorandum in 1972 in which they asserted that, "the International Olympic Committee has made its own definition of sex" and recommended that, "the use of the test should be cancelled" (50). Noted geneticist Albert de la Chapelle called the test "not only inaccurate but also discriminatory in that it excludes women who should be allowed to participate" (8). Even so, these condemnations did little to shake the IOC's confidence in the procedure, and sex testing persisted for the next 30 years.

It is impossible to know how many women have been disqualified by the results of their sex tests. In the wake of Ewa Kłobukowska's humiliation in 1967, officials pledged to keep the results confidential. Experts estimate that the examinations have eliminated one or two women at each Olympic Games, but this does not accurately represent the number of women athletes with DSDs – only those who make it to the Olympic stage. It says nothing of women in the lower or recreational echelons of sport. Potential female Olympians who do not neatly align within the sporting parameters of femaleness are likely to be ruled out at the local, regional, or national levels and do not make it to the international stage. Even women not directly affected by the tests might avoid sport if they suspect they might not pass.

Because organizations pledged confidentiality, it was only when a woman openly criticized or challenged her results that the public learned of her sex-test "failure." This was the situation for Spanish hurdler María José Martínez-Patiño, who received her "GV card" in 1983 but neglected to bring it to the 1985 World University Games in Kobe, Japan. Authorities tested her again and were troubled by the results (which backed critiques that the tests were unreliable). They advised Martínez-Patiño to fake an injury and drop out of the race. She complied. Two months later, she received a letter reading, "Karyotype is decided 46, XY" (30). Genetically speaking, and much to her astonishment, the IAAF had classified Martínez-Patiño as male.

Upon further testing, Martínez-Patiño learned – for the first time – that she also has complete androgen insensitivity syndrome (CAIS), in which her cells do not have typical androgen receptors and, consequently, cannot respond to circulating testosterone secreted by internal testes. There may be high or "male" levels of androgens in her body, but this does not affect her athletic aptitude. Although women with CIAS appear to be genetically male, they do not develop the strength, musculature, or body types associated with male levels of testosterone; neither can they benefit from the use of anabolic steroids or exogenous testosterone (that is, testosterone that originates outside an individual's body). "I could hardly pretend to be a man," Martínez-Patiño wrote of the ordeal. "I have breasts and a vagina. I never cheated. I fought my disqualification" (30). After nearly three years, and with the support of Dr. de la Chapelle, the European Athletics Association allowed her to compete as a woman, though the trial significantly and irreversibly damaged her life and athletic career (31).

As a result of Martínez-Patiño's case and other mounting objections, the IAAF dropped the sex chromatin test in 1988 and substituted in its place a "medical examination for the health and well-being of all athletes (men and women)." This would, according to IAAF-affiliated researchers, "ensure satisfactory physical status for competition and would, of course, include simple inspection of the external genitalia" (29). Four years later, the IAAF recognized that contemporary sports clothing and urine samples, collected in the presence of anti-doping officials, made the "health screen" unnecessary for identifying anomalous or ambiguous genitalia. As of May 1992, a federation spokesperson declared, "We have no femininity list—the file is closed" (53). And yet, the file was not entirely closed, but rather left ajar for officials "to be able to address the occasional anomalies that do surface," the policy explained (21).

The search for *SRY*, 1991–1999

Despite the IAAF's change in protocol, IOC officials remained "wedded to the notion that gender testing was necessary to prevent masquerading males from infiltrating female-only events" (49). In 1991, members of the IOC's Medical Commission replaced the sex chromatin test with DNA analysis of the Y chromosome using polymerase chain reaction amplification, looking specifically for the *SRY* gene (sex-determining region Y) to define an individual's sex. In other words, female athletes could have a Y chromosome, but not a specific gene located on that chromosome if they wanted to compete in women-only events. As before, experts criticized the efficacy of this test – indeed, of any test – for determining sex (7, 41).

Genetic testing did not last long. At the 1996 Centennial Olympic Games in Atlanta, Georgia, 8 women out of 3387 (1 in 423) expressed the *SRY* gene.[3] Additional examinations found that seven of the women had androgen insensitivity syndrome (four complete, three partial), and one woman had 5α-reductase deficiency, a disorder in which testosterone cannot be converted to its active metabolite, dihydrotestosterone; she had also undergone a gonadectomy (10). Authorities cleared all eight women to compete as women at the 1996 Games.

That all of the *SRY* women ultimately competed, in addition to the considerable costs and time the analyses required, added support to those who called for the elimination of sex-testing procedures. The Norwegian medical community collectively refused to administer the examinations at the 1994 Winter Games in Lillehammer, and the Norwegian parliament subsequently banned genetic testing for the purpose of sex verification in sport (11). By 1996, nearly every major medical society had called for the end of these practices. Additional recommendations from the IOC World Conference on Women and Sport and the IOC's Athletes' Commission finally convinced the IOC's Executive Board to concede. The 2000 Summer Games in Sydney, Australia, marked the first the first time in more than three decades that female Olympians could compete without first proving their sex.

Suspicion-based testing, 2000–2011

Still, officials could resurrect the tests at any time. Like the IAAF before it, the IOC resolved to intervene when someone cast aspersions on the sex of a female competitor. In the event of "any 'suspicion,'" according to the guidelines, "or if there is a 'challenge' [to her sex] then the athlete concerned can be asked to attend a medical evaluation" (21). Instead of comprehensive sex testing, authorities targeted only those women of ambiguous femininity. This became standard operating procedure for most national and international sports organizations until 2011.

Shortly after India's Santhi Soundarajan finished second in the 800-meter race at the 2006 Asian Games in Doha, Qatar, she found herself ensnared in this very procedure. Although her birth certificate affirmed her as female and she identified and lived her entire life as such, the Indian Olympic Association determined that Soundarajan "did not possess the sexual characteristics of a woman" (20). Without explaining what those characteristics were, officials stripped her of her silver medal and banned her from future competitions for what they called a "Games rule violation." Soundarajan attempted suicide not long after her expulsion. As she explained to reporters, "I am physically and mentally totally broken" (5).

South Africa's Caster Semenya likewise found herself caught in the crosshairs of suspicion-based testing at the 2009 track and field World Championships in Berlin, Germany. As the 18-year-old Semenya cruised to victory in the 800-meter race, Australian journalists published unsubstantiated rumors that she "has a chromosomal abnormality that gives her both male and female characteristics" and that her "testosterone levels were three times the normal level for a woman" (15). IAAF officials did not comment on the specifics of Semenya's case, but they did confirm that they had subjected her to "gender verification" procedures amid "concerns that she does not meet the requirements to compete as a woman" (44). The federation allowed Semenya to retain her 800-meter title and prize money, but requested she withdraw from subsequent competitions while a medical committee, which included a gynecologist, endocrinologist, psychologist, internal medicine specialist, and a "gender expert" reviewed her tests (43).

In July 2010, nearly a full year after Semenya's last race, IAAF administrators announced they had accepted "the conclusion of a panel of medical experts that she can compete with immediate effect" (22). She was noticeably slower upon returning to the track, leading to speculation that, in the interim, she had undergone some type of treatment to reduce her testosterone (44). Although Semenya has never addressed that rumor, the IAAF's succeeding policy on hyperandrogenism seemed to support the theory.

The testosterone question

In April 2011, an IAAF-appointed panel of experts, working closely with the IOC's Medical Commission, released a 28-page document titled *Regulations Governing Eligibility of Females with Hyperandrogenism to Compete in Women's Competition.* The new policy replaced "the IAAF's previous Gender Verification Policy and the IAAF has now abandoned all reference to the terminology 'gender verification' and 'gender policy' in its Rules" (23). The test was no longer about sex, the federation maintained; it was about health, fair play, and testosterone.

Hyperandrogenism, as defined in the IAAF's document, is "the excessive production of androgenic hormones (Testosterone)." It quantified "excessive" as women with 10 or more nanomoles of functional testosterone per liter of serum (nmol/L). This threshold is above the "normal" reference range for women (0.12–1.79 nmol/L) and at the low end for "normal" men (7.7–29.4 nmol/L) (2). Hyperandrogenic women (those who were not androgen insensitive) had two options: drop out of sport or agree to a "prescribed medical treatment" that would "correct" their "disorder" (23).

Indian sprinter Dutee Chand refused both. Instead, she challenged the Sports Authority of India's 2014 decision that disqualified her based on a diagnosis of hyperandrogenism. Chand took her case before the Court of Arbitration for Sport (CAS), where adjudicators ruled that there was "insufficient evidence about the degree of advantage that androgen-sensitive hyperandrogenic females enjoy over non-hyperandrogenic females." CAS gave the IAAF 2 years to produce a conclusive "correlation" between high endogenous testosterone and enhanced athletic performance. Failure to provide evidence to this effect would void the Federation's policy (9).

In 2017, scientists declared that they had found the evidence. In a study funded by the IAAF and the World Anti-Doping Agency (WADA), researchers divided track and field competitors – men and women – into three groups based on their testosterone. No significant patterns emerged for men, but women with the highest levels of testosterone outperformed women in the lowest tertile in five events: the 400-meter race (in which high-testosterone females performed 2.7% better than low-testosterone females), 400-meter hurdles (2.8%), 800-meter race (1.8%), pole vault (2.9%), and hammer throw (4.5%) (2).

Based on this study, the IAAF approved new regulations in 2018 that only apply to "relevant athletes" who compete internationally in "restricted events": the 400 meters, 400-meter hurdles, 800 meters, 1500 meters, and 1-mile races. Curiously, the 2017 study did not find that testosterone affected performance in the 1500-meter and mile races. Even more curiously, the two events that showed the widest performance gaps, the pole vault and hammer throw, are not included in the restricted events. "Relevant athletes," as stipulated in the 2018 regulations, are women with testosterone >5 nmol/L (half the threshold of the 2011 policy) who are diagnosed with a specific DSD, including 5α-reductase type 2 deficiency, partial androgen insensitivity syndrome, 17β-hydroxysteroid dehydrogenase type 3 deficiency, congenital adrenal hyperplasia, 3β-hydroxysteroid dehydrogenase deficiency, ovotesticular DSD, or any other genetic condition involving disordered gonadal steroidogenesis. These athletes must lower their testosterone to below 5 nmol/L for 6 months prior to competition. Those who refuse or fail to do so can compete in a nonrestricted event, in male events, or in "any applicable intersex or similar classification that may be offered" (24).

The logic is even more confounding when juxtaposed with testosterone-related regulations for trans athletes. In 2015, the IOC released a document that outlined the results of a *Consensus Meeting on Sex Reassignment and Hyperandrogenism.* It is important not to conflate women with hyperandrogenism and DSDs with transgender athletes. Still, the proposed eligibility requirements both isolate testosterone levels as the determining factor for who counts as a woman. The IOC no longer requires "surgical anatomical changes as a pre-condition" for trans athletes to compete as the sex with which they identify. But a trans woman athlete (one who transitions from male to female) "must demonstrate that her total testosterone level in serum has been below 10 nmol/L for at least 12 months prior to her first competition." She must remain below that threshold throughout her athletic career (26). The effect of this seemingly progressive rule is to reinforce the idea that testosterone levels define sex, which strengthens the proposed policy on hyperandrogenism.

Whereas officials wrestle over the "requirements to compete as a woman," they appear unconcerned with identifying any requirements to compete as a man. According to the IOC's 2015 consensus, trans male athletes (who transition from female to male) "are eligible to compete without restriction." The document provides no exclusionary provisions for trans men, including the use of exogenous testosterone (26). Under different circumstances, the use of exogenous testosterone is illegal; it is doping. But WADA, which guides most organizations' policies on performance-enhancing drugs (including the IOC's), allows athletes to take a banned substance if they can prove they have a medical necessity through what is called a Therapeutic Use Exemption (TUE).

To that end, WADA's 2016 policy recognizes that "androgen therapy is essential for completion of the anatomical and psychological transition process in FtM [female-to-male] athletes." As such, "FtM athletes may be granted a TUE," though the specific eligibility criteria "is entirely left to the different sporting federations and organizations" (54). Hyperandrogenic and trans women must suppress their endogenous testosterone, but trans men are permitted the use of exogenous testosterone.

What is more, cis men (those affirmed male at birth and who identify as men) who drop below the "normal" male-typical testosterone threshold can petition for a TUE for exogenous testosterone if a physician diagnoses them with an "androgen deficiency." And although most men fall within the expansive 7.7–29.4 nmol/L range, sports organizations do not impose an upper limit for male athletes' endogenous testosterone in the same way they do for hyperandrogenic and trans women.

At the same time, WADA's policy makes it clear, in bold font, that a "TUE for androgen deficiency should not be approved for females" (54). Even if a woman's functional testosterone registers below the female-typical range, she is not granted the same opportunity as a man to raise her testosterone to levels commensurate with her same-sex competitors. This becomes not just an issue of sport performance, but can also present significant health concerns.

The impossibility of fair

The discussion of endogenous and exogenous testosterone highlights the complexities of defining sex for the purpose of elite sport competition (2, 17, 27). It also underscores the complexities, perhaps the impossibilities, of determining what is fair. Authorities have long argued that sex testing is necessary "to insure fair play" and "to create a level playing field in female sport" (16, 19). Yet, sport is inherently unfair. The playing field is irredeemably unlevel. As other authors in this book point out, there are genetic variations that predispose athletes for enhanced performance, but authorities do not rule these athletes ineligible to compete or ask them to suppress any potentially advantageous condition those variations might confer. It is only when a condition challenges the ways we define sex that policymakers intervene.

On the issue of inequality, we might further consider the social, environmental, and class-based inequities that advantage certain athletes over others. Even on the specific issue of hyperandrogenism, a number of women diagnosed with the condition come from "rural or mountainous regions of developing countries," as one study concluded (12). These women may not have the same access to healthcare, much less the advanced sport training, facilities, equipment, or competitive opportunities as their international peers. Is that fair?

Debates about the need for sex testing invariably lead to considerations about the necessity of sex segregation in sport. Researchers estimate that there is, on average, a 10% performance gap between elite male and female athletes – that men perform about 10% better than women in the highest ranks of competition. This varies according to the sport. The difference between the best men and women's times in the 800-meter freestyle swimming event is 5.5%, but in weightlifting the top men outperform the top women by 36.8% (51). To eliminate sex segregation would put most women athletes at a disadvantage. Still, the dilemma remains: By what criteria should we define sex? Even more, do those criteria account for the performance gap?

There are no conclusive answers to these questions. Some researchers have proposed that instead of sex segregation, we divide competitors by "sports sex" that would be "determined by biological parameters … and not linked to gender categories, but rather only focused on valid in relation to athletic performance" (32). The word "sex" in "sports sex" is misleading, then. Instead, the proposal might amount to something akin to the use of "sport classes" in parasport, whereby evaluators classify athletes according to impairment and activity limitation. But there are problems with this system as well. Any attempt to equalize the field of play will cause controversy. This much is evident in the history of sex testing, and it is a history that is unlikely to be brought to a conclusion any time soon.

Notes

1 Sex testing goes by several alternative terms, including sex control, sex determination, gender testing, gender verification, and femininity control. In this chapter, I refer to *sex* as the biological characteristics associated with male and female, and *gender* the culturally constructed characteristics associated with masculinities and femininities.
2 Administrators at the 1967 Pan American Games in Winnipeg, Manitoba, also subjected women to a "nude parade," an experience 16-year-old American shot putter Maren Seldler described as "hideous" and "humiliating" (28).
3 At the 1992 Olympic Games in Barcelona, Spain, technicians screened 2406 female athletes. Five women tested positive for the *SRY* gene, but the IOC provided no further information about the women's eligibility (45).

References

1. **Berg S**. How Dora the man competed in the women's high jump. Spiegel, 15 Sept. 2009. www.spiegel.de/international/germany/1936-berlin-olympics-how-dora-the-man-competed-in-the-woman-s-high-jump-a-649104.html. [Accessed 13 Nov. 2017.]
2. **Bermon S, Garnier P**. Serum androgen levels and their relation to performance in track and field: mass spectrometry results from 2127 observations in male and female elite athletes. *British Journal of Sports Medicine* 51: 1309, 2017.
3. **Bermon S, Garnier PY, Hirschberg AL, Robinson N, Giraud S, Nicoli R, Baume N, Saugy M, Fénichel P, Bruce SJ, Henry H**. Serum androgen levels in elite female athletes. *Journal of Clinical Endocrinology Metabolism* 99: 4328–4335, 2014.
4. **Bermon S, Ritzén M, Hirschberg AL, Murray TH**. Are the new policies on hyperandrogenism in elite female athletes really out of bounds? *American Journal of Bioethics* 13: 64, 2013.
5. **Bhowmick N, Thottam J**. Gender and athletics: India's own Caster Semenya. *Time* 1 Sept. 2009. www.time.com/time/world/article/0,8599,1919562,00.html. [Accessed 24 Jan. 2010.]
6. Change of sex. *Time* 28: 39–40, 1936.

7. **Cotinot C**, **Pailhoux E**, **Jaubert F**, **Fellous M**. Molecular genetics of sex determination. *Seminars in Reproductive Medicine* 20: 157–68, 2002.
8. **de la Chapelle A**. The use and misuse of sex chromatin screen for "gender identification" of female athletes. *Journal of the American Medical Association* 256: 1920–1923, 1986.
9. Dutee Chand *v*. Athletics Federation of India and the International Association of Athletics Federation, CAS 2014/A/3759.
10. **Elsas LJ**, **Hayes RP**, **Muralidharan K**. Gender verification at the centennial Olympic games. *Journal of the Medical Association of Georgia* 86: 50, 1997.
11. **Elsas LJ**, **Ljungqvist A**, **Ferguson-Smith MA**, **Simpson JL**, **Genel M**, **Carlson AS**, **Ferris E**, **de la Chapelle A**, **Ehrhardt AA**. Gender verification of female athletes. *Genetics in Medicine* 2: 249–254, 2000.
12. **Fénichel P**, **Paris F**, **Philibert P**, **Hiéronimus S**, **Gaspari L**, **Kurzenne JY**, **Chevallier P**, **Bermon S**, **Chevalier N**, **Sultan C**. Molecular diagnosis of 5α-reductase deficiency in 4 elite young female athletes through hormonal screening for hyperandrogenism. *Clinical Endocrinology Metabolism* 98: E1055–E1059, 2013.
13. **Ferris EA**. Gender verification testing in sport. *British Medical Bulletin* 48: 692, 1992.
14. **Hanson SK**. *The Life of Helen Stephens: The Fulton Flash*. Carbondale, IL: Southern Illinois University Press, 2004.
15. **Hart S**. Caster Semenya "is a hermaphrodite," tests show. *Sydney Herald* 11 Sept. 2009. www.tele-graph.co.uk/sport/othersports/athletics/6170229/Caster-Semenya-is-a-hermaphrodite-tests-show.html. [Accessed 13 Nov. 2017.]
16. **Hay E**. Sex determination in putative female athletes. *Journal of the American Medical Association* 4: 39–41, 1972.
17. **Healy ML**, **Gibney J**, **Pentecost C**, **Wheeler MJ**, **Sonksen PH**. Endocrine profiles in 693 elite athletes in the postcompetition setting. *Clinical Endocrinology* 81: 294–305, 2014.
18. **Heggie V**. Testing sex and gender in sports; Reinventing, reimagining and reconstructing histories. *Endeavour* 34: 157–63, 2010.
19. **Ingle S**. Sebastian Coe: IAAF right to seek court ruling over hyperandrogeism issue. *Guardian* 12 Aug. 2017. www.theguardian.com/sport/2017/aug/12/sebastian-coe-iaaf-hyperandrogenism. [Accessed 13 Nov. 2017.]
20. Indian runner fails gender test, loses medal. *ESPN*, 18 Dec. 2006. http://sports.espn.go.com. [Accessed 16 Jan. 2007.]
21. **International Association of Athletics Federations**. IAAF Policy on Gender Verification (Technical Report). 2006. www.iaaf.org.
22. **International Association of Athletics Federations**. Caster Semenya may compete. 6 July 2010. www.iaaf.org/news/iaaf-news/caster-semenya-may-compete. [Accessed 12 July 2012.]
23. **International Association of Athletics Federations**. IAAF Regulations Governing Eligibility of Females with Hyperandrogenism to Compete in Women's Competition (Technical Report). 2011. www.iaaf.org/medical/policy/. [Accessed 12 July 2012.]
24. **International Association of Athletics Federations**. Eligibility Regulations for the Female Classification (Athletes with Differences of Sex Development). 23 April 2018. www.iaaf.org/about-iaaf/documents/rules-regulations#collapseregulations. [Accessed 1 Sept. 2017].
25. **International Olympic Committee**. The work of the Medical Commission. *Olympic Review* 10: 269, 1968.
26. **International Olympic Committee**. IOC Consensus Meeting on Sex Reassignment and Hyperandrogenism (Technical Report). Nov. 2015 https://stillmed.olympic.org/. [Accessed 17 July 2017.]
27. **Karkazis K**, **Jordan-Young R**. Debating a testosterone "sex gap." *Science* 348: 858–869, 2015.
28. **Larned D**. The femininity test: a woman's first Olympic hurdle. *WomenSports*, July: 9, 1976.
29. **Ljungqvist L**, **Simpson JL**. Medical examination for health of all athletes replacing the need for gender verification in international sports: The International Amateur Athletic Federation plan. *Journal of the American Medical Association* 267: 850–852, 1992.
30. **Martínez-Patiño MJ**. Personal account: a woman tried and tested. *Lancet* 366: S38, 2005.
31. **Martínez-Patiño MJ**, **Mateos-Padorno C**, **Martínez-Vidal A**, **Sánchez Mosquera AN**, **García Soidán JL**, **Díaz Pereira MD**, **Touriño González CF**. An approach to the biological, historical and psychological repercussions of gender verification in top level competitions *Journal of Human Sport and Exercise* 5: 307–321, 2010.

32. **Martinez-Patiño MJ**, **Vilain E**, **Bueno-Guerra N** The unfinished race: 30 years of gender verification in sport. *Lancet* 388: 541–543, 2016.

33. **Moore KL**. The sexual identity of athletes. *Journal of the American Medical Association* 205: 163–164, 1968.

34. Olympic Games. *Time* 28: 46, 1936.

35. Olympics require sex test. *New York Times* 30 June: 48, 1968.

36. **Peters M** with **Wooldridge I**. *Mary P.: Autobiography*. London: Paul, 1974, pp. 55–56.

37. **Pieper LP**. *Sex Testing: Gender Policing in Women's Sports*. Urbana, IL: University of Illinois Press, 2016, 29–31.

38. Preserving la difference. *Time*, 16 Sept.: 74, 1966.

39. **Rand FR**. Olympics for girls? *School & Society* 30: 194, 1929.

40. Records of Polish girl sprinter who flunked sex test barred. *New York Times* 26 Feb.: 50, 1968.

41. **Ritchie R**, **Reynard J**, **Lewis T**. Intersex and the Olympic Games. *Journal of the Royal Society of Medicine* 101: 395–399, 2008.

42. Russians win sex-check track meet. *Washington Post* 16 Sept.: D2, 1967.

43. **Schultz J**. Caster Semenya and the "question of too": sex testing in elite women's sport and the issue of advantage. *Quest* 1: 228–43, 2011.

44. **Schultz J**. *Qualifying Times: Points of Change in U.S. Women's Sport*. Urbana, IL: University of Illinois Press, 2014.

45. **Serrat A**, **García de Herreros A**. Determination of genetic sex by PCR amplification of Y-chromosome-specific sequences. *Lancet* 341: 1593, 1993.

46. Sex test disqualifies athlete. *New York Times* 16 Sept.: 28, 1967.

47. **Simpson JL**. Gender verification in competitive sports. *Sports Medicine* 16: 305–315, 1993.

48. **Simpson JL**, **Ljungqvist A**, **Ferguson-Smith MA**, **de la Chapelle A**, **Elsas LJ**, **Ehrhardt AA**, **Genel M**, **Ferris EA**, **Carlson A**. Gender verification in the Olympics. *JAMA* 284: 1568–1569, 2000.

49. **Stephenson J**. Female Olympians' sex tests outmoded. *JAMA* 276: 178, 1996.

50. **Strömgren E**. A memorandum on the use of sex chromatin investigation of competitors in women's divisions of the Olympic Games. 3 Feb. 1972, IOC files folder: "Danish Report, "Sex Tests," 1972. The International Olympic Committee's Historical Archives, Lausanne, Switzerland.

51. **Thibault V**, **Guillaume M**, **Berthelot G**, **El Helou N**, **Schaal K**, **Quinquis L**, **Nassif H**, **Tafflet M**, **Escolano S**, **Hermine O**, **Toussaint JF**. Women and men in sport performance: the gender gap has not evolved since 1983. *Journal of Sports Science and Medicine* 9: 214–223, 2010.

52. **Teitel J**. Faster, higher, stronger. *Toronto Life* Dec.: 73, 1983.

53. **Vines G**. Last Olympics for sex test? *New Scientist* 135: 39–42, 1992.

54. **World Anti-Doping Agency**. TUE Physician Guidelines, Medical Information to Support the Decisions of TUE Committees: Female-to-Male (FtM) Transsexual Athletes (Technical Report). March 2016. www.wada-ama.org. [Accessed 13 Nov. 2017.]

SECTION 7

Conclusions

35

EXERCISE GENOMICS, EPIGENOMICS, AND TRANSCRIPTOMICS: A REALITY CHECK!

Claude Bouchard

Over the last three decades or so, several books have dealt with the highly specialized topic of genetics and exercise. The first effort was more than 20 years ago when there was only minimal data to report across a range of topics of relevance to exercise (8). Since then, a few other volumes have appeared, reflecting an incremental growth in content but with only a modest paradigm shift in the underlying science (5, 20, 22). As one could expect, the present effort under the editorial guidance of Drs. Timothy Lightfoot, Monica Hubal, and Stephen Roth is the most up-to-date and comprehensive of these publications. It allows us to understand the progress we have made but also the territory that has been only superficially explored as well as the many issues and research questions that we have not even begun to address.

The editors have asked me for a commentary and concluding remarks probably because I have been an actor and a witness of the evolution of research in the field of exercise genetics. I launched my first study in the area in 1978. It took the form of several fitness and exercise-related traits that were measured in nuclear families and some of their extended relatives, pairs of monozygotic and dizygotic twins, adopted siblings, and foster parents who were recruited as part of the Quebec Family Study (6, 16). This was followed by several exercise training experiments performed on pairs of identical twins (9, 15, 21, 23). Two major conclusions that have stood for the last three decades were reached in these studies: first, the heritability of cardiorespiratory fitness and exercise-related traits is moderate and not as high as was suggested by earlier studies; and second, there is a genetic component to human variability in trainability. Incidentally, these conclusions were later strongly supported by the findings of the multicenter HERITAGE Family Study (2, 4).

However, the research landscape became more complicated when, beginning around 1980, my laboratory tried to identify DNA variants associated with cardiorespiratory fitness and other exercise-related traits in the sedentary state or their responsiveness to exercise training (3, 7, 10, 11). Our efforts followed closely the progress at the time in research designs and technologies used in human genetics to illuminate the genetic architecture of complex traits. Soon, it became clear that association studies based on candidate genes or restriction fragment length polymorphisms, or linkage studies based on panels of microsatellite markers to identify quantitative trait loci were insufficient to conclude about genes and alleles of relevance to complex, multifactorial exercise phenotypes. The reasons for these failures to deliver in a reproducible manner were not originally obvious. It took the advances in genome-wide association studies (GWAS) and the Encyclopedia of DNA Elements Consortium (ENCODE) project to highlight how challenging the genomic architecture of human complex traits truly is and to define the major reasons the earlier research paradigms failed to deliver (1). This view has been reenforced by the recently launched human cell initiative (www.humancellatlas.org) and advances in the Genotype-Tissue Expression (GTEx) project (www.gtexportal.org).

The early exercise genetic studies assumed that the relation between genotype and phenotype was rather direct and simple, that the regulation of gene expression in a given tissue was dependent on a small number of regulatory elements, and that an allele of interest would have a large effect size on a relevant exercise trait. In the end, it turned out that none of these three assumptions were true. Thus complex traits are influenced by genes and alleles with small effect sizes; the regulation of transcription, translation, and other cellular processes is widely distributed and highly complex; and pervasive redundancy at gene, protein, and pathway levels makes prediction even more challenging.

The human genome in numbers

An illustration of this enormous degree of genomic complexity can be obtained from the findings of the ENCODE project, resulting from the contributions of hundreds of scientists from around the world (www.genome.gov/10005107/the-encode-project-encyclopedia-of-dna-elements). As partially summarized elsewhere (1), less than 2% of the human genome sequence encodes an estimated 20,687 protein-coding genes and about 80% of the genome is transcribed into other encoded products involved mainly in the regulation of gene expression and other cellular events. Interestingly, only about 10% of the single nucleotide polymorphisms (SNPs) commonly genotyped in GWAS reside within protein-coding sequences. The human genome harbors almost 3 million protein-binding sites along its DNA, which include transcription factor-binding sites, recombination sites, and restriction sites, but only a few thousands may be relevant to a given cell type. The more than 1600 or so transcription factors identified to date have been shown to bind at DNA sites representing about 8% of the genome. There are about 8800 small RNAs, including greater than 2000 miRNAs targeting large numbers of mRNAs, and more than 9600 long noncoding RNAs of more than 200 nucleotides in length being transcribed variously depending on cell type, and most participate in the regulation of transcription and translation. One last set of numbers to illustrate the inherent structural complexity of the genome: human DNA encodes about 70,000 promoter regions, 400,000 enhancer regions, and multiple repressor sites. These numbers are lower for a given cell type or tissue, and the relevant sequences are often at a substantial genomic distance from the genes they are thought to regulate. However, DNA is twisted and folded in ways that sequences located at long physical distance away from each other on the linear DNA can be actually physically close to one another when wrapped around nucleoproteins. Thus, in the aggregate, a complex network of regulatory molecules and DNA binding sequences are involved in the widely distributed regulation of less than 21,000 protein-coding genes.

A few additional numbers can help us appreciate the extraordinary complexity of the human genome. There are on average as many as 250 DNA protein-binding sites per protein-coding gene, each transcription factor could relate to an average of 15 protein-coding genes, and there are on average about 23 promoter and enhancer regions per protein-coding gene. The biological instructions encoded in the human genome are vastly more complex than we thought. This fact alone should give us pause when designing new studies or when attempting to conclude about the functional relevance of DNA variants, epigenetic marks, or transcript abundance, taken in isolation, for a given exercise trait.

Additionally, cytosines in CpG dinucleotides can be methylated to form 5-methylcytosine under the action of DNA methyltransferases. Altering the methylation status of cytosines in a gene promoter region has the potential to influence gene expression. There is growing evidence that there is a dose–response relation between the number of methylated CpG dinucleotides in a given promoter/regulatory region and the expression level of the targeted gene. It has been shown that there are about 28 million CpG sites and more than 30,000 genomic regions where these sites are concentrated into CpG islands of up to 1500 base pairs long in the human genome. Of course, one also needs to incorporate the array of histone chemical modifications to cytosine methylation levels in order to draw a more complete picture of the impact of given epigenetic signatures on gene expression.

Genomic architecture of complex traits

The impetus provided by the impressive wave of GWAS publications on complex traits over the last decade or so has nurtured a major shift in our understanding of the genomic architecture of these traits. Unfortunately, adequately powered GWAS data are not yet available for most exercise-related traits, mainly because it is very difficult to generate appropriately large samples of subjects in which laboratory-based exercise trait measurements were obtained. Despite the lack of solid data on exercise-related traits, there are many lessons that we can borrow from large studies of other complex traits to appreciate what is in all likelihood the genomic architecture landscape of exercise traits of interest. One excellent case from which we can derive useful lessons is in the biology of the body mass index (BMI) as illuminated by GWAS.

For decades, it was assumed in some quarters that the heritability of BMI was quite high, over 80% by some estimates. There were divergent views but they did not receive much attention. More recently, two studies conducted on large sample sizes with large panels of SNPs have reached the conclusion that the BMI heritability based on hundreds of SNPs was of the order of 27% with small standard errors (13, 25). Common variants characterized by minor allele frequencies greater than 0.4 accounted for about 80% of the heritability (25). One study from Iceland showed that by combining information on close and distant relatives with a panel of SNPs, the heritability of BMI reached 42% with a standard error of about 2%. Such data are not available yet for exercise traits measured in the sedentary state or in response to standardized exercise programs but it would not be surprising if the true heritability of exercise traits would be lower than originally reported from genetic epidemiology and statistical genetics approaches.

Recent reports have begun to define pathways and biological systems represented by the many SNPs associated with individual differences in BMI (14, 18, 24). As is typically observed for complex traits, BMI common variants are characterized by small effect sizes, but they still account for most of the SNP heritability. In the largest study to date, Turcot et al. searched for rare (minor allele <1%) and low (minor allele <5%) frequency variants associated with BMI in 718,734 individuals from 125 studies (24). They observed 14 rare coding variants in 13 genes, with effect size about ten times larger than what is typically seen in common SNPs. However, because these variants are not very prevalent in human populations, they account for only a very small fraction of the variance in BMI in populations, but they can have a large impact on individuals who happen to be carriers of these high-risk BMI alleles. These findings are concordant with what has been reported for rare, low, and common frequency variants affecting human height (19).

Unpublished findings based on the HERITAGE Family Study strongly suggest that the most important effects of common genomic variants can be imputed to alleles in noncoding regions of the genome (Ghosh S, Bouchard C, et al, unpublished). A bioinformatics exploration of the biology underlying a panel of SNPs associated with VO_2max in the sedentary state (at $P <10 \times 10^{-5}$) reveals that DNA variants located in transcription factor binding sites, promoter and enhancer sites, and CpG-rich areas were substantially more prevalent compared to variants in other genomic regions.

Epilogue

Overall, these observations and our current understanding of the extraordinary complexity of the human genome support the view that the trilogy of DNA sequence variants, epigenetic signatures, and transcript abundance of relevant genes are all participating in the modulation of cardiorespiratory fitness and other exercise traits of interest. However, in spite of all the progress made in genomics and bioinformatics, it remains an extraordinary challenge to define causal relationships between DNA variants, epigenetic events or gene expression profile, and a relevant phenotype. This is true even when adequate statistical power, strong research designs, and state-of-the-art physiological and behavioral phenotyping combined with cutting-edge molecular and high-throughput omics technologies are used. Establishing a clear and unambiguous genotype–phenotype connection is fraught with difficulties.

We believe that the field of exercise biology and genetics must urgently address two key questions. First, are there DNA sequence variants, epigenetic marks in specific cell populations, or gene expression profiles in some tissues that influence the intrinsic level of activity in children and adults? In a nutshell, having a reasonable picture of the biology and genetics of the intrinsic and spontaneous levels of activity would go a long way in advancing efforts to develop more comprehensive explanations for the fact that some people enjoy being physically active whereas most adults do not care about exercising regularly. One cannot rule out, depending on the nature of the biological and genetic explanations, that compensatory approaches aimed at enhancing the interest for a physically active lifestyle could arise from such advances. This topic is of great importance and it does not receive the attention it deserves as we have been arguing recently in a consensus paper (17).

The second question can be framed as follows: What are the molecular transducers of adaptation to acute and chronic exposures to exercise and are they influenced by DNA sequence variants, epigenetic marks, and other molecular substrates? The global topic of the molecular transducers of adaptation to exercise (endurance and resistance exercise) is currently being addressed by the Molecular Transducers of Physical Activity Consortium (MoTrPAC), comprising more than 20 laboratories working in an integrated and coordinated manner with funding support by the Common Fund of the US National Institutes of Health (www.motrpac. org). The research is based on animal models and human experimentations with a focus on acute and chronic endurance exercise, and acute and chronic resistance exercise programs. A sample of children and sets of trained endurance and resistance athletes are also incorporated in the research program of MoTrPAC.

To conclude: we have made progress. But in some areas, the progress is superficial and will not endure the test of time. Given the complexity of the human genome and the overarching principles stipulating that DNA variants are characterized by small effect sizes, that the regulation of gene expression is heterogeneous and widely distributed, and that biological redundancy is pervasive, it should not be surprising that the science of exercise genomics is still in its infancy. In fact, one should not be surprised if most of the observations reported in this volume turn out to be partially wrong or totally false once all the evidence is in. However, this is not as bad as it may look and should not be a source of discouragement: if exercise genomics lags behind, it is likely to be caused by the fact that it is underfunded in general and that it has been next to impossible to put together the resources necessary to investigate a myriad of questions and test hypotheses with appropriate study designs, under adequate experimental and reproducible conditions.

Another reason not to be discouraged by contradictory facts and negative observations is that, as a community of scientists, we should be thriving in the presence of the unknown. Scientists are by definition striving to reduce the level of ignorance regarding a specific topic. Ignorance is the driver of science as creatively proposed by Stuart Firestein from Columbia University, New York City (12). Greater progress is achieved when an experimental observation contradicts the prevailing theory or view. It forces a revision of the theory and encourages the formulation of new hypotheses. Fully accepting that exercise scientists are best positioned to recognize the level of ignorance characteristic of exercise genomics in its current incarnation could actually be a productive stand. It could lead to a greater level of doubt on isolated and perhaps poorly reproducible facts so that the focus shifts to higher-order levels of generalization and theoretical models. So, let's collectively focus on eradicating what is poor science and on identifying clearly what is unknown in exercise genomics with the aim of devising stronger and more comprehensive models that we can submit to experimentation aimed at reducing our level of ignorance.

References

1. **Bouchard C**. Exercise genomics – a paradigm shift is needed: a commentary. *Br J Sports Med* 49: 1492–1496, 2015.
2. **Bouchard C, An P, Rice T, Skinner JS, Wilmore JH, Gagnon J, Perusse L, Leon AS**, and **Rao DC**. Familial aggregation of VO(2max) response to exercise training: results from the HERITAGE Family Study. *J Appl Physiol (1985)* 87: 1003–1008, 1999.
3. **Bouchard C, Chagnon M, Thibault MC, Boulay MR, Marcotte M, Cote C**, and **Simoneau JA**. Muscle genetic variants and relationship with performance and trainability. *Med Sci Sports Exerc* 21: 71–77, 1989.
4. **Bouchard C, Daw EW, Rice T, Perusse L, Gagnon J, Province MA, Leon AS, Rao DC, Skinner JS**, and **Wilmore JH**. Familial resemblance for VO₂max in the sedentary state: the HERITAGE Family Study. *Med Sci Sports Exerc* 30: 252–258, 1998.
5. **Bouchard C** and **Hoffman EP**. *Genetic and Molecular Aspects of Sports Performance, Vol. XVIII of the IOC Encyclopeadia of Sports Medicine, an IOC Medical Commission Publication*. Chichester, West Sussex: Wiley-Blackwell, 2011.
6. **Bouchard C, Lortie G, Simoneau JA, Leblanc C, Theriault G**, and **Tremblay A**. Submaximal power output in adopted and biological siblings. *Ann Hum Biol* 11: 303–309, 1984.
7. **Bouchard C** and **Malina RM**. Genetics of physiological fitness and motor performance. *Exerc Sport Sci Rev* 11: 306–339, 1983.
8. **Bouchard C, Malina RM**, and **Perisse L**. *Genetics of Fitness and Physical Performance*. Champaign, IL: Human Kinetics, 1997.
9. **Bouchard C, Tremblay A, Despres JP, Theriault G, Nadeau A, Lupien PJ, Moorjani S, Prudhomme D**, and **Fournier G**. The response to exercise with constant energy intake in identical twins. *Obes Res* 2: 400–410, 1994.
10. **Chagnon YC, Allard C**, and **Bouchard C**. Red blood cell genetic variation in Olympic endurance athletes. *J Sport Sci* 2: 121–129, 1984.
11. **Dionne FT, Turcotte L, Thibault MC, Boulay MR, Skinner JS**, and **Bouchard C**. Mitochondrial DNA sequence polymorphism, VO2max, and response to endurance training. *Med Sci Sports Exerc* 23: 177–185, 1991.
12. **Firestein S**. *Ignorance: How It Drives Science*. Oxford: Oxford University Press, 2012.

13. **Ge T, Chen CY, Neale BM, Sabuncu MR**, and **Smoller JW**. Phenome-wide heritability analysis of the UK Biobank. *PLoS Genet* 13: e1006711, 2017.

14. **Ghosh S** and **Bouchard C**. Convergence between biological, behavioural and genetic determinants of obesity. *Nat Rev Genet* 18: 731–748, 2017.

15. **Hamel P, Simoneau JA, Lortie G, Boulay MR**, and **Bouchard C**. Heredity and muscle adaptation to endurance training. *Med Sci Sports Exerc* 18: 690–696, 1986.

16. **Lesage R, Simoneau JA, Jobin J, Leblanc J**, and **Bouchard C**. Familial resemblance in maximal heart-rate, blood lactate and aerobic power. *Hum Hered* 35: 182–189, 1985.

17. **Lightfoot JT, De Geus EJC, Booth FW, Bray MS, M DENH, Kaprio J, Kelly SA, Pomp D, Saul MC, Thomis MA, Garland T**, Jr., and **Bouchard C**. Biological/genetic regulation of physical activity level: consensus from GenBioPAC. *Med Sci Sports Exerc* 50: 863–873, 2018.

18. **Locke AE, Kahali B, Berndt SI, Justice AE, Pers TH, Day FR, Powell C, Vedantam S, Buchkovich ML, Yang J, Croteau-Chonka DC, Esko T, Fall T, Ferreira T, Gustafsson S, Kutalik Z, Luan J, Magi R, Randall JC, Winkler TW, Wood AR, Workalemahu T, Faul JD, Smith JA, Zhao JH, Zhao W, Chen J, Fehrmann R, Hedman AK, Karjalainen J, Schmidt EM, Absher D, Amin N, Anderson D, Beekman M, Bolton JL, Bragg-Gresham JL, Buyske S, Demirkan A, Deng G, Ehret GB, Feenstra B, Feitosa MF, Fischer K, Goel A, Gong J, Jackson AU, Kanoni S, Kleber ME, Kristiansson K, Lim U, Lotay V, Mangino M, Leach IM, Medina-Gomez C, Medland SE, Nalls MA, Palmer CD, Pasko D, Pechlivanis S, Peters MJ, Prokopenko I, Shungin D, Stancakova A, Strawbridge RJ, Sung YJ, Tanaka T, Teumer A, Trompet S, van der Laan SW, van Setten J, Van Vliet-Ostaptchouk JV, Wang Z, Yengo L, Zhang W, Isaacs A, Albrecht E, Arnlov J, Arscott GM, Attwood AP, Bandinelli S, Barrett A, Bas IN, Bellis C, Bennett AJ, Berne C, Blagieva R, Bluher M, Bohringer S, Bonnycastle LL, Bottcher Y, Boyd HA, Bruinenberg M, Caspersen IH, Chen YI, Clarke R, Daw EW, de Craen AJM, Delgado G, Dimitriou M**, et al. Genetic studies of body mass index yield new insights for obesity biology. *Nature* 518: 197–206, 2015.

19. **Marouli E, Graff M, Medina-Gomez C, Lo KS, Wood AR, Kjaer TR, Fine RS, Lu Y, Schurmann C, Highland HM, Rueger S, Thorleifsson G, Justice AE, Lamparter D, Stirrups KE, Turcot V, Young KL, Winkler TW, Esko T, Karaderi T, Locke AE, Masca NG, Ng MC, Mudgal P, Rivas MA, Vedantam S, Mahajan A, Guo X, Abecasis G, Aben KK, Adair LS, Alam DS, Albrecht E, Allin KH, Allison M, Amouyel P, Appel EV, Arveiler D, Asselbergs FW, Auer PL, Balkau B, Banas B, Bang LE, Benn M, Bergmann S, Bielak LF, Bluher M, Boeing H, Boerwinkle E, Boger CA, Bonnycastle LL, Bork-Jensen J, Bots ML, Bottinger EP, Bowden DW, Brandslund I, Breen G, Brilliant MH, Broer L, Burt AA, Butterworth AS, Carey DJ, Caulfield MJ, Chambers JC, Chasman DI, Chen YI, Chowdhury R, Christensen C, Chu AY, Cocca M, Collins FS, Cook JP, Corley J, Galbany JC, Cox AJ, Cuellar-Partida G, Danesh J, Davies G, de Bakker PI, de Borst GJ, de Denus S, de Groot MC, de Mutsert R, Deary IJ, Dedoussis G, Demerath EW, den Hollander AI, Dennis JG, Di Angelantonio E, Drenos F, Du M, Dunning AM, Easton DF, Ebeling T, Edwards TL, Ellinor PT, Elliott P, Evangelou E, Farmaki AE, Faul JD**, et al. Rare and low-frequency coding variants alter human adult height. *Nature* 542: 186–190, 2017.

20. **Pescatello LS** and **Roth SM**. Exercise genomics. In: *Molecular and Translational Medicine*, edited by Pescatello LS and Roth SM. New York: Humana Press, 2011, p. 179–230.

21. **Prud'homme D, Bouchard C, Leblanc C, Landry F**, and **Fontaine E**. Sensitivity of maximal aerobic power to training is genotype-dependent. *Med Sci Sports Exerc* 16: 489–493, 1984.

22. **Roth SM**. *Genetics Primer for Exercise Science and Health*. Champaign, IL: Human Kinetics, 2007.

23. **Simoneau JA, Lortie G, Boulay MR, Marcotte M, Thibault MC**, and **Bouchard C**. Inheritance of human skeletal muscle and anaerobic capacity adaptation to high-intensity intermittent training. *Int J Sports Med* 7: 167–171, 1986.

24. **Turcot V, Lu Y, Highland HM, Schurmann C, Justice AE, Fine RS, Bradfield JP, Esko T, Giri A, Graff M, Guo X, Hendricks AE, Karaderi T, Lempradl A, Locke AE, Mahajan A, Marouli E, Sivapalaratnam S, Young KL, Alfred T, Feitosa MF, Masca NGD, Manning AK, Medina-Gomez C, Mudgal P, Ng MCY, Reiner AP, Vedantam S, Willems SM, Winkler TW, Abecasis G, Aben KK, Alam DS, Alharthi SE, Allison M, Amouyel P, Asselbergs FW, Auer PL, Balkau B, Bang LE, Barroso I, Bastarache L, Benn M, Bergmann S, Bielak LF, Bluher M, Boehnke M, Boeing H, Boerwinkle E, Boger CA, Bork-Jensen J, Bots ML, Bottinger EP, Bowden DW, Brandslund I, Breen G, Brilliant MH, Broer L, Brumat M,**

Burt AA, Butterworth AS, Campbell PT, Cappellani S, Carey DJ, Catamo E, Caulfield MJ, Chambers JC, Chasman DI, Chen YI, Chowdhury R, Christensen C, Chu AY, Cocca M, Collins FS, Cook JP, Corley J, Corominas Galbany J, Cox AJ, Crosslin DS, Cuellar-Partida G, D'Eustacchio A, Danesh J, Davies G, Bakker PIW, Groot MCH, Mutsert R, Deary IJ, Dedoussis G, Demerath EW, Heijer M, Hollander AI, Ruijter HM, Dennis JG, Denny JC, Di Angelantonio E, Drenos F, Du M, Dube MP, Dunning AM, Easton DF, et al. Protein-altering variants associated with body mass index implicate pathways that control energy intake and expenditure in obesity. *Nat Genet* 50: 26–41, 2018.

25. **Yang J, Bakshi A, Zhu Z, Hemani G, Vinkhuyzen AA, Lee SH, Robinson MR, Perry JR, Nolte IM, van Vliet-Ostaptchouk JV, Snieder H, LifeLines Cohort S, Esko T, Milani L, Magi R, Metspalu A, Hamsten A, Magnusson PK, Pedersen NL, Ingelsson E, Soranzo N, Keller MC, Wray NR, Goddard ME**, and **Visscher PM**. Genetic variance estimation with imputed variants finds negligible missing heritability for human height and body mass index. *Nat Genet* 47: 1114–1120, 2015.

36

AFTERWORD – CLOSING THE LOOP: OBSERVATIONS AND CONCLUSIONS

J. Timothy Lightfoot, Monica J. Hubal, and Stephen M. Roth

Introduction

As we close this volume, we believe that a few points need to be made – a sort of summary if you will. Because the authors in each chapter have done such a great job of summarizing the field in each of their areas, this chapter will be rather more of a 30,000′ overview of the whole field. It was not long ago that many of us hoped that understanding the underlying systems genetics of any trait would be as easy as understanding the gene polymorphisms present in different individuals, a view captured and forever immortalized in pop culture in the movie "Gattaca." However, one thing that is clear from the previous chapters is that we are not working in the "genetics" of 40 years ago; i.e., to paraphrase an automobile advertisement from several years ago, "This is not your Father's (or Gattaca's) genetics!"

As succinctly summarized by Dr. Bouchard's closing words (Chapter 35) and as demonstrated in almost every chapter, complexity reigns supreme in the systems genetics of exercise and sport. The literature has roundly dispensed with the idea that only one or a few genes control any one exercise-related phenotype; rather, it has become widely accepted that because all exercise phenotypes are complex traits that are made up of numerous different physiological pathways, the genetic mechanisms that control most – if not all – exercise phenotypes are made up of hundreds, if not thousands, of genes, each contributing a small amount to the overall regulation. Adding to this complexity, as mentioned in Chapters 7 and 9, Xu and Garland, Jr. have provided experimental proof (10) that some exercise phenotypes may be the result of multiple different genetic architectures – a confirmation of the "multiple independent evolutionary solution" hypothesis in genetics. Thus, the exercise scientist who is interested in studying exercise and sport systems genetics must know that the potential genetic mechanisms influencing exercise and sport phenotypes are likely to be complex, and will be difficult to not only understand, but also to translate and apply in practice. In short, the world presented in the movie "Gattaca" is now viewed as hopelessly naïve and outdated, especially considering the new findings and concepts in systems genetics that are being added to the literature on an almost daily basis. But as David Epstein pointed out in the Foreword, there are cases where a single gene variant can markedly affect sport performance, and as such, there will probably always be a few exceptions to the "complexity rule" that we are seeing in exercise and sport systems genetics.

Writing during a time in history where politicians routinely question whether science is truthful or relevant, scientists often take offense at any critique of their findings. However, it is often forgotten that science only thrives when "what we think we know" is heavily scrutinized and respectfully challenged within the scientific community. As an example of examining carefully what we think we know, early in the development of this project, in one of the numerous outlines that we composed, one of us wrote the following sentence, "There is no doubt that genetics plays a role in all exercise behaviors and little doubt that exercise behaviors are driven by numerous genes with small effect sizes." With the paragraphs of this chapter and throughout much of this volume, you would think that the previous sentence would be entirely defensible. However, as is appropriate, there have been several articles recently (5, 7) and at least one formal scientific debate that have questioned whether genetics is actually involved in determining exercise phenotypes (in particular, these articles question the "nonresponder to training" phenotype established originally by Bouchard and Rankinen (3) and covered extensively in Section 3 of this volume). While the editors of this volume believe that the authors of those questioning papers do not appreciate or allow for the complexity of genetic regulation, nonetheless, these types of discussions are invaluable to ensure that the science within this field is on a solid foundation (and we look forward to including in the next edition of this volume the upcoming published debates regarding this topic). In short, debate, critique, and examination of our ideas and findings are critical to advancement of the field.

Along the lines of a 30,000′ overview, we would be remiss if we did not recognize what may be tremendous advances coming to the field in the next few years (and probably before the next edition of this volume) due to the rapid embrace of clustered regularly interspaced short palindromic repeats (CRISPR)-Cas9 technologies (4). While the final impact of CRISPR-Cas9 on all systems genetics is unknown at this point, the potential of such a low-cost, precise, and relatively easy system of altering genomes will certainly be applied to exercise phenotypes soon, if not being applied already. For example, early results were recently announced that CRISPR technologies reversed a form of muscular dystrophy in a canine model (1). Additionally, given that some countries are already allowing CRISPR-Cas9 experimentation on nonviable embryos (e.g., 9), one can easily imagine that this technology may be applied to viable embryos in the future. This development will potentially forever change sport and exercise systems genetics, and may bring sport gene-doping (or -editing) to the forefront quicker than we can philosophically deal with it. Readers and scientists alike should continue to watch the literature for developments in this exciting area.

It is a given that within each of the exercise phenotypes that have been covered within this volume, there are specific nuances, findings, and conclusions that can be made. Certainly, progress within each of the phenotypes covered (loosely grouped into the book sections) have been uneven, probably because of the scientists involved and the resources within each area that have been brought to bear on the topic. As such, we have provided an overall summary below of each section of the book, to provide overall take-home messages for each of the exercise/sport phenotypes that have been covered in this volume.

Summary – Section 1: General systems genetics

The biggest take-home messages of the first section of the book – which dealt with a general overview of current systems genetics knowledge – begin with the thought that systems genetics is rapidly advancing with new ideas, techniques, and concepts being added to the literature almost daily. Systems genetics is a dynamic field and marrying it with exercise and sport science should provide fertile research grounds for many years. While many exercise scientists may want to ignore systems genetics of exercise and sport, it is incredibly important that we consider systems genetics so that we can further understand how activity, exercise, and sport provide positive health outcomes. As Dr. Booth and colleagues noted in Chapter 1, understanding the "genetic symphony" underpinning physiology is critical as we all continue to face health challenges brought about by our improving quality of life and the concomitant reduction in physical activity/exercise in our daily lives. As such, translational efforts can serve to identify those who are at higher risk of being inactive with a potential of providing differing exercise prescriptions to those who are at risk. Further, there are already robust human modeling techniques that can be used to study these types of genetic interventions to aid in the application of systems genetics results to human physiology.

From a general systems genetics standpoint, the next 5 years should be exciting. The application of CRISPR-Cas9 approaches to a wide variety of physiological questions (4) promises to illuminate many pathways that may play major roles in exercise and sport responses. However, the complexity of understanding how all the systems genetics pieces "fit" together to influence a phenotype will remain a challenge to those who are interested in determining how physiology is regulated by systems genetics mechanisms. Even the new appreciation for the role of exosomes and their ability to deliver miRNA to sites other than where they are produced promises to provide potential mechanisms controlling many of the normal physiological responses. The professional interested in studying or applying systems genetics needs to watch the literature closely for additional concepts that may apply to their physiological interests.

Summary – Section 2: Systems genetics of physical activity

Some would argue that the most critical health-related issue currently facing humanity is the increase in the number of chronic conditions and diseases caused by physical inactivity. The major take-home messages from the chapters relating to physical activity are that: 1) there is a significant amount of literature – well over 50 papers at this point – that conclusively show, in both humans and animal models, that systems genetics play a large role in regulating physical activity and physical inactivity; 2) physical activity and physical inactivity have genetic underpinnings which may be different depending upon whether one is studying activity or inactivity; and 3) the systems genetics influence on physical activity/inactivity likely has both peripheral (e.g., skeletal muscle) and central (e.g., brain) control components, with environmental factors such as diet and exposure to toxicants altering the underlying systems genetics control of activity/inactivity. There can be little argument that, as noted in a recent consensus paper (6), "choosing not to investigate these mechanisms would be irresponsible and would hinder the science or understanding the causes of this critical health issue."

The primary challenge facing investigators considering the systems genetics of physical activity is the need for more hypothesis-driven, causative studies. Correlational/associative studies have provided critical observations, including the suggestion of multiple genes and/ or other genetic factors involved in regulating physical activity. However, there have been few attempts to validate the suggested genetic factors and provide causative data supporting many of these factors. Providing causative data is incredibly difficult and may be nearly impossible in human studies; however, the number of solid animal models available provides an avenue through which to provide initial causative data. In this same vein, there needs to be translational studies that include both humans and animal models. There have been minimal attempts using this approach, with the existing data significantly flawed; however, this issue does not predicate future, well-designed, and properly interpreted translational studies. In fact, the lack of translational data available to bridge the voluminous animal data and the voluminous human data is a critical gap in the literature.

Another challenge that has faced investigators in this area has been the relative lack of funding. Scientific reviewers have been reluctant to accept that systems genetics plays a significant role in the determination of physical activity/inactivity levels; however, given the extensive literature basis cited in Chapters 5–10 as well as recent efforts to provide consensus statements in the area (e.g., 6), we hope that scientists seeking funding in this area will be able to more easily make a convincing case that these mechanisms are worth funding and investigation.

Within the next 5 years, we believe that several different avenues within the systems genetics of physical activity/inactivity will begin to be investigated. As mentioned previously, we anticipate that the application of CRISPR-Cas9 systems will be used to supplement the minimal amount of *in vivo* gene silencing that has already been done in the area to provide more causative data and better gene targets. These types of approaches will not only provide more causative data, but will help investigators further understand the role of newer concepts that have not been investigated in the field such as the role of exosomes and epigenetics in determining physical activity/inactivity. Further, as noted in both Chapters 4 and 6, there are already initial efforts to examine the genetics of affective mood and the role that these pathways might play in physical activity/inactivity. We anticipate that these efforts toward understanding the genetics of affective mood will surely blossom over the next 5 years and the topic will deserve a chapter of its own in future editions of this volume. Lastly, and maybe most critically, we believe that over the next 5 years there will be efforts to understand why there has been variability in the genetic results related to physical activity to date – especially in the human genome wide association study (GWAS) results – and whether this variability is a result of multiple independent evolutionary solutions for physical activity (10) or if there are other factors that need to be considered in the research paradigms used.

In summary, it is clear that systems genetics play a role in regulating physical activity and physical inactivity. Research efforts in these areas have thrived over the past 20 years and new concepts and tools will only increase the progress in this area into the future.

Summary – Section 3: Systems genetics of exercise endurance and trainability

Exercise traits related to endurance are highly complex even at the organ level, integrating organ systems such as lung, skeletal muscle, and the cardiovascular system. Much of Section 3 is devoted to explaining endurance-related traits from a multitude of perspectives, from a general phenotype primer in Chapter 12 to more focused chapters on the anthropological evolution of the endurance phenotype (Chapter 11) and underlying mitochondrial physiology and genetics (Chapter 16). Two chapters explore heritability estimates of endurance-related traits, splitting the literature into animal- (Chapter 13) and human-based (Chapter 14) evidence, both providing high estimates of heritability of baseline endurance, with lower estimates of heritability for response to training, indicating that contributions of environmental factors to variance in training responses are substantial.

There is great interest in optimizing aerobic fitness across many different populations, as it is so tightly linked to overall health, longevity, and athletic performance. At one end of the spectrum, there is always pressure on elite athletes to find any advantages over their competitors. Recently, Kenya's Eliud Kipchoge smashed the world record for the marathon, running 2:01:39 in the 2018 Berlin Marathon. A year earlier, Kipchoge had run 2:00:25 as part of Nike's Breaking 2 project, running with several advantages impossible in a real marathon (such as staggered pacing). After the Berlin marathon, there was much press about what factors limit human performance capacity, such as lactate threshold, VO$_2$max, and mechanical efficiency in a given task. Obviously, genetic variation plays a role in endurance performance, but not in a simplistic way. An example of a simplistic view would be the influence of a mutation in the angiotensin-converting enzyme (a key part of blood flow regulation) on endurance performance. Despite over 1000 studies on the *ACE* I/D variant, there is still no consensus about its effects on overall endurance performance (summarized in Chapter 17). Most likely, there are thousands of genetic variants affecting endurance components that sum to affect performance, many of which likely interact among the key biological pathways related to endurance. Initial efforts to identify gene variants specific to elite athletes have fallen short, likely due to lack of statistical power.

At the other end of the spectrum are people with low cardiorespiratory fitness due to aging, lack of activity, or other reasons. This end of the spectrum is much more populated than the elite athlete end, and diseases and disabilities related to low fitness drive most healthcare costs in many developed countries. There is a great deal of interest in understanding endurance-related traits at the genetic and molecular levels to drive the generation of new therapeutics, such as exercise "mimetics" that may help treat these inactivity-related diseases and help reduce the incredible healthcare costs associated with them. Though there is great debate about whether an exercise mimetic could provide all the positive benefits of actual exercise (e.g., 2), therapeutics, such as AICAR, that affect systems related to endurance exercise have been used to promote health (8). It is hoped that with current efforts such as the National Institutes of Health Molecular Transducers of Physical Activity Consortium (MoTrPAC; www.MoTrPAC.org), which was described extensively by Dr. Bouchard in Chapter 35, we will better understand the molecular and genetic determinants of endurance-related traits and will be better able to develop and deliver targeted therapeutics.

Summary – Section 4: Systems genetics of muscle mass, strength, and trainability

Section 4 explored exercise-related traits generally associated with resistance (strength) training, highlighting strength and size variability among people at baseline and following training. These traits fall into the general pattern we see with many exercise-related phenotypes, in that classic heritability studies tell us that they should be strongly linked to genetic background. This concept is summarized expertly by Dr. Martine Thomis in Chapter 18, stating that "twin and family studies have indicated that genetic factors significantly (>0.50–0.70) contribute to the observed differences in muscle mass and strength characteristics." Each of the authors in Section 4 were tasked with exploring both strength and size at baseline and these responses following exercise training. Similar to the endurance-related traits highlighted in Section 3, heritability estimates are higher for baseline size and strength compared to responses to training.

At least from traditional SNP studies, associations between candidate gene variants and strength or size traits sometimes overlap between baseline and post-training changes, but often do not, suggesting a partially unique genetic basis of training response. However, we have mentioned many times throughout the book that there are many limitations within the traditional SNP association studies (including lack of power, varied intervention parameters, lack of ethnic diversity, etc.) that limit our ability to extrapolate their findings, meaning that we still do not fully understand genetic versus environmental drivers of strength and size.

One thing that we can be sure of is that determinants of strength and size, whether at baseline or following training, are much more complex than we once thought, as are the traits themselves (Chapters 19 and 20 provide primers for strength and size, in addition to an excellent review of neuroendocrine drivers of these traits in Chapter 21). Given a 50–70% heritability for strength and size, much work was devoted in the 2000s to identifying a few gene variants that could explain large amounts of variation in each phenotype. A prime example of these efforts are the findings regarding mutations in the myostatin gene, which provide dramatic changes in muscle size and body composition in animal models. Dr. Dustin Hittel summarizes the exploration of myostatin to date, highlighting the complexity of regulation of myostatin-related pathways (see Figure 22.1) and noting that common variants of the myostatin gene with large effect sizes simply don't exist in humans, though modification of myostatin's effects pharmacologically could be of use in certain clinical populations. It is possible that newer efforts like MoTrPAC will identify new gene variants associated with muscle strength and size, but efforts to date have explained only a fraction of the variation present among humans. MoTrPAC and other efforts are emphasizing multiscale omics approaches that should shed more light on the molecular underpinnings of strength and muscle size.

Summary – Section 5: Systems genetics of sports performance

In the bulk of Section 5, we see the challenges of expanding our genetic analysis to the level of "performance" rather than specific underlying traits. Performance is arguably the hardest trait to measure and study, because it represents the contributions of many underlying traits that combine in specific ways for a specific outcome in a specific activity. What equates as "maximal performance" in sprinting varies from soccer, which varies from cricket, which varies from wrestling, and on and on. Moreover, measuring elite-level performance has the added challenge that elite performers, by definition, are rare and thus unique, making research studies difficult to pursue and far-reaching conclusions difficult to come by. Researchers are addressing these questions through consortia and other means, but there is a clear conundrum facing researchers focused on the systems genetics of exercise and sport: how to address the remarkable complexity of performance while necessarily focusing on the "narrower" analyses of specific traits, be it grip strength, stroke volume, or lactate threshold. Those detailed studies are needed, but they may not enhance the broader understanding of performance as they are done independently of the broader gene networks and other variables impacting the more complex performance traits.

While the studies to date clearly support a genetic contribution to performance, in particular from the twin and family studies outlined, we've made little progress in identifying the underlying systems genetics factors involved. More complex GWAS and direct DNA sequencing approaches are beginning to emerge and will require replication and extension. The many environmental contributors to performance will necessarily complicate this task, but that makes replication even more important. What remains to be seen is whether, as outlined in the conclusion of Chapter 26, E.O. Wilson was right those many years ago when he effectively argued that there are so many possible combinations of exceptional genes that predicting their appearance in an individual is nearly impossible. And the corollary to that thought is knowing whether there are so many unique combinations that looking for similarities across even hundreds of elite athletes within the same sport may ultimately yield hundreds of specific, unique, genetic patterns, all of which predispose to elite performance and which may be reflective of the "multiple independent evolutionary solutions" hypothesis mentioned earlier.

In considering the chapters across Sections 2–5, the field appears to be caught in the middle space between the single gene studies of the 2000s and the more advanced genome-wide omics techniques of present day, with an inherent desire to identify specific genes while knowing we are pursuing variation in extensive genomic networks instead. Those latter studies are remarkably complex, requiring the combined power of multiple omics analyses within a carefully studied (and sufficiently large) cohort. While these studies are emerging in a variety of fields (e.g., cancer and diabetes), our ability to successfully pursue systems genetics studies in exercise and sport is particularly challenged by the nature of our complex exercise interventions, differences in measurement techniques, and inherently small sample sizes. That funding agencies in some countries are less inclined to support sport-related research is an added barrier to the establishment of large studies and international consortia capable of addressing these complex issues. But these constraints are being addressed in a variety of ways and the number of consortia to emerge in the past few years is remarkable. There is clearly optimism that the emerging tools in genomic analysis coming primarily from disease-oriented fields will be equally beneficial to the field of exercise and sport.

Although slightly unique in context from the other chapters, Chapters 27 and 28 are notable for their implications for our field to better identify individuals predisposed to sport-related injury, as well as improve prevention and treatment approaches. That genetic predisposition exists in both brain and soft tissue injuries is clear, though the details (as with all other traits in the field) remain to be clarified. And yet these findings yield additional complexities for sport; while genetic testing and genetic technologies to improve performance are generally frowned upon (as shown in Section 6), their potential use for injury prevention and recovery often result in an opposite perspective. Navigating those different viewpoints won't be easy, as one person's injury recovery is another's performance enhancement.

One area that is clearly lacking in this volume is an examination of epigenetics in exercise and sport. While we recognized the importance of the topic, we felt the state of the literature was too underdeveloped to warrant a dedicated chapter at the time we designed the book. That will surely change over the next few years and the findings may illuminate unique aspects of systems genetics in exercise that will help dissect the unique interaction of genes and environment in sport, perhaps with implications for heritability.

Summary – Section 6: The ethics of systems genetics in exercise and sport

While the previous sections have focused on the discovery of new insights into the systems genetics of exercise and sport sciences, Section 6 of the book takes a much different approach and examines some of the ethical considerations stemming from those research findings. Despite scientists' best intentions (or lack of interest), their findings in the field of genetics have the potential to impact broad aspects of society and human culture, perhaps even humanity itself. So, it is important that the readers of this volume who may otherwise simply be interested in learning about the latest findings and future directions of scientific inquiry in their particular area of focus should at least be aware of these broader implications.

Genetic testing of athletes (and potential athletes) emerged as a controversial topic in the early days of the field, as soon as the testing technology became less expensive and Internet-based companies became more common. Despite the science of the field being less than conclusive (as we've seen from the previous sections of the book), companies are generously employing the existing science and marketing testing products of questionable scientific validity. Because sports performance traits typically fall outside the stringent oversight requirements of testing for health-related traits, the companies have very little restriction on their ability to produce and market such tests. While savvy consumers may have access to much of the same literature as scientists, few are likely to delve deeply enough into that literature to understand the limitations and consequences of genetic testing for sport performance and will instead rely on the companies carefully selected (and limited) reference lists to judge the validity of a testing product. We would do well as a field to consider the implications of our findings around specific genes and specifically mention the limitations of the use of such information for genetic testing in our published papers. In this way, companies bent on marketing products with limited scientific evidence will at least have to ignore our explicit cautions about such uses.

The authors in Section 6 also challenge us in several ways to consider the broad implications of our work on society more generally. Consider the implications of studying genetic aspects of performance in specific race groups. While such work is a natural extension of the basic question, "Why is this group disproportionately represented on the leaderboard?", the pursuit of the research may inadvertently support the notion of biological determinism and racial superiority. Any carefully controlled research study limits the number of variables examined to better ensure clear, valid conclusions; examination of a question as broad as that posed above would require inclusion of social, cultural, economic, and other factors, which would clearly overwhelm a typical research team and muddy an otherwise straightforward hypothesis and research study. But we would be wise to tread carefully into such domains without clearly identifying for ourselves and our audience the limits and limitations of our research.

Similarly, examination of sex and performance is fraught with challenge. As shown in Section 5's Chapter 29, sex differences appear in a variety of sports and appear linked to biological and physiological differences. Defining those differences and ensuring equity in the sports arena, however, is remarkably difficult. Defining the clear biological underpinnings of sex seems as if it should be straightforward, but the varied attempts over the years at finding such a definition (for determining an equal playing field) have only failure in common. Scholars in biological fields recognize the importance of "exceptions" to every rule, and the varied nature of human biology becomes more evident with every attempt at categorizing "men" and "women." Genetic analysis will surely shed light on this variation in our species, but will simultaneously wreak havoc on our ability to categorize people for the purposes of parity and fairness in sport competitions.

Perhaps most important of all the challenges raised by the authors of Section 6 are the implications that genetic engineering has for human biology and society. Mind you, the potential for genetic engineering to alter humanity is not specifically tied to the world of sport, as much of the work and technical innovation are being driven by the study of disease treatment and elimination (e.g., CRISPR-Cas9, as outlined above). Nevertheless, athletes' willingness to pursue such technologies for performance enhancement makes the implications evident to a broader swath of society and enables both different questions and a wider pool of discussants. And, as Chapters 32 and 33 demonstrate, we have a long way to go before reaching any semblance of consensus about the role of genetic engineering in sport, let alone society more broadly. Do we allow somatic-cell genetic engineering, but outlaw gamete manipulation to prevent "permanent" changes to the human genome? What forms of genetic therapy should be allowed for athletes, or are such athletes destined to be categorized separately? Where such manipulation can even be measured in an athlete, how much testing should we require (e.g., regular biopsies)? Where might genetic technologies be allowed for injury treatment? Many questions remain to be considered and addressed as genetic manipulation becomes more commonplace in our society.

Final conclusions

This volume represents an exciting look into one of the more dynamic research areas in exercise and sport sciences. Within this volume we have worked to show where the field has been, where it is currently, and maybe more importantly, where we think the field is going in the near future. We hope that with this book as a spring-point, you will choose to continue to journey with us and the investigators in this book, as we all continue to work to understand the systems genetics of exercise and sport. As we close this volume, we again want to thank all the authors who have so kindly contributed chapters to this book; simply put, without their contributions, this volume would not exist.

References

1. **Amoasii L, Hildyard JCW, Li H, Sanchez-Ortiz E, Mireault A, Caballero D, Harron R, Stathopoulou TR, Massey C, Shelton JM, Bassel-Duby R, Piercy RJ**, and **Olson EN**. Gene editing restores dystrophin expression in a canine model of Duchenne muscular dystrophy. *Science* 362: 86–91, 2018.
2. **Booth FW** and **Laye MJ**. Lack of adequate appreciation of physical exercise's complexities can pre-empt appropriate design and interpretation in scientific discovery. *J Physiol* 587: 5527–5539, 2009.
3. **Bouchard C** and **Rankinen T**. Individual differences in response to regular physical activity. *Med Sci Sports Exerc* 33: S446–S451, 2001.
4. **Doudna JA** and **Charpentier E**. Genome editing. The new frontier of genome engineering with CRISPR-Cas9. *Science* 346: 1258096, 2014.
5. **Joyner MJ** and **Lundby C**. Concepts about VO2max and trainability are context dependent. *Exerc Sport Sci Rev* 46: 138–143, 2018.
6. **Lightfoot JT, De Geus EJC, Booth FW, Bray MS, den Hoed M, Kaprio J, Kelly SA, Pomp D, Saul MC, Thomis MA, Garland T**, and **Bouchard C**. Biological/genetic regulation of physical activity level: consensus from GenBioPAC. *Med Sci Sports Exerc* 50: 863–873, 2018.
7. **Lundby C, Montero D**, and **Joyner M**. Biology of VO2 max: looking under the physiology lamp. *Acta Physiol (Oxf)* 220: 218–228, 2017.
8. **Narkar VA, Downes M, Yu RT, Embler E, Wang YX, Banayo E, Mihaylova MM, Nelson MC, Zou Y, Juguilon H, Kang H, Shaw RJ**, and **Evans RM**. AMPK and PPARdelta agonists are exercise mimetics. *Cell* 134: 405–415, 2008.
9. **Tang L, Zeng Y, Du H, Gong M, Peng J, Zhang B, Lei M, Zhao F, Wang W, Li X**, and **Liu J**. CRISPR/Cas9-mediated gene editing in human zygotes using Cas9 protein. *Mol Genet Genomics* 292: 525–533, 2017.
10. **Xu S** and **Garland T**. A mixed model approach to genome-wide association studies for selection signatures, with application to mice bred for voluntary exercise behavior. *Genetics* 207: 785–799, 2017.

INDEX

Printed in the United States
by Baker & Taylor Publisher Services